COMPUTED TOMOGRAPHY AND MAGNETIC RESONANCE OF THE THORAX

Second Edition

COMPUTED TOMOGRAPHY AND MAGNETIC RESONANCE OF THE THORAX

Second Edition

David P. Naidich, M.D.
Professor of Radiology
Department of Radiology
Bellevue Hospital
New York University Medical Center
New York, New York

Elias A. Zerhouni, M.D.
Associate Professor of Radiology
Director, Thoracic Imaging and MRI
Department of Radiology and Radiologic Science
Johns Hopkins Medical Institutions
Baltimore, Maryland

Stanley S. Siegelman, M.D.
Professor of Radiology
Department of Radiology and Radiologic Science
Johns Hopkins Medical Institutions
Baltimore, Maryland

Contributing Author

Jerald P. Kuhn, M.D.
Professor of Radiology
State University of New York at Buffalo
Director, Department of Radiology
The Children's Hospital of Buffalo
Buffalo, New York

Raven Press ❧ New York

Raven Press, 1185 Avenue of the Americas, New York, New York 10036

Made in the United States of America

Library of Congress Cataloging-in-Publication Data
Naidich, David P.
    Computed tomography and magnetic resonance of the thorax / David
P. Naidich, Elias A. Zerhouni, Stanley S. Siegelman; contributing
author, Jerald P. Kuhn. — 2nd ed.
        p. cm.
    Rev. ed. of: Computed tomography of the thorax. c1984.
    Includes bibliographies and index.
    ISBN 0-88167-567-9
    1. Chest—Tomography.   2. Chest—Magnetic resonance imaging.
I. Zerhouni, Elias A.   II. Siegelman, Stanley S., 1932–
III. Naidich, David P. Computed tomography of the thorax.
IV. Title.
    [DNLM: 1. Magnetic Resonance Imaging.   2. Thoracic Radiography.
3. Tomography, X-Ray Computed. WF 975 N155c]
RC941.N27   1991
617.5'40757—dc20
DNLM/DLC
for Library of Congress   89-10488

The material contained in this volume was submitted as previously unpublished material, except in the instances in which some of the illustrative material was derived.

Great care has been taken to maintain the accuracy of the information contained in the volume. However, neither Raven Press nor the authors can be held responsible for errors or for any consequences arising from the use of the information contained herein.

9 8 7 6 5 4 3 2 1

To my wife, Jocelyn,
my son, Zachary
and my mother, Edith
D.P.N.

To Nadia,
Djillali, Yasmin, and Adam
E.A.Z.

To the memory of Charles Siegelman
S.S.S.

Contents

Preface to the First Edition

Diagnostic imaging has undergone a profound and astonishingly rapid transformation over the last decade, paralleling the rapid evolution of modern computer science. The first CT unit, conceived and developed by Godfrey Hounsfield, underwent initial clinical testing at the Atkinson Morley Hospital, Wimbledon, England, in 1971. This early scanner employed two sodium iodide crystals and produced an image based on an 80 × 80 matrix. The scan time of four and one half minutes effectively limited the machine to examination of intracranial pathology.

Within three years, Ledley developed a CT unit capable of imaging the body. In 1974 and 1975, whole body scanner prototypes were installed first at the Cleveland Clinic, and then at the Mallinckrodt Institute of Radiology, and the Mayo Clinic. Initial reports from these institutions were enthusiastic about the role of CT in the evaluation of the pancreas, liver, and retroperitoneum but pessimistic about the value of CT in the thorax.

Further improvements in instrumentation were necessary in order to assess the clinical role of thoracic CT. The pace of technological innovation was such that by 1977, scanners capable of scan times shorter than breath-holding had been developed. Additional improvements, including more detectors to increase resolution and finer collimation allowing a reduction in slice thickness to minimize partial volume averaging, soon became standard. As a result, initial pessimism about the role of CT in the thorax quickly gave way to considerable enthusiasm. This first became apparent as reports of the value of CT in analyzing mediastinal disease were published. Thereafter, an ever-expanding range of uses for thoracic CT has evolved and continues to evolve.

In December 1977, a CT scanner was installed at the Johns Hopkins Hospital. At that time, Drs. Naidich and Zerhouni were residents under the tutelage of Dr. Siegelman, under whose auspices the three authors of this volume enthusiastically began a series of studies concerning the utility of thoracic CT in a wide range of clinical settings. In July 1980, Dr. Naidich joined the staff at New York University Medical Center, and in January 1981, Dr. Zerhouni moved to the East Virginia Medical Center. Despite this separation, the team continued their collaborative endeavors, and in 1982 and 1983, presented instruction courses in chest CT at the annual meeting of the American Roentgen Ray Society. From these presentations, the need for a volume representing the current status of thoracic CT became apparent.

This textbook has been organized primarily around the major anatomic subunits of the thorax. These include: the mediastinum, the airways, the hila, the pulmonary parenchyma, the pleura and chest wall, the pericardium, and the diaphragm. Additional chapters have been added specifically on the role of CT in evaluating lobar collapse and the pulmonary nodule, as these represent discrete topics best addressed apart. This organizational scheme represents the authors' views that CT is primarily an anatomic imaging modality. Specifically excluded from consideration is the use of CT in evaluating the heart. It is only appropriate to consider cardiac CT in comparison to other cardiac imaging modalities, including angiography, echocardiography, and nuclear cardiology. It is the authors' feeling that this is outside the intended scope of the present volume as initially conceived.

Thoracic CT has become an integral part of the daily practice of radiology. With the ever-increasing number of diagnostic modalities, the task of deciding which diagnostic test is the most appropriate for a given clinical problem has become a significant part of medical practice. The authors believe that an adequate understanding of clinical issues is necessary for practicing radiologists to best help the referring physician. Consequently, throughout the text, a strong emphasis has been placed on discussing CT as it relates to clinical issues, especially as compared to other routine imaging modalities.

It is to be anticipated that further technologic advances in diagnostic imaging will further compli-cate the role of radiologists. It is hoped that this text will prove valuable in assisting this process.

DAVID P. NAIDICH

ELIAS A. ZERHOUNI

STANLEY S. SIEGELMAN

Preface

Seven years have passed since the original publication of *Computed Tomography of the Thorax.* In this period, remarkable advances have been made in our understanding of the use of CT to evaluate thoracic disease. In the preparation of the Second Edition, we have focused on three primary goals. First, update images to reflect the dramatic improvements in the quality of CT scans that have occurred over the past several years. In this regard, nearly all the images used in the First Edition have been replaced. Second, thoroughly review the avalanche of data that has been published not only in the radiologic literature, but throughout the general medical and surgical literature in order to provide as definitive a list of references as possible. Third, review current indications for the use of CT in light of this vast expansion of reported experience.

As if this were not a sufficiently daunting task, in the interim magnetic resonance imaging has become a practical reality as well, available to an increasingly large number of radiologists. Although the utility of MR as a method for imaging the thorax has lagged behind other applications, a sufficient body of knowledge has already been amassed to warrant in-depth analysis of the potential applications of this technology. In our judgment, these have been sufficiently significant to warrant renaming our text *Computed Tomography and Magnetic Resonance of the Thorax.*

As before, this volume has been organized primarily around the major anatomic subunits of the thorax, including the mediastinum, the airways, the hila, the pulmonary parenchyma, the pleura and chest wall, the diaphragm, and the heart and pericardium. Most of the chapters have been thoroughly revised. In the case of the chapter on diffuse lung disease, the change has been nearly total, reflecting the development of high-resolution computed tomographic imaging of the pulmonary parenchyma. In addition, in order to correct what we now perceive as substantial oversights, additional chapters have been added on lung cancer and on pediatric imaging.

Each chapter has been organized similarly, with special emphasis placed first on optimization of scan technique, followed by an in-depth analysis of pertinent anatomy. Attention is then focused separately on the indications and limitations of CT and MR in the evaluation of specific disease entities. As before, considerable emphasis has been placed on clinical correlation, in the belief that accurate radiologic interpretation is based on more than simple familiarity with pattern recognition. It is hoped that general adherence to this scheme will simplify the use of this text.

As described in the Preface to the First Edition, thoracic CT has indeed "become an integral part of the daily practice of radiology." It is also true, as before, that "it is to be anticipated that further technologic advances in diagnostic imaging will further complicate the role of radiologists," especially given the continued rapid technical advances of magnetic resonance imaging. Again, it is hoped that the current edition will prove of value to all radiologists challenged by the need to diagnose thoracic disease.

DAVID P. NAIDICH

ELIAS A. ZERHOUNI

STANLEY S. SIEGELMAN

Acknowledgments

One singular pleasure in the preparation of a manuscript is the chance afforded to express our thanks to the innumerable individuals without whose friendship and advice this project would never have been completed.

At The Johns Hopkins Medical Institutions we especially thank Janet Kuhlman, M.D., for her many and varied contributions. We also thank Keith Penn-Jones, chief MR technologist, as well as Mary McAllister and Nola Miller for their help in the preparation of many portions of this manuscript.

At New York University Medical Center, we are deeply indebted to Drs. Dorothy McCauley and Barry Leitman for their tireless patience and considerable input into almost all phases of this project. We express our deep appreciation to Norman Ettenger, M.D., at the Manhatten V.A. Hospital for his extraordinary willingness to share cases and assist in any and all requests for data, no matter how inconvenient. A particular debt of gratitude is owed to Dr. Jeffrey Weinreb, Director of Body MR, without whose enthusiasm, expertise, and material this textbook would not have been possible in its current form. We also thank the many technologists, both in CT and MR whose patience in re-loading and re-imaging cases was invaluable; in particular we thank Roy Thompson, supervisor extraordinaire, Carolyn Tyson, Ladislav Kamenar, Michael Harbeson, Fred Indiviglia, Mel Gilliard, Debbie Harrigan, Jennifer McNew, Tania Yeargin, and Carolyn Gomez. We also thank Ellis Nicholas for his superb darkroom skills.

In addition, our deeply felt thanks is extended to Martha Helmers and Tony Jalandoni, whose photographic talents have contributed so much to the quality of this edition. We acknowledge Tom Xanakis and Lois Fischman whose elegant illustrations have contributed so much to enhancing our frequently inadequate attempts at verbal description. We express a much belated but no less deeply-felt thanks to Marge Gregorman whose enormous contribution as medical illustrator for the First Edition of this text unfortunately went unremarked.

Finally, special mention is owed to two individuals at Raven Press: Kathy Cianci, whose enthusiasm and patience has been an inspiration; and Mary Rogers, without whose faith and commitment in the face of constant delays this book would never have been published.

COMPUTED TOMOGRAPHY AND MAGNETIC RESONANCE OF THE THORAX

Second Edition

Chapter 1

Principles and Techniques of Thoracic CT and MR

Following several years of progressive technical improvements, computed tomography (CT) has evolved to a phase of relative technological maturity. Refinements and further sophistication of equipment have made possible the general use of techniques such as CT densitometry and high-resolution CT, which are playing an increasingly important role in assessing focal and diffuse pulmonary parenchymal diseases.

An appreciation of the role of technical parameters such as slice thickness, reconstruction software, and the physiology of intravenously administered contrast media in the depiction of complex anatomical structures and pathologies has led to the development of new imaging strategies. These strategies have been made possible by the development of automated contrast injectors and robust dynamic imaging modes with automated table incrementation. Improvements in computer hardware and software now permit immediate reconstruction of images. On-line tailoring of examinations is thus a practical proposition on most scanners. These advances, combined with newer high-heat capacity x-ray tubes and high-sensitivity solid state detectors,

have significantly improved patient throughput and reduced the unit cost of CT examinations. In inflation-corrected terms, the cost of CT studies has decreased significantly since the early 1980s. The combination of these technical advances (including very fast scan times of 1–3 sec) has made thoracic CT, once a minor application, one of the most commonly used cross-sectional imaging tests. In this chapter we will describe the impact of these advances on the techniques and imaging strategies necessary to maximize the diagnostic value of the CT thorax examination.

Since the publication of the first edition of this book, another modality, magnetic resonance imaging (MR), has been introduced to our diagnostic armamentarium. As in the early phases of CT development, thoracic applications of MR have lagged behind applications to the nervous system because of inherent technical difficulties related to cardiac and respiratory motion. However, recent technological developments as well as clinical experience presage an increasingly important role for thoracic MR. It is now possible to obtain superb diagnostic studies of all major vascular structures in the thorax, and

MR is quickly replacing alternative modalities for assessing vascular pathology. Consequently, the thoracic radiologist should develop an adequate understanding of flow phenomena, relevant pulse sequences, and imaging protocols. The informed radiologist understands that MR signals provide information fundamentally different from CT about the composition of normal and pathologic tissues. Although initial enthusiasm regarding the diagnostic value of relaxation time measurements has waned, MR can help characterize certain processes, such as mediastinal cysts and hemorrhage. It also can assess the response of certain tumors to therapy. Consequently, the radiologist should have a working knowledge of the basic meaning of tissue signals in MR. In this chapter the reader will find what we believe to be the essentials needed to optimally perform and interpret MR examinations of the thorax.

TECHNIQUES AND STRATEGIES IN CHEST CT

With improvements in technology and increasing clinical experience, the indications for thoracic CT have expanded. The two basic attributes on which the effectiveness of CT is based, however, remain unchanged. First, CT is used to overcome the problem of superimposition of anatomic structures inherent to chest radiography. The cross-sectional depiction of anatomy provides an additional dimension to conventional radiology and helps detect or clarify suspected pathology. Second, a difference in radiographic density of 0.5% can be detected with CT, whereas conventional methods require a 10% change for differentiation. CT thus achieves a much higher contrast that, with the judicious adjustment of window settings, increases the conspicuity of lesions. Diagnostic interpretation is consequently easier and less observer-dependent with CT.

Indications

The chest radiograph remains the most effective study in diagnostic radiology owing to the naturally high contrast of thoracic structures. CT is used as a second-line diagnostic study for problems unresolved by plain films. Examples of this role for CT are:

A mediastinal or hilar contour abnormality. This raises the possibility of vascular pathology such as dissection, aneurysm, congenital anomaly, normal variant, or distortion by tumor.

A pulmonary parenchymal nodule, mass, or infiltrate. In these cases, CT characterization through densitometric analysis or more precise morphologic analysis may be required. When a carcinoma is suspected, complete staging can be performed.

Complex cases of combined pleural and parenchymal pathology. On plain films, it is often difficult to dif-

ferentiate pleural from parenchymal components. In such cases contrast-enhanced CT is indicated.

Chest wall and spinal pathology. Because of the curvature of the chest wall, no single plain film projection is adequate for full evaluation. The transaxial format of CT permits better analysis of the location and extent of such processes.

Pathology involving the cervicothoracic or thoraco-abdominal junctional regions. Because plain films are not effective in the upper abdominal and cervical regions, CT is often indicated to clarify pathology spanning these junctional anatomic regions.

CT can be used to screen patients whose chest radiographs are negative but whose clinical condition leads to a high suspicion of occult intrathoracic pathology. CT is indicated when the following conditions are suspected:

Metastatic nodules in patients with extrathoracic malignancies, especially those with a high propensity for pulmonary metastases.

Endocrinologic or biochemical abnormalities that may be related to intrathoracic pathology, e.g., patients with myasthenia gravis to rule out a thymoma; patients with endocrine abnormalities that raise the possibility of a parathyroid adenoma following negative neck exploration; or patients with an endocrinologically active tumor such as an ectopic pheochromocytoma or a hormonally active bronchial neoplasm.

Underlying cancer in patients with hemoptysis, positive sputum cytology, or hypertrophic pulmonary osteoarthropathy.

Unknown source of infection, especially in the immunocompromised population.

Evaluation of the pulmonary parenchyma in patients with abnormal pulmonary function tests but normal or near normal chest x-rays.

Clearly, the expanding array of indications for CT and the boundless variations of pathologic presentations make it necessary to tailor each CT examination to the particular diagnostic task at hand. The radiologist should always review the available radiologic and clinical data to determine precisely which components of the thoracic anatomy need to be clarified and to determine the best examination strategy. With modern scanners, instant reconstruction times have eased these tasks, and a firm diagnosis should be established before the patient is removed from the CT gantry. Obviously, no single technique is optimal for all indications in thoracic CT. The best approach to an effective use of thoracic CT is to develop a working knowledge of the various scanner-related and patient-related parameters that affect the diagnostic quality of the study. Once understood, these basic parameters can be combined into a strategy that embodies the principle of "maximum diagnostic value at minimum risk and cost."

Technical Parameters

The operations of a CT scanner are complex and highly automated. However, several technical parameters remain operator-dependent and can significantly affect the diagnostic value of the thoracic CT examination.

Slice Thickness

The CT image is a two-dimensional representation of a three-dimensional slice of space. Although the third dimension, or thickness, of the cross-section is not displayed, it directly affects the quality of the image in the other two dimensions. All structures within the unit volume of space represented by the slice, also known as *voxel,* are averaged and represented by a single CT number for the unit surface of the image, also known as *pixel.* Thus, the attenuation values for each pixel represent the average of the attenuation values of all structures present within the voxel (Fig. 1). The thicker the slice, the more averaging of adjacent structures occurs. This phenomenon is known as the partial volume effect. To correct for this effect, an obvious solution is to reduce slice thickness. Thicknesses varying from 1–10 mm are commonly available. However, one should not conclude that the partial volume effect is necessarily deleterious. Paradoxically, thick slices have favorable attributes in thoracic CT. For example, the detection of a lesion by CT or any other modality depends essentially on the density gradient between the lesion and the surrounding normal tissue. In the lung, because normal parenchyma has a very low CT number [about -800 Hounsfield Units (HU)], even a small nodule in only a portion of the slice can be detected. This is because there is enough density difference between the voxels containing the nodule and the surrounding normal lung. Simple calculations show that a 1–2 mm lung nodule can easily be detected in a 10-mm–thick slice. In the mediastinum, when enough contrasting fat is present, 10-mm sections allow detection of lesions as small as 3 mm (Fig. 2). Thus, 10-mm sections are sufficient for routine thoracic CT, requiring fewer scans and less x-ray exposure per examination than other applications.

In addition to differences in density between lesions and surrounding normal tissue, detection and recognition of lesions depend on the ability to differentiate features intrinsic to the normal background of tissue versus features of the lesion. In this regard, thick sections offer another specific advantage in the lung parenchyma. Structures such as vessels, which run obliquely to the plane of the scan, are much better appreciated using thick sections because they can be followed over a longer portion of their course, even though they fill only a small portion of each voxel. Their branching nature can therefore be readily appreciated, and the round appearance of a small nodule is easily differentiated from vessels. On the other hand, if a thin section is used through the lungs, the vessels will be more difficult to recognize because their foreshortened cross-sections do not allow the recognition of their characteristic branching pattern. Thus, thick sections are advantageous in the lung pa-

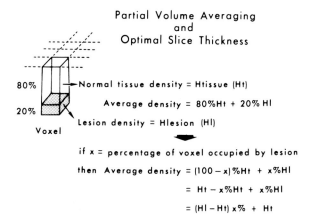

$$\text{Partial Volume Averaging}$$
$$\text{and}$$
$$\text{Optimal Slice Thickness}$$

80% / 20% Voxel

Normal tissue density = Htissue (Ht)

Average density = 80%Ht + 20%Hl

Lesion density = Hlesion (Hl)

if x = percentage of voxel occupied by lesion

then Average density = (100 − x)%Ht + x%Hl

= Ht − x%Ht + x%Hl

= (Hl − Ht) x% + Ht

FIG. 1. The partial volume effect. The detectability of a lesion partially occupying a voxel of normal tissue depends on the difference in CT density between the lesion (Hl) and surrounding tissue (Ht), or (Hl-Ht) multiplied by the percentage (x) of the slice thickness occupied by the lesion. Let us assume, for example, that a 2-mm lesion of density +50 HU is present within a 10-mm slice of lung tissue measuring −750 HU. Since the lesion occupies 20% of the slice thickness, the CT number difference generated by the mass will be equal to [50 −(−750)] × 20% = 160 HU. Since current scanners detect changes of 10–20 HU between voxels, this lesion will be easily visualized. Thus, the minimum size of lesions detectable by CT in any given organ is primarily dependent on the density difference between pathologic and normal tissues.

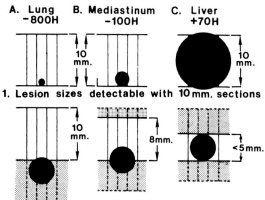

A. Lung −800H   B. Mediastinum −100H   C. Liver +70H

10 mm.

1. Lesion sizes detectable with 10 mm. sections

10 mm.   8mm.   <5mm.

2. Section thickness requirement to detect 5mm. lesion

FIG. 2. Relationship between slice thickness, lesion size, and tissue density. **1 (Top):** Minimum lesion size detectable in lung (**A**), mediastinum (**B**), and liver (**C**) are illustrated for a 10-mm section. With the large density gradient between aerated and pathologic lung, lesions as small as 1 mm can be easily detected. In the mediastinum with sufficient background fat, a 3-mm lesion is the smallest size detectable with a 10-mm section. In the liver, unless contrast is used, a lesion has to be 10 mm in size for detection with a 10-mm slice thickness. **2 (Bottom):** Slice thickness requirements to detect 5-mm lesions are illustrated for lung, mediastinum, and liver. Ten-mm sections are very adequate in the lung; however, 8-mm slice thicknesses are more appropriate for detecting mediastinal lymph nodes of 5 mm in diameter. In the liver it is necessary to have a slice thickness equal to the lesion size for optimal detection.

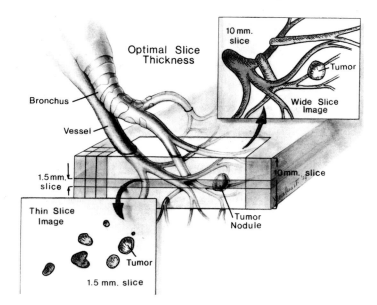

FIG. 3. Advantage of thick slices in lung imaging. In 10-mm thick sections, bronchovascular structures are imaged over a longer portion of their course. Thus, the branching nature of vessels and bronchi is easily recognized in thick slices (*upper right, inset*). With thinner sections, vessels and bronchi appear as round rather than tubular structures (*lower left, inset*). A tumor nodule, as illustrated, is easier to recognize against the background of branching structures in the thicker slice. See also Fig. 4.

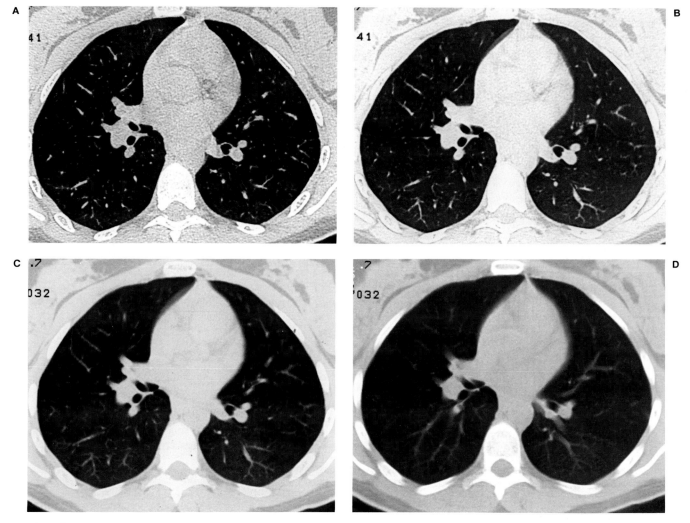

FIG. 4. Slice thickness and lung imaging. A series of four slices was obtained at the same anatomic level with 1-mm (**A**), 2-mm (**B**), 4-mm (**C**), and 8-mm (**D**) slice thicknesses. Technical parameters were kept identical except for slice thickness. Note that the branching nature of bronchial structures and vessels is progressively better appreciated as the slice thickness is increased from 1 to 8 mm. Note also the graininess of the image on the 1- and 2-mm slice thicknesses due to higher noise levels. For routine evaluations of the pulmonary parenchyma and mediastinum, 8-mm sections offer a definite advantage since focal lesions are easily recognizable against the background of branching structures. Very thin sections should be reserved for detailed analyses of the pulmonary parenchyma. Note that even though the noise levels appear high in the chest wall and mediastinal structures on the thin-section scans, the noise level does not affect the lung parenchyma with its low radiographic density.

renchyma owing to its high natural tissue contrast and because pulmonary vascular features are easier to recognize (Figs. 3 and 4).

Conversely, partial volume effects may be detrimental in areas of the thorax where tissue densities are not as contrasted as they are in lung parenchyma, such as the mediastinum or chest wall. More important, *the orientation of the anatomy* relative to the transaxial plane determines how much structure averaging and attendant loss of boundaries will be observed. For example, when two structures run in a course perpendicular to the plane of scanning, they are much easier to separate than when they run obliquely. The interpreter should be keenly aware of this problem in anatomic areas where structural boundaries are running in a course parallel or oblique relative to the scanned plane (Fig. 5A–E). The main areas in which this effect can be seen are the cervicothoracic junction, especially at the apex of the lungs; the aorticopulmonary window; the hilar regions; the subcarinal region; and the peridiaphragmatic areas. In such regions, thinner sections should be used.

Thus, 8 to 10-mm–thick sections, which are standard on current scanners, are generally adequate to examine the thorax. Thinner sections on the order of 3–5 mm are indicated when studying areas of anatomy oriented obliquely to the plane of scanning.

Thinner 1 to 2 mm sections are indicated to study fine details of the pulmonary parenchyma in association with high-resolution techniques (see below).

Slice Spacing

A general guideline for slice spacing is to use contiguous spacing throughout the regions of interest. With current technology, there is no need to scan the patient in a noncontiguous fashion because scan times, throughput, patient exposure, and costs have all been effectively reduced. An exception to this is sampling for diffuse lung disease. With very thin sections, collimation of the x-ray beam reduces the number of photons reaching the detectors. This increases noise, which is perceived as a graininess in the image (1,2). This noise will degrade resolution to a varying extent, depending on the density of the tissues examined. For example, thin-section scans demonstrate a much higher noise level in the mediastinum and chest wall regions than in the lung parenchyma, which is much less dense and requires less exposure to achieve adequate image quality (Fig. 4). Thus, when the primary intent for a thin-section scan is to examine the lung parenchyma, there is only a minimal need to increase exposure factors unless graininess

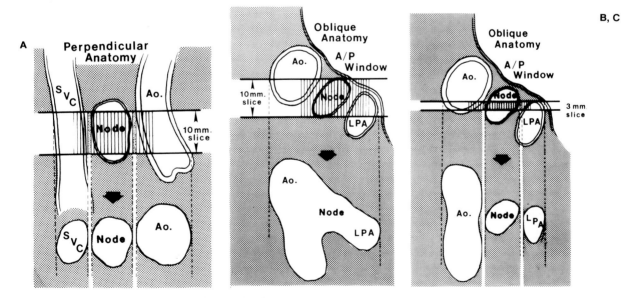

FIG. 5. Importance of anatomic orientation in defining optimal slice thickness. To illustrate the importance of anatomic orientation the mediastinal region, between the superior vena cava (*SVC*) and ascending aorta (*Ao*), which are perpendicular to the axial plane, is illustrated in **A**. The node located between the aorta and the superior vena cava is easily detectable provided a minimum amount of mediastinal fat is present. Image voxels located between the node, the superior vena cava, and the aorta contain only fat and thus allow separation of the node from surrounding structures in the resultant CT image (*lower half* of A). In **B** and **C** a coronal section obtained at the level of the aortico-pulmonary window (*A/P*) is represented. Since the arch of the aorta and the left pulmonary artery (*LPA*) run an oblique course relative to the axial plane, a node located between these two structures is likely to be undetectable on a thick section scan because all pixels represent a mixture of mediastinal fat, nodal tissue, and vascular tissue, thus preventing a separation of the node from the surrounding structures on the resultant CT image. When the slice width is reduced (C), the node becomes visible as a distinct structure, since pixels containing only fat are now present. It is therefore important to reduce slice thickness in areas of complex anatomy oriented obliquely to the axial plane such as the hila, anteroposterior window, thoracic inlet, and peridiaphragmatic regions.

D 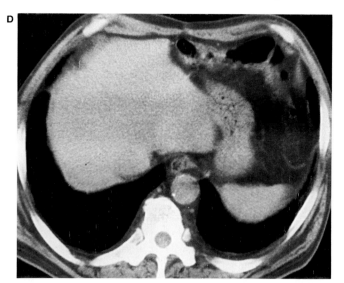 E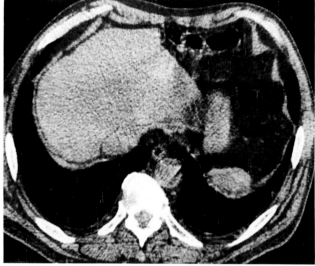

FIG. 5. (*Continued.*) Partial volume effect in thin-section scanning. As demonstrated in A–C, regions of oblique anatomy may require thinner section scans for delineation of structures. In **D** no separation is possible between the diaphragm and liver or the diaphragm and spleen on this 10-mm section. In **E**, a 2-mm section clearly demonstrates the separation between the diaphragm and the liver and provides a better appreciation of the anatomy of the diaphragm.

of the image is perceived, especially in the posterior paraspinal regions.

The most important consideration when studying the mediastinum or chest wall is to correct for the increasing noise levels of thin slices by increasing the milliamperage or scan time (2). Large patients will require more exposure than small or thin patients. Unlike underexposure, which is characterized by noisy images, overexposure is difficult to perceive on CT images. As opposed to standard radiography where the blackness of the film cannot be manipulated and overexposure is easily detected, CT images are digitized and the appearance of the image can be easily manipulated through window setting adjustments. Overexposure can, however, be recognized because it degrades image quality by generating streak artifacts near pulsatile structures like pulmonary arteries or the left heart border. Whenever streak artifacts are seen near such borders, the radiologist should make a point of verifying exposure factors and reduce them appropriately. As a guideline, adequate thoracic images can be obtained with about one-half to one-third of the exposure factors used in the abdomen (3).

Scan Time

Effective scan times have been greatly reduced over the past few years. For thoracic imaging, a short scan time is necessary to reduce the effect of respiratory motion. Furthermore, with scan times in the 1-sec range, images are more often obtained within the longer and quieter diastolic period of the cardiac cycle, thereby improving visualization of cardiac structures. Whenever possible, and to the extent that short scan times are not

obtained at the expense of reduced image quality, it is advisable to use scan times on the order of 2 sec or less. It should be remembered, however, that shorter scan times are often achieved by decreasing the number of sampling projections. A loss of resolution can occur with very short scan times because the amount of data used to reconstruct the image is itself reduced. This is not correctable by using higher photon fluxes, i.e., by increasing beam intensity. For studies in which high resolution is needed, it may be necessary to increase the scan time to allow for more data to be collected by the detectors.

With the short scan times currently available, scans at suspended respiration can be easily obtained in virtually every patient. Even with fast scan times, respiratory motion can degrade image quality and suspended breathing remains mandatory. In most cases, scanning the thorax is performed at full lung capacity (end-inspiratory volume). This is the most commonly used way of suspending respiration. The instructions are simple: "Take a deep breath and hold your breath." Full inspiration promotes separation of pulmonary structures. However, the reproducibility of inspiratory breathing is less than that of breathing at resting lung volume (end-tidal volume). Thus, reproducibility of lung position when needed, e.g., when measuring the CT density of pulmonary nodules, is best achieved at resting lung volume. The instructions to the patient in such a case are: "Breathe in, breathe out, relax and hold your breath." Lack of breathing reproducibility can sometimes create significant problems such as totally missing a known pulmonary nodule (4). Spirometric devices that control breathing have been proposed but have not yet been proven to be of definite clinical value (5,6).

A potentially important trend is the development of scanners capable of acquiring multiple scans within one breath-holding period. Recently, continuous spiral acquisition of slices within a single breath-hold has been proposed as a method of correcting for lack of respiratory reproducibility (7). The advent of cine-CT methods with acquisition times on the order of 50–100 msec also offers the potential for imaging the entire thorax within a single breath-hold. This is particularly helpful in children and critically ill patients (8).

Field of View

Another important parameter is the choice of an appropriate field of view for image reconstruction. Although not often appreciated, the diameter of the field of view has a profound effect on the image quality achieved with CT. This is because CT images are the representation of a 512 × 512 matrix of numbers. This matrix is the mathematical support of the computer calculations used to represent the space examined within the aperture of the scanner. The portion of space represented by an individual pixel depends on the size of the field of view as indicated to the computer by the operator. Because the total number of pixels in each image is limited, if we select a large area of interest, each pixel represents a proportionately larger volume of space. Resolution is then limited to the size of that pixel. For example, if we choose a 51-cm field of view, each pixel would be about 1 mm × 1 mm in size. Clearly then, it is most appropriate to adjust the field of view size to the size of the anatomic area we wish to examine. Ideally, pixels should be smaller than the minimum distance resolvable by a scanner. On current scanners, resolutions on the order of 0.3–0.45 mm can be achieved. Thus, maximum resolution is obtained only when fields of view of about 15 cm are used (15 cm ÷ 512 = 0.3 mm pixels).

In practice, it is sufficient to adjust and match the diameter of the field of view to the size of the transverse diameter of the thorax. It should also be noted that simple magnification of CT images is not effective in improving details, because the pixel size is not changed with magnification (Fig. 6). On the other hand, retrospectively reconstructing selected areas of the object from raw data, a process known as "targeted reconstruction," is the best way to achieve a high level of anatomic detail for high-resolution studies.

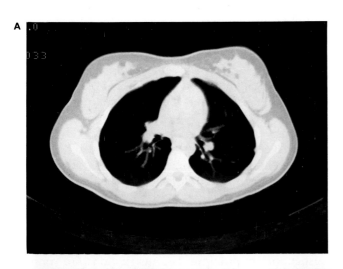

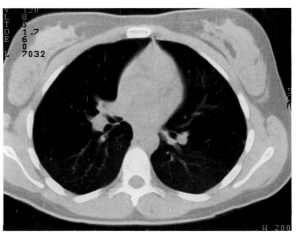

FIG. 6. Field of view. **A:** Selection of field of view too large for the patient's size results in suboptimal images and a loss of anatomic detail and diagnostic information. In this example, less than half of the image matrix is used to image the patient. **B, C:** To correct for the inadequate image in A, simple magnification was applied (B) and the raw data was reconstructed with a smaller field of view (C). Note the difference in quality between B and C. Simple magnification does not improve spatial resolution. Structure edges are not sharp, whereas with image reconstruction with a field of view adjusted to the patient's size, better detail is seen.

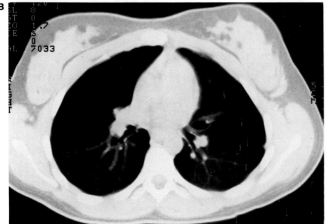

Window Settings

The full scale of CT numbers cannot be displayed in a single image because a limited number of gray shades is available for electronic display. The operator must select a portion of the CT number range to be displayed. This is done by using electronic windows and defining the width and level at which the window will be active. Because the range of CT numbers in the thorax is the greatest of those for all body parts extending from the almost air density of the lungs (-800 HU) to the high density of bones ($+600$ HU), no single window setting can properly display all the information available on a thoracic CT study. Each thoracic CT examination should be viewed with at least two and, in selected cases, three sets of window settings: one for the lung parenchyma, one for the mediastinal and chest wall structures, and, whenever needed, one for the bony structures. Although the precise window settings are often a matter of subjective preference, certain guidelines should be followed to avoid suboptimal representation of anatomic structures. It has been shown that the most accurate representation of an object is achieved when the window level is placed at a value midway between the CT number of the structure to be measured and the

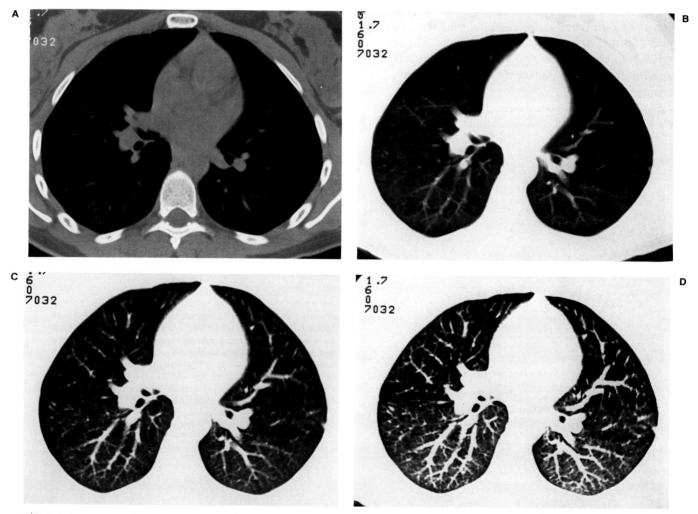

FIG. 7. Influence of window settings on visibility of pulmonary structures. An 8-mm thick scan in the mid-thoracic region is represented at different window settings. In **A**, small pulmonary vessels cannot be appreciated. However, at this window setting of -375 window level (WL) and 2,000 window width (WW), a good compromise is achieved between visualization of anatomic structures of the chest wall and mediastinum and those of the pulmonary parenchyma. The interface between the pulmonary parenchyma and the pleura is well delineated. Even though fine detail of the parenchymal structures is not observable, the relatively clear background helps identify focal lesions. This window setting is appropriate for routine evaluations. In **B**, the effect of lowering window level and width is demonstrated. More peripheral and smaller branches of the pulmonary arteries are demonstrated. These small branches were not visible on the prior scan because their density was averaged with that of the surrounding air and was too low. However, by reducing the window width more image contrast is achievable and reducing the window level permits a better matching with the low density of these peripheral vessels. Note, however, the associated loss of visualization of the chest wall and mediastinal structures. The interface between pulmonary parenchyma and pleura is difficult to define. **C** and **D** illustrate the effect of further reducing window width. More contrast is now present between pulmonary vascular structures and lung parenchyma. Vessels appear more prominent in size and very small structures in the range of 0.5 mm can be detected with such window settings even though slice thickness is 8 mm. However there is complete loss of detail in the mediastinum, hila, and chest wall. Note also that central vessels and bronchial walls appear falsely prominent.

CT number of the surrounding tissue (9,10). For example, if a lung nodule measures 50 HU and the surrounding parenchyma measures −800 HU, the proper window level should be about −375 HU. In the lung parenchyma, as vessels become smaller from the center to the periphery of the lung, their CT density decreases proportionately because of partial volume averaging of vessel and surrounding air. To represent the smaller vessels in the lung parenchyma, it is thus necessary to use low window levels and widths (Fig. 7). Because of lesser partial volume effects, the density of vessels is greater. Therefore, on thin-section scans, the window levels to be used for representing small vessels and parenchyma need to be higher than those used to represent the same structures on a thick-section scan (Fig. 8). Suggested window settings for different slice thicknesses and sizes of pulmonary structures are presented in Table 1.

It is important to remember that the apparent size of structures is markedly affected by the choice of window settings. This is due to the relative blurring of edges inherent to the CT scanning process. As shown in Figure 9, this edge blurring will affect the apparent size of structures depending on the window settings used. More important, when an inappropriate window setting is used, the apparent size of smaller structures (e.g., blood vessels in the lung parenchyma) is much more affected than that of larger structures (e.g., the aorta). For example, a blood vessel can be magnified 300–400% if too low a window level is used, whereas the thoracic aorta will be magnified at most 20–30%. This effect is critically important in the interpretation of diffuse parenchymal processes.

Window width should be chosen so as to encompass at least the entire range of densities present within the scan. For example, in the mediastinum the range would be −100 HU for fat to +400 to +500 HU for bony structures of the sternum or spine. Thus a window width of about 500–600 HU is recommended. In the pulmo-

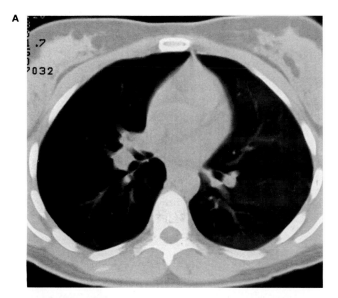

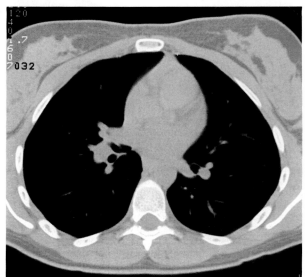

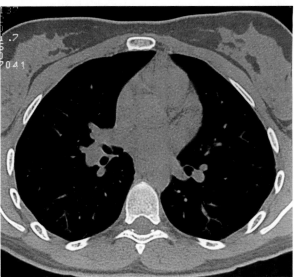

FIG. 8. Effect of slice thickness on window settings. Because partial volume effects are reduced with thinner section scans, the density of peripheral vessels increases on such scans. Thus, the appropriate window level will be proportionately higher on thinner section scans than with thicker section scans. Examples of a scan obtained with 8-mm (**A**), 4-mm (**B**), and 2-mm (**C**) slice thicknesses at the same anatomic level illustrate this effect. In A, at −675 WL and 2000 WW, a good compromise is achieved between visualization of parenchymal structures, chest wall, and mediastinal structures. To achieve the same degree of relative visualization of parenchymal, mediastinal, and chest wall structures the level of −545 WL and 2,000 WW is appropriate for a 4-mm thick scan (B), whereas a window level of −375 HU and a window width of 2,000 HU are needed to achieve the same degree of vascular visualization in a 2-mm thick scan (C). WL, window level; WW, window width.

TABLE 1. *Appropriate window settings as a function of slice thickness and size of pulmonary structures*

				Structure size			
	10 mm	5 mm	3 mm	2 mm	1 mm	0.5 mm	0.3 mm
Slice							
10 mm L	−375	−587	−673	−715	−757	−780	−788
W	2,000	2,000	2,000	1,360	688	320	192
5 mm L	−375	−375	−545	−630	−715	−757	−775
W	2,000	2,000	2,000	2,000	1,360	688	400
2 mm L	−375	−375	−375	−375	−587	−694	−736
W	2,000	2,000	2,000	2,000	2,000	1,700	1,024
1 mm L	−375	−375	−375	−375	−375	−587	−672
W	2,000	2,000	2,000	2,000	2,000	2,000	2,000

Assumptions: Lung density is −800 HU, structure density is 50 HU. Window width is given as maximum needed to differentiate structure from surrounding lung by at least one level of gray. L, window level; W, window width.

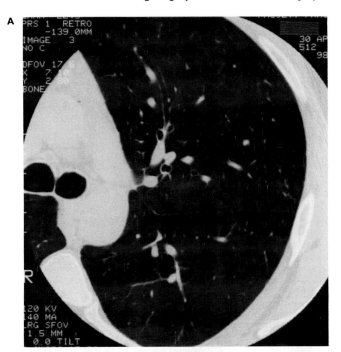

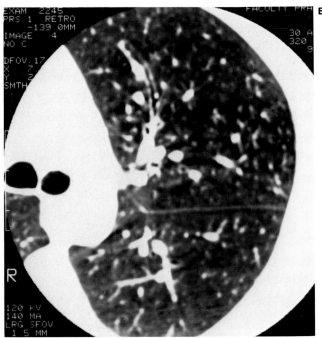

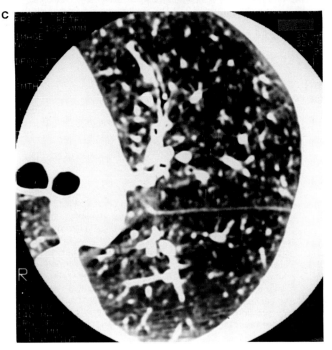

FIG. 9. Effect of window settings on apparent size of structures in the pulmonary parenchyma. At appropriate window levels and width of −375 WL/2,000 WW in **A**, accurate display of the size of pulmonary parenchymal structures is achieved. In **B**, window width was narrowed to 1,000 and window level was decreased to −650. Note that the interlobar fissure is now more prominent and vessels appear larger. In **C**, by further reducing window level and width, higher contrast is achieved. However, the vascular structures which appear very delicate in A now appear abnormally prominent. Note also that the smallest structures are magnified proportionately more than larger structures. For example, note how thickened the bronchial walls appear in C as compared to A. This nonlinear preferential magnification of small structures may lead the unwary observer to over diagnosis of diffuse pathology. WL, window level; WW, window width.

nary parenchyma, the range extends from −800 HU for the lung parenchyma to 400–500 HU for bone, thus a range of at least 1,300 HU and preferably 1,800 to 2,000 HU should be used. To increase conspicuity of pulmonary features, narrow window widths can be used in selected instances. The radiologist should be aware of the influence of window settings on the appearance of pulmonary and mediastinal structures.

Algorithm of Reconstruction

The computer software used to reconstruct a CT image from raw data can markedly affect the characteristics of the image. For the purposes of this chapter, we will consider computer reconstruction algorithms as falling into two general classes: those designed for ana-

tomic structures with inherently low contrast, or so-called high *contrast* resolution algorithms; and those designed for high-contrast anatomic structures, generally high *spatial* resolution algorithms. In general, CT software designers achieve high contrast resolution by "smoothing" the image, using so-called reconstruction filters that average the density of neighboring pixels (11). This is advantageous in the brain or liver because it reduces the apparent image noise, permitting the recognition of underlying lesions that are generally less dense than normal tissue by only 20–30 HU. However, in the thorax, this type of algorithm tends to blur the definition of small pulmonary structures. In the lung, since natural contrast is high, it is more desirable to use high spatial resolution software, which best preserves sharp edges and detail (12,13) (Fig. 10).

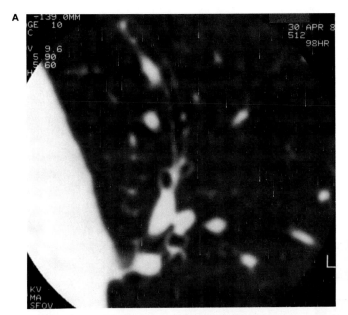

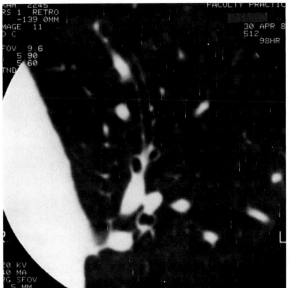

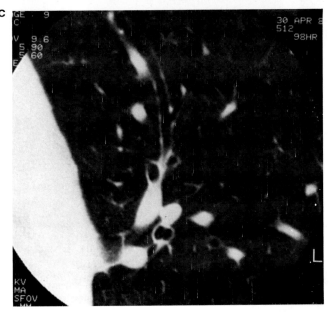

FIG. 10. Influence of reconstruction algorithm on image quality in high-resolution CT. High-resolution study of a left upper lobe in a normal patient with a low spatial resolution and high-contrast resolution or so-called "smoothing" algorithm in **A**, intermediate spatial resolution and contrast resolution in **B**, and high spatial resolution with low-contrast resolution in **C**. Note clear-cut improvement in detail in C compared to B and A, which exhibit blurring. Note also that the image in C appears noisier than either A or B. This example illustrates the trade-offs between various algorithms of reconstruction. High spatial resolution software as in C is more appropriate for analyzing fine lung parenchymal detail.

A drawback of the high spatial frequency algorithms is their tendency to enhance image noise. If excessive, this "enhanced" noise may hinder the interpretation of fine details of the lung parenchyma, especially in high-resolution studies (14). This is particularly true in the paraspinal areas where noise is higher because of the increased attenuation of the x-ray beam by the vertebral bodies. To determine the most appropriate algorithms of reconstruction in a given scanner, we recommend that a single normal CT scan be reconstructed with all available reconstruction filters. By comparing the scans obtained, it is generally easy to select the most appropriate by simply comparing the visual quality of the images, as illustrated in Figure 10.

Multi-planar Reconstruction and Three-Dimensional Volume Rendering

Sagittal, coronal, or oblique reconstructions of transaxial sections are sometimes helpful in thoracic CT. This is especially true in evaluating pathology located in the cervicothoracic or thoraco-abdominal regions (14). Obviously, the quality of multi-planar reconstructions is directly related to the slice thickness, which determines the pixel height in the reformatted image. In the past, multi-planar reconstructions were time consuming. The use of increasingly powerful computers, however, now allow these reconstructions to be performed rapidly. Ideally, thin contiguous sections should be obtained. In practice, 4-mm thick sections obtained every 3 mm, i.e.,

overlapping by 1 mm, offer the best compromise because they achieve reasonable resolution in sagittal, coronal, or oblique planes of reconstruction and prevent discontinuity between slices. When performing a multiplanar study, it is important to coach the patient to breathe in a reproducible manner between scans to avoid slice-to-slice gaps. More recently, powerful computer hardware and software have been developed to achieve true three-dimensional volume rendering of a stack of CT images (15–17). With advances in image analysis and automated structure recognition, these techniques may become important tools in the management of intrathoracic disease, allowing very precise three-dimensional staging for eventual surgery or planning customized therapy (Fig. 11).

High-Resolution Computed Tomography

One of the main limitations of conventional radiography in the evaluation of diffuse pulmonary parenchymal disease is the superimposition of structures due to the two-dimensional projectional format of that imaging method. Over the past few years, high-resolution computed tomography (HRCT) has been used increasingly as a powerful technique in the investigation of diffuse pulmonary processes (18–20).

HRCT simply represents the combination of 1–2-mm thick CT slices reconstructed with pixel sizes in the range of 200–300 μ, i.e., fields of view of 10–15 cm. By using a very thin section, structural superimposition

A
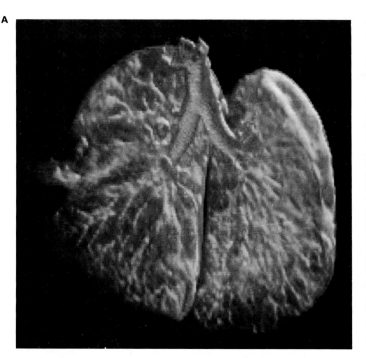
B
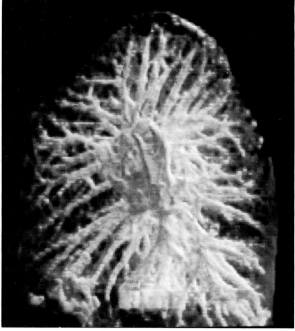

FIG. 11. 3-D reconstruction of a lung specimen imaged with 3-mm thin scans is illustrated. These images can be analyzed in three dimensions on specialized computers and may help in better delineating the relationship of pulmonary and mediastinal pathology. From Ney Derek et al., ref. 15, with permission.

within the thickness of the scan is greatly reduced, permitting optimal evaluation of lung details. The reduction of the field of view allows optimal resolution. This technique can be performed on any modern CT scanner. As mentioned above, it is critical to use appropriate high spatial resolution reconstruction algorithms with HRCT (see Fig. 10). These algorithms are standard on all current scanners. HRCT can therefore be routinely implemented, provided proper technique is used.

Some technical considerations should be kept in mind. With thinly collimated sections, the signal-to-noise ratio of the image may be degraded because of the reduced number of photons reaching the detectors. Because the reconstruction software used in HRCT tends to enhance the noisiness of the image, it is important to increase exposure levels to achieve optimal image quality. However, for HRCT applications, the critical factor is the noise level within the lung parenchyma, not that in the mediastinum or chest wall. The observer should not only adjust the exposure levels to reduce apparent noise (especially in the posterior regions of the lung parenchyma near the thoracic spine), but also not attempt to reduce noise in the chest wall or mediastinal structures. Using such an approach, the increase in exposure can be kept to a minimum, and no increase is usually necessary in thinner patients (3).

Proper window settings are critical for accurate displays of diffuse pathology. Using an inappropriate window level can make structures appear larger or smaller than they truly are. These magnification or minimization effects are much more pronounced for the fine parenchymal structures essential to the interpretation of HRCT (see Fig. 9).

Contrast Media

By definition, contrast agents are the means by which subject contrast can be improved to bring it within the detection range of a particular imaging modality. The thorax is the part of the body with the highest natural tissue contrast. Ribs and vessels are of markedly different density than the surrounding aerated lungs. Mediastinal structures are usually embedded in sufficient amounts of fat, so the role of contrast agents is limited in thoracic CT. In most cases, sufficient information is available without contrast enhancement. Knowledge of mediastinal and hilar anatomy is generally sufficient to determine whether a particular structure is pathologic. Contrast enhancement, however, may be necessary when mediastinal fat is lacking, when a vascular abnormality is suspected, or when patients have complex pleuroparenchymal disease.

Physiologic Considerations

Defining sensible strategies of contrast agent utilization requires a brief review of the physiology of intravenous contrast distribution in the body. First and foremost, intravenous contrast media used in CT distribute freely from the vascular compartment into the extravascular, extracellular compartment and vice versa (21–25). The only tissue of exception is the brain, where the vascular compartment is not permeable to contrast agents when the blood-brain barrier is intact. The depiction of the vascular compartment is easily achieved in the brain but not in the rest of the body. Rapid passage of contrast from the intravascular space into the extracellular, extravascular space occurs within seconds. Within one or two minutes after intravenous injection, equilibrium is reached. Because the extravascular space is several times larger than the vascular compartment, the majority of iodine molecules will be distributed in the extravascular space of tissues (21). Also, renal excretion actively decreases the concentration of the contrast agent. Therefore, the differentiation and characterization of a lesion depends on all of the following factors with contrast-enhanced CT: (a) the timing of the scan relative to the amount and speed of contrast delivery; (b) the vascularity of the lesion during injection and for a few seconds thereafter, while most contrast molecules are still in the vascular space; (c) the relative size of the extravascular space of the lesion compared to normal tissue, which determines the density difference between lesion and tissue for scans obtained beyond the early vascular phase of injection; (d) the permeability of the vascular space both for exit and re-entry of contrast molecules, since it determines the rate of contrast agent exchange between intra- and extravascular compartments; and (e) renal excretion.

Contrast Injection Techniques

Understanding the dynamics of contrast media distribution has important implications for selecting techniques of contrast delivery (25). For example, a bolus injection will provide sufficient vascular characterization for only the first few scans after injection, with progressively decreasing differentiation thereafter. Bolus injection combined with rapid scanning is essential when evaluating vascular processes (26). Nonvascular structures such as nodes and masses also can progressively increase in density over time depending on the amount of extravascular space present in these lesions. On occasion, we have observed nonvascular masses becoming as dense as nearby vascular structures when imaged several minutes after injection (Fig. 12). Because the determination of the vascular nature of an abnormality is usually made by comparing the density of a known vessel with that of the abnormality, it is important for the interpreter to define the exact mode and timing of injection used for a given scan. It should be remembered that the extravascular space is several times

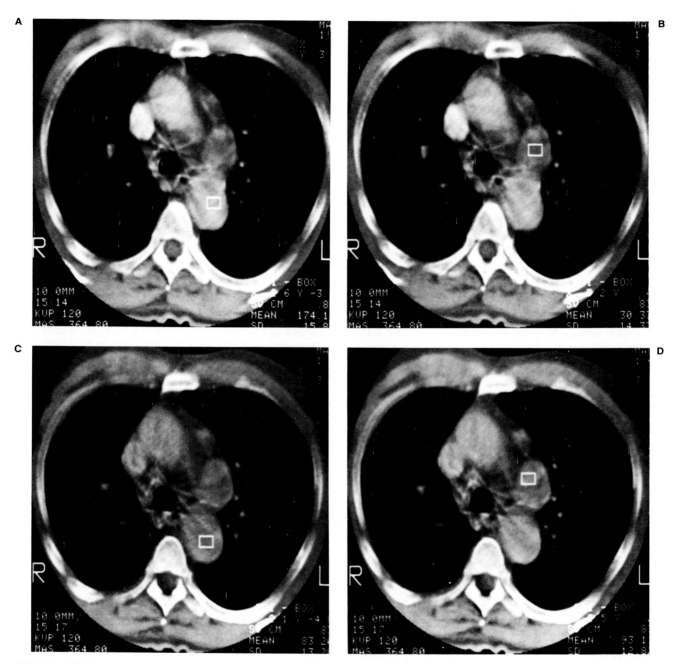

FIG. 12. A, B: Same section, at the level of the aorticopulmonary window, immediately following a bolus of contrast agent (note time reference in the lower left corner—15:14). The descending aorta has a mean density of 174 HU; the well-defined mass in the aorticopulmonary window has a mean density of 30 HU. **C, D:** Same section, at the same level as in (**A**) and (**B**), obtained 3 min later (note time reference in lower left corner—15:17). There has been a decrease in the density of contrast medium within the descending aorta, which now measures 83 HU [compare with (**A**)]. However, there has been a substantial increase in the density of the mass, which now measures 93 HU [compare with (**B**)]. The marked increase in density within this mass suggested the erroneous diagnosis of a saccular aneurysm of the undersurface of the aortic arch. This patient had known small cell carcinoma involving the left hilum. Following chemotherapy, a repeat scan showed total disappearance of the mass in the aorticopulmonary window, confirming this mass to be mediastinal adenopathy. Density within masses is a function of the total dose of contrast agent, the vascularity of a lesion, and the relative size of its extravascular space compared to normal tissue, the permeability of the capillaries within the mass, and the time elapsed from the end of the contrast medium injection.

larger than the intravascular space, and marked dilution of contrast occurs very rapidly after the end of injection.

A better understanding of these physiologic points, along with the availability of faster scanners and automated injectors, has popularized strategies combining an extended bolus injection of contrast with rapid scanning and automated table incrementation (27–32). This technique is extremely effective in evaluating vascular structures, especially in the hilar and perihilar regions. Indeed, the ideal method of contrast medium delivery for the mediastinum should provide a high level of vascular enhancement at the time of scanning, and only at that time. On the other hand, when evaluating pleuroparenchymal abnormalities, information relative to the postvascular phase is also important. In such cases, the start of scanning may be delayed by 20–30 sec to permit the distribution of some contrast agent to the extravascular space. This is helpful in differentiating inflammatory pleural processes from parenchymal infiltrates (see Chapter 9).

A working knowledge of the transit times of the intravenous bolus in the various vascular structures of the chest greatly helps in the timing of bolus injections and scans. To define this range of transit times, we have studied a series of patients to determine the average times of bolus arrival in the major vascular structures (Table 2). In hemodynamically normal individuals, antecubital vein to right heart transit is about 3 sec, 6 sec to pulmonary arteries, 9 sec to left heart, and 12–15 sec to major arteries. Another important consideration in contrast enhancement is to use agents with a lower concentration of iodine to avoid streak artifacts related to

marked differences in density between the concentrated agent and surrounding structures. Thus, agents with concentrations of 30–40% rather than 60% are recommended. In our experience, non-ionic contrast agents have been associated with a lower incidence of minor reactions, such as nausea and vomiting, when used with rapid, high-volume bolus injection techniques. Automatic contrast injectors coupled with dynamic scan programs now allow the complete evaluation of all thoracic vascular structures with a total dose of 100–150 cc of contrast. A rate of injection between 1.5–2 cc per sec is usually adequate.

Patient Factors

Studies of the lung parenchyma are best performed at full inspiration to promote separation of vascular structures. Scans obtained at lesser degrees of inspiration may demonstrate areas of increased densities in the dependent regions of the lung parenchyma. On conventional CT scans, these areas of dependent densities appear featureless, but on HRCT a pseudoreticular and often misleading appearance can be seen (Fig. 13). Classically, dependent densities have been attributed to fluid accumulation due to gravitational effects. More recently it has been shown that these dependent densities are due to areas of atelectasis (33,34). The best explanation for this process is that the pressure gradient needed to expand air spaces is lower in the nondependent regions of the lungs than in the dependent regions, which are subject to the weight of the lung above them. Thus, in the recumbent position, air space expansion does not occur homogeneously. Rather, it progresses from nondependent to dependent regions during inspiration. With incomplete inspiration, partially collapsed air spaces are likely to be present in the dependent regions of the lungs. Dependent densities may simulate or obscure underlying pathology. The best way to correct for this problem is to obtain a deep inspiration scan. If the abnormality does not disappear, it is necessary to place the patient in a prone position and re-scan the area after vigorous coughing and deep inspiration maneuvers have been attempted (see Fig. 13). Another often unrecognized patient-related artifact is the presence of atelectatic regions of lung due to processes compressing the lung focally, such as pleural plaques, pleural masses, chest wall masses, and large osteophytes (Fig. 14).

Patient Positioning

Patients are usually scanned in the supine position. To prevent streak artifacts from appearing on skeletal

TABLE 2. *Average thoracic transit times*[a]

	Bolus in (sec)	Bolus out (sec)
Superior vena cava	3.7 ± 1.5	9.0 ± 2.5
Pulmonary arteries	6.5 ± 2.5	10.0 ± 3.0
Ascending aorta	10.5 ± 3.0	17.8 ± 3.5
Descending aorta and neck vessels	12.3 ± 3.8	19.4 ± 3.8
Jugular vein	17.8 ± 5.0	27.0 ± 5.0
Inferior vena cava	16.0 ± 5.5	ND

[a] 2-sec i.v. bolus of 10 cc total volume in antecubital vein.
Data were obtained by measuring transit times with a gamma camera set at one image per sec from start of an injection of 20 mCi of technetium-99m methylene diphosphonate. The data of 35 consecutive patients of ages varying between 19 and 72 years were averaged. These average times should be taken into consideration when setting up dynamic scan programs or when obtaining individual scans of particular areas. Scans should start at the time of bolus arrival in the structures investigated. ND, not done.

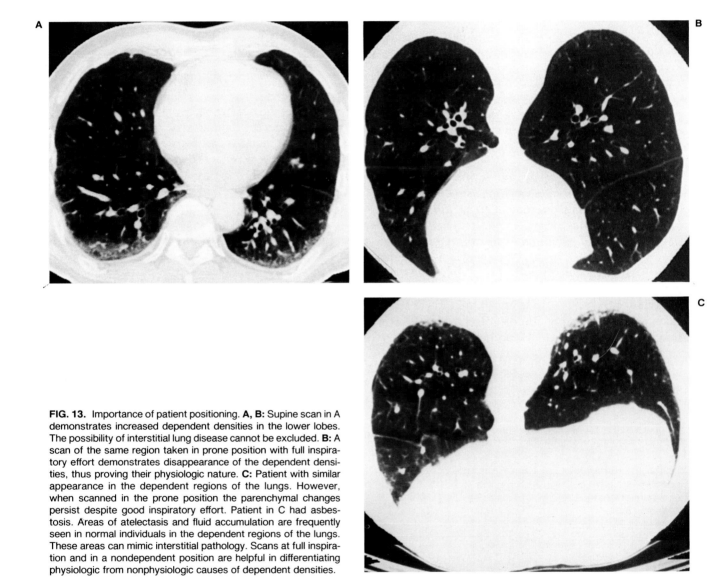

FIG. 13. Importance of patient positioning. **A, B:** Supine scan in A demonstrates increased dependent densities in the lower lobes. The possibility of interstitial lung disease cannot be excluded. **B:** A scan of the same region taken in prone position with full inspiratory effort demonstrates disappearance of the dependent densities, thus proving their physiologic nature. **C:** Patient with similar appearance in the dependent regions of the lungs. However, when scanned in the prone position the parenchymal changes persist despite good inspiratory effort. Patient in C had asbestosis. Areas of atelectasis and fluid accumulation are frequently seen in normal individuals in the dependent regions of the lungs. These areas can mimic interstitial pathology. Scans at full inspiration and in a nondependent position are helpful in differentiating physiologic from nonphysiologic causes of dependent densities.

A

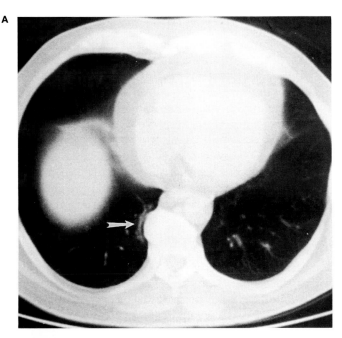

B

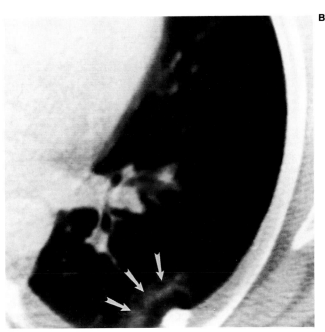

C

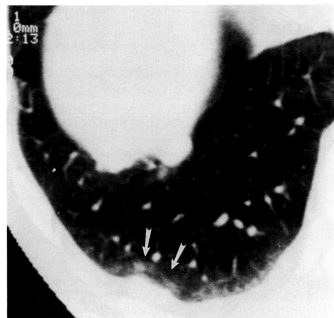

FIG. 14. Effect of focal pressure on lung parenchyma. Abnormal density of the lung parenchyma is often seen near processes that compress the lung. These changes are nonspecific and presumably represent areas of focal atelectasis. **A:** A focal lung compression due to large osteophyte. Linear area of atelectasis is seen in the subpleural region adjacent to the osteophyte (*arrow*). **B:** Example of focal subpleural atelectasis. The patient with a large callous from prior rib fracture (*arrows*). **C:** Example of same phenomenon near pleural plaque from asbestos exposure (*arrows*). Note absence of similar parenchymal changes in the regions immediately adjacent to the process that compresses the lung. These changes should not be interpreted as pathologic.

structures of the upper extremity, patients should be scanned with arms elevated above the head. In patients with pleural or parenchymal fluid collections, scanning in positions other than supine is useful. The effect of gravity may help to differentiate loculated from free effusion and pulmonary edema from other causes of infiltrates (35). Displacement of fluids by the use of lateral decubitus or prone positioning can also help define any underlying pathology.

CT PLANNING AND GUIDANCE OF PERCUTANEOUS NEEDLE BIOPSIES

CT is increasingly used to guide needle biopsy procedures in the thorax.

Biopsy of Pulmonary Lesions

Biplane fluoroscopic guidance is still the method of choice for pulmonary masses (36). Fluoroscopy has the unique advantage of visualizing the tip of the needle in real time. Observing the motion and the relationship of the needle tip to the lesion during the biopsy is the best way to ensure effective sampling. CT cannot provide such assurance. However, when lesions are poorly visualized under fluoroscopic guidance or when the lesion is seen in only one plane, CT can be used to provide in-depth information. CT can also be used to enable fluoroscopic guidance in a single plane, or to help decide whether CT should be the guiding modality. Using CT with thin sections, if necessary, can define the optimal path for needle penetration. It is important to define the relationship of lesions to surrounding pulmonary emphysema because the risk of pneumothorax is greatly increased if the needle traverses areas of emphysema. In addition, the risk of pneumothorax increases as the number of pleural leaflets crossed by the needle increases. Needle paths crossing fissures should be avoided whenever possible.

Certain technical factors should be kept in mind when performing CT-guided needle biopsy. First, the CT slice has a given thickness, and the needle position cannot be defined with an accuracy greater than the slice thickness. To increase the accuracy of needle placement, we strongly recommend the use of external visual landmarks. These landmarks can help to maintain a plane of penetration exactly parallel to the scanned plane (37). This is accomplished most simply by having an aide use a piece of cardboard with a vertical edge to guide the operator and ensure that the path of the needle is parallel to the scanned plane. Likewise, when an oblique angle of penetration is necessary because of intervening ribs, such an angle should be calculated from the CT image and then physically simulated with an appropriately cut cardboard edge to help the operator achieve the proper angle. The importance of such technical details cannot be underestimated, especially for deep-seated lesions. An error of a few angular degrees at the entry point can translate into an error of several centimeters at the lesion level. It is important to verify and document the needle tip penetration of a lesion before sampling, and a CT scan should be obtained for that purpose.

Biopsy of Mediastinal, Pleural, and Chest Wall Lesions

Unlike lung lesions, mediastinal lesions are almost always sampled under CT guidance (38,39). Uncomplicated pleural lesions are more appropriately sampled or drained under ultrasound guidance, but complex pleural or chest wall lesions are best managed with CT guidance. To avoid the risk of hemorrhage, precise identification of chest wall vascular structures is necessary. This is especially true for the subclavian and internal mammary vessels when an anterior approach is planned. Generally, anterior mediastinal lesions are best approached at the level of the second to the fourth intercostal space anteriorly and laterally to the internal mammary vessels. To avoid errors of localization, markers should always be placed on the surface of the thorax at the time of scanning. The most practical markers are made of radiopaque angiographic catheters cut at progressive lengths and taped perpendicular to the plane of scanning on the skin surface. With such an arrangement, the number of catheters visualized precisely indicates the level of the scan on the patient's thorax.

Hilar and posterior mediastinal lesions are best sampled via a posterolateral approach (38). Likewise, lesions located in the superior mediastinum are also best approached posteriorly because the anterior approach runs the risk of damaging subclavian vessels. Pleural and chest wall lesions are ideally suited for CT guidance because they are difficult to visualize under fluoroscopic control (due to the curvature of the chest wall). In addition, the superficial location of pleural and chest wall lesions allows precise and easy placement of percutaneous needles.

The most important technical point to remember is that the optimal route for sampling chest wall or pleural lesions is not necessarily the direct perpendicular approach, but rather is an obliquely oriented course along the main axis of the lesion. An oblique approach allows sampling of more of the pathology without the risk of penetrating the lung. This is particularly important in rib lesions and for chest wall and pleural lesions located near the diaphragm. A coaxial technique, using a needle with a larger bore to guide repeated sampling passes with a thinner needle, is useful in reducing procedure time (39).

TECHNIQUES AND STRATEGIES IN THORACIC MRI

Because of technical limitations, MRI has not been used extensively in the investigation of thoracic pathology. There are several drawbacks to the use of MR in the thorax. Motion artifacts generated by cardiac and respiratory movements are difficult to control. Only 10–20% of lung parenchyma represents tissue and circulating blood; consequently, expanded lung has insufficient protons capable of generating an MR signal. The parenchyma is difficult to image by MR because of magnetic susceptibility effects related to the numerous air-tissue interfaces inherent to the structure of lung. Finally, because the magnetic field is made heterogeneous by the different magnetic susceptibilities of air and tissue, the T2 relaxation time of lung tissue is short and reduces further the available signal. These characteristics mean that unless the lung becomes abnormal as a consequence of edema, consolidation, or fibrosis, it is difficult to image by MR. On the other hand, certain characteristics of MR enhance its usefulness for thoracic imaging. These characteristics include the ability to demonstrate flow without the use of contrast agents, the multiplanar capability of the modality, and its high tissue differentiation.

Recent technological advances have permitted the routine acquisition of nearly artifact-free images of the thorax. These images permit exquisite demonstration of all cardiovascular structures. With the advent of newer pulse sequences for MR angiography, MR imaging is fast becoming the preferred modality to initially evaluate primary cardiovascular pathology and to define the relationship of a mass to vascular structures. Because of its multi-planar imaging capability, MR is well-suited to evaluate processes located near the apex of the lung. This is especially true of Pancoast tumors, processes involving mediastinal structures (especially near the hila), and pathology located at or near the thoraco-abdominal junction (40,41). Because MR can also provide some degree of tissue characterization, it can help to differentiate fibrosis from other processes (42,43).

Indications

MR has very limited indications in evaluating parenchymal pathology except in cases of extensive combined pleural and parenchymal disease. The high tissue differentiation capability of MR provides an easy way to differentiate in a single examination pleural collections from areas of consolidation and associated mediastinal and chest wall involvement. This obviates the need for contrast injection. MR is appropriate for those patients in whom respiratory motion is generally absent or very reduced in the affected hemithorax (Fig. 15). MR is particularly useful in patients with impaired renal function. MR is also indicated for evaluating chest wall processes that may variably involve bones, muscles, fat, and pleural surfaces (44). It provides the best tissue differen-

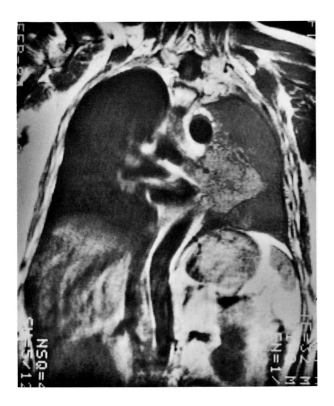

FIG. 15. Patient with opacified left hemithorax on chest radiograph. Coronal MR shows excellent delineation of pathology in the left lung. The left lung is collapsed. There is obstruction of the left main-stem bronchus by tumor. Associated left pleural effusion is present with shift of the mediastinum to the left side. Note the sharp demonstration of the left hemidiaphragm as compared to that of the right hemidiaphragm. MR is well suited to evaluate the opacified or partially opacified hemithorax because respiratory artifacts are nil in such cases and tissue differentiation afforded by MR permits a reliable and rapid diagnosis.

tiation and better defines involvement of chest wall structures (45,46). Likewise, invasion of the mediastinal structures and heart by tumors is optimally defined with MR because of its multi-planar and vascular visualization capabilities (Fig. 16) (47).

MR is quickly becoming the primary noninvasive modality in evaluating thoracic aortic dissection and aneurysms as well as in evaluating the postoperative aorta. Congenital anomalies of the aorta and major vessels are easily examined by MR. It provides exquisite demonstration of the pulmonary arteries and is accurate in the detection of central pulmonary emboli. A further indication for MR is the evaluation of the neck and upper mediastinal veins in patients with indwelling venous catheters for chemotherapy, parenteral nutrition, and long-term antibiotic therapy.

The major clinical indications of MR for cardiac applications are currently limited to the investigation of congenital heart disease and the evaluation of suspected intracardiac masses. Evaluation of pericardial disease is generally limited to the differentiation of constrictive pericarditis versus restrictive cardiomyopathy. The above indications reflect the current status of MR applications in thoracic imaging according to our experience. The recent advent of echoplanar imaging, which permits the acquisition of images in less than 100 ms, may enhance the prospects for thoracic applications in MR (48). Recent work detailing extremely short echo times on the order of 250 μsec appears capable of demonstrating pulmonary parenchymal structures and may be of eventual use in assessing the nature of parenchymal processes (49).

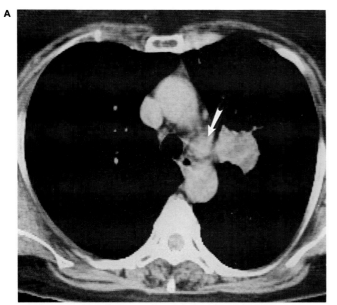

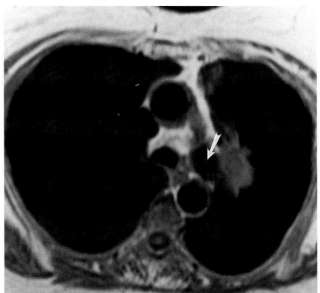

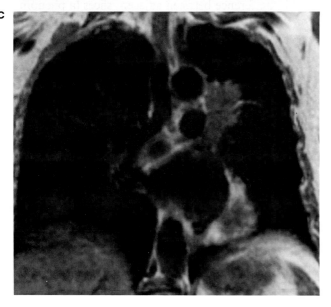

FIG. 16. Advantages of vascular and multi-planar imaging of MR. **A:** CT scan of a patient with a left upper lobe bronchogenic carcinoma interpreted as demonstrating a large node in the aorticopulmonary window (*arrow*). **B:** MR study demonstrates characteristic vascular flow void thus proving that the suspected lymph nodes on CT in fact represent the superior aspect of the left pulmonary artery which is unusually high in position (*arrow*). **C:** Coronal image in the same patient demonstrates absence of large node in aortico-pulmonary window.

Safety Considerations

There are no documented, lasting, harmful effects from MR. In high field strength magnets, RF-power deposition has the potential to raise body core temperature, especially in children. MRI is absolutely contraindicated in patients with cardiac pacemakers. Even at very low field strengths, the operation of a pacemaker can be modified by the magnetic field. In addition, pacing leads can act as antennas and receive the RF pulses from the imaging sequence, thus pacing the heart at a very high rate. Even with inactive pacemakers, examining patients with pacing leads in place is not recommended. Multiple instances of first and second degree burns of the thorax due to the proximity of looped electrocardiogram (ECG) wires have been reported. It is thus very important to avoid contact of looped ECG wires with the patient's skin. Because the magnetic field induces torque on ferromagnetic intracranial aneurysm clips, patients with such clips should not be studied. However, nonferromagnetic clips or prosthetic materials are not dangerous. All heart valves can be imaged except for the older Starr-Edwards type which are highly ferromagnetic. MR is also contraindicated in the presence of metal objects within the eye or near the spinal cord, cochlear implants, and neurostimulators connected to the patient.

Technical Parameters

The basic physics of MR is beyond the scope of this volume and will not be reviewed here. Only the principles relevant to the performance of optimal thoracic MR examinations will be stressed.

The thorax is probably the most difficult area of the body to examine with MR. Good image quality is difficult to achieve. MR is an imaging method characterized by a low signal level arising from tissues. Thus, any loss of signal or inappropriate increase in noise will degrade the image. Consequently, one should know at all times what steps have been taken (or not taken) to ensure an optimal signal-to-noise ratio (SNR). Another source of problems is the technique's sensitivity to motion artifacts.

Adequate Pre-scan Tuning

The MR signal is first generated by an RF excitation pulse and is received afterward by an antenna called a receiver coil. Because the MRI system is not absolutely stable, the resonance frequency may drift. In addition, the presence of the patient's body within the magnet changes the magnetic field slightly in a manner that varies from patient to patient. Consequently, the exact resonance frequency varies slightly for each patient. In addition, RF penetration is different from patient to patient and the RF pulse strength needed to maximize the signal will be different for each patient. It is therefore essential to perform a pre-scan procedure to define the exact resonance frequency and the appropriate level of RF exposure for each patient, each region of the body, and before each image sequence. Although it is tempting to save time by avoiding pre-scan procedures, we strongly recommend against such an approach because it is very likely to degrade the image quality. Most newer scanners now offer efficient automated pre-scan routines.

Signal-to-Noise Considerations

Several important steps are needed to ensure an adequate SNR for a thoracic MR examination. Optimizing SNR without increasing examination time is also an important factor. Because background noise is constant over the entire tissue volume but signal is proportional to the amount of tissue included in a voxel, it is not possible in MR to obtain the same spatial resolution as with CT. To maintain an adequate SNR, voxels in MRI have to be made larger than with CT. The most effective strategies to improve SNR relate to geometric factors such as slice thickness, pixel size, diameter of the field of view, and size of the receiving coil.

Slice Thickness

In MR, very thin slice thicknesses are not achievable for large body parts, and slices less than 5 mm in thickness should be avoided. Increasing slice thickness increases SNR in a linear fashion, i.e., if slice thickness is doubled, the SNR is doubled. Unlike CT slices, the boundaries of slices in MR are not exactly defined. To avoid interference between adjacent slices (a phenomenon known as *cross talk*), it is important always to keep a gap between adjacent slices, thereby avoiding signal reduction. Even though some manufacturers claim that gapless images can be obtained, this is not always true for all sequences. It is good practice to leave an interslice gap of about 20–30% of the slice thickness.

Pixel Size

A frequent bias of radiologists trained in other cross-sectional imaging methods is to use the finest matrix available. This lowers the SNR since each voxel is the smallest possible. In addition, scan times in MRI are directly proportional to the number of pixels in the phase-encoding direction. Generally, the spatial resolution of MR for large body parts is less than that achieved by CT. To maintain SNR, the user can select a number of image matrices, usually 256 frequency encoding steps by 256, 192, or 128 phase encoding steps. In our experience a 256 × 192 matrix is generally adequate for T1-weighted pulse sequences. A 256 × 256 matrix is reserved for cases in which maximum resolution is important. For proton density-weighted and T2-weighted images, fine matrices are almost never needed, and a 256 × 128 matrix is largely sufficient. These latter sequences are relied on mostly for their ability to provide information on tissue composition, and not for detail. In addition, since the repetition time (TR) of these latter sequences is long, using a coarser matrix reduces the need for averaging and shortens scan time. By reducing the matrix size, SNR is improved as a function of the increase in volume in the corresponding voxels. For example, changing from a 256 × 256 to a 256 × 128 matrix doubles the pixel size and doubles the SNR.

Field of View

The most powerful way to affect SNR short of changing receiver coil size is to modify the field of view (FOV). Ideally, FOV should be equal to the size of the region of interest. However, one should remember that when the FOV is reduced, the size of the pixel is reduced in both the X and Y directions. Therefore, in MR a reduction of the FOV by a factor of two reduces pixel size by four, thus decreasing SNR by four. This problem most commonly occurs with small patients, especially children. Too often, a large body receiver coil (40–50 cm in diameter) is used, and when the FOV is reduced to accommodate the patient's size, a drastic reduction in SNR occurs. As a general rule, avoid using an FOV of less than half the diameter of the receiving coil. A slight increase in FOV is a good way to improve SNR.

Receiver Coil

The best way to improve SNR is to place the patient in a smaller receiver coil, which enhances the reception of the signal. For example, a child may be placed in the head receiver coil. Small infants can sometimes be examined in extremity coils with outstanding results.

Short TE

Short echo-time (TE) is an important though not always available option. The MR signal decays as an exponential function of the T2 relaxation time. Since the T2 of tissues is relatively short (about 30–70 msec), a reduction in the TE time of a few milliseconds makes a potentially large difference. For example, for TE = T2, 63% of the signal is lost but if TE = 0.25 T2, only a 21% loss is observed, a 2 to 1 improvement. With current scanners TEs on the order of 15 msec are routinely achievable.

Improving SNR with Increased Scanning Time

Averaging signal from the same pixels by increasing the number of RF excitations (Nex) leads to a square root improvement in SNR. For example, by doubling the number of excitations, SNR improves by the root of two, or 1.44 or 44%, and for three averaged excitations it improves by the root of three, or 1.71 or 71%. It is clear that this is a time-inefficient way of improving SNR and should be avoided whenever possible. Another potential approach is to increase the TR. In the thorax, since all examinations are gated, this entails an even greater time penalty for little improvement in SNR.

Prevention and Correction of Motion Artifacts

There are three major sources of motion artifacts in thoracic MR: the beating heart, blood traveling through vessels, and respiratory excursions of the anterior chest wall. A series of correcting steps needs to be taken to achieve optimal image quality.

Cardiac Gating

In thoracic MRI, we strongly recommend the systematic use of cardiac gating. By synchronizing the acquisition of the images to the heart cycle, the cardiac walls can be imaged in reproducible positions. ECG gating entails only a 10–15% increase in scan time but significantly improves image quality (50). An important technical consideration that is often overlooked is the fact that ECG gating is most reliable in the early phase of the cardiac cycle between the QRS and the T-wave of the ECG tracing (systole). The later part of the cardiac cycle is the most variable. It is, therefore, better to scan the thorax in a caudal to cranial direction, rather than from the thoracic inlet to the abdomen as usually performed in CT. This ensures that the scans obtained over the heart are acquired during the early and most reproducible portion of the cardiac cycle (Fig. 17). For patients with irregular cardiac rhythms, ECG gating may not be feasible. In such cases, averaging a large number of echoes by shortening TR and increasing the number of excitations to 8–10 is effective.

Elimination of Artifacts Related to Blood Motion

Blood traveling in a pulsatile fashion through the major mediastinal vessels can generate variable degrees of signal, provoking ghost artifacts in the phase direction

A

B

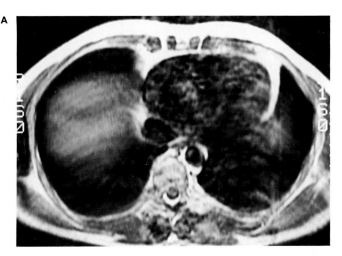
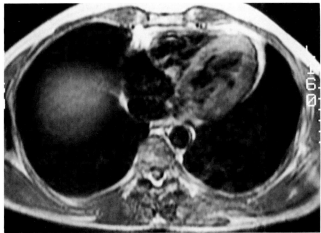

FIG. 17. Cranio-caudal versus caudo-cranial scanning with ECG gating. **A:** ECG-gated image of the heart obtained with a cranio-caudal prescription where first scan is obtained near the thoracic inlet and last scan is obtained in the cardiac region. Note absence of detail and major artifacts over the heart region. **B:** Same patient, same ECG-gating except that the scans were prescribed in a caudo-cranial direction with the early scans being obtained in the cardiac region. Intracardiac detail is now available with much decreased motion and flow artifacts. In ECG-gated thoracic scanning, scans where maximum image quality is desired should be prescribed first to correspond with the systolic phase.

of the image (Fig. 18). The most effective technique for reducing this effect is to destroy any signal that may arise from moving blood, thereby preventing the creation of ghost artifacts. This is best achieved by saturating, i.e., destroying the magnetization of incoming blood, by repeatedly imposing radiofrequency pulses to the areas adjacent to the imaged volume (51). This method greatly reduces flow artifacts, especially in high field strength magnets. Gradient moment-nulling techniques, also called flow compensation techniques, have been advocated to reduce motion artifacts in the abdomen (52). However, these techniques tend to increase blood signal and are less effective in thoracic MR.

Respiratory Motion Artifacts

Respiratory gating is never used because the cycle time of respiration is too long, necessitating excessively lengthy examination times (53). However, respiratory compensation techniques that change the order of acquisition of the phase encoding steps of the image can be quite effective. These techniques match the motion of the anterior chest wall to the acquisition and reconstruction of the image, significantly reducing respiratory artifacts. This method, known as respiratory-ordered phase encoding, is quite effective if the anterior chest wall motion of the patient is properly recorded. Thus, special attention should be given to the placement of the sensing device, usually a pneumatic belt or nasal thermistor.

Pulse Sequences

The thorax is best examined with pulse sequences that are less motion sensitive. In addition, mediastinal fat is

an ideal contrasting tissue. Thus, sequences with long TR and long TE, which decrease the contrast between fat and surrounding tissues and are extremely motion sensitive, should be reserved for purposes of tissue characterization.

T1-weighted sequences with shorter TR and TE are extremely effective in the thorax and form the backbone of the thoracic MR study. Since all studies are gated, the TR is equal to the RR interval. The TE should be short, about 15 to 20 msec. For spin echo images, it is not necessarily productive to use TE shorter than 15 msec because it tends to increase blood signal, thereby generating ghost artifacts. With a normal heart rate of 60–80 beats per minute, ECG gating produces pulse sequences with a TR of 700–1,000 msec. Thus, simultaneous acquisition in a multi-slice mode of 14–20 images can easily be achieved.

In practice, it is most advantageous to first perform a coronal T1-weighted series of images with a 10 mm slice thickness, 3–5 mm gap, 256 × 192 matrix, 1 Nex, 42–48 cm FOV (54). This series of images requires 192 heartbeats. Based on the first sequence, a series of T1-weighted axial scans can then be prescribed. As mentioned above, it is important to acquire scans in the cardiac region early in the RR interval. Slice thickness should be 7 to 10 mm with a 256 × 192 matrix, TE 15 or 20 using respiratory compensation and presaturation above and below the imaging volume. The field of view should be adjusted to the patient's size, and, whenever possible, the arms should be elevated over the head to avoid wraparound artifacts. In patients with excessive respiratory motion or cardiac instability, a 256 × 128 matrix with 4 Nex is more advantageous. In patients with severe cardiac arrhythmias, an ungated T1-weighted series with TR = 300, TE = 15, and 10 Nex is recommended in the cardiac region. This is quite effective in obtaining diagnostic quality studies in the absence of gating.

Role of T2-Weighted Sequences

In our experience, the coronal and transaxial T1-weighted sequences are the most effective. If no pathology is found on these sequences, it is unlikely that a T2-weighted sequence would reveal additional information. T2-weighted sequences are often necessary to characterize pathology already detected or suspected on the T1-weighted scans. The quality of T2-weighted scans is heavily dependent on the TR of the sequence. The TR should be at least 2,000 msec in a low- or mid-field magnet and 2,500 msec for high field strength magnets. Consequently, it is imperative to match these TR times with the heart rate of the patient. Cardiac gating programs are now available that allow for gating every third or fourth beat if necessary. A double-echo sequence is preferable for tissue characterization and provides proton density as well as T2 information in a single sequence. A minimum TE time of 80 msec for the second echo is recommended. The T2-weighted sequence is best performed in the axial plane with 10 mm sections, 256×128 matrix, 2 Nex, 30% gap. Coronal, sagittal, or oblique T2-weighted images are indicated to evaluate chest wall invasion near the apex or diaphragmatic regions.

Oblique Planes

In thoracic MR there are two major indications for acquiring images in nonorthogonal axes. The first is to study the thoracic aorta. In such cases, a T1-weighted parasagittal scan intersecting the ascending and descending aorta can assist in evaluating dissections and aneurysms. The second indication is to study tracheal processes. In these cases, a paracoronal scan parallel to the long axis of the trachea and the main-stem bronchi is often helpful.

Gradient Echo Pulse Sequences

Gradient echo recalled techniques are a class of pulse sequences that do not rely on the acquisition of a spin-echo (55,56). The main advantages of these sequences are: (a) a very short TR that enables acquisition of images in less than 12 sec, thus permitting breath holding; (b) marked contrast between flowing blood, which appears bright, and static tissues. These sequences are, however, very sensitive to motion artifacts and field inhomogeneity. Nevertheless, they are extremely effective in evaluating vascular structures of the upper thorax and

mediastinum, where they help define the patency and flow pattern of major vessels.

We prefer to use gradient echo recalled sequences with suspended respiration in the mediastinum. To define flow and motion dynamics in the cardiac region, ECG gating is needed to obtain either a series of images at several levels or a series of 8–32 images obtained throughout the cardiac cycle at one or two selected levels. These latter sequences are most useful when evaluating intracardiac pathology or pathology involving the proximal aorta or pulmonary arteries.

RELATIONSHIP OF MR SIGNAL AND FLOW

Several phenomena explain why the presence of flow alters signal intensity in MRI. These phenomena can be classified into three broad categories: time-of-flight effects, saturation effects, and phase effects (57,58). Interpretation of MR studies requires familiarity with the appearance of flow effects.

Time-of-Flight Effects

To generate an MR signal, protons first need to be excited with a radiofrequency pulse. In spin-echo images, this initial pulse is followed at a variable interval of time by a refocusing 180° RF pulse to generate the spin-echo. A plug of flowing blood traveling through the slice may then be excited by the initial RF pulse but may leave the slice before the spin-echo signal can be recorded. Likewise, protons flowing into the slice after the initial RF pulse will not generate a signal as they have not been pre-excited (58). Therefore, in areas of flow there will be signal loss. The amount of signal loss depends on the velocity of flow. If flow is fast and if all protons have completely left the slice before being imaged, there will be a complete flow void effect (Fig. 16). If flow is slow, some signal may be generated (Fig. 18). If flow is very slow an almost normal, static, tissue-like signal will be seen. The presence of signal in vessels is therefore most likely to occur during diastole, the phase of the cardiac cycle when blood has the slowest velocity. With long TE times, blood has time to exit the excited slice. With short TE, blood protons will still be in the excited slice and will therefore generate signal. This is why better flow void effects are seen with relatively long echo times (in the range of 20–30 msec) than with shorter echo times.

Saturation Effects

Time-of-flight effects are complicated in clinical practice by the fact that multiple slices are excited in rapid succession. Therefore, blood traveling through a set of

A 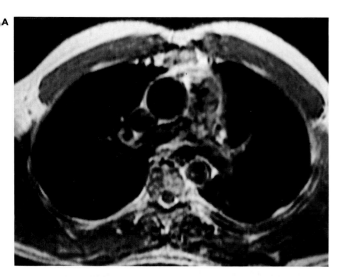 B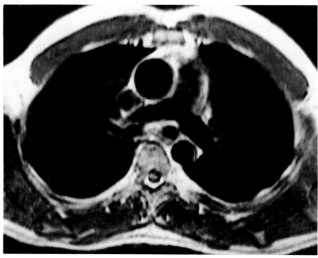

FIG. 18. Flow-related artifacts. **A:** Image obtained during diastolic phase shows presence of signal in most vessels due to nearly stationary flow during diastole. Note visualization of pulmonary vessels. **B:** Same scan level obtained during systolic phase. Better flow void effect is observed due to the higher velocity of blood during systole. Note also that pulmonary vessels are not visualized on this scan.

multiple adjacent slices is likely to be exposed to many more RF pulses per unit of time than are static tissues. The resulting effect is the destruction of longitudinal magnetization and a reduced signal from flowing blood. This also explains the entry slice phenomenon—the presence of high blood signal often seen in the first few slices at the edge of the imaged volume. As a traveling proton enters the first slice, it is fully relaxed and can generate a strong signal. Consequently, on the first and last few slices of an imaging sequence, high signal can be seen in vessels in which flow is directed toward the imaging volume. As blood protons further penetrate the imaging volume, they are exposed to more RF pulses and the flow void effect is always better in slices located in the middle of the imaged volume. This entry slice phenomenon can be eliminated. If saturation pulses that destroy all residual magnetization are applied above and below the imaging volume, blood protons are completely saturated and signal is eliminated (51).

Phase Effects

Phase effects can either enhance or decrease blood signal depending on the pulse sequence used (59). The best way to understand phase effects is to remember that the signal in an imaged voxel is due to the sum of the minute signals generated by protons. If the protons are in phase with each other, a strong additive signal is generated. If the protons are not in phase, there will be cancellation of signal. Moving protons precess at slightly different resonant frequencies during their displacement along the magnetic field gradients. These differences in resonant frequencies generate dephasing; unless compensation gradients are used to null these effects (also

known as gradient moment-nulling or flow compensation techniques), signal is destroyed.

Differentiation of Thrombus from Slow Flow

Based on the above discussion, it is clear that the signal of flowing blood can vary and may overlap with the signal of intravascular thrombus. Differentiation of the two entities is a common problem in thoracic MR. Several approaches have been proposed. First, in spin-echo imaging, slow flow enhances in signal intensity on the second echo of a symmetrical double spin-echo sequence. This phenomenon, known as even-echo rephasing, is manifested as an increase in intravascular signal intensity from the first echo to the second echo image (60). In contrast, fixed material, such as thrombus or tumor, usually displays a decrease or very minimal increase in signal intensity. However, this method is not always reliable because the appearance of thrombi depends on the age of the process. Old thrombi produce a medium signal intensity on first echo images and low signal intensity on second echo images. They are, therefore, easily differentiated. However, recently formed thrombi have substantially higher signals on both first and second echo images. Subacute hematomas can also produce a high signal intensity on T1-weighted as well as T2-weighted images.

Another method of differentiating slow flow from thrombus is the use of phase display images (61,62). As protons moving along gradients accumulate phase differences relative to static tissue, a phase image provides a way of differentiating moving from nonmoving tissues. Phase display imaging demonstrates high or low signal intensity for moving objects, whereas static objects have a constant signal intensity. However, any structure that is moving during the imaging sequence (e.g., the base of the heart, the aortic root, or a mobile thrombus) can produce an observable phase change that may lead to an incorrect diagnosis.

Other practical signs can help differentiate slow flow from intravascular tumor or thrombus. First, tumors and thrombi should appear identical on orthogonal images. Slow flow often appears different on axial and coronal views due to dephasing effects and changes in cardiac timing (62). Another aid to differentiation is the presence of a zone of low signal intensity between the vessel wall and the slow flowing blood. The wide range of velocities of the traveling blood near the vessel wall also leads to phase differences and tissue signal loss.

In our experience, the most effective and simplest method is to use a gradient echo recalled sequence with flow compensation. These sequences are extremely sensitive to the presence of flow. It is best to acquire a single slice at a time to prevent any saturation effects from adjacent slices and to allow for breath holding. Flowing blood appears very bright, whereas tumors or thrombi demonstrate lower signal intensity. However, even with gradient echo techniques, thrombi age affects signal intensity. In addition, when flow is parallel to the scan plane, as is commonly the case in subclavian vessels, blood is exposed to multiple RF pulses. This reduces its signal, potentially simulating thrombi. Acquiring a scan perpendicularly oriented relative to the vessel in question is the best way to resolve the ambiguity.

TISSUE CHARACTERIZATION BY MRI

The differences in signal intensity patterns of human tissues are based essentially on differences in proton density and T1 and T2 relaxation times (63). Tissue differentiation and contrast in images also depends on the particular pulse sequence used. One of the most difficult tasks for the diagnostic radiologist analyzing MR images is to develop an understanding of the meaning of signal intensity changes. Unlike CT, where image contrast is essentially determined by atomic attenuation of x-rays, the tissue characteristics that determine MR relaxation times are more complex. In this section we will present the most important concepts underlying the interpretation of signal differences in MR images.

Role of Molecular Motion on Relaxation Times

Relaxation times are essentially determined by the size, motional characteristics, and degrees of motional freedom of the various molecules making up tissues.

T1 Relaxation

The first step in generating an MR image is to excite hydrogen nuclei with an RF pulse. After excitation, the nuclei progressively return to rest by giving off energy to the surrounding molecules. This is known as the spin lattice, or T1 relaxation process. When the exchange of energy between the proton and the molecule on which it is located is efficient, the T1 time is short. When this exchange of energy is inefficient, the T1 time is long. The most important factor in determining efficiency of T1 relaxation is whether the resonance frequency of the MR scanner is close to the frequency of motion of the surrounding molecules.

Indeed, all molecules move or "tumble" at a given frequency. This motional frequency basically depends on the size of the molecule. For example, large tissue molecules, such as proteins or DNA, have a very slow tumbling frequency of about 1,000 cycles/sec. On the other hand, water molecules, which are very small, have a much higher frequency of motion—in the range of 100 billion to 1 trillion cycles/sec. Between these extremes are tissue molecules of various sizes and varying frequencies of motion.

When molecules move at a rate equal to or near the resonance frequency of the magnet, energy exchanges between the resonating protons and their carrier molecules are enhanced. In human tissues, fat molecules or triglycerides have molecular motional frequencies close to the resonance frequencies of clinical scanners. Thus, fat exhibits the shortest T1 relaxation time, ranging from 250–400 msec. For molecules larger or smaller than fat with respectively lower or higher frequencies of motion, relaxation times are less efficient than for fatty molecules (Fig. 19). This explains why water molecules have a much longer T1 than fat. It also explains why large macromolecules, such as those found in fibrous tissue, exhibit long T1 times. This is simply because their motional frequencies are not matched to the resonance frequencies of current clinical scanners. This also explains why T1 times of tissues are different for magnets of different field strengths. In general, as the resonance frequency increases with higher field strength, T1 relaxation becomes less efficient and T1 times increase. As a rule of thumb, there is an increase of about 500 msec for each Tesla of increase in magnetic field strength.

Influence of Degree of Molecular Freedom on T2 Relaxation

T2 relaxation depends primarily on interactions between nuclei. In a general way, T2 depends on the degree of freedom between molecules in a particular tissue.

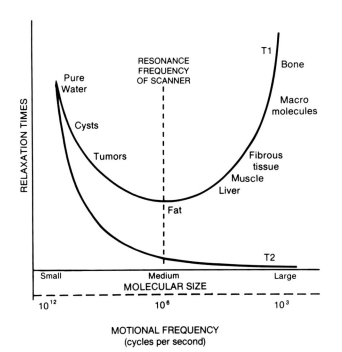

FIG. 19. Relaxation times. Idealized curve of relaxation time for various tissues is represented as a function of molecular size. For molecules such as fat, which have a motional frequency close to the resonance frequency of clinical scanners, T1 relaxation is most efficient and the T1 time is shortest. For smaller molecules such as pure water or larger molecules such as macromolecules, the T1 times will be much longer because they are not matched to the resonance frequency of the scanner. T2 times relate mostly to degree of freedom between molecules. For pure water, where molecules are freely mobile, the T2 time is long. For macromolecules or bone where atoms are restricted in motion, the T2 times are short. These factors are the main determinant of relaxation times.

For example, water molecules move freely and very little restrictions or interactions exist. Hence, the T2 relaxation of pure water is long. In larger molecules, spin interactions are so restricted that rapid dephasing of the magnetic vectors of nuclei is observed after RF excitation, leading to a short T2 time. One can then simplify the understanding of relaxation times by relating them to molecular size, which is itself related to molecular motion for T1, and relative freedom between molecules for T2. This concept is summarized in Figure 19. For tissues that have very short T2 times, the MR signal decays very fast and cannot be recorded within the TE time. As a consequence, macromolecules, proteins, cell membranes, and all tissues where molecules are restricted in motion are not usually visible by MR. In essence, only mobile water and fat molecules generate signal in clinical MR. However, this does not mean that MR is simply a water/fat imaging technique. Water molecules do interact with surrounding proteins and macromolecules that make up the structure of live tissues. Thus, the motional frequency and degrees of freedom of water can be affected by the nearby molecules, thereby changing the relaxation time of water.

Influence of Macromolecular/Water Interactions on Relaxation Times

Water molecules that come close to the larger MR "invisible" molecules may be slowed in their motional frequency by temporary bindings near the surface of such molecules (Fig. 20). Therefore, relaxation times of

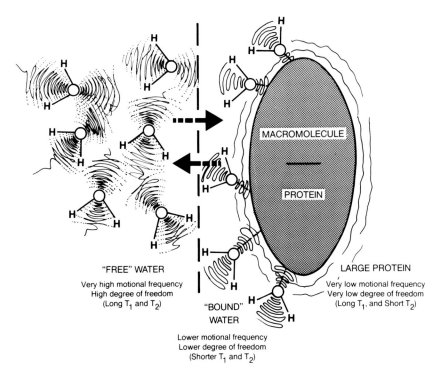

FIG. 20. Macromolecular/water interactions. The main determinant of relaxation times in tissues is the interaction of water with large macromolecules which are not normally visible in MR. When water is "free," long T1 and T2 times are observed due to the high motional frequency and the high degree of freedom observed in free water. However, when water molecules come close to larger biological molecules such as proteins, its motional frequency and degree of freedom are reduced, thus the T1 and T2 relaxation times are proportionately reduced. The degree of slowing down of water by the various biological molecules is what ultimately determines in great part the appearance of tissues on MR images.

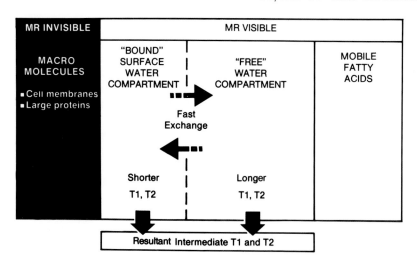

FIG. 21. Fast exchange two-state model (F.E.T.S.) tissue signals in MR. Tissues can be conceived of as containing two major components: an MR invisible component made up of macromolecules and an MR visible component made up of water and fat. Water interacts variably with the MR invisible molecule, thus modulating the T1 and T2 times of a given tissue.

water are modulated by the presence of the various macromolecules of tissues. Even though large tissue molecules are not directly visible by MR, their effect on the water molecules surrounding them can actually be seen as a change in the relaxation time of water. This is the mechanism by which tissue contrast and tissue characterization are achieved in MR. For the purposes of diagnostic radiology, an approximate model of what determines MR signal is simplified by thinking of tissues as follows:

There is an MR *invisible* part of biological tissues made up of macromolecules, proteins, cell membranes, bone, etc.

There is an MR *visible* portion of tissues made up essentially of water and fat.

Fat molecules are organized in such a way that they do not interact with other molecules.

Water molecules, on the other hand, interact with the surrounding "MRI invisible" compartment and the T1 and T2 of water is modulated by such interactions.

At the basic level, this model implies that increases in free water, as well as decreases in protein concentration, lead to lengthened T1 and T2 relaxation times. High protein content and paramagnetic substances in contrast media (or natural processes such as hemorrhage) decrease T1 with a variable effect on T2. More structured tissues, such as fibrosis and connective tissues, exhibit short T2 times. The two-state fast exchange model, is, in our opinion, the one with which we should become familiar because it allows us to understand tissue contrast in clinical images (Fig. 21).

At the tissue level, MR signal reflects the averaged contribution of the histologic constituents of normal and pathologic processes. Components of tissues with

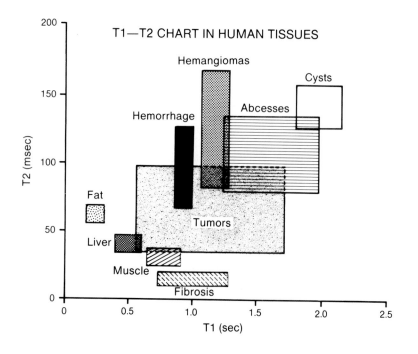

FIG. 22. T1/T2 chart of normal and pathologic tissues in humans. This chart summarizes current data on the range of T1 and T2 times observed in various pathologies. Note that fibrosis and tumors overlap in their T1 time but not in their T2 time, thus providing the potential for differentiation.

high free-water content (edema, inflammation, necrosis, glandular fluids, cysts, retained secretions, hemorrhage, and actively growing malignant cells) contribute to high signal intensity on T2-weighted images and to low signal intensity on T1-weighted images. Tissue components rich in structured collagen, elastic fibers, and large proteins exhibit a low signal on T2-weighted scans and a low to intermediate signal on T1-weighted images. Clearly, the MR signal of any given tissue is the complex sum of the signals of its basic constituents. Because identical pathologic processes may differ in the relative amount of their constituents, they may exhibit different MRI signal characteristics. Conversely, dissimilar pathologic processes may generate the same signal if the sum effect of their basic elements (necrosis, edema, connective tissue, etc.) is identical. Clearly, the MR signal of any given tissue cannot be very specific and overlap is observed across tissues (Fig. 22). However, if the histologic composition of a tissue changes over time, MR signal is likely to change as well. This ability to track

histologic modification is unique to MR and has been proposed as a mechanism for monitoring various tumors (see Chapters 2 and 6).

Influence of Paramagnetic Agents

The above-mentioned model of relaxation time does not take into account the effect of paramagnetic substances. However, paramagnetic substances are capable of shortening relaxation times by similar mechanisms. Indeed, when a paramagnetic substance is present, the main effect by which it reduces T1 times is locally varying the magnetic field and increasing the range of resonance frequencies of protons at the local level. This permits more effective matching between the motional frequencies of a greater range of tissue molecules and those of the hydrogen nuclei they carry.

Processes with paramagnetic properties, such as subacute hemorrhage or contrast-enhanced tissues, exhibit

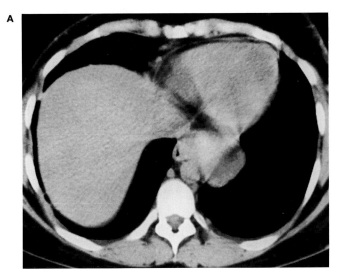

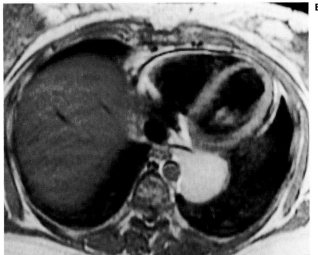

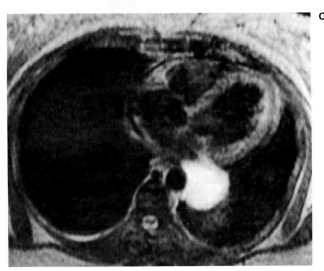

FIG. 23. Tissue characterization by MR. **A:** CT scan of a patient demonstrated a mass of soft-tissue density near the gastro-esophageal junction. **B:** Proton density weighted scan, TR 2,700/TE 20, and **C:** T2-weighted scan, TR 2,700/TE 80 demonstrated a high signal intensity characteristic of fluid. At surgery a duplication cyst with a high protein content was found. Such cysts can appear very dense with CT. However, with MR, their cystic nature can easily be determined.

a relatively higher signal on T1-weighted images with no effect on the T2-weighted scans. When a superparamagnetic substance such as ferrite is present in tissues, magnetic field heterogeneity is created. This is also true when tissues are made of components with markedly different magnetic susceptibility properties, such as air spaces and interstitium of lung. Consequently, T2 is reduced and the signal intensity of these tissues is decreased on both T1- and T2-weighted scans.

Implications for Tissue Differentiation

As demonstrated in Figure 22, experience with clinical MR shows significant overlap between various types of pathologies. Since differentiation of MR signal depends on the interaction of water and surrounding molecules, limited characterization can be expected. The major differentiating tissue in the thorax is mediastinal and chest wall fat, which has a high signal intensity on T1-weighted scans because of its short T1 time. Vessels, airways, and pathologic lesions are easily contrasted against the fat background. MR may be useful in differentiating cysts from solid masses (64,65). With CT, it is common to observe high density cysts indistinguishable from solid masses. With MR, these cysts tend to have longer T2 relaxation times than solid masses and are therefore of very high intensity on T2-weighted scans, permitting differentiation (Fig. 23). MR has been disappointing in distinguishing inflammatory from neoplastic lymphadenopathy (66). *In vivo* and *in vitro* studies both demonstrate a significant overlap between bronchogenic carcinoma, nodal metastasis, lymphoma, and granulomatous diseases (67). Even though T1 and T2 relaxation times have been shown to be longer for nodes involved with bronchogenic carcinoma than for nodes involved with sarcoidosis, the clinical value of these differences is negated by considerable overlap.

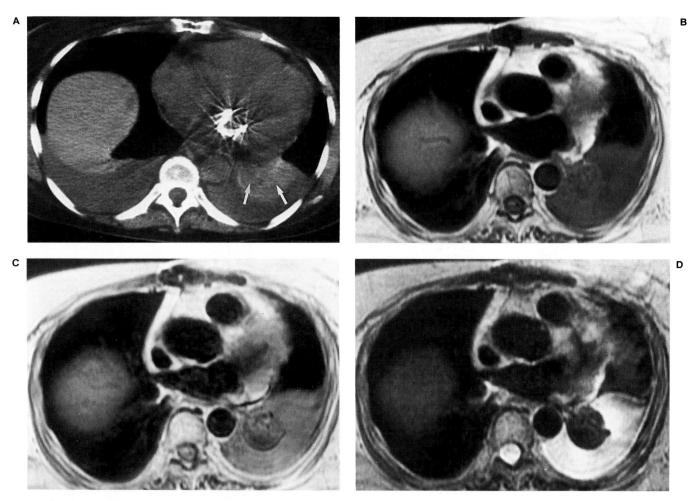

FIG. 24. Tissue differentiation on MR. Nonobstructive atelectasis. **A:** CT scan in a patient with large bilateral pleural effusions demonstrates compressed left lower lobe (*arrows*). **B:** On T1-weighted scan obtained several days later, effusion is again noted and compressed lung is seen with a signal intensity similar to that of the surrounding effusion. Note small areas of low signal intensity in the compressed lung represent flow void effect in small pulmonary vessels and not air bronchograms. **C:** Proton density weighted image. Compressed lung parenchyma is now slightly less intense than surrounding pleural effusion. **D:** T2-weighted scan. Compressed lung demonstrates very low signal intensity whereas pleural effusion demonstrates high signal intensity. The low signal intensity of the compressed lung is probably due to residual air not appreciable on CT scan or T1- or T2-weighted scans. (From Herold et al., ref. 72, with permission.)

MR is capable of differentiating fibrosis from tumors by virtue of the marked differences in T2 relaxation time of these two processes (42,43,68,69). Therefore, when a question of tumor versus fibrosis is raised, MR will demonstrate a low signal intensity for the fibrotic components of the tumor and a high signal intensity for the neoplastic tissue. This may be helpful in differentiating radiation fibrosis from recurrent or residual bronchogenic carcinoma and is a useful adjunct in the management of patients with residual lymphomatous masses (see Chapter 2).

MR is valuable and specific in the diagnosis of hemorrhage and hematoma (70). Subacute hemorrhagic lesions characteristically show high signal intensity on T1-weighted images. This is due to a shortened T1 relaxation time, resulting from the paramagnetic effects of desaturated hemoglobin and methemoglobin, which occurs as a result of the oxidation of ferrous iron to a high-spin ferric state. Except for hemorrhagic, fatty, cystic, and possibly fibrotic lesions, MR offers little in the differentiation of other malignant or benign processes.

Likewise, MR is limited in the differentiation of pul-monary parenchymal processes. The tissues involved in pulmonary consolidation exhibit substantial overlap in signal characteristics. However, alveolar proteinosis is notable for short T1 value. Pulmonary hemorrhage may also demonstrate a short T1 behavior at some point in its evolution. Some studies suggest that active severe interstitial lung disease is associated with high signal intensity on T2-weighted scans, probably due to alveolitis with edema. Experimental studies on rats show that MR signal intensities are elevated in alveolitis and early fibrosis, and T1 and T2 values are significantly decreased in chronic, more advanced fibrotic lung disease. It would appear that T1 and T2 values in the lung parenchyma correlate with changes in water content of the diseased lung (71).

More recently we have shown that obstructive atelectasis can be distinguished from nonobstructive atelectasis on T2-weighted images. Nonobstructive atelectasis characteristically demonstrates a very low signal intensity on T2-weighted scans (Fig. 24), whereas obstructive atelectasis demonstrates high signal intensity (Fig. 25). These may be indistinguishable from each other on ei-

A
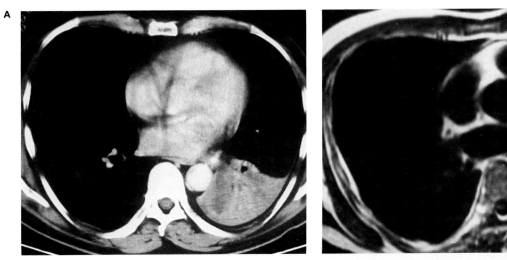

B
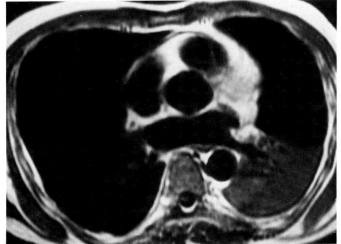

C
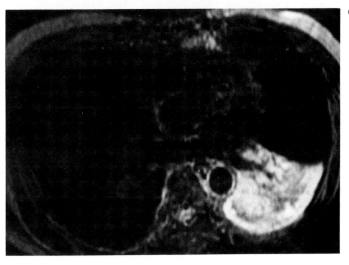

FIG. 25. Tissue differentiation by MR. Obstructive atelectasis. Patient with centrally located bronchogenic carcinoma with obstructive atelectasis of the left lower lobe. **A:** CT scan demonstrates collapsed left lower lobe with minimal residual air in some bronchi. **B:** T1-weighted scan demonstrates relatively low signal intensity atelectatic lung. **C:** T2-weighted scan shows high signal intensity consistent with a high water content. At surgery, the lung was found to contain a large amount of retained secretions and exhibited changes of postobstructive pneumonitis. (From Herold et al., ref. 72, with permission.)

TABLE 3. *Patterns of tissue signal*

	Pulse sequence				Appearance
	T1-weighted	Proton density	T2-weighted	Gradient echo	
Cyst	Low	Medium	High	Variable	Homogeneous sharp border round
Abscess	Low-medium	Medium	High	Variable	Heterogeneous ill-defined border
Seroma	Low	Medium	High	Variable	Same as cyst
Lipoma	High	High	High	Medium	Sometimes brighter than normal fat
Neurofibroma	Medium	Medium	High	Medium	Often with central area of low signal on T2
High-protein content collections (bronchogenic cyst)	Medium-high	Medium	High	Variable	Initially homogeneous
Obstructive atelectasis	Low-medium	Medium	High	Variable	
Nonobstructive atelectasis	Low-medium	Medium	Low	Low	
Bronchogenic carcinoma	Low-medium	Medium	Medium-high	Medium-low	Mixed patterns are most common
Pulmonary secretions	Low	Medium	High	Variable	
Alveolar proteinosis (before lavage)	Medium-low	Low	Medium-low	Low	
Hemorrhagic collections					
Acute	Low	Medium	High	Medium-high	Homogeneous
Subacute	Medium-high	Medium	High	Low	Heterogeneous fluid-fluid level
Chronic	Low	Medium	Medium-high	Low-medium	Homogeneous with dark rim
Blood clot					
Acute	Medium	Medium	Medium-high	Medium	
Chronic	Medium	Medium-low	Medium-low	Low-very low	Gradient echo signal void is larger than clot (magnetic susceptibility)
Arteriovenous malformation	Very low	Low	Medium-low	High	Appearance depends on flow rate

ther CT scans or T1- and proton density-weighted images. We presume that with obstructive atelectasis, accumulation of secretions and disappearance of residual air increase the T2 time of the collapsed lung. In nonobstructive atelectasis, collateral ventilation and clearance of secretions are still active. Presumably, the magnetic susceptibility effects of microscopic residual air lead to a low T2 relaxation time. The behavior of several tissues of interest is summarized in Table 3.

REFERENCES

1. Trefler M, Haughton VM. Patient dose and image quality in computed tomography. *AJR* 1981;137:25–27.
2. Haaga JR, Miraldi F, Macintyre W, Lipuma JP, Bryan PJ, Wiesen E. The effect of MAs variation upon computed tomography image quality as evaluated in vivo and in vitro studies. *Radiology* 1981;138:449–454.
3. Naidich DP, Marshall CH, Gribbin C, Arams RS, McCauley DI. Low-dose CT of the lungs: Preliminary observations. *Radiology* 1990;175:729–731.
4. Gorich J, Beyer-Enke SA, Muller M, van Kaick G. The influence of breathing technic on the visualization of lung metastases in computed tomography. *Rontgenblatter* 1989;42(4):170–171.
5. Jones KR, Robinson PJ. Organ volume determination by CT scanning: reduction of respiration induced errors by feedback monitoring. *J Comput Assist Tomogr* 1986;10(1):167–171.
6. Kalender W, Seissler W, Vock P: Single-breath-hold spiral volumetric CT by continuous patient translation and scanner rotation. *Radiology* 1989;176(1):181–183.
7. Shaffer K, Pugatch RD. Small pulmonary nodules: dynamic CT with a single-breath technique. *Radiology* 1989;173(2):567–568.
8. Brasch RC. Ultrafast computed tomography for infants and children. *Radiol Clin North Am* 1988;26(2):277–286.
9. Baxter BS, Sorenson JA. Factors affecting the measurements of size and CT number in computed tomography. *Invest Radiol* 1981;16:337–341.
10. Koehler RP, Anderson RE, Baxter B. The effect of computed tomography viewer controls on anatomical measurements. *Radiology* 1979;130:189–194.
11. Joseph PM, Sadek KH, Schulz RA, Kelcz F. Clinical and experimental investigation of a smoothed CT reconstruction algorithm. *Radiology* 1980;134:507–516.
12. Zwirewich CV, Terriff B, Muller NL. High-spatial-frequency (bone) algorithm improves quality of standard CT of the thorax. *AJR* 1989;153(6):1169–1173.
13. Mayo JR, Webb WR, Gould R, Stein MG, Bass I, Gamsu G, Goldberg HI. High-resolution CT of the lungs: an optimal approach. *Radiology* 1987;163(2):507–510.
14. Bar Ziv J, Solomon A. The use of a modified direct coronal computed tomographic technique for assessing thoraco-abdominal problems. *Gastrointest Radiol* 1989;14(3):205–208.
15. Ney Derek R, Kuhlman JE, Hruban RH, Ren H, Hutchins GM, Fishman EK. Three dimensional CT-volumetric reconstruction and display of the bronchial tree. *Invest Radiol* 1990;25:736–742.
16. Stern RL, Cline HE, Johnson GA, Ravin CE. Three dimensional imaging of the thoracic cavity. *Invest Radiol* 1989;24(4):282–288.
17. Wu X, Latson LA, Driscoll DJ, Ensing GJ, Ritman EL. Dynamic

three-dimensional anatomy of pulmonary arteries in pigs with aorto-to-pulmonary artery shunts. *Am J Physiol Imaging* 1987;2(4):169–175.

18. Webb WR. High-resolution CT of the lung parenchyma. *Radiol Clin North Am* 1989;27(6):1085–1097 (Review).

19. Zerhouni EA, Naidich DP, Khouro NF, Stitik FP, Siegelman SS. Computed tomography of the pulmonary parenchyma: interstitial disease. *J Thorac Imaging* 1985;1:54–64.

20. Murata K, Khan A, Rojas KA, Herman PG. Optimization of computed tomography technique to demonstrate the fine structure of the lung. *Invest Radiol* 1988;23(3):170–175.

21. Kormano M, Dean PB. Extravascular contrast media: the major component of contrast enhancement. *Radiology* 1976;121:379–382.

22. Newhouse JH. Fluid compartment distribution of intravenous iothalamate in the dog. *Invest Radiol* 1977;12:364–367.

23. Newhouse JH, Murphy RX. Tissue distribution of soluble contrast: effect of dose variation and changes with time. *AJR* 1981;136:463–467.

24. Gardeur D, Lautrou J, Millard JC, Berger N, Metzger J. Pharmacokinetics of contrast media: experimental results in dog and man with CT implications. *J Comput Assist Tomogr* 1980;4:178–185.

25. Ono N, Martinez CR, Fara JW, Hodges FJ. Diatrizoate distribution in dogs as a function of administration rate and time following intravenous injection. *J Comput Assist Tomogr* 1980;4:174–177.

26. Young SW, Turner RJ, Castellino RA. A strategy for the contrast enhancement of malignant tumors using dynamic computed tomography and intravascular pharmokinetics. *Radiology* 1980;4:137–147.

27. Godwin JD, Webb WR. Dynamic computed tomography in angiography. *J Comput Assist Tomogr* 1977;1:405.

28. Glazer GM, Francis IR, Gebarski K, Samuels BL, Sorenson KW. Dynamic incremental computed tomography in evaluation of the pulmonary hila. *J Comput Assist Tomogr* 1983;7:59–64.

29. Reese DF, McCullough EC, Baker HL. Dynamic sequential scanning with table incrementation. *Radiology* 1981;140:719–722.

30. Godwin JD, Herfkens RL, Skjoldebrand CT, Federle MP, Lipton MJ. Evaluation of dissections and aneurysms of the thoracic aorta by conventional and dynamic CT scanning. *Radiology* 1980;136:125–133.

31. Passariello R, Salvolini U, Rossi P, Simonetti G, Pasquini U. Automatic contrast media injector for computed tomography. *J Comput Assist Tomogr* 1980;4:278–279.

32. Shepard JO, Dedrick CG, Spizarny DL, McLoud TC. Dynamic incremental computed tomography of the pulmonary hila using a flow-rate injector. *J Comput Assist Tomogr* 1986;10(2):369–371.

33. Tokics L, Hedenstierna G, Strandberg A, Brismar B, Lundquist H. Lung collapse and gas exchange during general anesthesia: effects of spontaneous breathing, muscle paralysis, and positive end-expiratory pressure. *Anesthesiology* 1987;66(2):157–167.

34. Hedenstierna G, Tokics L, Strandberg A, Lundquist H, Brismar B. Correlation of gas exchange impairment to development of atelectasis during anaesthesia and muscle paralysis. *Acta Anaesthesiol Scand* 1986;30(2):183–191.

35. Zimmerman JE, Goodman LR, St. Andre AC, Wyman AC. Radiographic detection of mobilizable lung water: the gravitational shift test. *AJR* 1982;138:59–64.

36. Westcott JL. TI percutaneous transthoracic needle biopsy. *Radiology* 1988;169(3):593–601.

37. Costello P, Onik G, Cosman E. Computed tomographic-guided stereotaxic biopsy of thoracic lesions. *J Thorac Imaging* 1987;2(2):27–32.

38. Williams RA, Haaga JR, Karagiannis E. CT guided paravertebral biopsy of the mediastinum. *J Comput Assist Tomogr* 1984;8(3):575–578.

39. van Sonnenberg E, Lin AS, Deutsch AL, Mattrey RF. Percutaneous biopsy of difficult mediastinal, hilar, and pulmonary lesions by computed tomographic guidance and a modified coaxial technique. *Radiology* 1983;148(1):300–302.

40. Swensen SJ, Ehman RL, Brown LR. Magnetic resonance imaging of the thorax. *J Thorac Imaging* 1989;4(2):19–33 (Review).

41. Spritzer C, Gamsu G, Sostman HD. Magnetic resonance imaging of the thorax: techniques, current applications, and future directions. *J Thorac Imaging* 1989;4(2):1–18.

42. Glazer HS, Lee JKT, Levitt RL, et al. Radiation fibrosis: differentiation from recurrent tumor by MR imaging. *Radiology* 1985;156:721–726.

43. Rahmouni AD, Zerhouni EA. Role of MRI in the management of thoracic lymphoma. *Contemp Issues CT* 1990;11:23–33.

44. Templeton PA, Zerhouni EA. MR imaging of the opaque hemithorax. *Radiology* 1989;173:209.

45. Bittner R, Schorner W, Sander B, Weiss T, Loddenkemper R, Kaiser D, Felix R. Malignant chest wall infiltration in MR: comparison with CT and surgical findings. *ROFO* 1989;151(5):590–596.

46. Haggar AM, Pearlberg JL, Froelich JW, Hearshen DO, Beute GH, Lewis JW Jr, Schkudor GW, Wood C, Gniewek P. Chest-wall invasion by carcinoma of the lung: detection by MR imaging. *AJR* 1987;148(6):1075–1078.

47. Fisher MR. Magnetic resonance for evaluation of the thorax. *Chest* 1989;95(1):166–173 (Review).

48. Firmin DN, Klipstein RH, Hounsfield GL, Paley MP, Longmore DB. Echo-planar high-resolution flow velocity mapping. *Magn Reson Med* 1989;12(3):316–327.

49. Bergin CJ, Pauly J, Glover G, Macovski A. High resolution MR imaging of the lung parenchyma. Abstract. SCBT meeting, Palm Springs, 1989.

50. Mark AS, Winkler ML, Peltzer M, Kaufmann L, Higgins CB. Gated acquisition of MR images of the thorax: advantages for the study of the hila and mediastinum. *Magn Reson Imaging* 1987;5(1):57–63.

51. Felmlee JP, Ehman RL. Spatial presaturation: a method for suppressing flow artifacts and improving depiction of vascular anatomy in MR imaging. *Radiology* 1987;164(2):559–564.

52. Pattany PM, Phillips JJ, Chiu LC, Lipcamon JD, Duerk JL, McNally JM, Mohapatra SN. Motion artifact suppression technique (MAST) for MR imaging. *J Comput Assist Tomogr* 1987;11(3):369–377.

53. Lewis CE, Prato FS, Drost DJ, Nicholson RL. Comparison of respiratory triggering and gating techniques for the removal of respiratory artifacts in MR imaging. *Radiology* 1986;160(3):803–810.

54. Webb WR, Jensen BG, Gamsu G, et al. Coronal MRI of the chest: normal and abnormal. *Radiology* 1984;153:729–735.

55. Haase A, Frahm J, Matthaei D, et al. FLASH imaging: rapid NMR imaging using low flip angle pulses. *J Magn Reson* 1986;67:258–266.

56. Wehrli F. Fast scan magnetic resonance imaging: principles and contrast phenomenology. In: Higgins C, Hricak H eds. Magnetic resonance imaging of the body. New York: Raven Press, 1987.

57. Axel L. Blood flow effects in magnetic resonance imaging. *AJR* 1984;143:1157–1166.

58. Bradley WG, Waluch V, Lai KS, et al. The appearance of rapidly flowing blood on magnetic resonance images. *AJR* 1984;143:1167–1174.

59. Valk PE, Hale JD, Crooks LE, et al. MRI of blood flow: correlation of image appearance with spin-echo phase shift and signal intensity. *AJR* 1986;146:931–939.

60. Bradley WG, Waluch V. NMR even echo rephasing in slow laminar flow. *J Comput Assisted Tomogr* 1984;8:594–598.

61. White EM, Edelman RR, Wedeen VJ, et al. Intravascular signal in MR imaging: use of phase display for differentiation of blood-flow signal from intraluminal disease. *Radiology* 1986;161:245–249.

62. White RD, Winkler ML, Higgins CB, et al. Magnetic resonance imaging of pulmonary arterial hypertension and pulmonary emboli: differentiation of intraluminal signal by multiphasic ECG-gated technique. *AJR* 1987;149:15–21.

63. Schmidt HC, Tscholakoff D, Hricak H, Higgins CB. MR image contrast and relaxation times of solid tumors in the chest, abdomen, and pelvis. *J Comput Assist Tomogr* 1985;9(4):738–748.

64. Webb WR, Gamsu G, Stark DD, et al. Evaluation of magnetic resonance sequences in imaging mediastinal tumors. *AJR* 1984;143:723–717.

65. Barakos JA, Brown JJ, Brescia RJ, Higgins CB. High signal intensity lesions of the chest in MR imaging. *J Comput Assist Tomogr* 1989;13(5):797–802.

66. Webb WR. Magnetic resonance imaging of the hila and mediastinum. *Cardiovasc Intervent Radiol* 1986;8(5–6):306–313.

67. Glazer GM, Orringer MB, Chenevert TL, Borrello JA, Penner MW, Quint LE, Li KC, Aisen AM. Mediastinal lymph nodes: relaxation time/pathologic correlation and implications in staging of lung cancer with MR imaging. *Radiology* 1988;168(2):429–431.

68. Nyman R, Rehn S, Glimelius B, et al. Magnetic resonance imaging for assessment of treatment effects in mediastinal Hodgkin's disease. *Acta Radiol Diagn* 1987;28:145–151.

69. Rholl KS, Levitt RG, Glazer HS. Magnetic resonance imaging of fibrosing mediastinitis. *AJR* 1985;145:255–259.

70. Swensen SJ, Keller PL, Berquist TH, et al. Magnetic resonance imaging of hemorrhage. *AJR* 1985;145:921–927.

71. Wexler HR, Nicholson RL, Prato FS, et al. Quantitation of lung water by nuclear magnetic resonance imaging: A preliminary study. *Invest Radiol* 1985;20:583–590.

72. Herold CJ, Kuhlman J, Zerhouni EA. MRI of pulmonary atelectasis. *Radiology* 1990;[In press].

Chapter 2

Mediastinum

The value of thoracic computed tomography (CT) is greatest in the study of the mediastinum. With conventional radiography, pathologic processes cannot be detected unless they produce a contour abnormality deforming the normal lung-mediastinal interfaces. With its superior contrast resolution, CT readily distinguishes vessels, lymph nodes, and masses from the surrounding fat. The transaxial plane of CT imaging generally is well-suited to the investigation of mediastinal structures, most of which are oriented perpendicularly to the axial plane. Confusing radiographic appearances due to superimposition of different structures are readily re-

solved. The site of origin and extent of lesions are clearly depicted. With CT, the traditional radiographic "blind spots" of the thoracic inlet, the intrapericardial vessels, and the diaphragmatic crura are no longer difficult to evaluate (1).

The indications for mediastinal CT can be subdivided into two broad categories:

1. To better define an abnormality detected by plain chest roentgenography. The chest radiograph remains the screening procedure of choice in the thorax. When a mediastinal abnormality is suspected, CT should be the

A,B

C,D

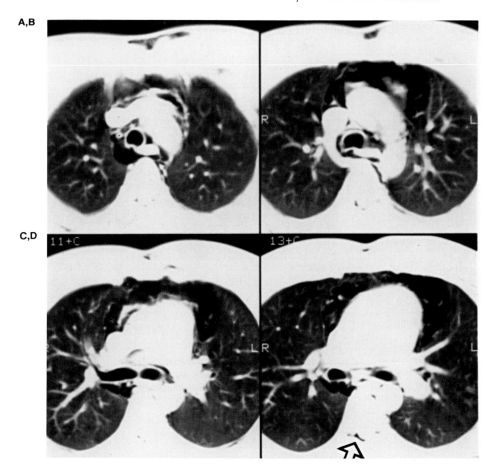

FIG. 1. Pneumomediastinum. **A–D:** Sequential sections through the mediastinum in a patient with extensive pneumomediastinum following trauma. Air has dissected throughout all mediastinal compartments and has even extended to the spinal canal (*arrow* in D). These sections illustrate the extensive intercommunication between mediastinal compartments as well as their truly capacious nature.

next procedure; in our opinion, there is no longer any use for conventional tomographic evaluation of the mediastinum. With CT, normal variations are easily identified as are most benign conditions, such as abnormal fat accumulations or water-containing cysts. If a pathologic condition is present, CT can precisely define its site of origin (vessels versus nodes versus adjacent lung) and direct further investigations (2,3).

2. To more critically evaluate the mediastinum in patients with an established clinical problem. CT may be indicated in these patients because of its high detection sensitivity. Radiographically occult pathology can be readily detected, which helps the staging, treatment planning, and follow-up of patients with known neoplasia, as well as the management of conditions potentially associated with a mediastinal abnormality, such as a thymoma in myasthenia gravis or an ectopic parathyroid adenoma in surgically resistant hyperparathyroidism.

Classically, the mediastinum is divided into several anatomic compartments. This facilitates interpretation of the conventional radiographic manifestations of mediastinal pathology (4). Although some entities are more commonly seen in certain subcompartments, most pathologic processes can express themselves in all (Fig.

1). Furthermore, CT can separately visualize the basic mediastinal anatomic components: fat, lymph nodes, veins and arteries, thymus, thyroid, parathyroid, esophagus, and the paraspinal tissues.

As a consequence, this chapter is organized so that each of these components is discussed separately; this provides a more unified and clinically relevant look at mediastinal CT than would the traditional compartmental approach. Additionally, in each section the potential contribution of magnetic resonance (MR) as it applies to mediastinal analysis will be addressed.

IMAGING TECHNIQUES

CT

As a general rule, CT technique varies according to the specific indication for scanning. For evaluating the mediastinum, the chest radiograph should always serve as the guide to the CT study. If the primary indication is to rule out a mediastinal mass, in a surprising number of cases, adequate images can be obtained without the use of intravenous contrast media (5). Consequently, an initial sequence of nonenhanced scans is recommended. In most cases, a slice thickness of 8–10 mm is generally

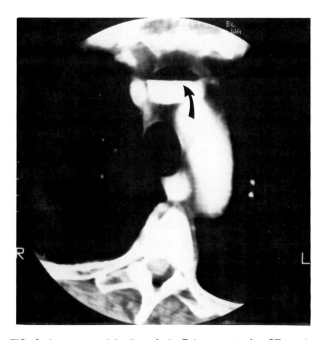

FIG. 2. Intravenous injection of air. Enlargement of a CT section obtained at the level of the aortic arch following a bolus of i.v. contrast media administered through a power injector. Note that an air-fluid level is present in the left brachiocephalic vein (*arrow*), the consequence of air within the injector. Despite the seemingly large volume of air, this patient remained asymptomatic.

sufficient. Thinner slices are required for the assessment of smaller abnormalities in areas where anatomic structures are not oriented perpendicularly to the scan plane (such as the aorticopulmonary window), and when mediastinal fat is lacking.

If contrast is required, optimally it should be administered in the form of a bolus, preferably utilizing a power injector at a rate of 1.5–2.0 cc per sec (6,7), taking care, of course, to minimize the risk of injecting air (8,9) (Fig. 2). Scans can then be obtained with or without table incrementation, as indicated. On most state-of-the-art scanners, interscan delays generally are in the order of 1.8 sec without table incrementation, and run about 3.8 sec with table incrementation. If 2-sec scans are used, therefore, a series of eight images obtained at a single level (so-called dynamic static scanning) takes approximately 30 sec, whereas an identical series of eight images obtained with table incrementation (so-called dynamic incremental scanning) takes approximately 42 sec (Fig. 3). Variations among manufacturers' specifications will result in some differences, although these generally are not very significant (with the obvious exception of scanners capable of subsecond imaging).

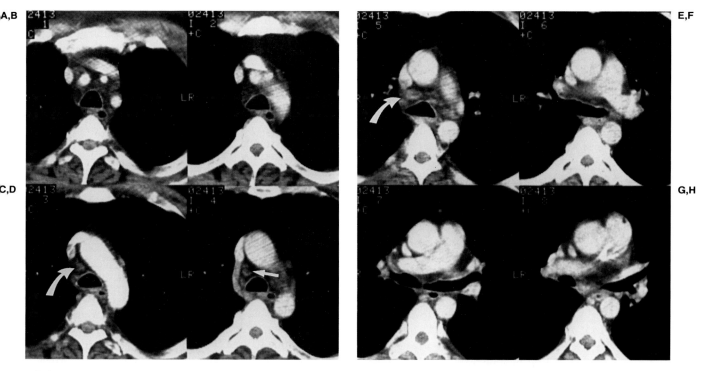

FIG. 3. Mediastinal imaging, dynamic incremental scanning. **A–H:** Coned-down views of sequential 10-mm CT sections through the mediastinum following the bolus injection of 120 cc of 60% iodinated contrast medium through a left-sided arm vein, using a power injector at a rate of 2 cc per sec. This provides dense opacification of all mediastinal vessels allowing easy identification of a few small nodes, especially in the retrocaval and pretracheal spaces (*arrows* in C, D, E). Using 2-sec scan times with a 3.8-sec interscan delay, this series of images was obtained in approximately 42 sec.

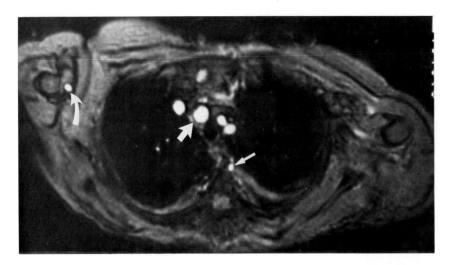

FIG. 4. Mediastinal MR imaging. Section through the great vessels using gradient-recalled echoes (TR = 25 msec, TE = 13 msec, flip angle = 20°). In these images, flowing blood results in considerable signal within vessels, not only in the mediastinum (*straight arrows*) but in the chest wall as well (*curved arrow at right*). TR, repetition time; TE, echo time.

MR

In our experience, MR is best utilized as a problem-solving modality, especially for cases in which CT cannot be performed, or is suboptimal. Each case is individualized; no standard algorithm is universally applicable. As discussed in Chapter 1, following acquisition of initial coronal scout images, cardiac-gated, T1-weighted axial sections are obtained through regions of interest. With gating, the effective repetition time (TR) is set by the heart rate. Coronal and sagittal images are generally best reserved for specific indications, such as analyzing the chest wall, the aorticopulmonary window, or subcarinal space.

T2-weighted images are reserved specifically for those cases for which tissue characterization is deemed necessary. These may be acquired either utilizing a prolonged TR (2,000 ms) without cardiac gating, or preferably utilizing cardiac gating (especially if the region of interest is near the heart or hila) with images obtained every second or third cardiac cycle. Increasingly, we have relied on single section, multi-echo imaging in order to obtain T2-weighted images. Although this technique restricts imaging to one image plane, the resultant data may be of greater reliance in tissue characterization. In select cases, for example, evaluating thoracic inlet and/or mediastinal veins to exclude thrombosis, gradient-refocused sequences with breath-holding can be employed to reduce scan time and optimize visualization of vascular pathology (Fig. 4).

AORTIC ARCH AND GREAT VESSELS: NORMAL ANATOMY AND VARIANTS

Accurate interpretation of mediastinal pathology requires detailed knowledge of normal cross-sectional anatomy, as well as an awareness of the wide range of normal anatomic variants and congenital anomalies that may involve the aortic arch and great vessels. This anatomy has been reviewed by numerous authors (4,5). The significance of recognizing normal anatomy and variants has been emphasized by Baron et al. (2): in an evaluation of 71 patients referred for CT examination because of widening of the mediastinum on plain radiographs, nearly 50% were found to have a vascular anomaly or abnormality.

Anatomy of the Arch and Great Vessels

The anatomy of the aortic arch and great vessels can be conceptualized as a series of characteristic sections. Figure 5 is a schematic drawing of the major arterial and venous structures of the mediastinum on which these characteristic levels have been drawn.

The aortic arch normally has an oblique course extending posteriorly and to the left (Fig. 6). Anteriorly, the aortic arch lies in front of the trachea and is inti-

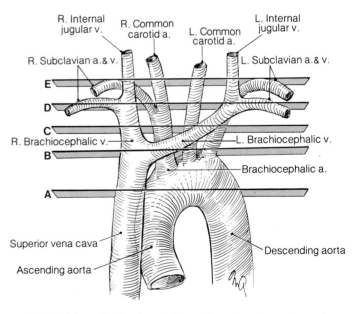

FIG. 5. Schematic drawing of the aortic arch and great vessels. Characteristic levels have been labeled A through E.

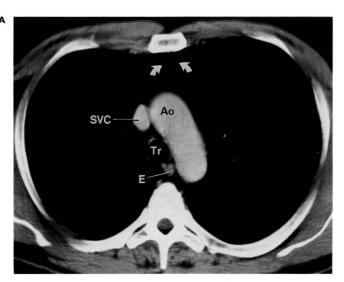
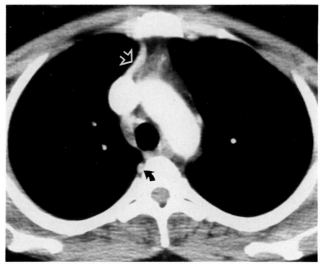

FIG. 6. **A:** CT section through the aortic arch (Ao), corresponding to level A in Fig. 5. SVC, superior vena cava; Tr, trachea; E, esophagus. At this level, the anterior mediastinum has a triangular configuration, with the apex pointing anteriorly (*arrows*). **B:** CT section at the level of the aortic arch shows a prominent right internal mammary vein draining into the superior vena cava (*open arrow*). This appearance should not be mistaken for residual thymic tissue. Curved arrow points to the right superior intercostal vein which characteristically lies in a paravertebral location.

mately related to the anteromedial aspect of the superior vena cava on the left side. As the arch extends posteriorly, it lies to the left of the trachea, and, more posteriorly, at the junction of the aortic knob and descending aorta, it is intimately related to the esophagus.

At this level, the anterior mediastinum has a triangular configuration, with the apex pointing anteriorly. In a normal adult, following regression of the thymus gland, the anterior mediastinum should contain only fat. Occasionally, the prominent internal mammary veins may be identified draining into the superior vena cava, an appearance that is usually easily differentiable from residual thymic tissue. The middle mediastinum is also well-defined by fat at this level, bordered posteriorly by the convexity of the trachea, anteriorly by the posterior and posterolateral aspect of the superior vena cava, medially by the arch of the aorta, and laterally by the mediastinal pleural reflections.

Frequently, sections at or just below the level of the aortic arch will also include the arch of the azygos vein, which crosses over the right upper lobe bronchus and courses anteriorly along the right wall of the distal trachea to join the superior vena cava. The arch of the azygos usually can be localized to the T5-T6 vertebral body level, and helps to define the pretracheal, retrocaval space (Fig. 7). This space is limited by the anterior convexity of the distal trachea, the medial wall of the aortic arch, the posterior and posteromedial borders of the superior vena cava, and the medial border of the azygos arch (10). Normally, the pretracheal, retrocaval space contains mediastinal fat, fibrous connective tissue, and lymph nodes (commonly referred to as azygos nodes). The clinical importance of this space derives from the critical role played by the azygos nodes that drain the subcarinal and bronchopulmonary-hilar nodes

efferently, and are afferent links with the paratracheal and middle mediastinal nodes superiorly.

Above the level of the aortic arch, through most of the superior mediastinum, five vessels can be identified routinely. These include the three major branches of the aortic arch (i.e., the brachiocephalic artery, the left common carotid artery, and the left subclavian artery) and the left and right brachiocephalic veins. The brachiocephalic artery is midline, in close proximity to the

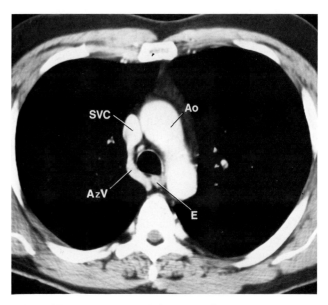

FIG. 7. CT section at the level of the arch of the azygos vein (AzV). Identification of the azygos arch helps to define the pretracheal, retrocaval space that is bounded by the anterior margin of the distal trachea, the posterior wall of the aorta (Ao), and the posteromedial border of the superior vena cava (SVC). Note the presence of a normal-sized lymph node in this location, embedded within mediastinal fat. E, esophagus.

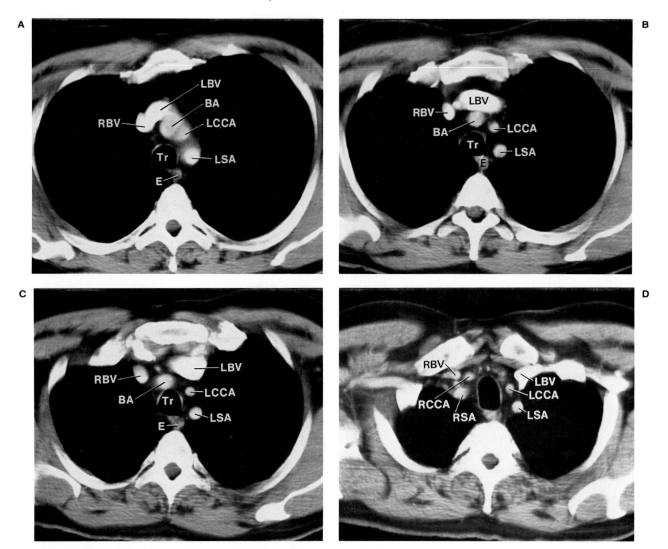

FIG. 8. Cross-sectional CT anatomy, great vessels. **A–D:** Sequential contrast-enhanced CT images through the great vessels, from below-upward, corresponding to levels B, C, D, and E in Fig. 5, respectively. Note that the left brachiocephalic vein (LBV) has a much more horizontal course than the right brachiocephalic vein (RBV) as it crosses the mediastinum. The left brachiocephalic vein is an important landmark, dividing the mediastinum into pre- and retrovascular compartments. Tr, trachea; LSA, left subclavian artery; LCCA, left common carotid artery; BA, brachiocephalic artery; RSA, right subclavian artery; RCCA, right common carotid artery; E, esophagus.

anterior wall of the trachea (Fig. 8). The left common carotid artery lies to the left and slightly posterolateral to the brachiocephalic artery; generally it has the smallest diameter of the three major arteries. Throughout most of its course, the left subclavian artery is a relatively posterior structure, lying to the left and frequently adjacent to the trachea. Additionally, the lateral border of the left subclavian artery lies adjacent to the mediastinal reflections of the left upper lobe, which it indents in a typically convex fashion (Fig. 8). Contact of the lung with the mediastinum anterior to the left subclavian vein has been noted to be the most common cause of a left paratracheal reflection when identified on routine chest radiographs (11).

The two brachiocephalic veins have fundamentally different configurations. The right brachiocephalic vein has a nearly vertical course throughout its length; the left brachiocephalic vein has a longer course, and, inferiorly, courses horizontally as it crosses the mediastinum from left to right (Figs. 3A–C, 5, and 8). The horizontal component of the left brachiocephalic vein is a convenient anatomic landmark, being the line of demarcation between the anterior mediastinum (the prevascular space) anteriorly and the middle mediastinum posteriorly. The precise configuration of this vein is highly variable; although generally illustrated at the level of the great vessels, the horizontal component of the left brachiocephalic vein can be found at almost any level of the superior mediastinum, including in front of the aortic arch where it may superficially mimic the appearance of an intimal flap (Fig. 3C). Because of the key role played by the horizontal component of the left brachiocephalic vein in dividing the compartments of the mediastinum, when intravenous contrast medium is employed it should be given, whenever possible, in a left-sided arm vein. This maximizes visualization of the full length of the left brachiocephalic vein (Figs. 3A–C, and 6).

The arch of the aorta is not a "flat" structure; instead, it has a general superoposterior configuration, and the three great arteries arise sequentially at different levels. The brachiocephalic artery arises first and at the most caudal level of the arch. The left common carotid artery arises next, at a higher level. The left subclavian artery is the last branch and arises from the posterosuperior portion of the aortic knob. As sequential images are obtained through the origins of the great vessels, progressively smaller portions of the aortic knob will be visualized posteriorly. At the level of origin of the left subclavian artery, the posterior portion of the arch should not be confused with a mediastinal mass (Fig. 3).

Above the level of the brachiocephalic artery bifurcation, the right subclavian and right common carotid arteries can be identified separately (Fig. 8). These vessels are essentially mirror images of the left subclavian and common carotid arteries. The exact position of the bi-

furcation of the brachiocephalic artery is variable, depending on the length and degree of tortuosity of this vessel. In a significant percentage of cases, the brachiocephalic artery bifurcates "late"; in these cases the right subclavian artery will have an oblique course, and if thin sections are not obtained near the thoracic inlet, it may not be visualized at all. When the right common carotid and right subclavian arteries are seen, they normally are found only in sections through the uppermost portion of the superior mediastinum. Visualization of these vessels in a more inferior position, just above the aortic arch, frequently indicates the presence of some type of vascular mediastinal anomaly, usually involving the aortic arch. This has been termed the "four vessel sign" by McLoughlin et al. (12).

Although the great vessels should be recognized by their characteristic configurations, tortuosity or ectasia of these vessels may present a confusing picture and be easily mistaken as pathologic. Use of intravenous contrast media will almost always resolve this problem.

The subclavian arteries and veins exit and enter the mediastinum by crossing over the first ribs, behind the proximal portions of the clavicles (Fig. 9) The subclavian vein lies anterior and the subclavian artery lies posterior to the anterior scalenus muscle, which attaches to the superior border of the first rib. Once it has crossed over the first rib, the subclavian vein courses toward the

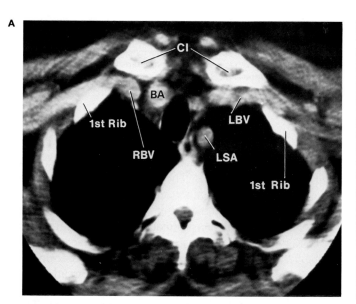
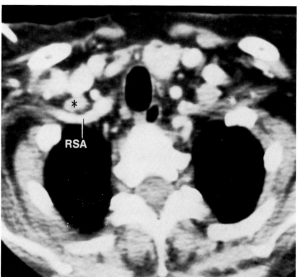

FIG. 9. A: Section through the sternal notch between the proximal portions of the clavicles. The subclavian veins cross into the mediastinum by passing over the first ribs, behind the clavicles (CI). There is continuity between the axillary portions of the subclavian veins lying posterior to the pectoralis minor muscles and the right and left brachiocephalic veins (RBV, LBV). The subclavian arteries generally have a more angled, oblique course as they exit the mediastinum, and frequently are not seen crossing the first rib. The axillary portions of the subclavian arteries lie posterior to the corresponding subclavian veins. LSA, left subclavian artery; BA, brachiocephalic artery. **B:** Contrast-enhanced section just above the clavicles shows characteristic relationship between the right subclavian artery (RSA) and the anterior scalene muscle (*).

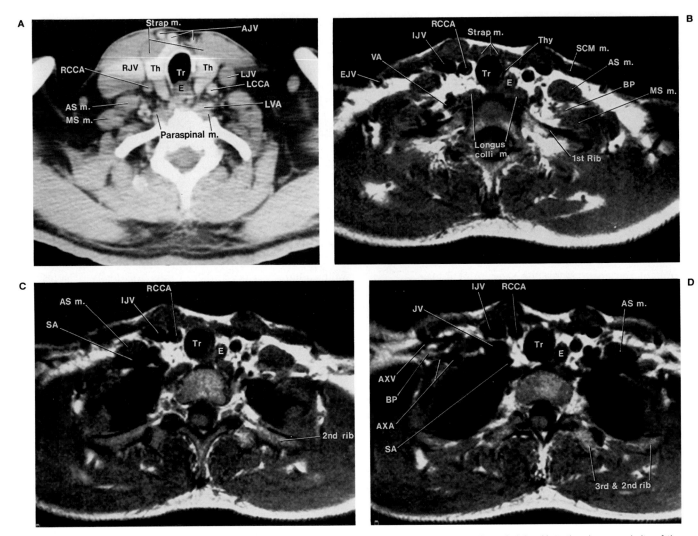

FIG. 10. Thoracic inlet, CT/MR evaluation. **A:** CT section through the lower neck, just above the thoracic inlet. Note the close proximity of the thyroid gland to the trachea. **B–D.** Sequential MR images from above-downward through the thoracic inlet. The anatomy of the thoracic inlet is especially well-visualized with MR. Note the relationship between the anterior scalene muscle and the subclavian artery which lies immediately posteriorly. The brachial plexus usually can be identified just above the subclavian artery as it passes behind the anterior scalene. AJV, anterior jugular veins; ASm, anterior scalene muscle; AXA, axillary artery; AXV, axillary vein; BP, brachial plexus; E, esophagus; EJV, external jugular vein; IJV, internal jugular vein; JV, jugular vein; LCCA, left common carotid artery; LJV, left jugular vein; LVA, left vertebral artery; MSm, middle scalene muscle; RCCA, right common carotid artery; RJV, right jugular vein; SA, subclavian artery; SCMm, sternocleidomastoid muscle; Th, Thy, thyroid; Tr, trachea; VA, vertebral artery.

axilla, which lies behind the pectoralis muscles. This line of continuity is easily traced with CT, allowing differentiation between mediastinal versus axillary venous obstruction. The transition from the mediastinal to the axillary portions of the subclavian arteries is more difficult to visualize because there is a sharper degree of angulation in the course these vessels take as they cross over the first rib. The axillary portions of the subclavian arteries lie posterior to the corresponding veins. The thoracic inlet demarcates the junction between the root of the neck and superior mediastinum (Fig. 10) (13). It characteristically follows an oblique plane, paralleling the first rib. The trachea at this level is surrounded on both sides by the inferior lobes of the thyroid gland; lateral to the trachea, the internal jugular veins and common carotid arteries can be identified. These structures are bounded circumferentially by strap muscles, including the sternocleidomastoid muscles anteriorly, the anterior scalenus muscles laterally, and the longus colli muscles posteriorly in the prevertebral area (Fig. 9).

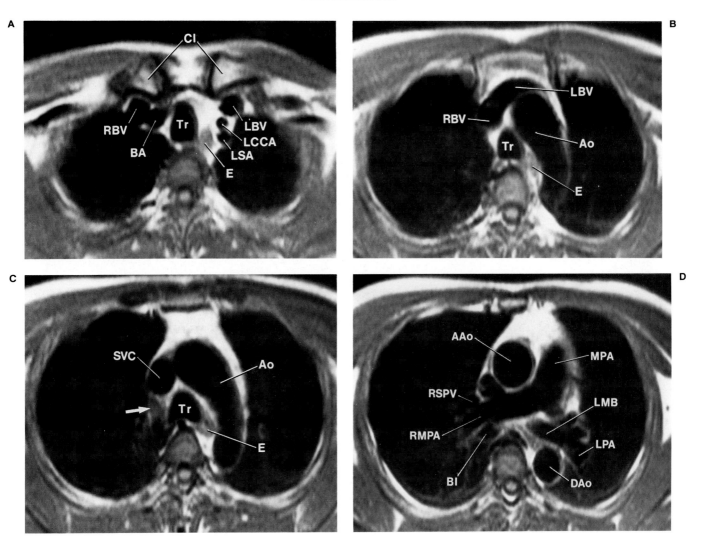

FIG. 11. Cross-sectional MR anatomy. **A–D:** Cardiac-gated MR images through the mediastinum from above-downward. A,B, and C correspond to levels C, B, and A in Fig. 5, respectively. Tr, trachea; LBV, left brachiocephalic vein; LCCA, left common carotid artery; LSA, left subclavian artery; E, esophagus; RBV, right brachiocephalic vein; BA, brachiocephalic artery; Cl, clavicles; Ao, aorta; SVC, superior vena cava; MPA, main pulmonary artery; LMB, left main-stem bronchus; LPA, left interlobar pulmonary artery; DAo, descending aorta; Bl, bronchus intermedius; AAo, ascending aorta; RSPV, right superior pulmonary vein; RMPA, right main pulmonary artery. Note that signal is present within the azygos vein, posterior to the SVC (*arrow* in C), presumably secondary to slow flow.

MR Evaluation of the Normal Mediastinum

In many respects, the MR appearance of mediastinal anatomy is strikingly similar to CT (Fig. 11). Although cross-sectional imaging of the mediastinum is generally adequate to visualize most pathologic processes, because of its ability to visualize structures in multiple planes, MR potentially can add to our understanding of the origin and extent of disease (Fig. 12). Utilization of multi-planar images, however, requires detailed knowledge of normal relationships between mediastinal structures in both standard coronal and sagittal planes (Figs. 13 and 14). Once familiar, these images can be augmented by use of select parasagittal planes that maximize visualization of select regions, such as the aorticopulmonary window (see Fig. 6, Chapter 5). Familiarity should also be gained with the appearance of the aorta and great vessels using gradient-recalled echoes (Fig. 4).

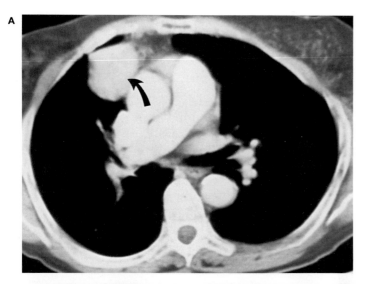

FIG. 12. Anatomic localization, CT/MR correlation. A: CT section at the level of the right main pulmonary artery following a bolus of i.v. contrast media. A well-defined soft-tissue mass is present on the right side (arrow). Despite the appearance of this lesion, accurate localization is difficult. The lesion could just as easily originate within the lung as from the mediastinum. Sections above and below were of no further assistance. B, C: T1- and T2-weighted coronal images through the mass, respectively. On the T1-weighted image, fat clearly marginates both the superior and inferior borders of the mass (arrows in B), indicative of a mediastinal origin. Note that anatomic localization is considerably more difficult on the T2-weighted image, although there has been a marked increase in the relative signal of the lesion. Biopsy confirmed noninvasive thymoma.

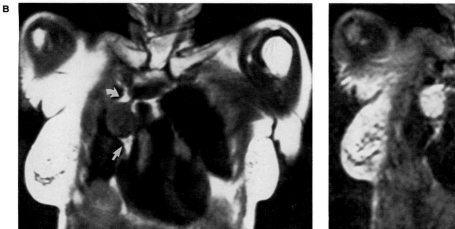

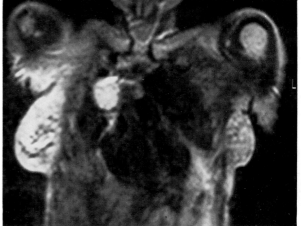

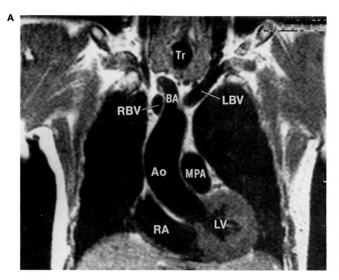

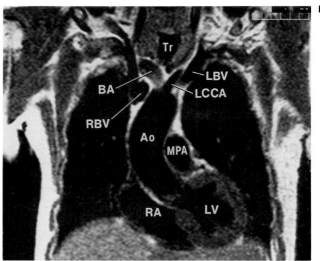

FIG. 13. Mediastinal anatomy, coronal MR images. A–H: Sequential coronal MR images from anterior to posterior. Identification of individual structures is easiest when comparison is made to the sections immediately adjacent, limiting potential problems of interpretation due to partial volume averaging. Ao, aorta, RA, right atrium; LV, left ventricle; MPA, main pulmonary artery; BA, brachiocephalic artery; RBV, right brachiocephalic vein; LBV, left brachiocephalic vein; Tr, trachea; LCCA, left common carotid artery; SVC, superior vena cava; RSPV, right superior pulmonary vein;

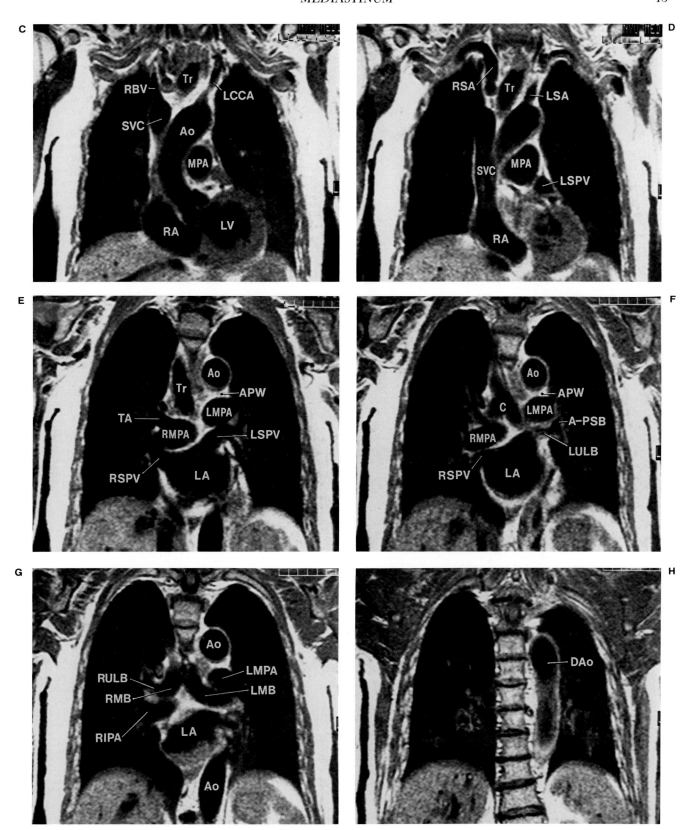

FIG. 13. *(Continued.)* RIPA, right inferior pulmonary artery; RSA, right subclavian artery; LSA, left subclavian artery; TA, truncus anterior; RMPA, right main pulmonary artery; LMPA, left main pulmonary artery; LSPV, left superior pulmonary vein; APW, aorticopulmonary window; RULB, right upper lobe bronchus; LMB, left main-stem bronchus; RMB, right main-stem bronchus; LA, left atrium; RMPA, right main pulmonary artery; LULB, left upper lobe bronchus; A-PSB, apical-posterior segmental bronchus; DAo, descending aorta. Note that the thyroid gland is easily identified adjacent to the trachea in A and B.

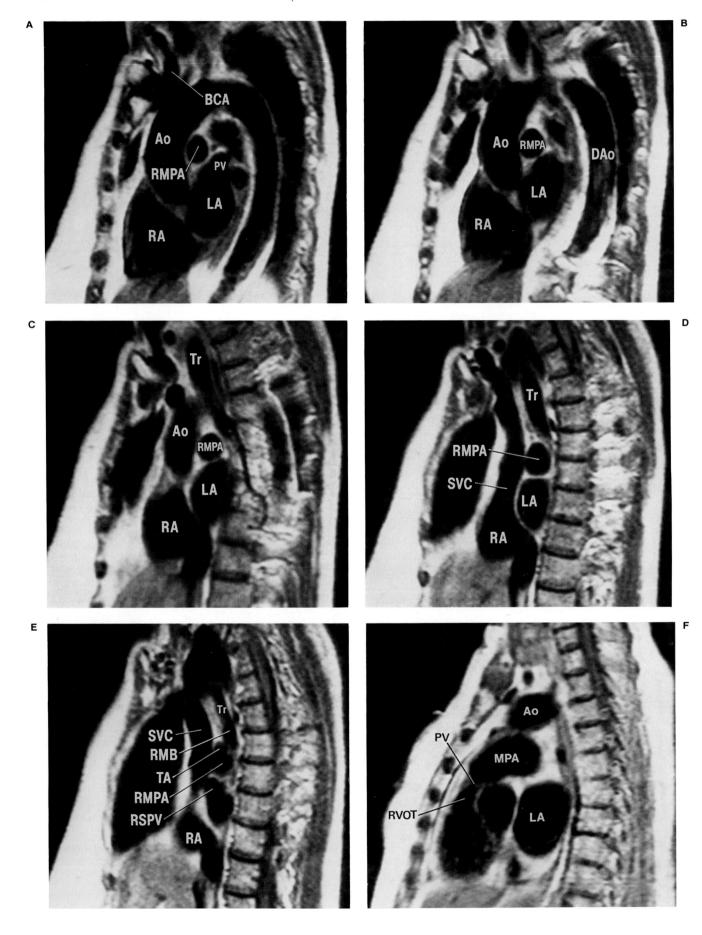

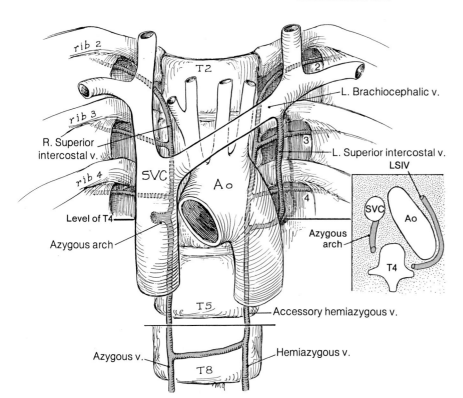

FIG. 15. Schematic drawing of the azygos, hemiazygos, and superior intercostal venous systems. *Inset* is a schematic cross-section at the level of the aortic arch.

Anatomy of the Azygos, Hemiazygos, and Superior Intercostal Veins

Cross-sectional anatomy of the azygos, hemiazygos, and superior intercostal venous systems has been described in detail (Fig. 15) (14–19). Inferiorly, the azygos and hemiazygos veins represent continuations into the thorax of the left and right ascending lumbar veins. The azygos vein parallels the esophagus to the right, and laterally is in contact with the medial pleural reflections of the right lower lobe, defining the medial border of the azygo-esophageal recess (Figs. 3F,G,H). The azygos vein drains the lower intercostal veins along its route (Fig. 16). On the left side, the hemiazygos vein parallels the descending aorta posteriorly, draining the lower intercostal veins on the left side. The hemiazygos vein itself generally drains into the azygos vein via communicating vessels that cross the midline in the vicinity of the T8 vertebral body. Normally, these are almost never seen on CT (18,19).

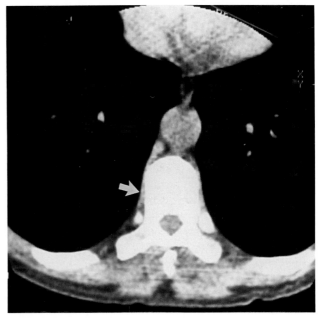

FIG. 16. Enlargement of a section through the lower thorax shows a normal-sized intercostal vein draining into the azygos vein (*arrow*).

FIG. 14. Mediastinal anatomy, parasagittal MR images. A–E: Sequential parasagittal images through the mediastinum, from the level of the aortic arch to the right hilum, respectively. Familiarity with this particular plane is especially important as it intersects both the ascending and descending aorta, thus allowing visualization of the entire aorta in a single plane (see A). Ao, ascending aorta; BCA, brachiocephalic artery; RA, right atrium; LA, left atrium; RMPA, right main pulmonary artery; PV, left superior pulmonary vein; DAo, descending aorta; Tr, trachea; SVC, superior vena cava; RSPV, right superior pulmonary vein; TA, truncus anterior; RMB, right main-stem bronchus. F: True sagittal MR image through the main pulmonary artery (MPA). Note that in this plane, the relationship between the MPA and the right ventricular outflow tract (RVOT) is especially well seen. As shown in this example, occasionally a section at this level allows visualization of the pulmonic valves.

A

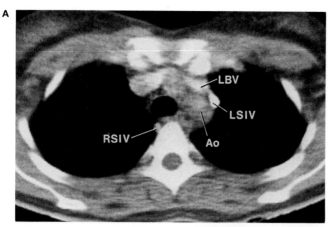

B

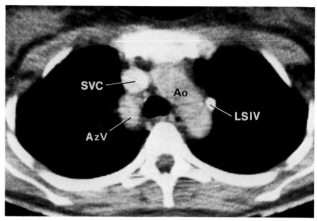

C

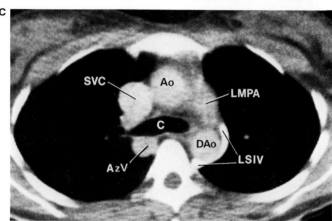

FIG. 17. Left superior intercostal vein, azygos continuation. **A–C:** Sequential contrast-enhanced images from below-upward. Dense contrast is present in the accessory hemiazygos vein, allowing it to be identified as it joins the left superior intercostal vein to arch around the aorta and drain into the left brachiocephalic vein. As the left superior intercostal vein (LSIV) winds around the aorta (Ao), it may assume a vertical configuration, in which case it may be mistaken for preaortic adenopathy. Note that in this case the azygos vein and arch (AzV) are markedly dilated in this patient, with azygos continuation of the inferior vena cava. SVC, superior vena cava; LMPA, left main pulmonary artery; DAo, descending aorta; C, carina; LBV, left brachiocephalic vein; RSIV, right superior intercostal vein.

Superiorly, the azygos vein terminates by arching over the medial aspect of the right upper lobe bronchus and then coursing anteriorly to join the posterior aspect of the superior vena cava (Fig. 6). Just prior to the formation of the azygos arch, the azygos vein is joined by the right superior intercostal vein (Fig. 15). This vein drains the right second to fourth intercostal veins, and then courses inferiorly in a paraspinal location.

On the left side, the accessory hemiazygos vein continues above the point of termination of the hemiazygos vein (the two are frequently in communication), ascending posterior to the descending aorta (Fig. 15). At the level of the aortic arch, the accessory hemiazygos is joined by the left superior intercostal vein (which drains the second to fourth intercostal veins), in approximately 75% of patients (16). The left superior intercostal vein forms a venous arch (also referred to as the arch of the hemiazygos vein) that courses anteriorly around the aortic arch to join the left brachiocephalic vein superiorly (Fig. 17). On routine radiographs, the left superior intercostal vein is most often seen end-on, adjacent to the aortic knob. Because of its appearance, it has been

termed the "aortic nipple," and can be seen in up to 10% of normal patients (16). Prominence of the aortic nipple has been reported secondary to congenital absence of the azygos vein (20); more importantly, enlargement of this vein may indicate impending superior vena caval obstruction (21).

The arch of the azygos is well-known radiologically, probably because of the frequent need to differentiate a prominent azygos vein from paratracheal adenopathy. The azygos arch is very variable in dimension. Dilatation of the arch may be caused by central venous hypertension (as may occur with right ventricular heart failure), obstruction of the superior or inferior vena cava, or azygos continuation of an anomalous inferior vena cava (IVC) (Fig. 17, Fig. 18). Idiopathic dilatation of the azygos arch may occur, in which case the arch may be mistaken for a pulmonary lesion (22).

The azygos and hemiazygos venous systems are important collateral systems when there is obstruction or interruption of blood flow through either of the brachiocephalic vessels or the superior or inferior vena cava (21) (Fig. 19).

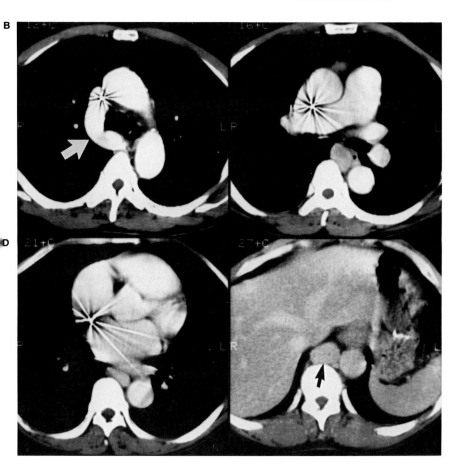

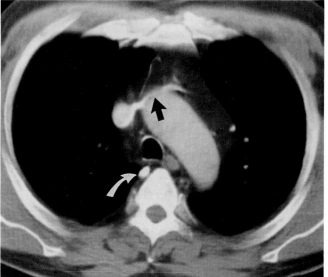

FIG. 18. Azygos continuation. **A–D:** Coned-down views of the mediastinum from the level of the azygos arch superiorly to the lower thorax. The dilated hemiazygos vein is easily identified, especially at the level of the azygos arch (*arrow* in A). Note that the azygos vein is as large as the descending aorta (*arrow* in D)

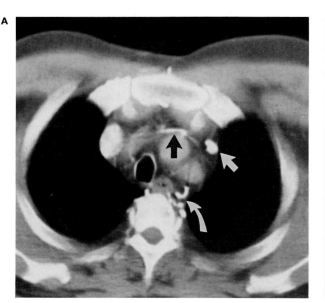

FIG. 19. Obstruction, left brachiocephalic vein. **A, B:** Sequential images through the great vessels and the aortic arch, respectively, following a bolus of i.v. contrast media administered through a left-sided antecubital vein. The left brachiocephalic vein is markedly attenuated, the result of a previous indwelling venous catheter (*black arrows* in A and B). Note that there is bright opacification of both the azygos (*curved arrows* in A and B) and hemiazygos systems (*curved arrow* in A), including the left superior intercostal vein beginning at the left brachiocephalic vein (*straight white arrow*). The azygos and hemiazygos venous system serves as an important collateral pathway when there is obstruction either of the brachiocephalic veins or the vena cavae.

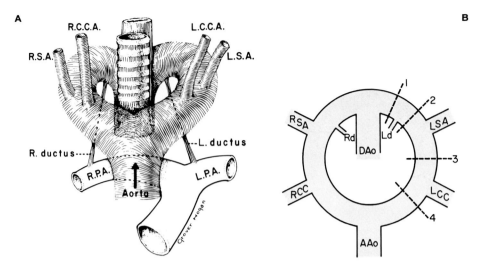

FIG. 20. A: Hypothetical double aortic arch of Edwards. (From: Shuford WH, and Sybers RG. *The Aortic Arch and Its Malformations,* 1974. Courtesy of Charles C Thomas, Springfield, Illinois.) **B:** Schematic representation of embryonic double aortic arch. Normally, there is interruption of the right arch distal to the right subclavian artery. The result is a normal left arch. Right aortic arches result when there is interruption of some portion of the left aortic arch. Five potential sites of interruption have been identified. If there is interruption distal to the left subclavian (at either 1 or 2), the result is a right aortic arch with mirror-image branching (types 1 and 2). If there is interruption between the left subclavian and left common carotid arteries (at 3), the result is a right aortic arch with an aberrant left subclavian (type 3). If the arch is interrupted proximal to the left common carotid artery (at 4), the result is a right arch with an aberrant innominate artery (type 4). Finally, interruption may occur both distal to the left subclavian artery and proximal to the left subclavian artery (at both 1 and 3); this results in an isolated left subclavian artery, connected to the left pulmonary artery via the left ductus arteriosus (type 5). DAo, descending aorta: AAo, ascending aorta, LSA, left subclavian artery; LCC, left common carotid artery; Ld, left ductus arteriosus; Rd, right ductus; RCC, right common carotid artery; RSA, right subclavian artery.

Dilatation of the azygos and hemiazygos veins is classically associated with anomalies of the inferior vena cava, although idiopathic aneursyms have been reported (23–28). When there is developmental failure of the hepatic or infrahepatic (prerenal) segment of the inferior vena cava, blood returns to the heart via the cranial portion of the supracardinal veins, i.e., the azygos and hemiazygos veins. This anomaly has been reported in up to 2% of cases in patients with congenital heart disease undergoing cardiac catheterization. The association between azygos continuation and the asplenia and polysplenia syndromes has been well-documented (19). Azygos continuation may also be present in otherwise asymptomatic patients, and in this setting may be misinterpreted as some other form of pathology, specifically, a right paratracheal mass, a posterior mediastinal mass (if the dilated azygos or hemiazygos vein is identified along the paravertebral pleural reflections), or a retrocrural mass or adenopathy.

The appearance of azygos continuation is easily defined on CT by the following constellation of findings: enlargement of the arch of the azygos, enlargement of the paraspinal portions of the azygos and hemiazygos veins (especially if confluent at higher sections with the azygos arch), and enlargement of the retrocrural portions of these same veins in the absence of a definable inferior vena cava (Fig. 18). It should be noted that once

an abnormality of the inferior vena cava is diagnosed, careful examination of the abdomen should be performed to further define and clarify its specific nature.

Anomalies of the Arch and Great Vessels

To recognize anomalies of the aorta and great vessels, it is essential to have some knowledge of embryology. These anomalies are most easily understood if the hypothetical double arch system, described by Edwards (29) as a basic pattern from which all aortic anomalies can be derived, is used (Fig. 20). In this system, there is an aortic arch and a potential ductus arteriosus on each side; the descending aorta is in the midline posteriorly. Interruption of this arch system at different locations can explain the various aortic arch anomalies. These may be divided into three main groups: left aortic arch anomalies, right aortic arch anomalies, and double arch anomalies.

Normally, there is interruption of the hypothetical right arch distal to the right subclavian artery. The right common carotid and subclavian arteries fuse to become the right brachiocephalic artery as the proximal portion of the embryologic right arch becomes incorporated into

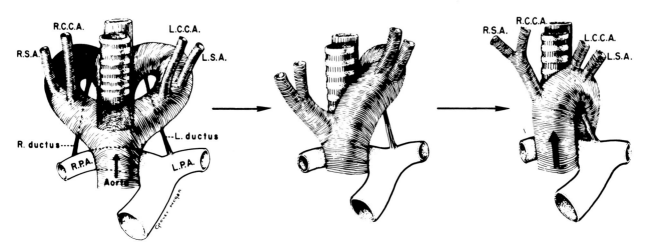

FIG. 21. Hypothesized embryologic development of the normal left arch. The shaded portion of the right arch, distal to the right subclavian artery, is interrupted. (From: Shuford WH, and Sybers RG. *The Aortic Arch and Its Malformations,* 1974. Courtesy of Charles C Thomas, Springfield, Illinois.)

the left arch. The result is the normal left-sided aortic arch. This series of events is illustrated in Fig. 21.

ported; this may be associated with an aberrant right subclavian artery (33).

Left Aortic Arch Anomalies

The most common congenital anomaly of the aorta is an aberrant right subclavian artery originating from an otherwise normal left-sided arch, occurring in approximately 0.5% of the normal population (29). Theoretically, this occurs when there is interruption of the embryologic right aortic arch between the right common carotid and the right subclavian arteries. The right subclavian then originates from the posterior portion of the left-sided arch and crosses the mediastinum obliquely from left to right, lying posterior to the trachea and esophagus (Fig. 20, Figs. 22 and 23) (30). Dilatation of the artery at its origin (the so-called diverticulum of Kommerell) is common, occurring in up to 60% of cases (31). If sufficiently large, this outpouching at the origin of the right subclavian artery may be mistaken as either a mediastinal mass, or aneurysm of the arch of the aorta (Fig. 24) (32). Although the aberrant right subclavian artery causes an impression on both the trachea and esophagus, symptoms rarely result from this anomaly, and other associated anomalies are never present. Other left aortic arch anomalies are rare. Left aortic arch associated with a right-sided descending aorta has been re-

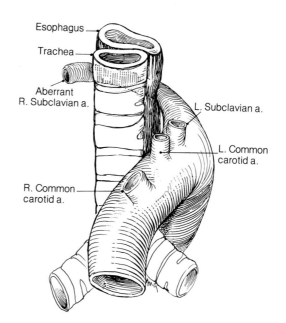

FIG. 22. Schematic representation of an aberrant right subclavian artery.

A,B,C

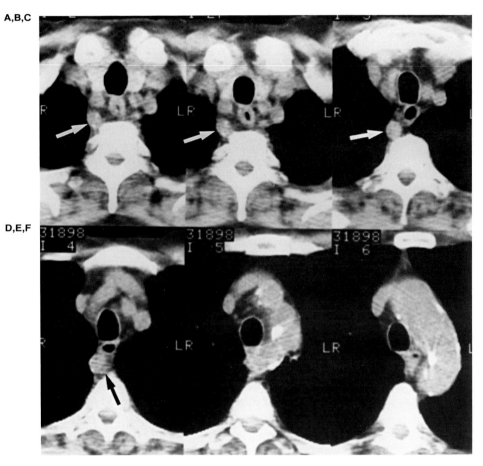

D,E,F

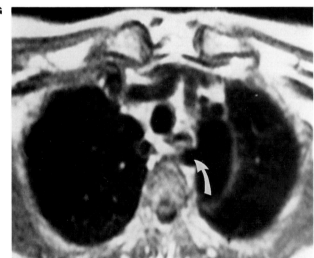

FIG. 23. Aberrant right subclavian artery. **A–F:** Enlargements of sequential CT images through the mediastinum from the great vessels to the aortic arch, inferiorly, respectively. An aberrant right subclavian artery is present, arising from the medial-posterior portion of the aortic arch on the left. This artery passes posterior to the esophagus and trachea (*arrow* in D) and then proceeds superiorly to eventually lie in a normal position in the superior mediastinum (*arrows* in A, B, and C). **G, H:** Axial and sagittal MR images, respectively, in another patient with an aberrant right subclavian artery. Again, the aberrant artery is easily identified arising from the aorta (*arrow* in G), posterior to the esophagus and trachea (*arrow* in H).

G

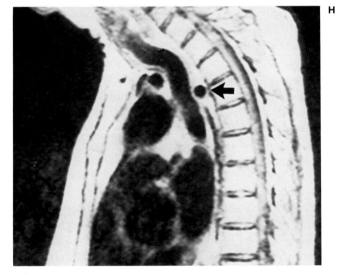

H

Right Aortic Arch Anomalies

Numerous variations in the classification of right aortic arch anomalies have been reported (34–36). Using Edwards' hypothetical double aortic arch model, five potential anomalies can be predicted, although only three are usually described and only two are relatively common (Fig. 20) (37,38). The type of anomaly encountered will depend on the exact point at which the left aortic arch is interrupted.

The two most common right aortic arch anomalies are right aortic arch with an aberrant left subclavian

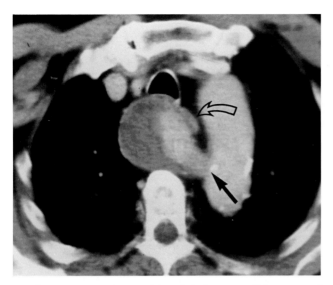

FIG. 24. Aneursym, aberrant right subclavian artery. Enlargement of a CT image through the aortic arch following a bolus of i.v. contrast media. An aneurysmally dilated aberrant right subclavian artery can be identified arising from the aortic arch (*arrow*) causing considerable compression of the adjacent esophagus (*curved arrow*). Note the presence of considerable thrombus within the aneurysm.

artery, and right aortic arch with mirror-image branching of the great vessels.

The most common right aortic arch anomaly is a right aortic arch with an aberrant left subclavian artery (type 3) (34). The sequence of events leading to the malformation is illustrated in Figure 25. In this case, there is interruption of the left arch between the left common carotid and left subclavian arteries. This leads to an anterior left common carotid artery as the first branch of the ascending aorta, and a retroesophageal left subclavian artery (Fig. 26). The distal portion of the left arch

(incorporated into the posterior portion of the right arch) frequently persists and may become aneurysmally dilated. This type of right arch anomaly is only infrequently associated with congenital heart disease.

A right aortic arch with mirror-image branching occurs if the hypothetical left arch is interrupted distal to the left subclavian artery (Fig. 27). The left innominate artery then arises as the first branch of the ascending aorta. Most frequently, this interruption is distal to the left ductus arteriosus. The result is a mirror image of normal (Figs. 20 and 27). This anomaly is significant because of the well-known association of congenital heart disease (especially tetralogy of Fallot) that is present in nearly 100% of cases (39).

In the usual case of right aortic arch with mirror-image branching, interruption of the left arch occurs distal to the ductus arteriosus (type 1). The result is that there is no structure posterior to the trachea or esophagus. More rarely, interruption occurs distal to the left subclavian artery but proximal to the ductus (type 2) (Fig. 20) (40). If the ductus on the left side persists, the result is a true vascular ring, formed by the right-sided aortic arch anterior and to the right, and the persistent left-sided ductus, originating from the distal right-sided arch, passing behind the trachea and esophagus, and joining the left main pulmonary artery. Symptomatology reflects the degree of constriction caused by the vascular ring. This type of malformation is only rarely associated with congenital heart disease. Although exceedingly rare, the appearance on CT of this anomaly has been reported (41).

Two other right aortic arch anomalies have been described. If the left aortic arch is interrupted proximal to the left common carotid artery, the result is a right aortic arch with an aberrant left brachiocephalic artery (type 4)

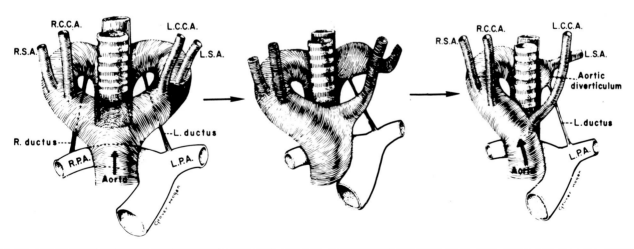

FIG. 25. Hypothesized embryonic development of a right aortic arch with an aberrant left subclavian artery. RSA, right subclavian artery; RCCA, right common carotid artery; LCCA, left common carotid artery; LSA, left subclavian artery; LPA, left pulmonary artery; RPA, right pulmonary artery. (From: Shuford WH and Sybers RG. *The Aortic Arch and Its Malformations,* 1974. Courtesy of Charles C Thomas, Springfield, Illinois.)

A

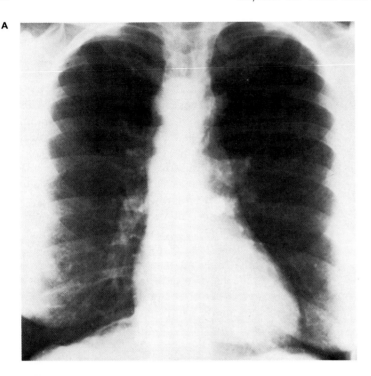

FIG. 26. Right aortic arch, aberrant left subclavian. **A:** Posteroanterior radiograph. **B–E:** Sequential sections—from below, then upward—starting at the level of the right-sided aortic arch. The trachea and esophagus are deformed and displaced anteriorly (B, C). There is aneurysmal dilatation of the posterior portion of the aortic arch (C). The left subclavian artery arises from this diverticulum and passes behind the esophagus coursing to the left (*arrow* in D). The left subclavian artery assumes a normal position at the apex of the mediastinum (*arrow* in E).

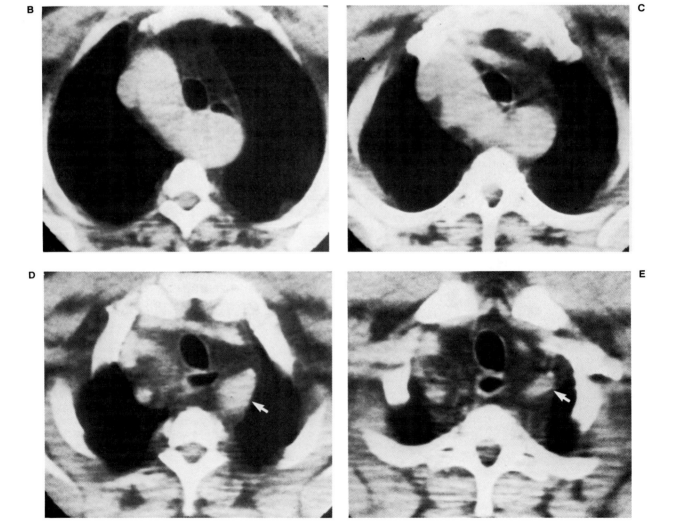

B   C

D   E

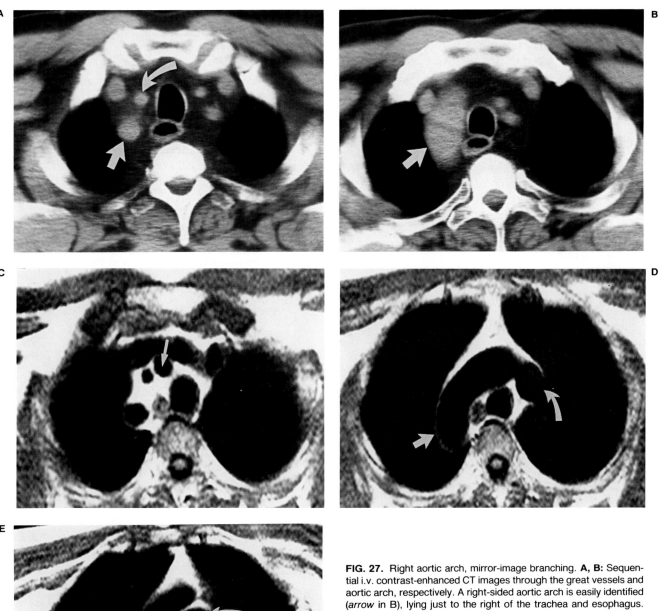

FIG. 27. Right aortic arch, mirror-image branching. **A, B:** Sequential i.v. contrast-enhanced CT images through the great vessels and aortic arch, respectively. A right-sided aortic arch is easily identified (*arrow* in B), lying just to the right of the trachea and esophagus. Mirror-image branching of the great vessels is present; a right brachiocephalic artery (not shown) has given rise to an otherwise normally positioned right subclavian artery (*arrow* in A) and a right common carotid artery (*curved arrow* in A). **C, D, E:** Sequential MR images through the great vessels, the aortic arch, and the aortico-pulmonary window, respectively, in a different patient than shown in A and B. Again note the presence of a right-sided aortic arch (*arrow* in D) with mirror-image branching, identifiable by the presence of a left brachiocephalic artery (*arrow* in C). Note that in this case there is complete situs, with a left-sided superior vena cava (*curved arrows* in D and E) as well as a reversal of normal lung segmentation, identifiable by the presence of an anatomic right upper lobe bronchus on the left (*arrow* in E).

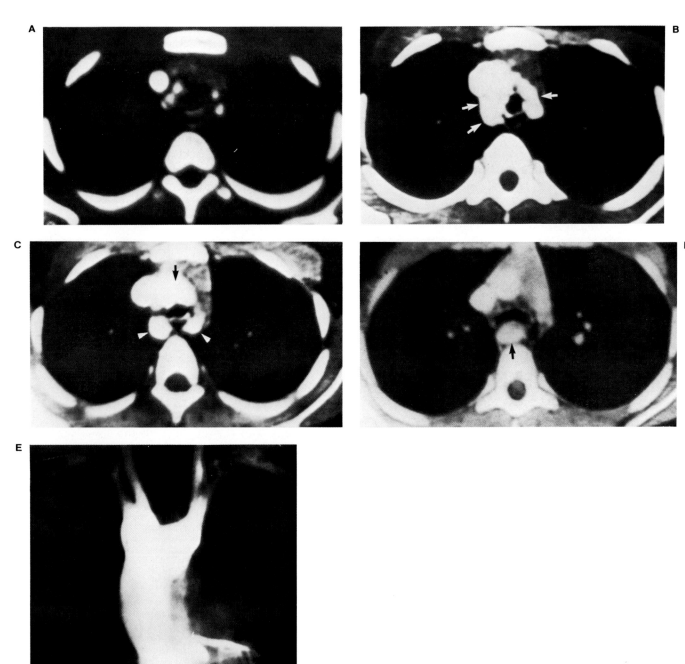

FIG. 28. Double aortic arch. **A–D:** Sequential images—from above, then downward—in a patient with a functional double aortic arch. In A, all four arteries can be identified at a level more caudal than normal, an important clue to the presence of an arch anomaly. B is a section through both arches; the right arch (*two arrows*) is larger than the left arch (*single arrow*). C is a section through the ascending aorta (*arrow*) and the posterior portions of both the right and left arches, which lie behind the trachea and esophagus in close proximity (*arrowheads*). Below this level, the descending portions of both arches fuse to form one descending aorta (*arrow* in D). **E** is the corresponding angiogram. (Case courtesy of Ina L. D. Tonkin, M.D., University of Tennessee Center for the Health Sciences. Images obtained by Bennett A. Alford, M.D., University of Virginia Hospital.)

(42). Its appearance is similar to that of a right arch with an aberrant left subclavian artery, except that both the left subclavian and left common carotid arteries are "replaced" to the posterior portion of the right arch, and derive from a common trunk.

Finally, the left arch may be interrupted in more than one place. Most typically, interruption occurs both proximal and distal to the left subclavian artery. The result is "isolation of the left subclavian artery" (type 5) (41). The left common carotid artery arises as the first branch of the right-sided aorta. The left subclavian attaches by a persistent ductus arteriosus to the left pulmonary artery. Although this anomaly is the third most frequent right aortic arch anomaly, it is still rare.

Double Aortic Arch Anomalies

Double aortic arches have been classified into two types, depending on the patency of the arches (43). The most frequent form is a "functional" double aortic arch (type 1). In this case, both arches remain patent; the right common carotid and subclavian arteries arise from the right arch, while the left common carotid and left subclavian arteries arise from the left arch. Both arches join posteriorly to form one descending aorta, which may be midline or, more usually, left-sided. The two arches may be of equal size, although the right arch is generally larger (Fig. 28; see also Fig. 21, Chapter 11).

More rarely, a double arch is present, with atresia of some portion of the left arch (type 3) (43). As may be anticipated, there is considerable similarity in appearance between a double aortic arch with atresia of some portion of the left arch and the right aortic arch anomalies. Theoretically the major difference is that with double aortic arches, some portion of the left arch persists

despite atresia, and a vascular ring around the trachea and esophagus is present. With right aortic arch anomalies there is true interruption of the left aortic arch, and a true vascular ring is only rarely formed. Practically the two may be impossible to differentiate even angiographically, although, as suggested by Garti et al. (44), a double aortic arch with atresia may be differentiated from a right aortic arch by noting that (a) double aortic arches cause both a right- and left-sided impression on the esophagram, and (b) with double aortic arches, the left common carotid and left subclavian arteries have independent origins. With right aortic arch anomalies, excepting those with an aberrant subclavian artery, there is always a left innominate artery.

Venous Anomalies

In addition to congenital (and acquired) abnormalities of the azygos-hemiazygos venous system, the most common, clinically significant venous anomaly is persistence of the left superior vena cava (45). The left superior vena cava forms from a confluence of the left subclavian and left jugular veins and courses inferiorly in a position analogous to the normal superior vena cava on the right side (Fig. 27, Fig. 30). Inferiorly, the left superior vena cava lies anterior to the left hilum and always drains into a markedly dilated coronary sinus. The anatomic course of the left superior vena cava reflects embryologic retention of the left anterior and common cardinal veins and the left horn of the sinus venosus, structures that ordinarily regress (Fig. 29). A right superior vena cava may or may not be present (Fig. 30; see also Fig. 20, Chapter 11).

The clinical significance of this anomaly is minimal unless there is an associated atrial septal defect, with a resultant left-to-right shunt.

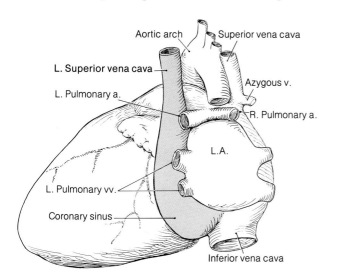

FIG. 29. Schematic drawing of a persistent left-sided superior vena cava, posterior view. The left-sided cava passes in front of the left hilum to drain inferiorly into an enlarged coronary sinus. LA, left atrium.

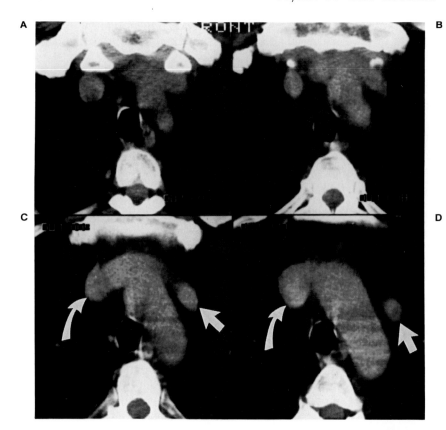

FIG. 30. Left-sided superior vena cava. **A–D:** Enlargements of sequential CT images from the great vessels superiorly to the aortic arch inferiorly, respectively. In addition to a left-sided vena cava (*arrows* in C and D), there is persistence of a right-sided vena cava as well (*curved arrows* in C and D).

CT/MR Correlations: Vascular Anomalies

Numerous reports have documented the value of CT in identifying anomalies of the aortic arch and great vessels (12,46,47). In addition to the abnormalities described above, other aortic anomalies, including coarctation, pseudocoarctation, cervical aortic arches, L and D transpositions, and truncus arteriosus have all been described in the CT literature (see Fig. 28, Chapter 5) (6,48–52). The most common anomalies, such as aberrant right and left subclavian arteries, are easily identified and should not be misinterpreted on routine scans as evidence of pathology. Despite the accuracy of CT in diagnosing these common abnormalities, however, CT has proven of somewhat less value in analyzing more complex abnormalities, especially those encountered in childhood or those associated with complex cardiac malformations. In our experience, a general paucity of mediastinal fat in children coupled with difficulties in the administration of an adequate bolus of intravenous contrast media have limited the effectiveness of CT.

MR has significant advantages for assessing cardiovascular pathology. These include, in particular, nondependence on intravenous contrast to visualize vascular structures, multi-planar imaging capabilities, and the lack of ionizing radiation. Numerous investigators have documented the applicability of MR to the diagnosis of anomalies of both the aortic arch and great vessels, including the pulmonary arteries (Figs. 31 and 32)

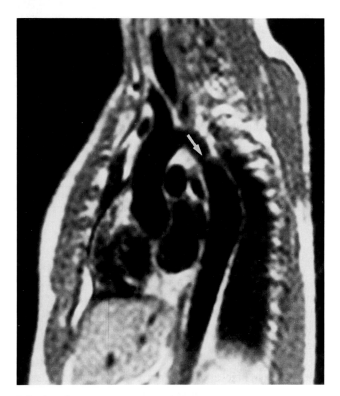

FIG. 31. Coarctation, postsurgical evaluation. Parasagittal MR image through the aorta shows characteristic appearance of narrowing of the aortic lumen just distal to the origin of the subclavian artery (*arrow*). Note that there is moderate poststenotic dilatation as well. In this population, MR has proven especially efficacious in assessing postoperative complications, including re-stenoses, postoperative aneurysms, and perianastomotic hematomas.

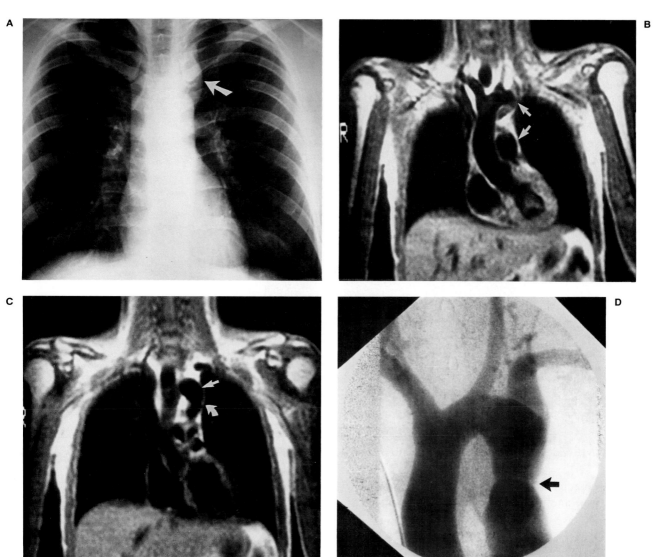

FIG. 32. Pseudocoarctation. **A:** Posteroanterior radiograph shows unusual configuration of the superior mediastinum on the left side (*arrow*). Differentiation between an aneurysm and a mediastinal mass is difficult. **B, C:** Sequential coronal MR images through the root of the aorta and posterior portion of the aortic arch, respectively. The ascending aorta is elongated as indicated by the considerable distance between the arch superiorly and the main pulmonary artery inferiorly (*arrows* in B). There is aneurysmal dilatation of the aorta (*arrow* in C), below which there is abrupt narrowing of the lumen, suggesting possible coarctation (*curved arrow* in C). **D:** Coned-down view from a subtraction aortogram shows characteristic kink in the course of the aorta (*arrow*), without actual narrowing. No pressure gradients could be measured across this region. (Case courtesy of Patricia Redmond, M.D., Staten Island, NY.)

(53–58). These findings have proven especially significant in older children and young adults, patients in whom two-dimensional echocardiography is more difficult to perform. Fletcher and Jacobstein in a study of 19 patients suspected of having either anomalies of the aorta or pulmonary arteries, found that in 11 patients, MR demonstrated lesions that echocardiography either failed to visualize or were interpreted as inconclusive, including three cases of coarctation and one case of a hypoplastic aortic arch (53). Similar findings have been reported by Gomes et al. (54). In their study of 34 patients with known or suspected congenital anomalies of the aortic arch evaluated with both MR and two-dimensional echocardiography, MR enabled diagnosis in

15 of 18 (83%) patients studied prospectively, as compared with only 13 of 20 (65%) patients evaluated prospectively with echocardiography.

MR has proven especially efficacious in the evaluation of coarctation of the aorta, both pre- and postrepair (Fig. 31) (59–64). In this setting, the ability to acquire parasagittal images through the aorta represents a clear advantage of MR as compared with CT. Preoperatively, MR has been shown to be comparable to angiography and more accurate than two-dimensional echocardiography both for accurate display of aortic anatomy, and delineation of enlarged collateral vessels (62). MR has proven especially valuable in assessing the results of both surgical and nonsurgical therapy. Postsurgical

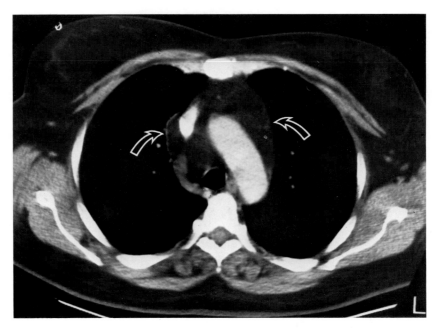

FIG. 33. Mediastinal lipomatosis. Contrast-enhanced CT image at the level of the aortic arch shows abundant fat throughout the mediastinum causing distortion of the normal pleuromediastinal interfaces (*arrows*). Note that the fat is similar in density to subcutaneous fat, and is exceedingly homogeneous. This patient had no history of either steroid therapy or Cushing's syndrome.

complications include re-stenosis (re-coarctation), postoperative aneurysms (especially following placement of a Dacron patch), perianastomotic hematomas, and hypertension, which frequently occurs in the absence of demonstrable pressure gradients. MR has been shown to provide good visualization of postoperative changes, including accurate assessment of the degree of re-stenosis (60). Although pressure gradients per se cannot be directly measured with MR, assessment of the degree of stenosis may still be valuable. As shown by Rees et al. in a study of 36 patients evaluated postoperatively in which MR was compared with the results of echocardiography including Doppler ultrasound and catheterization, a reduction of lumen diameter correlated well with the measured gradient. The authors concluded that re-stenosis at the site of repair can be suspected when there is a 50% stenosis (64).

Of even greater interest is the potential of MR to predict the response of patients who might be candidates for balloon angioplasty (62,63). In these cases, balloon angioplasty works best when the stenosis is short and is located just distal to the left subclavian artery. When the stenosis involves the proximal arch or is long, balloon angioplasty proves less successful. As documented by Bank et al. in their study of 12 children with suspected coarctations evaluated both pre- and postsurgical repair, MR proved accurate in identifying those patients who were unlikely to benefit from balloon angioplasty. Additionally, MR proved valuable by determining the appropriate balloon size for angioplasty (62).

FATTY LESIONS

Fat is specifically recognized by its low CT numbers, which vary from -70 to -130 Hounsfield units (HU). Fat is normally present in the mediastinum and its amount may increase with age. Normal fat is unencapsulated and equally distributed throughout the connective tissue matrix of the mediastinum. Most of the fat in the anterior mediastinum is contained within the fibrous skeleton of the involved thymus. The contours of the mediastinum are not affected by normal amounts of fat.

Abnormalities of fat distribution can be diffuse, as in lipomatosis, or focal, as in lipomas or fat-containing transdiaphragmatic hernias.

Mediastinal Lipomatosis

Lipomatosis is a benign condition in which overabundant amounts of histologically normal, unencapsulated fat accumulate in the mediastinum. The excess deposition is most prominent in the upper mediastinum, with resulting smooth mediastinal widening on chest radiographs and convex-bulging pleuromediastinal interfaces of CT images (Fig. 33). Tracheal compression or displacement is uniformly absent (65–67). Less commonly, fat will also accumulate in the cardiophrenic angles and paraspinal areas (Figs. 34 and 35)

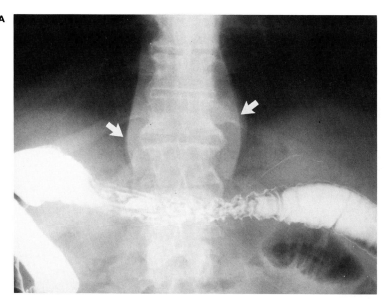
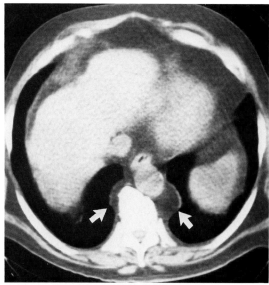

FIG. 34. Mediastinal lipomatosis. **A:** Coned-down anteroposterior radiograph of the lower thoracic spine in a patient undergoing a barium enema. The paraspinal interfaces are abnormally convex bilaterally (*arrows*), the appearance of which is nonspecific. **B:** CT section at the level of the distal esophagus unequivocally confirms that the abnormality seen in A is due to excessive fat in the posterior mediastinum (*arrows*). Note again the homogeneous nature of the fat, confirming this as lipomatosis.

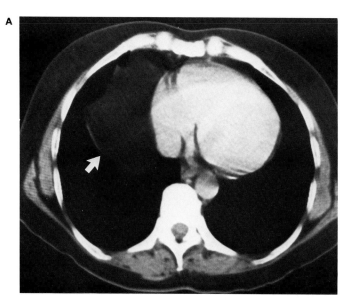
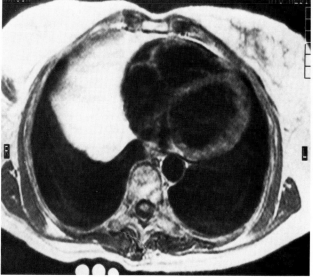

FIG. 35. Cardiophrenic lipomatosis. **A:** Contrast-enhanced CT image through the heart demonstrates a large accumulation of fat adjacent to the right heart border (*arrow*). Note the similarity in appearance between paracardiac and subcutaneous fat. **B:** T1-weighted MR image at the same level as shown in A. On T1-weighted sequences fat appears bright (compare with the signal intensity of adjacent subcutaneous fat).

(68–70). The fat in lipomatosis should appear homogeneously lucent. If inhomogeneity is noted, superimposed processes such as mediastinitis, hemorrhage, tumor infiltration, postradiation fibrosis, and postsurgical changes should be considered. Lipomatosis may be associated with Cushing's syndrome, but these factors are absent in up to one-half of cases (71). The diagnosis, therefore, should not be excluded in the absence of predisposing factors. CT is the definitive diagnostic modal-

ity for lipomatosis, which is now diagnosed with surprising frequency.

Rarely, multiple symmetrical lipomatosis may mimic the appearance on CT of simple lipomatosis; however, this entity often produces compression of surrounding structures, the trachea in particular, and does not involve the anterior mediastinum, cardiophrenic angles, or paraspinal regions. In addition, periscapular lipomatous masses are almost always present (72).

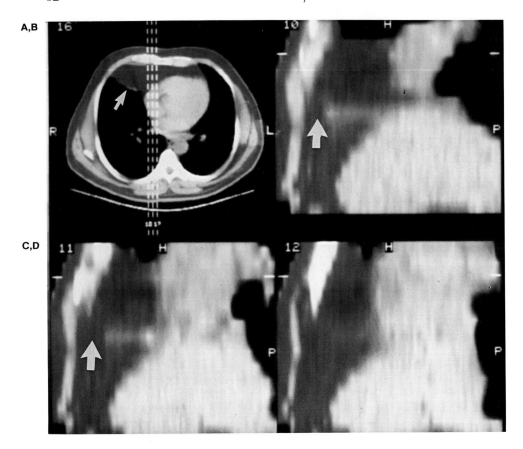

FIG. 36. Morgagni's hernia. A: CT section at the level of the cardiophrenic angle. This study was performed to further evaluate a patient with a prominent paracardiac density of uncertain etiology (not shown). Excessive homogeneous paracardiac fat is present (*arrow*), accounting for the radiographic abnormality. B–D: Sequential sagittal reconstructions at the levels indicated by the *dotted lines* in A. Note that the paracardiac fat in this case is continuous with fat below the diaphragm which appears discontinuous (*arrows* in B and C). Surgically confirmed Morgagni's hernia. (Case courtesy of Deborah Reede, M.D., Long Island College Hospital, New York, NY.)

Fatty Masses

In the large majority of cases, discovery of the fatty nature of a mass indicates benignancy. In our experience, most fatty masses are seen in the peridiaphragmatic areas and they most often represent herniation of abdominal fat (Figs. 36 and 37). Although true lipomatous tumors are much less common, as will be discussed, fat is commonly identifiable as a component of mediastinal germ cell tumors.

Fatty Herniations

There are several direct connections between the abdomen and mediastinum that permit passage of intraabdominal fat into the thorax.

Omental fat can herniate through the foramen of Morgagni to create the appearance of a cardiophrenic angle mass, almost always located on the right side (Fig. 36) (73,74). The omentum is freely mobile and does not always carry the transverse colon with it into the hernia. Fine linear densities can sometimes be seen within herniated omental fat and probably represent omental vessels. When seen within a fatty mass, these linear densities should suggest fat herniation rather than a lipoma.

Fat herniation through the foramen of Bochdalek occurs most often on the left side since the liver limits the frequency of its occurrence on the right (75,76).

Herniation of perigastric fat through the phrenicoesophageal membrane surrounding and fixating the esophagus to the diaphragm is the first step in the pathogenesis of hiatus hernias (77). The herniated fat can extend along the aorta and widen the paraspinal line or it can appear as a retrocardiac mass (Fig. 38). Although multi-planar reconstructions are sometimes helpful for demonstrating the connections of the fatty hernia with abdominal fat (Figs. 36 and 37), due to its multi-planar imaging capabilities, MR may be better suited to the evaluation of such lesions (78).

FIG. 38. Lipoblastoma. An 8-month-old boy with large mass discovered on chest radiograph. A, B: CT scans show a large mass with low CT numbers compatible with a fatty tumor. The suggestion of chest wall invasion anteriorly in B, the patient's age, and the minimal inhomogeneity would be unusual for a simple lipoma. Surgery was therefore recommended. A lipoblastoma, a rare benign tumor of childhood made of immature adipose tissue with rapid growth and local recurrence potential, was removed.

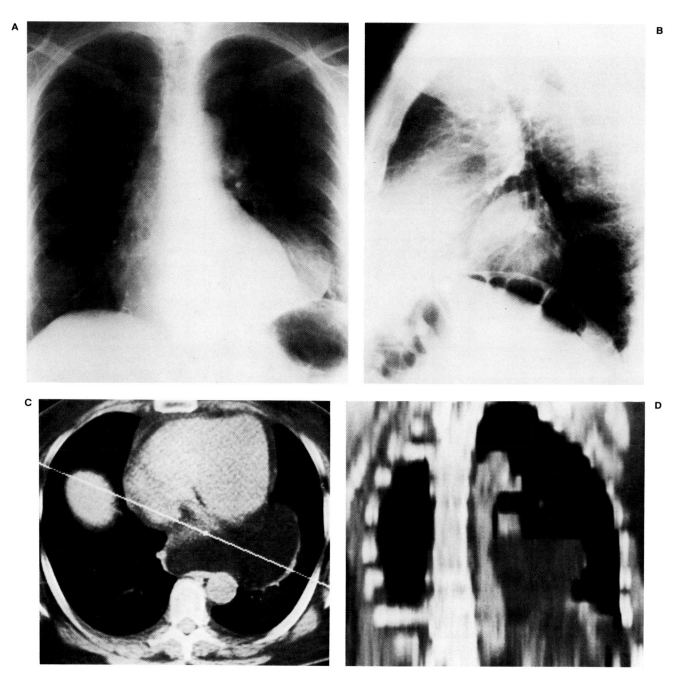

FIG. 37. Large paraesophageal omental hernia. A 39-year-old woman with dysphagia. **A, B:** PA and lateral radiographs. **C:** CT scan at level of mass. **D:** Oblique reconstruction through axis of line seen in C. A large, smooth retrocardiac mass is identified. The axial CT image shows an entirely fatty mass. Note again the faint linear densities within the mass, most probably representing omental vessels. A planar reconstruction shows the true intra-abdominal origin of the mass, found at surgery to represent omental fat extending into the mediastinum via a large esophageal hiatus. Peridiaphragmatic fatty masses are much more likely to represent hernias containing fat than lipomas.

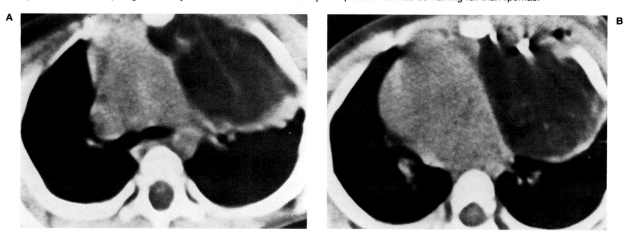

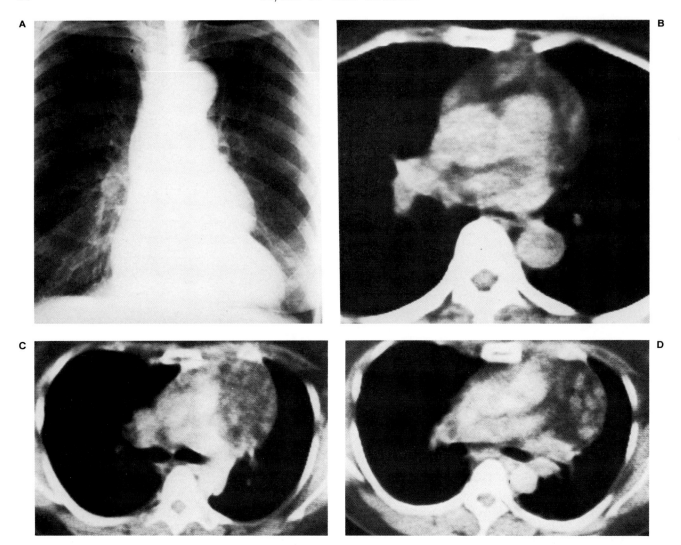

FIG. 39. Thymolipomas. **A, B:** A 71-year-old asymptomatic woman. PA chest radiograph (A). A smooth mass deforms the contour of the left heart border. CT at level of mass (B). The mass is mostly fatty, but areas of soft-tissue density are identified within it. It is therefore unlikely to represent a simple lipoma. However, its sharp borders, the lack of compression of the nearby vessels, and its location point to benign lesion. Thymolipoma is a benign fatty tumor of the thymus that is usually of no clinical consequence. No surgery was performed. **C, D:** Another example of thymolipoma in a 51-year-old woman. Note again the inhomogeneous appearance of the mass (C). Note in D the round areas of increased density that were found to represent lymph nodes on pathologic examination. No thymic tissue was identified.

Lipomas

Mediastinal lipomas are uncommon, constituting approximately 2% of all mediastinal tumors (79,80). They are soft and do not produce compressive symptoms unless they are large enough to compress surrounding structures. They may or may not be encapsulated. Although they contain variable amounts of fibrous septa, they appear to have homogeneously low CT numbers. Their boundaries are smooth and sharply defined, with no blurring, thickening, or invasion of surrounding structures. If inhomogeneity or invasion of the surrounding structures are seen, a benign lipoma cannot be confidently diagnosed. A superimposed process should be suspected, with consideration given to the rare possibility of a liposarcoma or lipoblastoma (81–83) (Fig. 38). Histologic differentiation between benign lipomas and well-differentiated liposarcomas depends on the pres-

ence of mitotic activity, fibrosis, neovascularization, atypia, and tumor infiltration, morphologic findings occasionally suggested on CT examination (84). As documented by DeSantos et al., however, the diagnosis of a liposarcoma is generally problematic with CT. In their series of 17 cases of documented liposarcomas, a preoperative diagnosis was made in only four cases (22%) (85).

Other rare, fatty lesions in the mediastinum have been reported; their diagnosis usually depends on a heightened sense of awareness. Inhomogeneous fatty masses of the anterior mediastinum, for example, raise the possibility of a thymolipoma (86) (Fig. 39). In the posterior mediastinum, spinal lipomas rarely may present as primary mediastinal masses (87). Other fat-containing masses that have been identified by CT in the posterior mediastinum include angiolipomas (88,89) and even fatty transformation of thoracic extramedullary hematopoiesis following splenectomy (90).

Germ Cell Tumors

Primary germ cell tumors arise from primitive germ cells that have arrested their embryological migration in the mediastinum, frequently within the thymus gland itself. Most cases occur during the second to fourth decades of life. They comprise dermoid cysts, benign and malignant teratomas, seminomas, embryonal carcinomas, endodermal sinus tumors, and choriocarcinomas. Fewer than 20% are malignant. Dermoid cysts and benign teratomas form the great majority of these lesions, and malignant teratoma is by far the most common of the malignant germ cell tumors. There is a strong preponderance of males in the group with malignancies, whereas benign lesions show equal sex distribution.

Dermoid cysts, which are said to contain elements of the ectodermal layer of germ cells only, and benign teratomas, said to contain elements of all germinal layers, have overlapping manifestations on CT (Figs. 40–42) (91–95). Commonly found in the anterior mediastinum, in nearly 5% of cases these tumors arise within the posterior mediastinum (96,97). They are well-demarcated and their benign character is suggested by this feature. Encapsulation, sometimes with an enhancing rim, is the

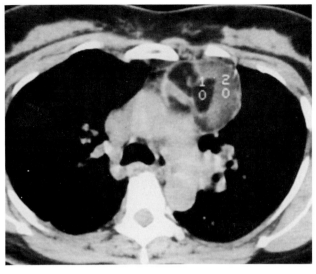

FIG. 40. Dermoid tumor. CT section through the carina shows a well-encapsulated mass anterior to the left pulmonary artery, within which fat elements are clearly discernible. This was confirmed by measurements obtained within the region of interest demarcated by *cursor number 1*. The remainder of the lesion was composed of soft-tissue elements.

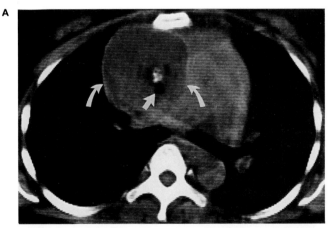

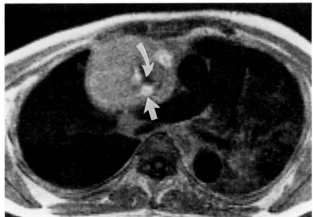

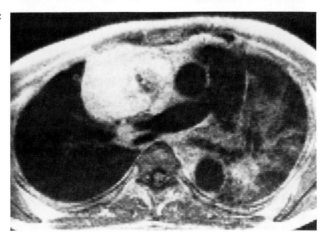

FIG. 41. Dermoid tumor. **A:** Non–contrast-enhanced CT section just below the carina shows a well-encapsulated mass anterior to the right main pulmonary artery (*curved arrows*). The mass is strikingly heterogeneous with fluid, fat (*arrow*), and calcific elements clearly discernible. **B, C:** T1- and T2-weighted MR images obtained at the same level as shown in A, respectively. On the T1-weighted image, regions of high-signal intensity correspond precisely to the fatty elements seen in A (*arrow* in B), while regions corresponding to calcium demonstrate signal void (*curved arrow* in B). Intermediate signal is present within the remainder of the mass, in this case presumably secondary to complex fluid within the tumor. Note that there is considerable signal enhancement within these regions on the T2-weighted image, consistent with the presence of fluid within the tumor. (Case courtesy of Jeffrey Weinreb, M.D., New York, NY.)

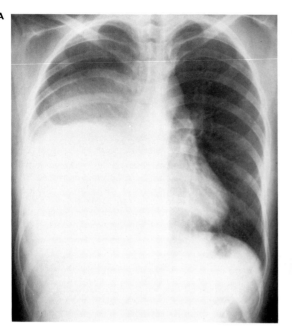
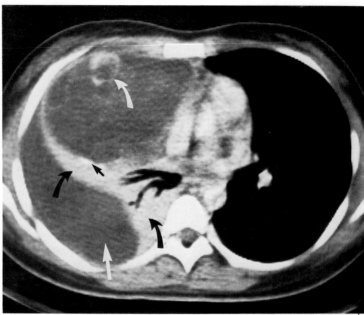

FIG. 42. Dermoid tumor. **A:** Posteroanterior radiograph shows extensive opacification of the mid- and lower right hemithorax in a teenage girl whose chief complaint was moderate dyspnea. The chest radiograph is nonspecific. **B:** Contrast-enhanced CT section through the midthorax shows a complex, cystic mass within which discrete septations can be recognized (*curved white arrow*), causing compression and posterior displacement of the adjacent lung (*curved black arrows*) as well as mediastinal shift to the left. Faint curvilinar calcifications can be identified posteriorly (*straight black arrow*). Although a pleural etiology was initially considered, the finding of multiple septations within this mass occurring in a young girl suggested the proper diagnosis. At surgery, the mass was found to extend posterior to the lung as well, accounting for the area of fluid density seen posteriorly (*straight white arrow*), otherwise mimicking the appearance of loculated pleural fluid.

rule. Calcifications are seen in one-third to one-half of cases (Figs. 41 and 42). The mixture of CT densities within the mass is varied; when fat is present the proper diagnosis can be strongly suggested, but only half demonstrate fat. The finding of a fat-fluid level within the mass is especially diagnostic (98,99). Rarely, a fat-fluid level may be identifiable within a pleural effusion secondary to presumed rupture of the primary tumor (100). The fluids within the cystic parts of the tumors also vary in their CT density and may reach soft-tissue density (Fig. 41).

Typically, teratomas contain a variable admixture of tissues that exhibit CT numbers in the range of fat, soft tissue, and calcium. This pleomorphic appearance is an important clue to the etiology of the lesion and makes possible its differentiation from thymoma and lymphoma. Malignant teratoma seems to be distinguishable from its benign counterpart in most cases. Its borders are poorly defined, and tumor molds and compresses surrounding structures (Fig. 43).

Although the other germ cell tumors are much less common, their CT appearance has been well described (101–104). Typically, primary mediastinal seminomas present as large, bulky, homogeneous soft tissue masses (Fig. 44), while nonseminomatous tumors have heterogeneous density, including ill-defined areas of low density secondary to necrosis and hemorrhage (Fig. 45). Confirmation that these lesions are indeed primary requires that there be no evidence of testicular or retro-

peritoneal tumor. Although frequently suggestive, the primary role of CT in evaluating patients with primary mediastinal germ cell tumors is defining disease extent, and especially monitoring response to therapy.

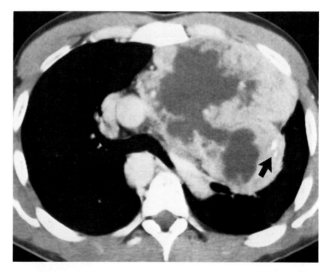

FIG. 43. Teratocarcinoma. Contrast-enhanced CT scan through the carina shows a large, poorly demarcated tumor within the anterior mediastinum causing compression and displacement of adjacent mediastinal structures. The tumor is markedly heterogeneous with areas of low density, presumably due to extensive tissue necrosis, as well as some punctate areas of calcification (*arrow*). These findings suggest a malignant etiology (cf. Figs. 40–42).

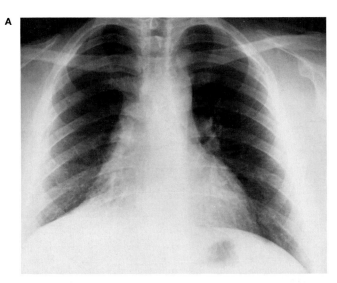

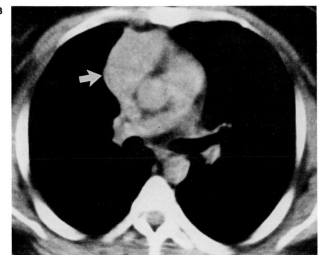

FIG. 44. Seminoma. A: Posteroanterior chest radiograph in a 35-year-old man shows poor definition of the right heart border and elevation of the right hemidiaphragm, findings initially thought to be secondary to middle lobe volume loss. B, C: Contrast-enhanced CT sections through the mid- and lower thorax, respectively, show a homogeneous soft-tissue mass to be present in the anterior mediastinum (arrows in B and C), marginating the right heart border. This appearance is entirely nonspecific. At surgery, this proved to be a seminoma.

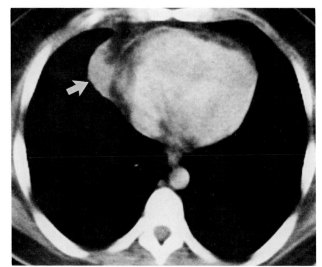

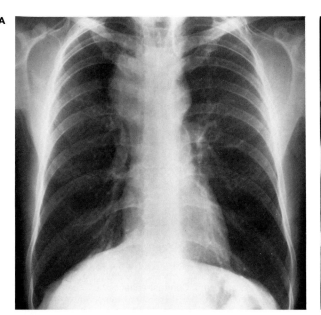

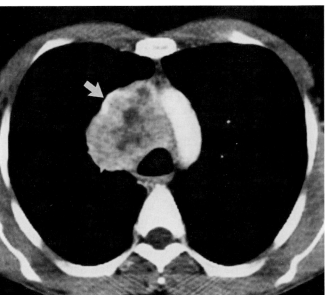

FIG. 45. Nonseminomatous germ cell tumor. A: Posteroanterior chest radiograph shows a mediastinal mass deforming the right pleuromediastinal interface. B: Contrast-enhanced CT section at the level of the aortic arch shows an irregular, heterogeneous tumor mass that is partially obstructing the superior vena cava (arrow). Although most germ cell tumors arise in the prevascular or anterior mediastinal compartment, these tumors may originate anywhere within the thorax. Surgery confirmed a nonseminomatous malignant germ cell tumor.

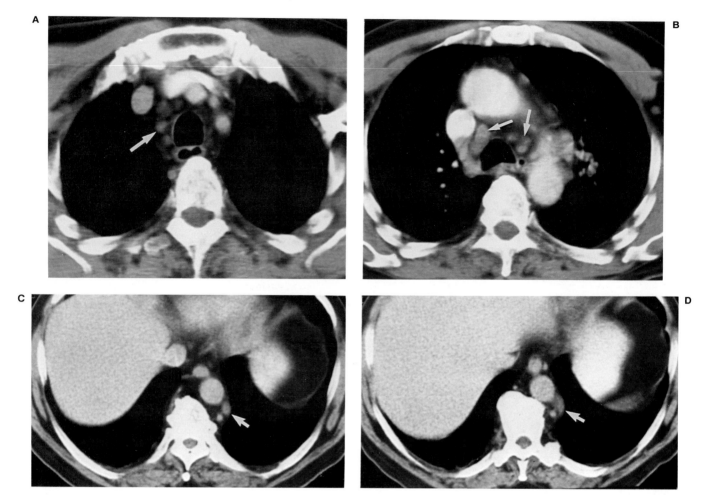

FIG. 46. Mediastinal lymphadenopathy, Hodgkin's disease. **A–D:** Contrast-enhanced CT sections at the level of the great vessels, the aortico-pulmonary window, and the lung bases, respectively. Mediastinal lymph nodes appear as round, oval, or triangular soft-tissue densities against the lower density background of mediastinal fat (*arrows* in A–D).

MR Evaluation of Fatty Lesions

The appearance of fatty tissue with MR has been well characterized (105,106). Typically, well-differentiated fat has a high signal intensity on both T1- and T2-weighted sequences, usually identical to subcutaneous fat (Figs. 35 and 41). Similar findings have been described, however, in patients with hematomas or tumors with hemorrhage. In an analysis of 17 patients with 18 lipomatous tumors, Dooms et al. reported that of 16 benign lesions, including 12 lipomas, the fatty components of the tumors were equally well visualized with both CT and MR (105). As reported by London et al. in an evaluation of 15 patients with documented liposarcomas, MR correctly identified the presence of fat in all eight cases in which it was pathologically present (106). Unfortunately, MR has proven no more accurate than CT in differentiating liposarcomas from benign lipomas. Although it might be anticipated that MR would

prove efficacious in diagnosing dermoid tumors and teratomas, especially those in which fat is demonstrable, experience with these tumors, in fact, is limited (107).

MEDIASTINAL LYMPH NODES

In autopsy series, the average number of mediastinal nodes is 64 (108). Almost 80% of the nodes are located immediately adjacent to the tracheobronchial tree and drain the lungs. Several systems of anatomic classification of the mediastinal nodes have been proposed, most recently by the American Thoracic Society (ATS) (109). This classification system attempts to define specific nodal stations in terms of well-recognized anatomic landmarks easily identifiable both before and during thoracotomy, specifically to facilitate both the staging and reporting of results in patients with non-small cell lung cancer. Despite limitations, its use in this setting should be encouraged (110) (see Chapter 6).

Numerous reports have addressed the issue of what constitutes the normal size, number, and appearance of mediastinal lymph nodes (10,111,112–117). As established both *in vivo* and by autopsy evaluation, the most useful definition of a normal-sized lymph node is 1.0 cm as measured in the short axis (114,115). Significant variations in node size exist, however, depending on their precise location. As shown by Glazer et al. in their evaluation of 56 patients without a known cause of mediastinal adenopathy, the largest normal-sized nodes are subcarinal (6.2 mm ± 2.2 SD) and lower right tracheobronchial (5.9 mm ± 2.1 SD) (corresponding to ATS nodal stations 4R and 10R, respectively), whereas upper paratracheal nodes (2R) are smaller than lower paratracheal nodes (4R), and right-sided nodes in general are smaller than those on the left side (113). Kiyono et al., in an evaluation of 40 adult cadavers, reported similar findings (114). In their series, mean short transverse nodal diameters ranged from 2.4 to 5.6 mm, with substantial variations noted depending on nodal station, subcarinal nodes again being largest. Based on these findings, these authors recommended using short axis measurements of 12 mm for subcarinal lymph nodes, 10 mm for right tracheobronchial and low paratracheal lymph nodes, and 8 mm for all other nodal groups.

With CT, nodes appear as round, oval, or triangular soft-tissue densities against the lower density background of mediastinal fat (Fig. 46). They are often found in clusters of two or three. The ability to see nodes is directly correlated to the amount of mediastinal fat. The manifestations on CT of nodal pathology are usually simple and nonspecific (128,129). Typically, four stages can be recognized in nodes involved by neoplastic as well as nonneoplastic diseases:

1. Normal nodes. The internal nodal architecture cannot be analyzed with CT. If no enlargement is present, pathology cannot be suspected or excluded with certainty.
2. Enlargement. With further progression of the disease, the nodes enlarge. Enlargement is recognized either by direct measurement of the cross-section of the affected nodes or by identifying bulging mediastinal contours, for example, replacing the normally concave azygoesophageal recess. Additionally, the node margins may lose their sharp definition and the surrounding fat may increase in density. These changes may be due to extension of the primary process through the nodal capsule or to an associated fibrotic or inflammatory reaction.
3. Coalescence. With further progression, the pathologic process may "burst" through the capsule of several adjacent nodes and fuse to form a single larger mass.
4. Diffuse spread. The connective tissue and fat may be diffusely invaded, with no recognizable nodes or focal mass.

TABLE 1. *Mediastinal adenopathy: CT evaluation*

A. Calcified lymph nodes
   Common:
      Infectious granulomatous diseases
         Tuberculosis
         Fungal infections (histoplasmosis)
      Sarcoidosis
      Silicosis
      Hodgkin's disease (following RT)
   Rare:
      Pneumocystis carinii pneumonia
      Metastases (mucinous adenocarcinoma of GI tract)
      Amyloidosis
      Scleroderma
      Castleman's disease
B. Low-density/necrotic lymph nodes
   Common:
      Infections
         Tuberculosis/fungal
      Metastases
         Lung cancer/seminoma
      Lymphoma
   Rare:
      Whipple's disease
C. Vascular lymph nodes
   Common:
      Metastases
         Renal cell cancer/lung cancer/thyroid/carcinoid
      Castleman's disease
   Rare:
      Sarcoidosis
      Angioimmunoblastic lymphadenopathy

RT, radiation therapy.

It should be emphasized that interpretation of contiguous CT scans is always necessary to differentiate nodes from vessels. Numerous pitfalls in the diagnosis of adenopathy have been described, including mistaking both normal and anomalous vascular structures such as aberrant right subclavian arteries and high-riding left pulmonary arteries as enlarged nodes (116,117), as well as prominent pericardial recesses, especially the superior recess of the pericardium (118). In difficult cases, use of a bolus of intravenous contrast material usually proves diagnostic.

The unique contributions of CT to the analysis of mediastinal nodes are twofold: (a) CT provides precise localization and delineation of the morphology of nodes, including identification of the secondary consequences of enlarged nodes on adjacent mediastinal organs such as the vena cava, pulmonary arteries, the airways, and the esophagus. (b) CT allows characterization of nodes based on their density, both pre- and post-intravenous contrast enhancement, as either homogeneous, necrotic low-density, calcified, or vascular. In combination, these findings frequently narrow the range of differential diagnoses; they also allow determination of the best approach, when necessary, to establish a histologic diagnosis (Table 1).

A,B

C,D

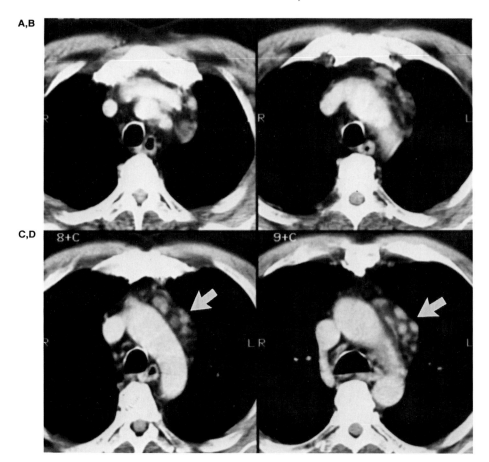

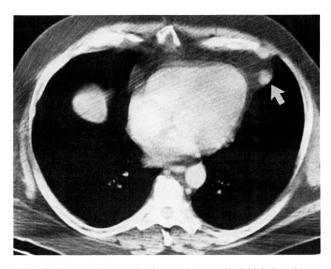

FIG. 47. Mediastinal lymphadenopathy, Hodgkin's disease. **A–D:** Contrast-enhanced CT sections at the level of the great vessels, aortic arch, and aorticopulmonary window, respectively. Clusters of enlarged prevascular lymph nodes are easily identifiable (*arrows* in C and D), while few if any enlarged nodes can be identified in the pre- or paratracheal spaces. This pattern of lymph node enlargement would be uncharacteristic of most granulomatous diseases and should instead suggest possible malignancy. Following therapy, these nodes regressed.

Localization and Morphology

Interpretation of the significance of mediastinal lymphadenopathy is usually influenced by the precise location of enlarged nodes. The range of diagnostic possibilities will vary depending on whether nodes are predominantly middle mediastinal (including pretracheal, subcarinal, and aorticopulmonary window nodes), and/or hilar, prevascular, paracardiac, or posterior mediastinal (Fig. 47). CT is clearly more accurate than plain radiography in establishing the presence of enlarged mediastinal nodes (119,120). The ability to define and precisely localize enlarged lymph nodes within the mediastinum has diagnostic significance. Of patients with sarcoidosis, for example, 80 to 90% develop lymphadenopathy at some time in the course of their disease. Typically, however, enlarged nodes are found in the hila bilaterally, often associated with either right paratracheal nodes or nodes in the aorticopulmonary window. Isolated enlarged nodes, or mediastinal adenopathy in the absence of hilar adenopathy, especially when localized either in the anterior or posterior mediastinum, is distinctly unusual (121–123).

Similarly, the finding of enlarged paracardiac nodes has diagnostic significance, as these generally prove malignant (Fig. 48). As shown by Vock and Hodler in their

study of 21 cases of cardiophrenic angle adenopathy, all proved to be due to malignancy, including 12 patients with malignant lymphomas, seven with metastatic carcinomas, and two with metastatic malignant mesotheli-

FIG. 48. Paracardiac lymphadenopathy, non-Hodgkin's lymphoma. Contrast-enhanced CT section through the lung bases shows a single, isolated, left paracardiac node (*arrow*).

omas (124). Similar findings have been reported by Sussman et al., who found that of 45 patients with paracardiac adenopathy, only two were found to have benign lymphadenopathy; the remaining patients had either lymphomas (40%), carcinomas, or sarcomas (125).

As will be discussed in greater detail in Chapter 6, the ability to localize enlarged nodes is especially important in the preoperative assessment of patients with lung cancer. Node location is predictive of the likelihood of malignancy. More importantly, accurate localization is usually of critical importance in determining the most

efficacious method for definitive staging (bronchoscopy with transbronchial needle biopsy versus mediastinoscopy versus mediastinotomy) (Fig. 49). CT may also be valuable in assessing node morphology. CT may allow differentiation between intra- and extranodal disease in those cases where tumor transgresses the capsule (Fig. 49). CT also may provide invaluable information concerning the secondary effects of enlarged mediastinal nodes on adjacent structures (see Fig. 39, Chapter 5). This frequently obviates the need for more invasive diagnostic procedures as in the assessment of patients

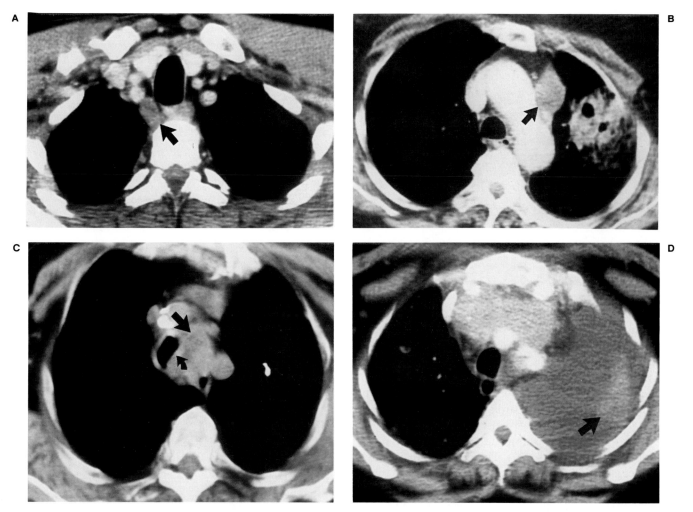

FIG. 49. Mediastinal adenopathy, lung cancer staging. **A:** Contrast-enhanced CT section through the superior mediastinum in a patient with known non-small cell lung cancer. An enlarged, 1.3 cm high right paratracheal lymph node can be identified just posterior to the right subclavian artery (*arrow*), corresponding to ATS nodal station 2R. Statistically, an enlarged node in this location is far more apt to be malignant than a similar sized lower paratracheal node. Surgery documented a metastatic lymphadenopathy. **B:** Contrast-enhanced CT section at the level of the aortic arch shows a markedly enlarged preaortic lymph node (*arrow*) in a patient with left upper lobe non-small cell carcinoma. Note that in this case there is an absence of pre- or paratracheal adenopathy (confirmed at other levels as well). This constellation of findings typifies the usual pattern of local lymph node metastases in patients with left upper lobe tumors. As clearly demonstrated by CT, in this case accurate staging is best accomplished by left parasternal mediastinotomy. **C:** Non–contrast-enhanced CT section at the level of the distal trachea in a patient with known non-small cell lung cancer associated with left vocal cord paralysis. An inhomogeneous soft-tissue mass is present (*arrow*) narrowing and displacing the trachea to the right (*curved arrow*). In this case CT not only provides the cause of the vocal cord paralysis, but additionally allows definitive noninvasive staging. **D:** Contrast-enhanced CT scan through the great vessels in a patient with an opacified left hemithorax. A large pleural fluid collection is present on the left, within which the tip of the collapsed left upper lobe can be visualized (*arrow*). Note that there is a poorly marginated soft-tissue mass extensively infiltrating throughout the mediastinum, resulting from extranodal spread of disease. This appearance in itself allows definitive CT staging, although in this case the presence of pleural fluid and contralateral metastases rendered this finding less significant.

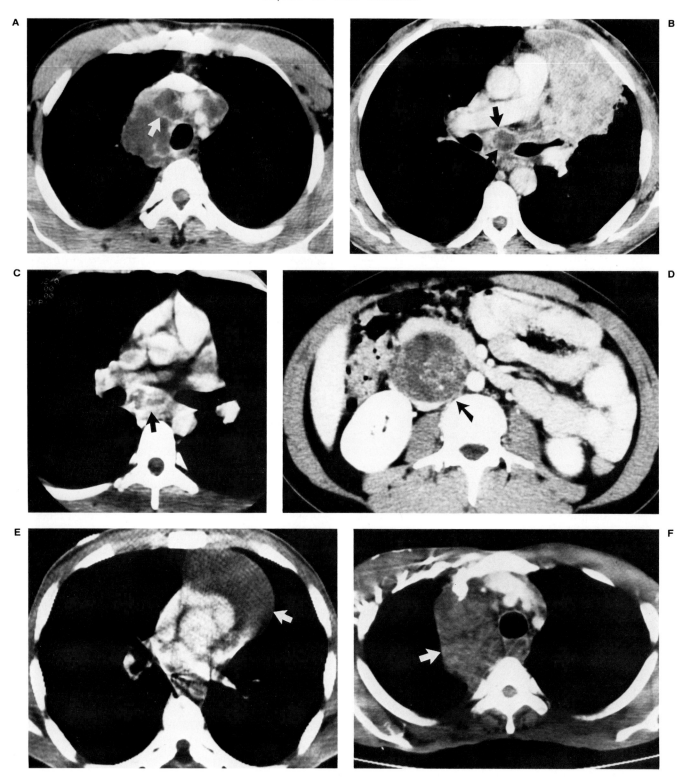

FIG. 50. Low-density masses/necrotic lymph nodes, CT assessment. **A:** Contrast-enhanced CT section through the great vessels. Massively enlarged low-density paratracheal and prevascular lymph nodes are present, many of which have a distinct vascular capsule (*arrow*). This appearance is especially suggestive of granulomatous infections such as tuberculous or cryptococcal infection, particularly in patients with AIDS. Tuberculous adenopathy in this case was established by mediastinoscopy. **B:** Contrast-enhanced CT section in a patient with malignant obstruction of the left upper lobe bronchus with associated left upper lobe atelectasis. An enlarged, low-density, necrotic subcarinal lymph node is present (*arrows*), surrounded by a vascular capsule. We have seen this type of necrotic lymph node in association with lung carcinomas of all histologic types. Transbronchial biopsy documented squamous cell carcinoma. **C, D:** Contrast-enhanced CT sections through the subcarinal space and the midabdomen, respectively, in a patient with known seminoma. Note the characteristic appearance of low-density, necrotic subcarinal (*arrow* in C) and retroperitoneal lymph nodes. A hypervascular rim can be identified around the subcarinal nodes. **E:** Contrast-enhanced CT scan through the heart shows a large, seemingly homogeneous low-density mass anteriorly (*arrow*) in a patient with documented non-Hodgkin's lymphoma. The appearance superficially resembles cystic lesions such as a pericardial or thymic cyst. **F:** Contrast-enhanced CT scan shows heterogeneous, low-density, right paratracheal mass. Biopsy proved lymphangioma.

presenting with signs of recurrent laryngeal nerve paralysis or airway compression, for example (Fig. 49) (126).

Density Discrimination

Of course, in a significant percentage of cases the location and morphology of mediastinal lymph nodes identified by CT prove nonspecific, necessitating evaluation of other associated features (127–129). In this regard, CT can also be used to define the density of lymph nodes, both pre- and post-injection of i.v. contrast media. This unique contribution of CT allows more precise characterization of the likely etiology of nodal enlargement (Table 1).

Although enlarged nodes typically have nonspecific soft-tissue density, nodes can frequently be classified as either low-density necrotic, calcified, or vascular, following administration of a bolus of intravenous contrast media. These CT findings can be shown to have histological counterparts.

Low-density Lymph Nodes

Low-density lymph nodes, with or without an enhancing rim following administration of intravenous contrast media, have been described as characteristic of a number of different pathologic entities (Fig. 50) (95). Typically, low-density nodes are due to necrosis. They are commonly seen in patients with tuberculous or fungal infections (130,131). In our experience, this has been particularly true in patients with acquired immune deficiency syndrome (AIDS). Low-density lymph nodes also occur as the result of metastatic seminoma, including patients evaluated both pre- and posttherapy. In these cases, low density usually results from extensive tissue necrosis, although low density may also correlate with the presence of numerous small epithelial-lined cystic spaces (Fig. 50) (132,133). Metastatic low-density nodes occur in patients with primary lung cancer, as well as ovarian, thyroid, and gastric neoplasia. Low-density nodes have also been described in patients with a variety of other entities, including lymphoma, both pre- and posttreatment, and even Whipple's disease (134,135).

The significance of low-density nodes in patients presenting with newly diagnosed lymphoma has been studied (Fig. 50). Hopper et al. in a study of 76 patients with newly diagnosed Hodgkin's disease found that 16 patients (21%) had low-density nodes at presentation. Significantly, no difference was found between those patients with and those without necrotic nodes with respect to stage, disease distribution, cell type, disease extent, the presence of bulk disease, or most importantly, prognosis (134).

Calcified Lymph Nodes

Calcification within nodes is most frequently identified in patients with granulomatous disease (Fig. 51). Typically, calcified granulomatous nodes are sharply defined. Even densely calcified nodes, however, are not inactive and can become involved with other processes, such as metastatic disease. Rarely, following initial infection fibrous healing may lead to complications such as vena caval or airway obstruction (136). In rare instances the fibrosis is not self-limited, but progressively encases all mediastinal structures resulting in fibrosing mediastinitis with replacement of the low-density mediastinal fat by higher density fibrous tissue and sometimes diffuse calcification (Fig. 52). The range of CT appearances of this entity has been well described, and include hilar and mediastinal masses, usually diffusely calcified, associated with compression and/or encasement of the tracheobronchial tree or mediastinal vessels (see Fig. 23, Chapter 5) (137). Rarely, these findings primarily affect the posterior mediastinum (138).

Histoplasmosis is the most commonly identified etiology but in the majority of cases the cause is not discovered (139). It has been suggested that fibrosis may result from seepage of yeast antigen from adjacent lymph nodes. Given the highly vascularized nature of the fibrous tissue within the mediastinum in these patients, coupled with the propensity for encasement of mediastinal vessels, CT may play an exceptionally important role in these patients by suggesting the proper diagnosis, and thus obviating the need for more invasive and potentially dangerous procedures.

Calcified lymph nodes may also be seen in patients with sarcoidosis (Fig. 50; see Fig. 37, Chapter 5). Typically described as eggshell, both central and peripheral calcifications may also be seen in patients with either silicosis or coal workers' pneumoconiosis, as well as in patients with Hodgkin's disease usually following but occasionally preceding radiation, and has even been described in patients with blastomycosis, histoplasmosis, amyloidosis, scleroderma, and Castleman's disease (140–143). Rarely, calcification may occur within nodes as a result of metastatic disease, typically from the colon (Fig. 51). Calcification may also be seen in patients with metastatic osteogenic sarcoma, as well as in patients with primary intrathoracic extraosseous osteogenic sarcomas (144). Calcified hilar and mediastinal lymph nodes have been observed in AIDS patients with *Pneumocystis carinii* infection, especially in patients receiving prophylaxis with aerosolized pentamidine, possibly as a result of a necrotizing vasculitis with resultant tissue infarction and dystrophic calcification (145).

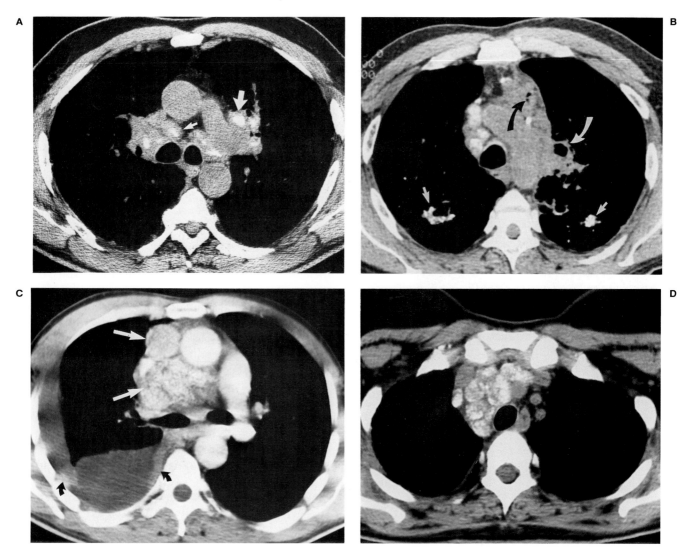

FIG. 51. Calcified lymph nodes, CT assessment. **A:** Non-enhanced CT section through the carina shows scattered calcified hilar and pretracheal lymph nodes in a patient with transbronchial, biopsy-documented sarcoidosis. Although these nodes frequently have been described as containing egg-shell calcifications, central or bull's eye calcifications can be identified within enlarged nodes (*arrows*) as frequently. **B:** Non-enhanced CT section through the aortic arch in a patient with documented silicosis. Calcified paratracheal nodes are easily identified, in this case associated with dense foci of parenchymal calcifications in the posterior segments of both upper lobes due to early progressive massive fibrosis (*arrows*). In addition, air can be seen in both enlarged left hilar and prevascular nodes (*curved arrows*). This unusual appearance is secondary to superimposed tuberculosis (silicotuberculosis). Air within these nodes is presumably secondary to necrosis of peribronchial nodes, with resultant fistulization to adjacent airways. **C:** Contrast-enhanced CT section just below the carina. Amorphous calcifications can be identified within markedly enlarged pretracheal and prevascular lymph nodes (*arrows*). A large, partially loculated pleural fluid collection is present on the right within which foci of soft-tissue density can be identified (*curved arrows*). This patient has known mucinus-producing colon carcinoma, metastatic to both the pleura and mediastinal nodes. Diagnosis was confirmed by mediastinoscopy. **D:** Non-enhanced CT section through the great vessels shows diffuse calcifications throughout pre- and paratracheal nodes. This patient had AIDS and was being treated prophylactically with aerosolized pentamidine. Mediastinoscopy revealed these nodes to be filled with *Pneumocystis carinii* organisms, a finding increasingly being observed in patients treated with aerosolized pentamidine.

Vascularized Lymph Nodes

Lymph nodes can be defined as highly vascularized when they substantially increase in density following a bolus of intravenous contrast media. The distribution of i.v. contrast medium within tumors and/or nodes is a reflection of several parameters, including blood flow, total quantity and concentration of contrast medium, distribution between the vascular and extravascular spaces, and renal function. The differential diagnosis of

enhancing mediastinal nodes is limited, and includes Castleman's disease and angioimmunoblastic lymphadenopathy, as well as vascular metastases, in particular, from renal cell carcinoma, papillary thyroid carcinoma, and especially small-cell lung carcinoma (Fig. 53; see Fig. 38, Chapter 5) (146). We have also observed considerable contrast enhancement within enlarged mediastinal and hilar nodes in some patients with sarcoidosis (Fig. 53). Differentiation between enhancing lymph nodes and vascular mediastinal masses may be problem-

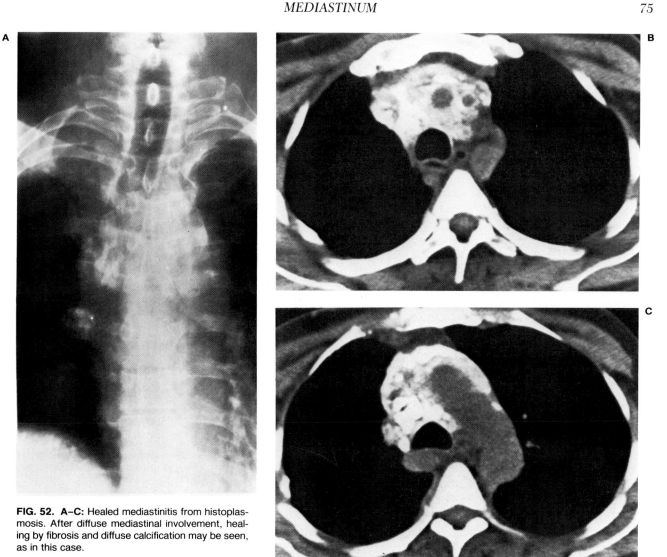

FIG. 52. A–C: Healed mediastinitis from histoplasmosis. After diffuse mediastinal involvement, healing by fibrosis and diffuse calcification may be seen, as in this case.

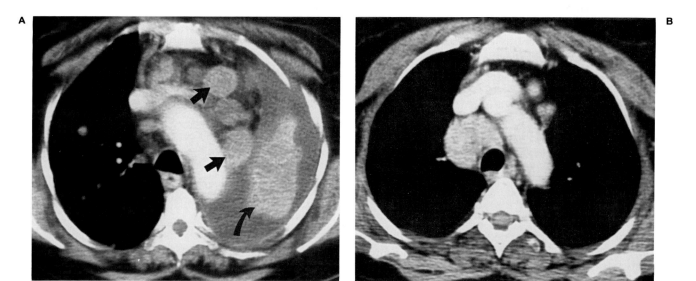

FIG. 53. Vascularized lymph nodes, CT assessment. **A:** Contrast-enhanced section through the aortic arch in a patient with obstruction of the left upper lobe bronchus due to non-small cell carcinoma. Note that there is considerable enhancement within several enlarged prevascular lymph nodes (*arrows*). A large pleural effusion is present on the left side within which a portion of the collapsed left upper lobe can be identified, also due to contrast enhancement of the still-vascularized parenchyma (*curved arrow*). **B:** Contrast-enhanced CT section through the aorta shows markedly enlarged, enhancing pre- and paratracheal and prevascular lymph nodes in a patient with documented sarcoidosis.

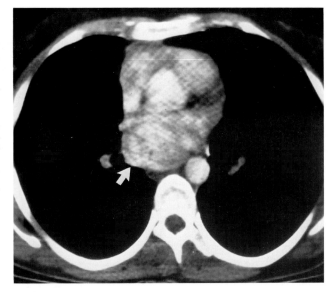

FIG. 54. Mediastinal pheochromocytoma. **A, B:** CT scans obtained at the level of the left atrium, both pre- and post-i.v. contrast enhancement, respectively. A large, homogeneous, low density mass can be identified causing marked compression of the left atrium (*arrows* in A and B). Note that following i.v. contrast administration there has been marked contrast enhancement within the mass. Without benefit of the precontrast image, this mass could easily be overlooked as representing a normal left atrium. (Case courtesy of Barry Gross, M.D., Detroit, MI.)

atic (146). These include substernal thyroid and para-thyroid glands, carcinoid tumors, hemangiomas, and paragangliomas, both intracardiac and mediastinal (147–149). Paragangliomas, in particular, are vascular tumors that originate from neuroectodermal cells within the autonomic nervous system, especially in the region of the aorticopulmonary window and the posterior mediastinum (Fig. 54). They have also been identified within the atria. Approximately 10% of these lesions are malignant. Identification of these lesions has been greatly aided recently by use of 131-I metaiodobenzyl-guanidine (131-I-MIBG) scintigraphy which localizes in catecholamine-producing tumors, including neuroblastomas and carcinoids (148,149).

Castleman's disease (also referred to by a host of other terms, including angiofollicular mediastinal lymph node hyperplasia, angiomatous lymphoid hamartoma, and giant mediastinal lymph node hyperplasia) is a disease of unknown etiology. Histologically, two forms of the disease have been described: the hyaline-vascular type and the plasma cell type (150,151). The hyaline-vascular type occurs in up to 90% of cases, and is characterized histologically by hypervascular hyaline germinal centers marked by extensive capillary proliferation. Typically, this form of the disease affects young people, and presents as a localized asymptomatic mediastinal mass in up to 70% of cases: in fact, any location within the body in which there are lymph nodes may be affected, especially within the retroperitoneum. Unlike the hyaline-vascular type of disease, the plasma cell type often presents as a multi-centric disease process, associated with

generalized lymphadenopathy and hepatosplenomegaly. Both forms may present with a wide range of systemic manifestations, including fever, refractory anemia, and hypergammaglobulinemia. When associated with localized disease, these findings usually disappear following total resection. The CT features of this form of the disease have been described, including the finding of marked contrast enhancement within well-defined mediastinal masses following a bolus of intravenous contrast medium; this corresponds with the highly vascular nature of these lesions as previously confirmed angiographically (146,152–157).

Similar findings have more recently been identified in patients with AIDS, including hypervascular follicular hyperplasia, indistinguishable from the plasma-cell type of Castleman's disease. This pattern has also been seen in association with Kaposi's sarcoma (KS), frequently within the same lymph node. This may account for the frequent observation of contrast enhancement in lymph nodes in patients with documented KS (158). Similar features have also been described in patients with angioblastic lymphadenopathy (AIL). This is especially significant given the propensity of AIL to evolve into malignancy.

Metastases to mediastinal lymph nodes from extrathoracic malignancies are rare. In a review of 1,071 cases of extrathoracic neoplasms, only 25 (2.3%) had evidence of hilar or mediastinal adenopathy (159). The extrathoracic tumors most likely to metastasize to the mediastinum originate from the head and neck, genitourinary tract, breasts (with a predeliction for the internal mam-

A
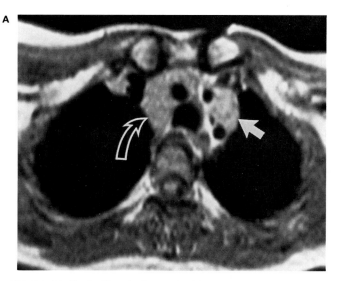
B
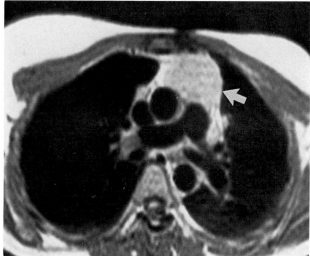

FIG. 55. Mediastinal lymphadenopathy, MR assessment. **A, B:** T1-weighted axial MR images through the great vessels and right main pulmonary artery, respectively. Enlarged, confluent, prevascular (*arrow* in A, B) and paratracheal (*curved arrow* in A) lymph nodes are easily identifiable as areas of intermediate signal intensity embedded in fat. Non-Hodgkin's lymphoma.

mary nodes), and skin with malignant melanoma. Most of these cause otherwise nondescript lymph node enlargement. Hypervascularity is the exception, most often secondary to metastatic leiomyosarcoma, neurofibrosarcoma, and melanoma. Enhancing lymph nodes also occur with some frequency in patients with primary lung cancer, metastatic to mediastinal nodes.

MR Evaluation of Mediastinal Lymph Nodes

MR has been reported to be comparable to CT in identifying mediastinal and hilar lymph nodes even though the spatial resolution of CT exceeds MR (160). This probably reflects the greater contrast resolution of MR which makes identification of mediastinal lymph nodes especially easy when they are embedded in mediastinal fat or adjacent to mediastinal or hilar blood vessels (Fig. 55, see Fig. 40, Chapter 5). MR, however, is no more specific than CT in differentiating hyperplastic from malignant lymph nodes (161). Furthermore, MR is unable to detect calcification, rendering identification of granulomatous nodes exceedingly difficult. Although MR has been used to diagnose fibrosing mediastinitis, recognition of this entity with MR is dependent on identifying secondary consequences such as vascular displacement and occlusion (see Fig. 23, Chapter 5) (162,163). Low signal intensity has been noted in calcified nodes on T2-weighted images in patients with fibrosing mediastinitis; however, this appearance is nonspecific (163). As will be discussed in greater detail later, a role for MR in assessing disease activity has been documented for patients with lymphoma following therapy.

VASCULAR PATHOLOGY

Technique

Accurate CT evaluation of the aorta requires meticulous scan technique (Table 2). As will be discussed, an initial sequence of non–contrast-enhanced scans through the aorta is mandatory in order to detect acute hemorrhage either within the wall of the aorta or within the mediastinum, evidence of acute dissection and/or rupture, respectively (Fig. 56). Other findings, including identification of displaced intimal calcifications, while less specific may still be of value, and are only reliably seen prior to the injection of intravenous contrast.

TABLE 2. *Aortic dissection: Technique*

A. Standard approach
   1. Initial nonenhanced sequence of 10-mm sections q15 mm through the thorax.
   2. 50- to 60-cc bolus of 60% iodinated contrast (± non-ionic).[a] 6–8 dynamic static scans (1.3 sec/q 3.5 sec) at the following levels: aortic arch/mid-ascending aorta/aortic root (optional).
   3. Between boluses: TKO. Following last bolus: 10-mm section q15 mm through chest and abdomen
B. Dynamic incrementation
   1. Initial nonenhanced sequence of 10-mm sections.
   2. 150-cc bolus of 60% iodinated contrast (± non-ionic).[a] Scan from approximately 2 cm above arch to the diaphragm using dynamic incrementation (1.3 sec/q 3.5 sec) at 2 cc/sec following 20-sec delay.

[a] ± power injector if available. TKO, to keep open.

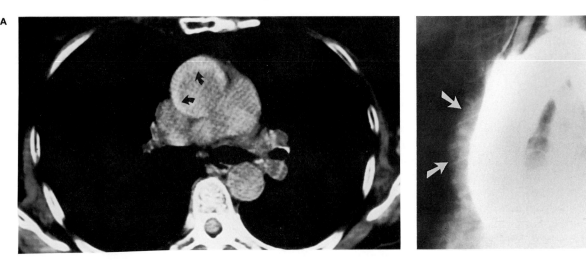

FIG. 56. Aortic dissection, acute hemorrhage. **A:** Non-enhanced CT section through the carina shows a crescentic area of markedly increased density in the ascending aorta (*arrows*) consistent with hemorrhage within an acute dissection. **B:** Corresponding aortogram confirms the presence of a Type A dissection (*arrows*). This case emphasizes the need to acquire an initial series of non–contrast-enhanced images when assessing patients for possible dissection.

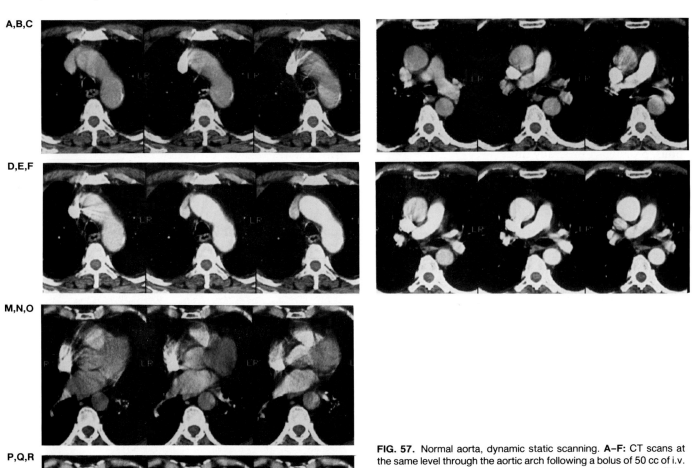

FIG. 57. Normal aorta, dynamic static scanning. **A–F:** CT scans at the same level through the aortic arch following a bolus of 50 cc of i.v. contrast media using a power injector at a rate of 2.0 cc per sec. With an interscan delay of 1.8 sec, these six images were obtained in approximately 30 sec. Note that the aorta is only densely opacified on the last two images. **G–L:** CT scans at the same level through the right main pulmonary artery using the identical technique described in A. Using this technique, the passage of contrast first through the superior vena cava, then the pulmonary arteries, and finally into the aorta is easily traced. **M–R:** CT scans at the same level through the root of the aorta using the identical technique described in A. At this level, images are usually partially degraded by adjacent heart motion, rendering them generally less helpful.

Following this, contrast enhancement is requisite. With minor variations, two general methods have been proposed to obtain adequate contrast enhancement of the aorta; both utilize bolus techniques, preferably utilizing power injectors (6,7).

1. Dynamic static scanning. Using this technique, a series of six to eight scans are obtained all at the same level following a bolus injection of intravenous contrast medium. This necessitates using two to three separate injections of between 50 and 60 cc's of contrast medium, with scans obtained at the level of the aortic arch, the mid-ascending aorta, and, if indicated, the aortic root, respectively (Fig. 57). Following the last injection, scans are then obtained sequentially to the level of the aortic bifurcation. This is necessitated by the very high frequency of associated abdominal aortic pathology, especially in patients with atherosclerotic disease.

The most important advantage of the static dynamic approach is that by acquiring sequentially timed scans at the same level, variations in cardiac output and hence concern over appropriate scan timing to obtain adequate aortic enhancement are minimized. Additionally, in patients with dissections, this technique optimizes visualization of differential flow rates between contrast in the true and the false lumens. The main disadvantage of this approach is the need for two to three separate injections, prolonging the study time.

2. Dynamic incremental scanning. Using this technique, a single injection of between 100 and 150 cc's of contrast material is utilized with scans obtained sequentially starting just above the level of the aortic arch and proceeding caudally to the level of the diaphragms (Fig. 58). In our experience, adequate visualization of the aorta can be obtained in almost all cases, especially when contrast is administered with a power injector. The main limitation of this technique is the variability of cardiac output, making it difficult to precisely determine the best time to initiate scanning following contrast administration. In our experience, a delay of about 20 sec from the onset of contrast administration to the initiation of scanning has proven adequate in most patients.

Regardless of the technique employed, it cannot be overemphasized that even with modern state-of-the-art scanners, adequate CT evaluation of aortic disease requires the use of large volumes of contrast medium, typically 100 and 150 cc's. Lesser degrees of contrast enhancement will lead to misdiagnoses in a significant percentage of cases, especially in patients with aortic dissection. The notion that there is value in obtaining low-dose contrast studies of the aorta should be discouraged. Ideally, iodine concentration should be sufficient to provide dense opacification of the aorta. The use of nonionic contrast agents has been suggested for patients with histories of either cardiac or renal disease.

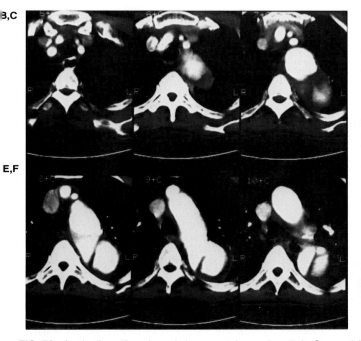
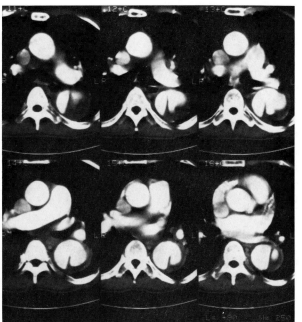

FIG. 58. Aortic dissection, dynamic incremental scanning. **A–L:** Sequential sections starting from a level approximately 2 cm above the aortic arch, ending at the level of the root of the aorta following a bolus of 150 cc of i.v. contrast media using a power injector at a rate of 2 cc per sec. With an interscan delay of 3.8 sec, these 12 images were obtained in just over 1 min. There is dense opacification of all mediastinal vessels, allowing easy recognition of a Type B dissection.

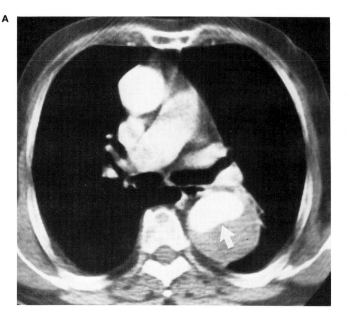

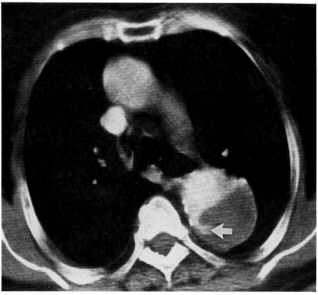

FIG. 59. Aortic aneurysm, CT assessment. **A:** Contrast-enhanced CT section through the carina shows characteristic appearance of a descending aortic aneurysm. Dense contrast enhancement identifies the residual, eccentric, kidney-shaped lumen as distinct from adjacent thrombus (*arrow*). **B:** Contrast-enhanced CT section through the carina in a different patient than shown in A. Again, characteristic features of a descending aortic aneurysm can be seen, including dense opacification of an eccentric residual lumen. Note that in this case, however, there is a focal area of ulceration that can be identified within the thrombus (*arrow*). Ulcerations of atheromatous plaques occur frequently, especially in patients with advanced atherosclerotic disease, and are generally confined to the intima. Rarely, extension to the media occurs leading either to a false aneurysm or transmural rupture.

Aortic Aneursyms

By definition, a true aneurysm involves all components of the vessel wall. Aneurysms are more common than dissections in the thoracic aorta, but acute aneurysmal rupture does not occur as frequently (164,165). Contrast-enhanced CT can demonstrate all the gross pathologic features of aortic aneurysms, including dilatation, intraluminal thrombi, displacement or erosion of adjacent structures, and perianeurysmal thickening and hemorrhage (Figs. 59–62; see Fig. 24, Chapter 5) (166–169). CT has also proven valuable in detecting unusual types of aneurysms, including mycotic and ductus aneursysms, as well as identifying complications arising from aneurysms, including those secondary to rupture (170–176). CT also plays an important role in distinguishing thoracic aortic aneurysms from pulmonary masses adjacent to the mediastinum (177).

Identification of a thoracic aortic aneurysm should not rest on absolute measurements of the aortic circumference. Although a minimal diameter of 4 cm has typically been used to diagnose aneurysmal dilatation, as documented by Aronberg et al., in a retrospective study of 102 chest CT studies in adults, significant variations in the aorta size occurred according to the individuals' age, sex, and thoracic vertebral body width (178). At a level just caudal to the aortic arch, for example, aortic diameters varied from 1.9 to 4.7 cm, with an average value of 3.51 cm. The ratio between the ascending and

descending aorta, in particular, varied markedly with age. These authors concluded that as a practical guide, on any given scan the descending aorta should never be larger than the ascending aorta, and that the ratio of the ascending to the descending aortic coronal diameter usually measured 1.5:1. The significance of these measurements lies in the fact that the maximal diameter of the aneurysm correlates with the incidence of rupture, which ranges from 2% for diameters of less than 5 cm to more than 50% for aneurysms larger than 10 cm (164–165). Overall, up to 50% of deaths from thoracic aortic aneurysms result from rupture.

The diagnosis of an aortic aneurysm can be made specifically when a dilated thin-walled lumen is identified. Identification of mural thrombus and calcification is also common, especially as the majority of aortic aneurysms are secondary to arteriosclerosis. These findings, however, are not specific as similar findings may be seen in patients with chronic aortic dissections with thrombosed false lumens (Fig. 63). The pattern of mural thrombi and calcifications within aortic aneursyms has been described (179–181). Typically crescentic in shape, thrombi often are circumferential, in which case the residual lumen appears circular. As a rule, the residual aortic lumen is smooth, although the aortic lumen may develop a very irregular contour, especially in larger aneurysms, depending on the extent of thrombus. Calcification within aneurysms is common, occurring in up to 85% of cases, both within the wall of the aorta (so-called mural calcifications) and within the thrombus itself (so-called thrombus calcification) (179). This latter type of calcification has been reported to occur in approximately 25% of patients both with thoracic and abdominal aortic aneurysms (180,181). The significance of calcification within thrombi is that this appearance can be mistaken for the displaced intimal calcifications seen in a patient with dissection. Additionally, it has been suggested that finding calcification within thrombus may presage impending rupture. Verification of this observation, however, must await further investigation (181).

CT can be used to follow up aneurysms, although this involves repeated use of intravenous contrast. An increasing diameter is readily detected with serial scans and helps prompt a surgical decision. It has also been suggested that CT may be valuable in assessing patients with posttraumatic or iatrogenic false aneurysms, as may occur following aortic valve replacement, cardiopulmonary bypass, or coronary artery bypass grafting (182–184).

Traumatic aneurysms occur most commonly at the level of the ligamentum arteriosum, just distal to the subclavian artery (60%). They may also occur near the aortic hiatus of the diaphragm (20%) and in the ascending aorta (20%). Of those few patients who survive long enough to reach a hospital, angiography is the procedure of choice. If the angiogram is negative and the patient unstable, CT may still be of value because in the early posttraumatic phase, a definite aneurysm may not yet have formed, even though significant damage to the

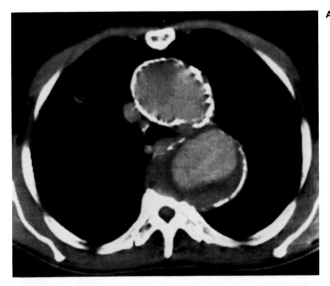

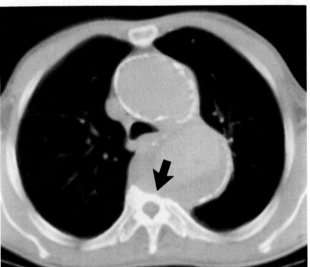

FIG. 61. Aortic aneurysm, CT assessment. **A, B:** Contrast-enhanced CT scans at the same level imaged with narrow and wide windows, respectively. There is dense calcification of the walls of both the ascending and descending aorta. An aneurysm is present within the proximal descending aorta, with considerable surrounding thrombus. The adjacent vertebral body has been significantly eroded (*arrow* in B).

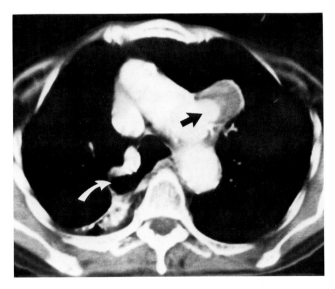

FIG. 60. Aortic aneurysm, CT assessment. Contrast-enhanced CT section shows typical appearance of a saccular aneurysm with contrast easily identified within the neck of the aneurysm (*arrow*). Note that the right upper lobe bronchus is displaced posteriorly (*curved arrow*). This is characteristic of cicatrization atelectasis within the right upper lobe secondary to previous granulomatous infection with resultant scarring.

aorta has occurred. CT signs of an acutely injured aorta have been described (185–187). As outlined by Heiberg et al., these include the presence of a false aneurysm, a linear lucency within the opacified aortic lumen caused by the torn edge of the aortic wall, marginal irregularity of the opacified lumen, periaortic or intramural hematoma, and dissection (185). In select cases, CT may be used as a surveillance modality in patients in whom surgery may be relatively contraindicated, or if a major artery such as the anterior spinal artery of Adamkiewickz arises from the traumatic aneurysm (188).

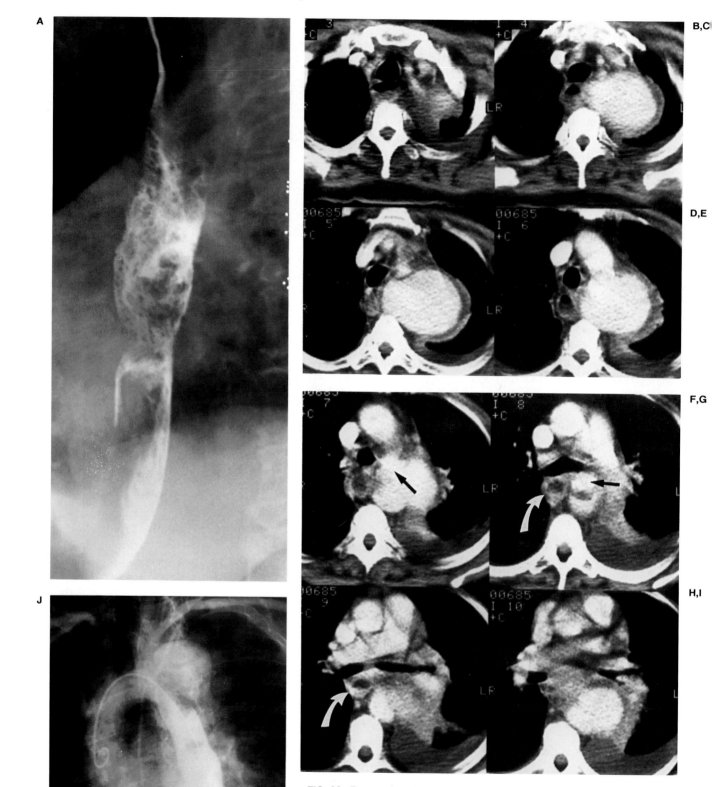

FIG. 62. Ruptured aortic aneurysm, CT evaluation. **A:** Coned-down view from an esophagram obtained in a patient who presented with hematemesis. A large filling defect is conspicuous within the esophageal lumen. **B–I:** Sequential contrast-enhanced CT sections from above-downward shows a large aortic aneurysm involving the proximal portion of the descending aorta. At the level of the distal trachea and carina, disruption in the wall of the aneurysm can be identified (*arrows* in F and G) with resultant mediastinal hematoma and associated left pleural effusion. A blood-fluid level can also be seen within the esophageal lumen (*curved arrow* in H). **J:** Corresponding aortogram showing a large aneurysm of the aorta without apparent leak. This patient expired shortly thereafter despite attempts at surgical repair.

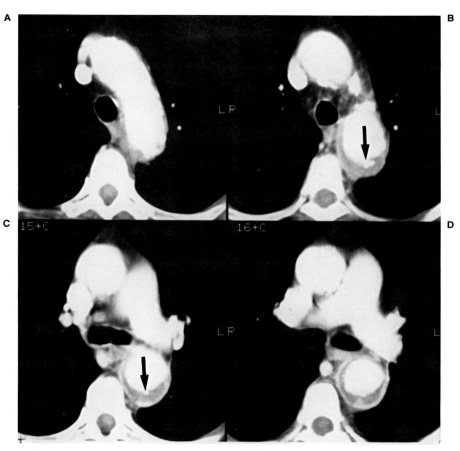

FIG. 63. Aortic aneurysm vs. chronic dissection, CT assessment. **A–D:** Sequential contrast-enhanced CT sections from the aortic arch to the carina. There is aneurysmal dilatation of the proximal descending aorta. Mural thrombus can be identified at multiple levels, as well as a suggestion of displaced intimal calcifications (*arrow* in B and C). Unfortunately, these findings are nonspecific as calcification can occur within thrombi. Luckily, differentiation between aneurysms with clot and thrombosed dissections is usually not a significant clinical problem.

Aortic Dissection

Dissection of the aorta most often presents as a clinical catastrophe, sometimes difficult to distinguish from myocardial infarction or pulmonary embolization. An insidious onset is, however, not infrequent. The chest radiograph usually demonstrates a widened aortic shadow; rarely, it may remain normal. The basic abnormality is hemorrhage within the aortic media, usually resulting from a localized intimal tear. The result is separation of the peripheral two-thirds from the central one-third of the media, rarely involving more than approximately one-half the circumference of the aorta (189). Although multiple conditions predispose to dissection, including Marfan's syndrome, pregnancy, syphilis, and coarctation with or without an associated bicuspid aortic valve, by far the most common association is with systemic hypertension. Indeed, it has even been suggested that dissection rarely if ever occurs in the absence of hypertension (189).

At present, evaluation of patients with aortic dissections revolves around answering two basic questions. (a) Does the dissection involve the ascending aorta? (b) Is the aorta aneurysmally dilated? These questions generally are easily evaluated with both CT and MR.

Type A dissections involve the ascending aorta with the intimal tear usually arising within a few centimeters of the aortic valve (Fig. 56). Without treatment, dissections within the ascending aorta are nearly always fatal. Proximal extension of the dissection to affect the aortic valve or rupture into the pericardium is the main pathophysiologic mechanism of death in these patients (189). Surgical intervention in Type A dissections significantly affects prognosis, unlike patients with Type B dissection, hence the rationale for early intervention. Recent surgical experience with repair of Type A dissections has made preoperative knowledge of the site of intimal tears, involvement of branch arteries, relative flow in the true versus the false lumen, and the presence and degree of aortic regurgitation less germane (190–192). Interestingly, in follow-up studies of operated patients, the false lumen is often seen to remain patent, which suggests that prevention of proximal extension by suturing or grafting rather than closure of the primary tear of the dissection is the main beneficial effect of surgery (193).

Type B dissections involve only the descending aorta, usually arising just distal to the origin of the left subclavian artery at the site of the ligamentum arteriosum (Fig. 58; Fig. 64). Characteristically, Type B dissections do not carry the risk of proximal extension; consequently,

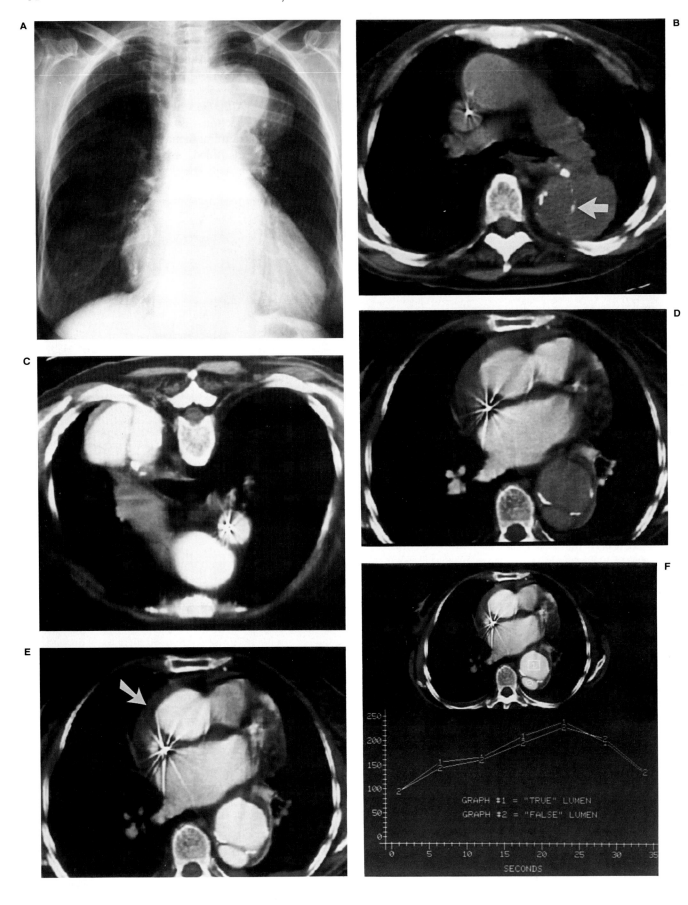

these are best treated medically by reducing peak systolic pressure to allow healing. However, in time, surgical intervention in Type B dissections may be mandated if the descending aorta becomes aneurysmally dilated. Other determinants of the outcome of patients with dissection include occlusion of major aortic branches and rupture of the aorta itself.

Type B dissection must be differentiated from a similar but distinct entity, so-called penetrating atheromatous ulcer with pseudoaneurysm (Fig. 65). In this condi-

tion, atheromatous disease of the aorta results in the formation of a penetrating ulcer (194,195). Typically involving the lower descending aorta, ulceration can result in the formation of an intramural hematoma that can progress to pseudoaneurysm formation and subsequent rupture. Although the clinical presentation may mimic aortic dissection, dissection is rarely present (Fig. 65). Instead, intramural hematoma and periaortic hemorrhage can be identified, provided that serial CT scans are obtained through the descending aorta following

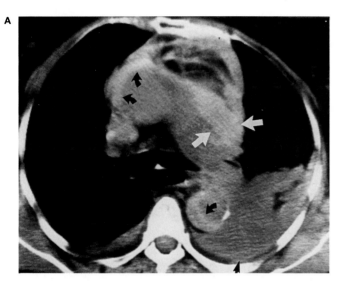
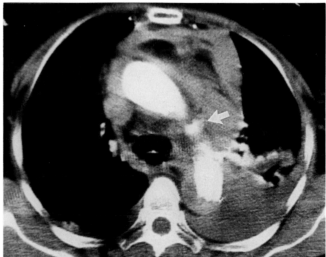
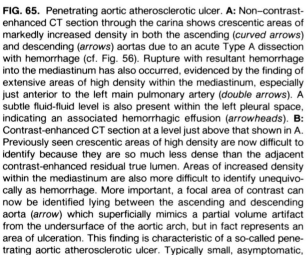
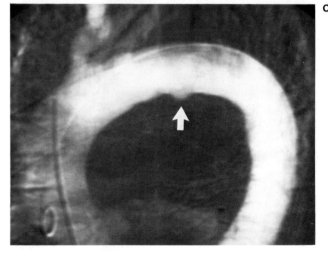

FIG. 65. Penetrating aortic atherosclerotic ulcer. **A:** Non–contrast-enhanced CT section through the carina shows crescentic areas of markedly increased density in both the ascending (*curved arrows*) and descending (*arrows*) aortas due to an acute Type A dissection with hemorrhage (cf. Fig. 56). Rupture with resultant hemorrhage into the mediastinum has also occurred, evidenced by the finding of extensive areas of high density within the mediastinum, especially just anterior to the left main pulmonary artery (*double arrows*). A subtle fluid-fluid level is also present within the left pleural space, indicating an associated hemorrhagic effusion (*arrowheads*). **B:** Contrast-enhanced CT section at a level just above that shown in A. Previously seen crescentic areas of high density are now difficult to identify because they are so much less dense than the adjacent contrast-enhanced residual true lumen. Areas of increased density within the mediastinum are also more difficult to identify unequivocally as hemorrhage. More important, a focal area of contrast can now be identified lying between the ascending and descending aorta (*arrow*) which superficially mimics a partial volume artifact from the undersurface of the aortic arch, but in fact represents an area of ulceration. This finding is characteristic of a so-called penetrating aortic atherosclerotic ulcer. Typically small, asymptomatic, and self-limited, occasionally these can penetrate into the media with resultant hematoma formation. This can subsequently lead to a pseudoaneurysm formation, aortic rupture, or as shown in this case, findings of acute dissection. **C:** Corresponding subtraction aortogram shows area of ulceration seen in B (*arrow*). On this image the dissection is difficult to identify.

←———

FIG. 64. Aortic dissection, CT assessment. **A:** Posteroanterior chest radiograph shows aneurysmal dilatation of the aorta. There is a suggestion of a possible soft-tissue mass adjacent to the arch. **B, C:** Pre- and postcontrast-enhanced images at the same level through the mid-ascending aorta. On the precontrast-enhanced section there is evidence of displaced intimal calcifications (*arrow*). Following the bolus administration of contrast, both the true and false lumens are easily identified, separated by a thin intimal flap. Note that the ascending aorta is normal and there is no evidence of a para-aortic mass. **D, E:** CT scans at the level of the left atrium obtained extremely early and then seconds later following another bolus administration of contrast. Displaced intimal calcifications and an intimal flap are again easily recognized. The apparent disparity in opacification of the ascending vs. the descending aorta in D reflects markedly slow flow in the aorta. A pericardial effusion can be seen on the right side (*arrow* in E). **F:** Same image as in E, with *cursors* placed on both the two lumens in order to generate time-density curves. Note that flow is equivalent in both channels. Despite the labeling, accurate differentiation between the true and false lumens is generally difficult.

contrast enhancement. Differentiation of this entity from classic Type B dissection is especially significant as surgery is requisite in these patients in order to avert aortic rupture.

CT is a reliable means for diagnosing or excluding aortic dissection (166,196–208). The diagnosis rests on findings observed both on non–contrast-enhanced and contrast-enhanced scans (Table 3).

On non–contrast-enhanced scans, a specific diagnosis of dissection can be made when a crescentic area of high density can be identified within the aortic wall (Figs. 56 and 65) (181,208). This sign has been reported to occur in up to 44% of cases, although in our experience it is seen far less frequently (161). It has been speculated that hyperdensity within the wall of the aorta represents intramural hemorrhage due to rupture of the vasa vasorum without intimal tear (208). Whatever its precise cause, this sign may only be recognized in the acute phase of dissection. After approximately 1 week, the hemorrhage begins to liquify with resultant decrease in CT density.

In addition to hyperdensity within the aortic wall, other findings on nonenhanced scans have been described. Rarely, an intimal flap itself can be identified within a nonopacified aortic lumen in patients with severe anemia (209). More commonly, displaced intimal calcifications are seen (Fig. 64). Unfortunately, although this finding may be helpful as a further confirmatory sign in patients with acute dissections also studied with contrast-enhanced images, in itself this finding frequently is problematic, especially when attempting to differentiate chronic thrombosed aortic dissections with displaced intimal calcifications from aortic aneurysms with calcification within thrombi (Fig. 63) (179–181). This differentiation may also be difficult when the aorta is extremely tortuous (210).

Following contrast enhancement, diagnosis of aortic dissection rests on identification of two lumens separated by an intimal flap (Figs. 58 and 64). Ancillary findings, such as differential flow through the two lumens, compression of and/or irregularity in the contour of the true lumen, increase in size of the aorta, and the presence of a hemopericardium, are less sensitive means for establishing the diagnosis (211).

Traditionally, the diagnosis of aortic dissection has required aortography. The major advantage of CT as compared with aortography is that CT is less invasive, obviating the need for catheterization. Additionally, there is no need to require precise positioning of the patient in order to project the intimal flap tangentially. CT also has the advantage of being able to simultaneously visualize periaortic structures, including the mediastinum and pericardium (211). However, the use of CT to evaluate aortic dissection is not without its limitations. Insufficient contrast enhancement is especially problematic, either as a result of improperly ad-

TABLE 3. *Aortic dissection: CT findings*

1. Pre-contrast:
    Displaced intimal calcifications
    Acute hemorrhage (identifiable as regions of high
        tissue density)
      Intramural
      Mediastinal
      Pericardial
    Aortic grafts
2. Post-contrast:
    Intimal flap
    Differential contrast opacification (true vs false lumen)
    Ulcerlike projections

ministered injections or difficulty in properly timing image acquisition following bolus administration of contrast medium. Streak artifacts and anatomic variants that caused difficulties in initial studies are less troublesome now (210,212). This is partly due to their familiarity, and partly due to the routine availability of current generation scanners with resultant improved image quality.

Numerous reports have compared the efficacy of CT to angiography in diagnosing aortic dissection. Overall, these support a primary role for the use of CT as the initial imaging procedure of choice (166,169,196–200,202,203,207). In most series, the accuracy of CT compares favorably with angiography, including documented cases in which the diagnosis of dissection was made only by CT (213). Nonetheless, it has also been documented that false negative CT scans do occur in a small percentage of cases (201,214,215). In a series of 137 patients with suspected acute aortic dissection reported by Vasile et al., there were seven false negative examinations (216). In three patients, CT was felt to be technically inadequate due either to artifacts or poor opacification following contrast administration. One of these patients subsequently was shown to have a Type A dissection, one patient was documented to have a Type B dissection, while another proved to have an aneurysm of the right coronary artery. In another four cases, CT failed to disclose an intimal flap in three patients with Type A dissections, one of which was subsequently verified at autopsy, and one patient with a Type B dissection. Similar examples have been published by others (201,214,215). Because the overall accuracy of CT in either diagnosing or excluding aortic dissection exceeds 90%, in our judgment CT should still be considered the initial procedure of choice. However, in select cases, a role for angiography clearly still exists, as will be discussed in detail later (215).

Patients who survive their initial dissection are prone to redissection, extension of dissection, aortic aneurysm,

A

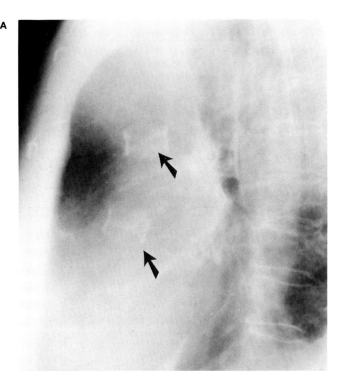

B,C

D,E

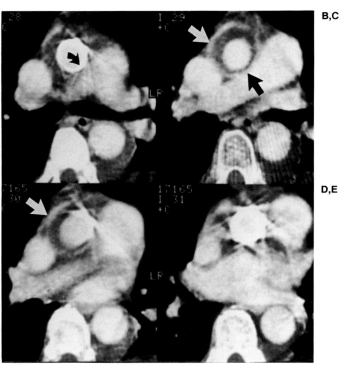

FIG. 66. Aortic repair, CT assessment. **A:** Lateral chest radiograph shows the presence of an aortic graft (*arrows*). **B–E:** Enlargements of contrast-enhanced CT sections through the ascending aorta, from above-downward. The graft is easily identified as a dense circular rim (*arrow* in B) surrounding the graft lumen which is perfectly round (*curved arrow* in C). Note that there is considerable low-density thrombus lying between the graft and the native aortic wall (*arrows* in C and D).

and aortic rupture. CT has proven valuable in detecting these complications (193,217–220). CT is also of considerable value in assessing postoperative changes (Fig. 66). Interestingly, a totally thrombosed false lumen appears to correlate well with a favorable response to medical therapy.

Aortic Disease: MR Evaluation

The advantages of MR for evaluation of the aorta include: (a) nonreliance on the use of intravenous contrast medium to image blood vessels; (b) the ability to acquire multi-planar images; and (c) a lack of ionizing radiation. These attributes make MR a particularly attractive method for imaging the aorta (221–224). Limitations of MR as compared with CT include: (a) inability to detect calcification; (b) decreased spatial resolution; (c) restriction in the numbers of patients eligible to be scanned due to the presence of various life-support systems and monitoring devices, such as pacemakers or ventilators; and (d) cost and availability.

Technique

The aorta usually is first studied using multi-section spin-echo technique. Electrocardiogram (ECG) gating should always be utilized as it improves anatomic detail.

For most cases, transaxial images should be acquired first, as these frequently provide adequate visualization of most cardiovascular structures (Fig. 67). Coronal

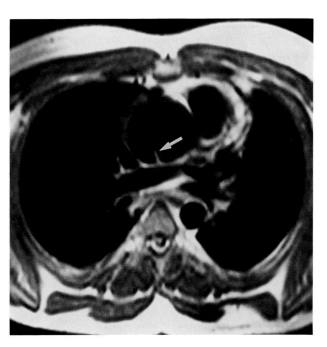

FIG. 67. Aortic dissection, MR assessment. ECG-gated, axial image through the ascending aorta demonstrates aneurysmal dilatation of the ascending aorta. An intimal flap is easily identified dividing the aortic lumen (*arrow*). The descending aorta is normal.

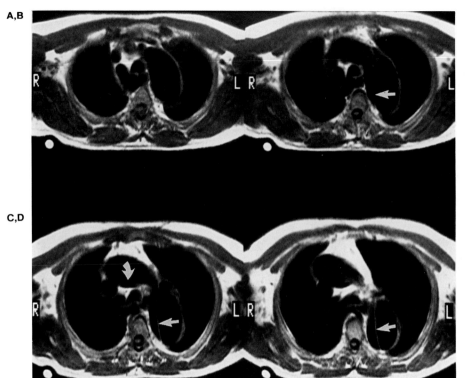

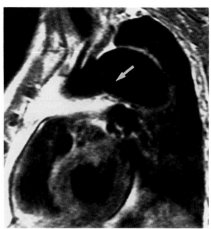

FIG. 68. Aortic dissection, MR assessment. **A–D:** Sequential axial images from above-downward through the great vessels, aortic arch, and ascending aorta. An intimal flap is clearly present within the descending aorta (*arrows* in B–D). Note small quantity of fluid in the superior pericardial recess, superficially mimicking an intimal flap in the ascending aorta (*curved arrow* in C). **E:** Sagittal MR image through the aortic arch shows the intimal flap arising just distal to the origin of the left subclavian artery (*arrow*).

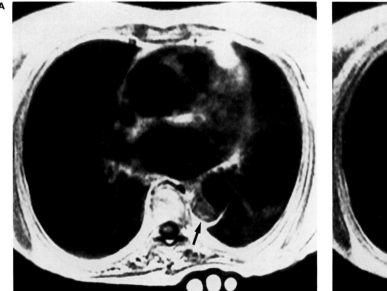

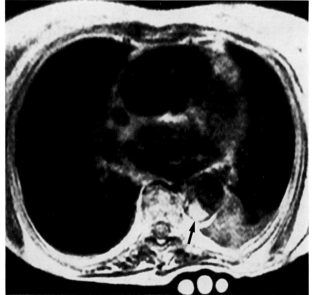

FIG. 69. Aortic dissection, MR assessment of slow flow vs. thrombosis. **A, B:** ECG-gated, axial MR images through the ascending aorta and arch with TEs of 30 and 60 msec, respectively. In A, an area of intermediate signal intensity can be identified adjacent to the descending aorta (*arrow* in A). Based on this image, differentiation between thrombus and dissection is difficult. In B, note that there is considerable signal enhancement within the same region (*arrow* in B), indicating the presence of slow flow within an aortic channel. Aortic dissection was surgically confirmed.

and/or sagittal images may be acquired as needed, as for example, when evaluating the aortic root or more precisely differentiating Type A versus Type B dissections (Fig. 68). Parasagittal images obtained through both the ascending and descending aorta are also frequently valuable, although their use is limited when there is marked tortuosity of the aorta (168,225–228).

In those cases in which signal is identified within the aortic lumen, acquisition of nongated spin-echo images with multiple symmetrical echoes can be of value in differentiating slow flow within a false lumen from thrombus within an aneurysm. Similar information

may be obtained by use of phase images, as well (Figs. 69 and 70) (229,230). Gradient-refocused sequences also may be valuable, especially when viewed in a cine mode, as these images may provide ancillary information in the assessment of patients with a wide diversity of aortic pathology (Fig. 71) (231,232). In select patients, gradient-refocused echoes may allow identification of intimal flaps otherwise difficult to define with routine spin-echo (SE) images (231). Potential additional advantages include determination of flow characteristics within true and false lumens, as well as evidence of aortic valvular regurgitation in patients with Type A dissections.

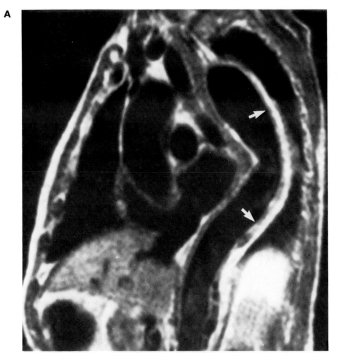

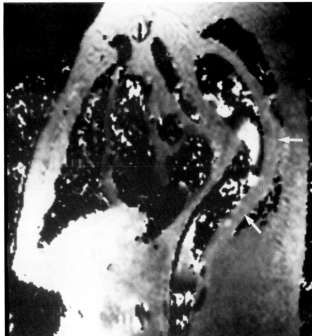

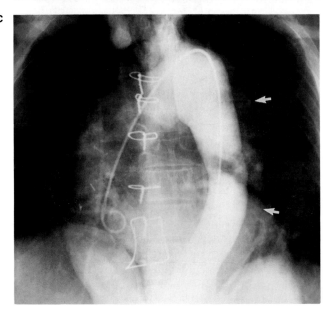

FIG. 70. Aortic dissection, MR assessment using phase images. **A:** Parasagittal MR image through the descending aorta (*arrows*) shows considerable signal paralleling the descending aorta. The appearance did not change on second-echo images. **B:** Phase image at the same level as A shows absence of phase shift in this region, suggesting chronic thrombosed dissection. **C:** Aortogram confirming a chronic Type B dissection (*arrows*). From Rumancik et al., ref. 250, with permission.

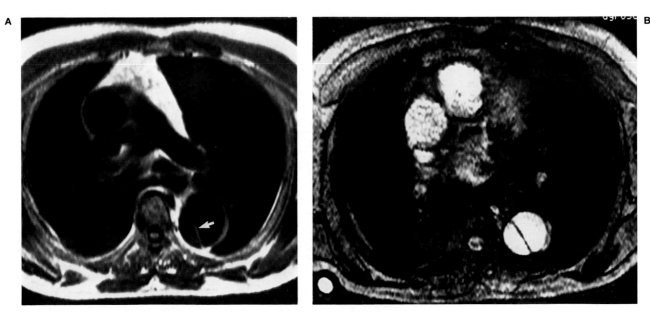

FIG. 71. Aortic dissection, assessment with gradient-refocused images. **A, B:** Spin-echo and gradient-refocused MR images at the same level through the carina show an intimal flap in the descending aorta compatible with Type B aortic dissection (*arrow* in A). With gradient-refocused sequences, flowing blood generates considerable signal, causing most vessels to appear white.

Aneurysms and Dissections

Aortic aneurysms are easily identified with MR because of the signal void usually associated with flowing blood (Fig. 72) (233–237). When present, organized thrombi within the lumen of aneurysms usually appear as areas of intermediate signal intensity, which characteristically show a decrease in relative signal intensity on second-echo images. In contradistinction, flowing blood within the residual aortic lumen typically either shows no change, or even more characteristically shows an increase in signal intensity on the second-echo image (168,224,236). As documented by Glazer et al., measurements of the maximum diameter of aneurysms with MR show near-perfect correlation with the same measurements obtained with CT scans (236). Additionally, MR provides accurate information concerning the relationships of aneurysms to surrounding mediastinal structures. As already noted, an important limitation of MR is its inability to detect mural calcifications. Although MR has been reported useful for assessing ruptured aortic aneurysms (238) as suggested by White et al., MR may in fact be limited in differentiating between mediastinal fat and subacute or chronic hemorrhage because of a leaking aneurysm, due to potential overlap in their signal intensity parameters (168).

The ability to obtain images in a variety of image planes with MR has proven especially valuable in detecting and characterizing thoracic aortic aneurysms in patients with cystic medial necrosis secondary to Marfan's syndrome (Fig. 73) (239–241). As reported by

Kersting-Sommerhoff et al., the aorta has a unique appearance in Marfan patients, characterized by enlargement of the aortic root and the caudal part of the ascending aorta, associated with a marked decrease to near normal values in the size of the aorta just proximal to the aortic arch (240). In distinction, aneurysms in patients without Marfan's syndrome typically involve the entire ascending aorta, frequently extending to the arch itself.

MR criteria for the diagnosis of aortic dissection are similar to those previously defined for CT (see also Chapter 12) (168,236,242–248). Characteristically, intimal flaps are identifiable by MR as a linear structure of intermediate signal intensity separating the true and the false lumens (Figs. 67–69 and 71). Identification of the site of intimal tears is usually not feasible. Flow characteristics within both the true and false lumens also can be characterized by MR. Characteristically, on second-echo images there is considerable signal enhancement within what is usually presumed to be the false channel due to the presence of slow moving blood (Fig. 69) (168,224,229,236,246,247). In fact, accurate differentiation of the true from the false lumen may not be possible, as theoretically, flow within the anatomic false lumen may actually exceed flow within a compressed residual true lumen. This differentiation may even be impossible at the time of surgery, although clinically this is usually insignificant given state-of-the-art surgical techniques.

Unfortunately, MR is no more sensitive than CT in differentiating those patients with completely throm-

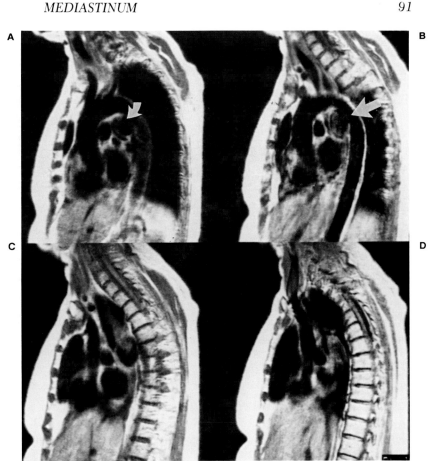

FIG. 72. Saccular aneurysm, MR assessment. **A–D:** Sequential sagittal MR images through the ascending and descending aorta show a large saccular aneurysm originating from the anterior aspect of the proximal descending aorta in the region of the ductus (*arrows* in A and B). Some signal is present within the aneurysm secondary to slow flow.

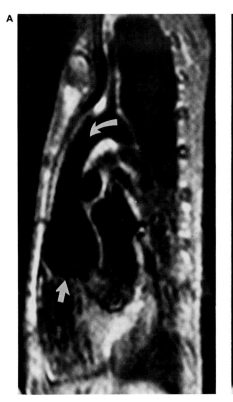

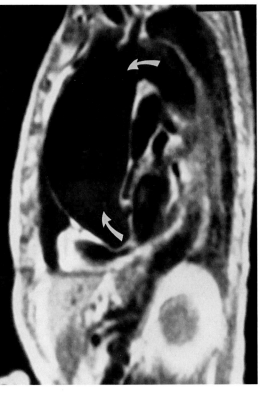

FIG. 73. Aortic aneurysms, MR assessment. **A:** Sagittal MR image through the ascending aorta in a patient with Marfan's syndrome shows characteristic appearance of dilatation predominantly affecting the aortic root and caudal portion of the ascending aorta (*arrow*) with near normal caliber of the ascending aorta just proximal to the arch (*curved arrow*). **B:** Sagittal MR image through the ascending aorta in a different patient shows characteristic appearance of a typical atherosclerotic aneurysm that involves the entire ascending aorta up to the level of the aortic arch (*arrows*).

A
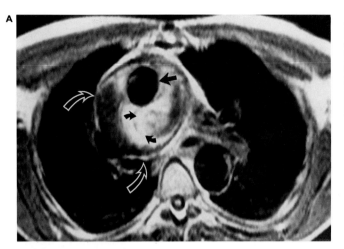

B
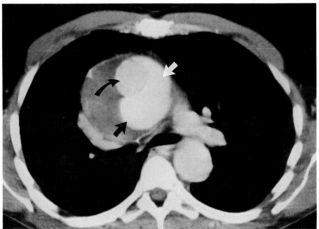

FIG. 74. Aortic dissection, postsurgical evaluation. **A:** MR section through the ascending aorta in a patient status-post repair of a Type A dissection. The graft itself is easily identified as a circular area of signal void (*arrow*). In normal postoperative patients, there is close approximation between the graft and the native aortic wall. In this case, the native aorta is aneurysmally dilated (*curved open arrows*). Between the native aortic wall and the graft there are distinct regions of heterogeneous signal intensity corresponding to thrombus, which appears as an area of relatively low signal intensity, and hemorrhage, which appears as an area of increased signal intensity (*curved black arrows*). Typically, hemorrhage results from anastomotic leaks and necessitates surgical exploration. **B:** Contrast-enhanced CT section at the same level as shown in A confirms all the same findings, including thrombus as well as an area of hemorrhage (*arrows*) adjacent to the aortic graft (*curved arrow*), indicating an anastomotic leak.

bosed false lumens from patients with thrombosed aneurysms. In fact, it has been suggested that MR may be somewhat less sensitive than CT in differentiating these entities because of its inability to detect displaced intimal calcifications (Fig. 70). As previously discussed, however, the value of this observation is problematic.

Numerous reports have compared the efficacy of MR with both CT and angiography in diagnosing aortic dissection (236,242–246). In most series, CT and MR have proven roughly comparable in identifying and/or excluding aortic dissection. In one report, the sensitivity of MR in detecting aortic dissection ranged from 84% to 96%, depending on the level of the interpreter's experience in accurately interpreting flow-related signal changes within the aorta (246). In our experience, one advantage of MR not adequately stressed in the literature is its ability to accurately differentiate Type A from Type B dissections. In select cases, this differentiation can be problematic when the aorta is viewed only in cross-section (Fig. 68).

MR is also of proven value in assessing the aorta following both aortic and cardiac surgery (248–250). Following surgery for aortic dissection, MR is especially useful in detecting either anastomatic leaks or aneurysmal dilatation beyond the graft site, findings that frequently necessitate surgical correction (Fig. 74). Additionally, MR can provide information concerning the status of the residual false lumen, which frequently remains patent after surgery. As documented by White et al., in their series of 11 dissections evaluated postoperatively, a residual intimal flap was identified in 10 cases, all of which were associated with at least partial patency of the residual false channel (249). Aneurysms develop-

ing in patients following aortocoronary bypass surgery as well as perivalvular infectious pseudoaneurysms complicating cardiac surgery in patients with infective endocarditis have also been described (251,252).

Like CT, there are pitfalls in MR interpretation. Confusion may arise, for example, in attempting to separate the aorta from adjacent structures that may simulate an intimal flap, such as the superior pericardial recess and

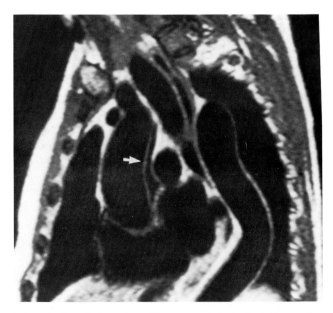

FIG. 75. Pseudodissection, MR assessment. Sagittal MR section through the ascending aorta. A fine line can be seen (*arrow*) that superficially mimics an intimal flap, but in fact represents a prominent superior pericardial recess marginating the posterior wall of the ascending aorta.

the left brachiocephalic vein (Fig. 68, Fig. 75). Other artifacts have been described as well (253). MR is also limited in its ability to visualize branch vessel involvement. Although identification of branch vessel abnormalities is possible in many cases, currently available scanners do not provide sufficient spatial resolution to reliably visualize small and medium-sized aortic branches, including the coronary arteries (248,254,255). Miller et al., in a prospective study of 10 patients with documented Takayasu's arteritis, compared the ability of MR to detect vascular abnormalities in the large arteries of the thorax and abdomen with angiography (255). MR proved only 38% sensitive on a patient-by-patient analysis and 54% sensitive with a lesion-by-lesion analysis.

CT/MR/Angiographic Correlation

Given the advantages and disadvantages of CT, MR, and angiography in the evaluation of aortic disease, it is possible to develop a logical approach to imaging the aorta. In our judgment, CT should be the procedure of choice for evaluating patients clinically suspected of having acute aortic dissection. The overall accuracy of CT coupled with its ease of performance, especially in extremely ill patients, mitigates against the routine use of angiography for assessing acute dissections.

Although precise definition of the role of MR is difficult because technological improvements continue to be rapidly made, in our judgment MR is currently indicated in the following clinical settings:

1. In any stable patient for whom there is either a relative or absolute contraindication for the use of iodinated contrast medium, such as a significant history of prior allergic reaction, or renal or cardiac insufficiency. Unstable patients present difficulties in monitoring that for the present preclude their routine evaluation with MR.

2. In the evaluation of patients requiring repeated cardiovascular assessment, as, for example, patients with aortic aneurysms, including patients with Marfan's syndrome, as well as most postsurgical patients. The overall accuracy of MR in assessing postoperative complications coupled with a lack of dependence on repeated injections of intravenous contrast medium strongly favors the use of MR in these settings when available.

3. MR is clearly the imaging procedure of choice in patients with suspected developmental abnormalities, including coarctation of the aorta, both pre- and postoperatively. In these cases, the combination of multiplanar imaging and the ability to visualize coexisting cardiac abnormalities coupled with the lack of nonionizing radiation and nondependence on intravenous

contrast agents, especially for pediatric cases, makes MR the logical choice for evaluating this select population.

Angiography should be considered the procedure of choice only in patients with a history of trauma in which an aortic tear or transsection is suspected, or for patients in whom a combination of aortic and great vessel injury is suspected. In these cases, the greater accuracy of angiography, especially for visualizing branch vessels, mitigates against the use of either CT or MR. Additionally, angiography should be considered in cases in which the CT or MR has been interpreted as equivocal. The incidence of false negative CT and MR studies, while small, is sufficiently high to warrant angiography when the clinical suspicion of dissection is great.

As previously emphasized, the status of these imaging modalities, MR in particular, continues to change, making definitive judgments concerning relative efficacy difficult. No doubt decisions regarding which modality to use will be affected by the state and availability of equipment as well as variations in levels of experience. It should also be noted that the status of CT, MR, and angiography may well be affected by the increased use of newer modalities including transesophageal echocardiography (256–258).

Acquired Venous Abnormalities

Venous obstruction due to extrinsic processes is easily detected with both CT and MR (107,259–265). Most often there is direct visualization of the cause of obstruction. Superior vena cava obstruction most often results from bronchogenic carcinoma (see Fig. 39, Chapter 5). Less frequently, obstruction results from either primary mediastinal tumors, including lymphoma, thymoma, or seminoma; from metastatic disease, especially breast cancer; or even from primary angiosarcomas (Figs. 76 and 77) (263,266). On occasion, the diagnosis of superior vena caval thrombosis actually may precede the diagnosis of lung cancer (Fig. 78). Other rare causes of venous obstruction include homocystinuria, which results in diffuse calcification of vessels (Fig. 79). Superior vena caval obstruction may cause a focal area of markedly increased density to occur, usually in the anterior aspect of the right lobe of the liver (Fig. 80) (267). It has been postulated that this occurs due to the development of focal systemic-portal collaterals. Indirect signs of superior vena caval obstruction such as collateral circulation in the veins of the chest wall or azygos vein also are useful. However, it should be emphasized that venous enlargement alone should not be relied on as a sign of obstruction because it is dependent on the respiratory cycle or a Valsalva maneuver, and sometimes represents a normal variant (Fig. 81) (268).

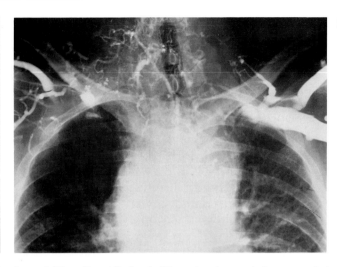

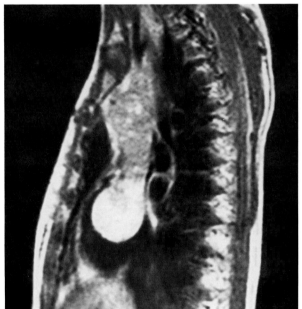

FIG. 76. Superior vena caval obstruction, thymic carcinoid. **A:** Contrast-enhanced CT section at the level of the carina shows a bulky, somewhat heterogeneous soft-tissue mass within the prevascular space obliterating the left brachiocephalic vein and invading the superior vena cava (*arrow*). There is dense opacification of the azygos vein (*curved arrow*) serving as a collateral. **B:** Coned-down view from simultaneous bilateral antecubital fossa venous injections shows complete obstruction of the brachiocephalic veins bilaterally. At surgery this proved to be a primary thymic carcinoid.

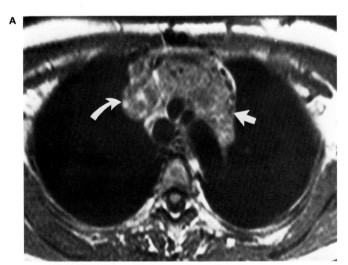

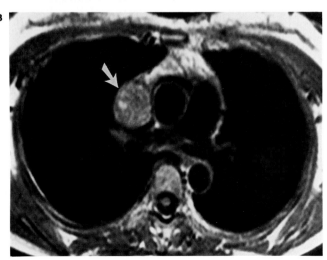

FIG. 77. Angiosarcoma. **A, B:** Axial MR images through the distal trachea and right main pulmonary artery, respectively, show a mass of intermediate signal intensity obliterating the left brachiocephalic vein (*arrow* in A), expanding the right brachiocephalic vein (*curved arrow* in A), and lying within the superior vena cava (*arrow* in B). **C:** Sagittal MR image through the superior vena cava confirms the presence of an intraluminal filling defect extending the length of the vena cava and projecting into the right atrium. At surgery this proved to be a primary angiosarcoma. A large hematoma was found covering the tip of the tumor, accounting for the difference in signal intensities between the filling defects in the brachiocephalic veins and superior vena cava, and the right atrium.

A

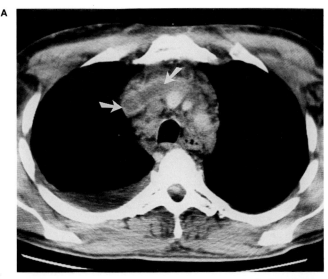

B

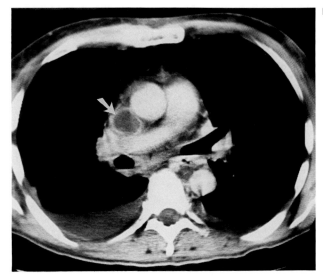

C

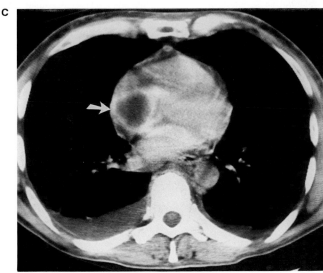

FIG. 78. Superior vena caval thrombosis, metastatic lung cancer. A–C: Sequential contrast-enhanced CT sections through the left brachiocephalic vein, the superior vena cava, and the right atrium, respectively. A well-defined filling defect is apparent (arrows in A–C) extending from the left brachiocephalic vein to the right atrium. There is considerable nodularity within the mediastinal fat, especially at the level of the great vessels. These were initially thought to represent dilated collateral mediastinal veins. Subsequent mediastinoscopy disclosed these to be metastatic lymph nodes consistent with a primary lung cancer.

Intrinsic obstruction due to thrombosis is becoming more common due to the increasing use of central venous catheters, larger bore catheters for hyperalimentation, and the increasing number of procedures involving passage of tubes into the upper body veins (Fig. 17). These include Swan-Ganz catheterization, pacemaker placement, and intravenous digital angiography (269–271). The classic signs on CT of venous thrombosis are (a) enlargement of the vein, (b) a lucent center, and (c) enhancing vein wall on contrast-enhanced studies (Fig. 77).

Initially, fresh thrombus can be as dense as flowing, contrast-enhanced blood and hence may be missed. Caution should be exercised so venous thrombosis is not diagnosed on scans obtained during or immediately after a bolus injection of contrast agent, since flow phenomena may mimic filling defects in mediastinal veins (272).

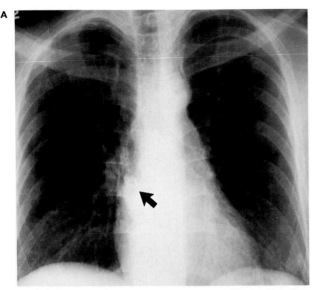

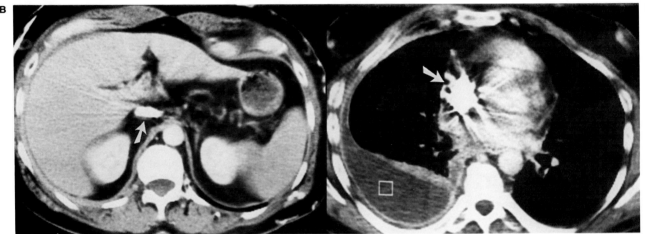

FIG. 79. Homocystinuria. **A:** Posteroanterior chest radiograph shows dense calcifications overlying the medial aspect of the right hilum, inferiorly (*arrow*). **B:** Contrast-enhanced CT section through the upper abdomen shows dense calcification with resultant obliteration of the inferior vena cava (*arrow*). Despite this, no obvious enlarged collateral veins are appreciated. **C:** Contrast-enhanced CT section through the aortic root shows dense calcification within the superior vena cava, causing streak artifacts (*arrow*). A moderate-sized right pleural fluid collection is present. This patient had documented homocystinuria.

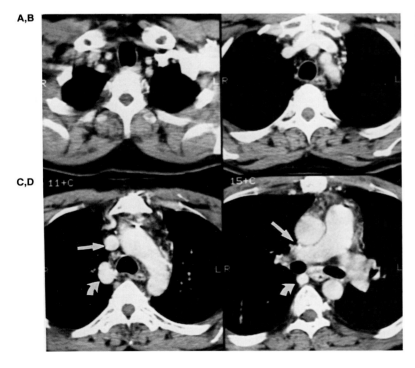

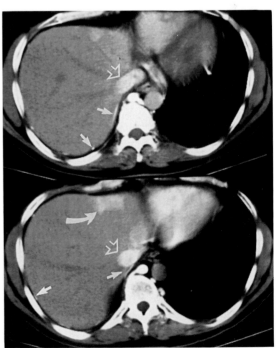

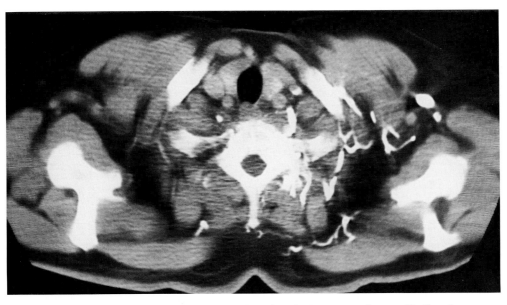

FIG. 81. Contrast-enhanced CT scan at the level of the first rib shows extensive opcaification of numerous chest wall veins. In this case there was no evidence of venous thrombosis or obstruction. Instead, contrast was administered as a bolus using a power injector. Visualization of otherwise normal chest wall veins frequently accompanies bolus administration of contrast, and need not be interpreted as abnormal.

THYMUS

Normal Thymus

CT offers an opportunity to view the thymus with much greater clarity than is provided by plain radiography or standard chest tomography. One must be aware, however, that (a) thymic morphology changes drastically with aging, and (b) in younger individuals (particularly those under the age of 25) there is a wide variation in the "normal" size and weight of the thymus gland. The CT appearance of the normal thymus has been well described for both the pediatric and adult population (273–277). (For a more detailed evaluation of the range of findings in the pediatric population, see Chapter 11.) The thymus is a bilobed structure fused at its apex near the thyroid gland and smoothly molded to the anterior aspect of the great vessels. It occupies the thyropericardic space of the anterior mediastinum and extends down to the base of the heart. The thymus is very rarely found in an ectopic location, usually the neck (278).

On conventional radiographs, the thymus seems largest in the neonate and young infant. In fact, the average weight of the thymus is 22 ± 13 g at birth and increases progressively to reach a maximum at puberty of ~34 g (279). The impression of a large thymus at younger ages stems from a higher ratio of thymic size to chest size.

Beginning at puberty, a phase of rapid involution takes place over a period of 5 to 15 years. The process of thymic involution is essentially one of progressive replacement of atrophied thymic follicles by fatty tissue. The proportion of thymic tissue to fat decreases progressively to become negligible after age 60 (280,281). In an autospy series of 20 patients over 60 years of age with myasthenia gravis, no thymus could be recognized with gross examination and only 11 had any thymic tissue seen histologically (281).

The appearances on CT of the thymus can be summarized as follows:

1. Birth to puberty: The thymus entirely fills the anterior mediastinum. It has a CT density equal to or slightly higher than muscle. Its borders are convex laterally. In this age group, it usually appears triangular or vaguely bilobed and molds the anterior aspect of the mediastinal vessels. Fat is notably lacking in this age group.

←——

FIG. 80. Superior vena caval ligation. **A–D:** Sequential contrast-enhanced scans through the mediastinum from the great vessels to the subcarinal space, respectively. The superior vena cava (*arrow* in C) has been surgically ligated just below the aortic arch (*arrow* in D). There is marked enlargement of the azygos vein (*curved arrows* in C and D) as well as enlargement of numerous small mediastinal veins, especially in the prevascular space anteriorly. **E, F:** Sequential images through the liver in the same patient as shown in A–D are shown. There is marked contrast enhancement of the azygos and hemiazygos veins. In addition, there is dense opacification of the inferior vena cava (*open arrows*) which is presumably filling through retrograde flow through intercostal and phrenic veins (*arrows* in E and F). Finally, there is an area of density in the anterior portion of the liver (*curved arrow*), probably the result of focal systemic-portal collaterals.

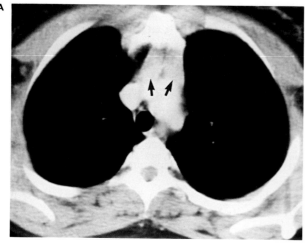

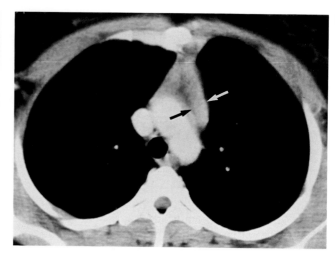

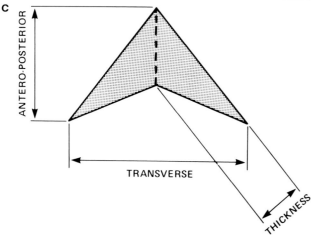

FIG. 82. Normal thymus gland, CT assessment. **A, B:** Sequential contrast-enhanced CT scans at the levels of the great vessels and aortic arch, respectively, show normal bilobed appearance of the thymus gland in a teenager (*arrows* in A). Measurements of the gland thickness are generally most useful, as indicated by the *arrows* in B. **C:** Schematic diagram of the thymus. (From Francis et al., ref. 276, with permission.)

2. Puberty to 25 years: During this phase of involution, fat appears in the anterior mediastinum. The thymus can now be recognized as a distinct triangular or bilobed structure. Typically convex with borders that are now flat or concave laterally, on occasion the thymus may still appear bilobed and slightly convex, even in this age group (Fig. 82). Its CT density usually decreases to less than that of muscle.

3. Over 25 years: With further involution, the well-defined soft-tissue–density structure previously recognized as the thymus will no longer be seen. Islands of soft-tissue density over the background of more abundant fat are noted. The speed and degree of involution are variable from subject to subject, and occasionally the thymus may still be recognized as an individual structure up to the age of 40. Finally, the anterior mediastinum appears entirely fatty. Most of the anterior mediastinal fat is contained within the fibrous skeleton of the thymus and may have a CT density slightly higher than that of subcutaneous fat.

Normal CT measurements have been defined for the thymus (Fig. 82) (273). The most meaningful is the thickness measured as the largest distance across the long axis of the gland on the CT image. Before age 20,

1.8 cm is the maximum normal for thickness, and 1.3 cm is the maximum normal thereafter. The accuracy of these dimensions recently has been confirmed by Francis et al., who also showed that although thymic thickness is a sensitive indicator of thymic abnormality, thymic shape was just as reliable in separating normal from abnormal glands, especially when the thymus was multi-lobulated (276). In fact, qualitative assessment of thymic shape alone should prove sufficient for diagnosing mass lesions of the thymus.

Thymic Enlargement

Since the thymus may weigh as much as 45–50 g in some normal younger individuals, it is difficult to certify mild degrees of thymic enlargement. However, when the thymus is manifested as a mediastinal mass readily detectable on plain chest roentgenography in older children or young adults, it can be considered to be enlarged. Hyperthyroidism is a condition that may be responsible for thymic enlargement (279). Less common associations are acromegaly, Addison's disease, and children recovering from burns (282). Occasionally a thymus weighing over 50 g will be biopsied or resected in a teenage subject (largely because malignant lymphoma cannot be excluded), only to discover an enlarged thymus with a normal histologic appearance.

Thymic Hyperplasia

Thymic germinal or lymphoid follicular hyperplasia (LFH) is a term used by pathologists to describe a gland that demonstrates numerous active, lymphoid germinal centers in the medulla (279). Although lymphoid follicles are often present in the medulla of the normal thymus, particularly in younger individuals, in myasthenia gravis the thymus often exhibits a distinctive proliferation of germinal centers. Unfortunately, although thymic enlargement may be identified in patients with LFH, the role of CT in detecting this abnormality is limited (283,284). Castleman and Norris have shown that in myasthenia gravis, total thymic weight of glands with germinal hyperplasia does not differ significantly from that of normal controls (285). Indeed, in our experience, it is not unusual for a thymus appearing entirely normal on CT surgically to contain germinal hyperplasia. In one large series with CT-pathologic correlation, glands with hyperplasia typically appeared larger than those of age-matched controls. However, based on diffuse enlargement of the gland, CT proved only 71% sensitive for diagnosing lymphoid hyperplasia (284).

Thymomas are rare before age 20. In patients aged 20–30, although theoretically it may not be possible to distinguish between thymic hyperplasia (with a slightly enlarged gland) and a small thymoma, to date, clinically, this has not proven to be a significant problem.

Thymoma

If glandular enlargement is grossly asymmetric (the left lobe is normally larger than the right and the gland is always slightly asymmetric) or if a lobular contour is seen, a thymic mass should be suspected. The most common primary thymic tumor is thymoma. This designation is limited to neoplasms originating from the thymic epithelium (286). The CT appearance of thymomas has been well described (276,284,287–294). On CT, thymomas appear as homogeneous soft-tissue density; oval, round, or lobulated mass; and usually sharply demarcated. Most often the tumor grows asymmetrically to one side of the anterior mediastinum (Fig. 83). Rarely, thymomas may actually be cystic, with discrete

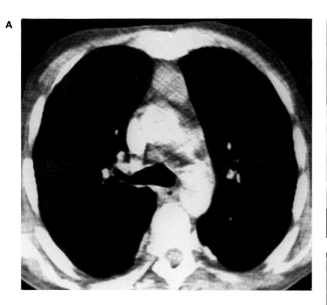
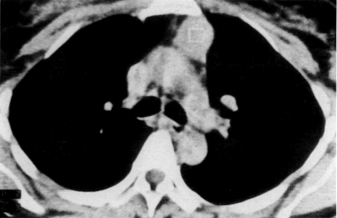
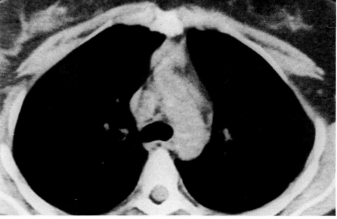

FIG. 83. Benign thymomas in patients with myasthenia gravis. **A:** 70-year-old man. There is an obvious solid, spherical mass in the anterior mediastinum surrounded by anterior mediastinal fat. **B:** 45-year-old woman. A solid, spherical mass can be identified bulging into the fat in the anterior mediastinum. The attenuation value within the mass is similar to that of the chest wall muscles. **C:** 39-year-old woman. The diagnosis of thymoma in this case is slightly more difficult because of a relative paucity of mediastinal fat. Key features are the spherical appearance of the lesion and the age of the patient.

A 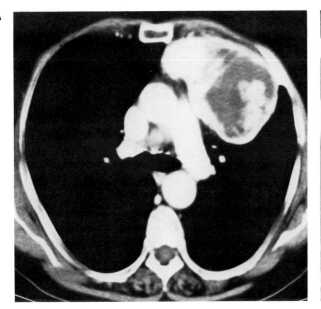 B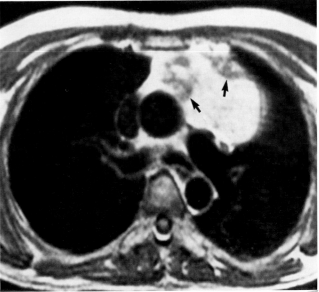

FIG. 84. Cystic thymoma. A: Contrast-enhanced CT scan shows a well-defined partially cystic mass in the anterior mediastinum within which distinct soft-tissue nodules can be seen. Biopsy proved cystic thymoma. B: MR image in a patient different than in A shows a heterogeneous high-signal intensity mass in the anterior mediastinum within which discrete nodules of intermediate signal intensity can be identified (*arrows*). Although most thymomas are solid, occasional thymomas prove to be at least partially cystic. High-signal intensity within the mass proved to be secondary to complex cystic fluid and not fat. Cystic thymoma was surgically documented.

nodular components (Fig. 84). The tumor usually enhances homogeneously after contrast medium injection, and not uncommonly may contain calcium. Despite some degree of initial controversy, using these criteria, CT has proven extremely accurate in diagnosing thymic neoplasms (Table 4). In the study reported by Chen et al. CT proved 91% sensitive and 97% specific in establishing the presence of a mass within the thymus (284). Of 34 patients with a CT diagnosis of a mass or neoplasm, all save one proved surgically to have either a thymoma (n = 31), thymic cyst (n = 1), or Hodgkin's disease (n = 1). Similar results have been reported by others (293,294).

Thirty percent of thymomas are malignant. Traditionally thymomas have been classified as predominantly epithelial, predominantly lymphocytic, and mixed lymphoepithelial, regardless of cytologic abnormalities identified within neoplastic epithelial cells (286,295). Using this classification, the histologic appearance of thymoma does not allow a reliable differentiation between benign and malignant thymoma; this can only be established by documenting the presence of tumor growth into or through the capsule. Recently, an alternate classification of thymoma has been suggested by Marino and Muller-Hermelink that categorizes thymomas as either cortical, medullary, or mixed, based on both morphology and histogenesis (296). This classification may have significant predictive value. As reported by Ricci et al., in their study of 74 cases of thymoma, those classified as medullary proved to be benign tumors arising late in life, with no associated mortality (297). In

distinction, cortical thymomas usually presented earlier in life and were associated with a 50% mortality at 5 years despite aggressive therapy.

Characteristically, malignant thymomas infiltrate adjacent structures or develop distal implants on the pleura or pericardium; malignant thymoma rarely metastasizes outside the thorax (Fig. 85). This neoplasm grows (a) to invade local mediastinal structures, including the superior vena cava, great vessels, and even the

TABLE 4. *Thymoma vs normal thymus: CT criteria*

Thymoma
1. Patient over 30
2. Mass spherical or lobulated with rounded margins
3. Attenuation of mass equals or exceeds muscle of chest wall
4. Lesion surrounded by fat
5. Calcified
6. Unilateral or midline

Normal thymus
1. Patient under 20
2. "Mass" elongated with length > width, as is typical of a normal lobe of thymus
3. "Mass" diffusely infiltrated with fat, seen much better with lower window setting
4. Paucity of thymic fat: hence lesion represents thymus with delayed involution
5. No calcification
6. Bilateral soft-tissue prominence (both lobes of thymus) seen in usual location of thymic lobes

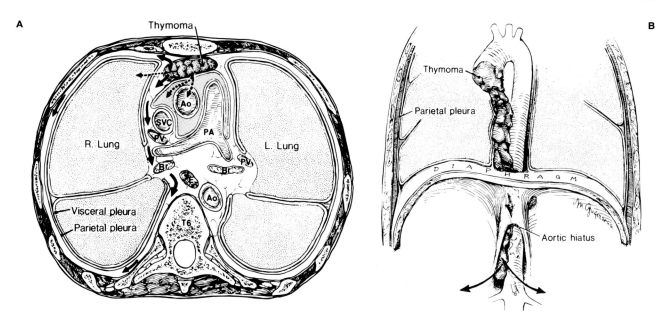

FIG. 85. A,B: The pattern of spread of invasive thymomas is graphically represented. In cross-section (f), the tumor can directly invade surrounding structures (*broken arrows*) or insinuate itself between the chest wall or mediastinum and the parietal pleura (*solid arrows*). Once the para-aortic—paraspinal area is reached (g), inferior extension through the aortic or esophageal hiatus can occur. With CT, such extension can be seen reliably and the study should always be extended to the upper abdomen. Ao, aorta; PA, pulmonary artery; PV, pulmonary vein; Br, bronchus; E, esophagus; SVC, superior vena cava. From Zerhouni et al., ref. 298, with permission.

airways; (b) to invade the adjacent lungs or chest wall; or (c) to spread by contiguity along pleural reflections, usually on one side of the chest cavity only, potentially seeding even the diaphragmatic surfaces with consequent direct extension into the abdomen (286,295,298–302). Thus, "invasive" is a more appropriate designation than "malignant" for this tumor.

Invasive thymomas can be classified into three stages: Stage 1, intact capsule or growth within capsule only; Stage 2, pericapsular growth into mediastinal fat; and Stage 3, invasive growth of surrounding organs and pleural implants at a distance from the primary mass. Surgery is indicated in all three stages, with supplemental radiotherapy in Stage 2 and radiotherapy plus chemotherapy in Stage 3 (303–305).

The spectrum of CT findings in patients with invasive thymomas is illustrated in Figure 86. With CT, caution should be used to avoid overdiagnosing invasion. As with other tumors, direct contact and absence of cleavage planes are not strictly reliable criteria to predict invasion. On the other hand, clear delineation of fat planes surrounding a thymoma should be interpreted as indicating an absence of extensive local invasion, especially when the study is performed with thin sections following a bolus of intravenous contrast medium (294). Invasive thymomas growing along pleural surfaces can reach the posterior mediastinum and extend downward along the

aorta to involve the crus of the diaphragm and the retroperitoneum. These areas are "hidden" in conventional studies, but CT excels at demonstrating these sites of involvement (Figs. 85 and 86) (298,299). A full CT examination of the thorax extended to the upper abdomen should be performed in these patients.

Metastases are apt to be silent since only a minority of patients with invasive thymomas present with symptoms from intrathoracic spread. CT provides invaluable guidance for the radiotherapist and chemotherapist to adjust their treatment plans.

Thymus and Myasthenia Gravis

The association of thymic pathology and myasthenia gravis is the clinical issue most relevant to thymic imaging.

Cures and remissions can be observed in patients with myasthenia gravis following thymic removal with or without a thymoma. To date, there is no convincing evidence to suggest that systematic removal of the thymus, whether normal or abnormal, improves outcome in patients who are medically well controlled. When medical therapy fails, it is generally agreed that surgery is indicated, regardless of thymic status. In this setting, effective therapy necessitates complete removal

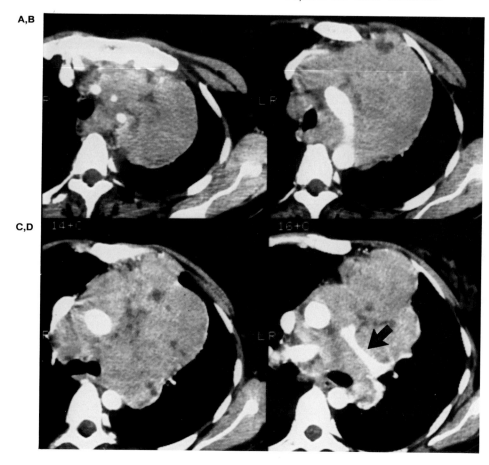

FIG. 86. The spectrum of invasive thymoma, CT findings. **A–D:** Sequential contrast-enhanced CT sections through the mediastinum show a bulky, nonhomogeneous soft-tissue mass deeply invading the mediastinum with encasement of all the great vessels as well as the left main pulmonary artery (*arrow* in D).

of all thymic tissue. Because surgical-anatomic studies have shown that gross and microscopic thymic tissue is widely distributed throughout the mediastinum, it has been suggested that en bloc transcervical-transsternal "maximal" thymectomy be performed (306).

Thymoma occurs in 15% of patients with myasthenia gravis. The patients most likely to benefit from thymectomy, in terms of disease control, are young females with a disease of short duration. Older patients rarely benefit from thymectomy. However, because thymoma is invasive in 30% of cases, surgical removal is indicated in all patients to eliminate the risk of malignancy, regardless of surgery's effect on the course of myasthenia.

The role of the radiologist, then, is to identify those patients with thymomas who require surgery. The apparent difficulty in this task is distinguishing hyperplasia from thymoma (Fig. 87). Sixty-five percent of patients with myasthenia gravis have thymic hyperplasia. This problem is compounded by the normally large thymic size in patients younger than 25 years old. However, thymomas are extremely rare in this population, and, unless very obvious, we would not make this diagnosis

in this age group (287,290,292,293,307,308). Over the age of 40, the diagnosis on CT of thymoma usually poses no problem. In the intermediate range, from 25 to 40 years, the thymus may be normally present and, unless a definite mass-like structure is seen (which is usually the case), a definite diagnosis cannot be made. It should be noted that invasive thymomas, our main concern, are such slow, locally growing tumors having little potential for distant metastases that, if in doubt, follow-up CT examinations can be safely recommended. The clinical information and CT features that are most helpful in distinguishing between a thymoma and a prominent but normal thymus are summarized in Table 4 and illustrated in Figures 83, 87, and 88.

A positive diagnosis on CT of hyperplasia is not very relevent to clinical decision-making since poor clinical response determines the need for thymic resection regardless of the presence of hyperplasia. Hyperplasia cannot reliably be excluded either, because it is a purely histologic diagnosis and the gland is not always enlarged. Up to 50% of the thymuses called normal on CT may prove to be hyperplastic at surgery (307).

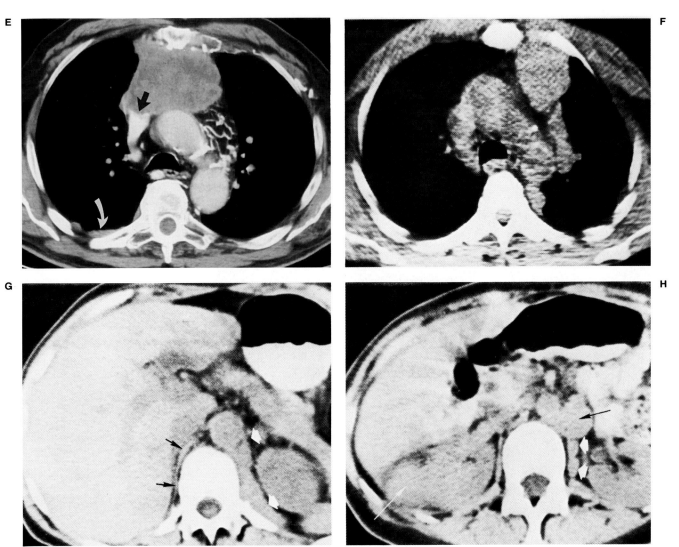

FIG. 86. *(Continued.)* **E:** Contrast-enhanced CT section through the carina in another patient shows a lobulated, slightly heterogeneous soft-tissue mass that is invading the adjacent superior vena cava *(arrow)*. Markedly enlarged collateral vessels can be identified in the region of the aorticopulmonary window draining into the hemiazygos and azygos veins. Pleural implants, not appreciated on the accompanying chest radiograph (not shown), are apparent on the right side *(curved arrow)* (cf. Fig. 76). **F–H:** CT sections at the level of the aortic arch and the hemidiaphragms, respectively, in another patient with documented invasive thymoma. The tumor has an irregular, lobulated contour. Poor definition of the interface between the tumor and the chest wall due to invasion is noted. Invasive thymomas grow by contiguous spread, and a tongue of tumor tissue extends along the pleuromediastinal surface on the left side to reach the para-aortic region. From there it can extend inferiorly to reach the diaphragm *(white arrows* in G [to be compared with the normal contralateral crus *(black arrows* in G)]). Further contiguous extension may lead to tumor growth into the retroperitoneum *(arrows* in H).

Thymic Masses: Differential Diagnosis

In addition to thymoma, a number of other malignancies may arise within the thymus gland, most notably lymphoma. In a recent review of a large series of patients with documented Hodgkin's disease, Heron et al. documented that the thymus is involved prior to therapy initiation in 30% and in patients with documented relapses in 38% (309). Significantly, however, thymic involvement was always accompanied by involvement of mediastinal lymph nodes; in no case did a patient with Hodgkin's disease present with thymic involvement alone.

Thymic cysts also frequently occur in association with mediastinal lymphoma. Usually reported following radiation therapy for Hodgkin's disease (310,311), it has been suggested that thymic cysts may arise as a consequence of primary thymic involvement, or alternatively that they are incidental preexisting lesions, probably congenital in origin (see Fig. 8, Chapter 11) (312–314). An association between thymic cysts and prior thoracotomy has also been noted (315).

In addition to lymphoma, other mediastinal tumors that may involve and/or arise from the thymus include neuroendocrine tumors, specifically thymic carcinoid tumors and metastases, especially from primary lung

A
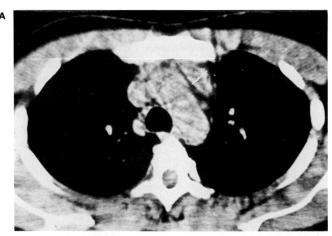

B
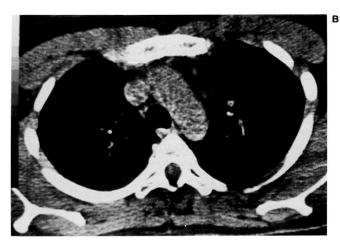

C
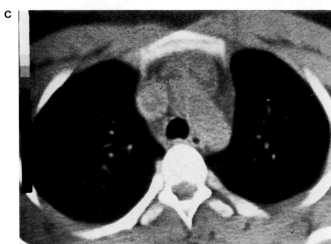

FIG. 87. Prominent thymus in patients with myasthenia gravis, no thymoma. **A:** 24-year-old man. The structure in the anterior mediastinum was considered to be a prominent left lobe of the thymus rather than a thymoma because of its elongated appearance. As determined from the image (*white line*), the width measured 1.5 cm. **B:** Same patient as in A, 1 year later. The left lobe of the thymus has been replaced by fat. **C:** Prominent thymus in a 21-year-old man. Thymoma was considered unlikely because of the patient's age and the lower attenuation of the thymus due to fatty infiltration. Note that the muscles of the chest wall have a higher attenuation than the thymus.

A
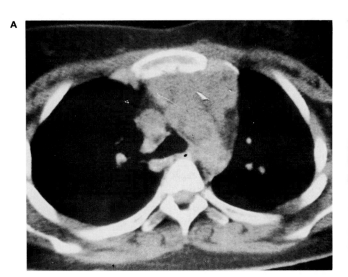

B
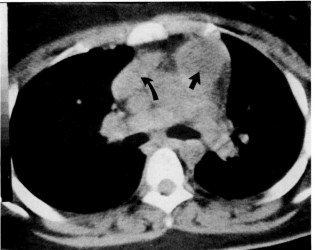

FIG. 88. Prominent thymus in myasthenia gravis due to hyperthyroidism. **A:** CT section at the level of the aortic arch shows a prominent thymus in a 28-year-old woman. The appearance initially suggests a possible thymoma. **B:** CT section just below that shown in A demonstrates prominence of both the right (*arrow*) and left (*curved arrow*) lobes of the thymus. Enlargement of both lobes would be distinctly unusual in thymoma. In this case, the enlarged thymus was attributable to concurrent hyperthyroidism.

and breast carcinomas (Fig. 76) (316). Rarer tumors, including lymphangiomas and hemangiomas, have also been reported, especially in children (see Fig. 8, Chapter 11) (317,318). Simple lymphangiomas and hemangiomas composed of capillary-sized, thin-walled channels may appear as solid masses; cavernous and cystic lymphangiomas or hemangiomas, in distinction, demonstrate a more complex anatomy, with cystic and solid areas allowing their differentiation from thymomas (Fig. 86).

Another unusual cause of thymic enlargement is a thymolipoma (Fig. 39). This rare, intrathymic neoplasm can grow down to involve the cardiophrenic angles and, as a rule, is asymptomatic. There is no known association with myasthenia gravis. On CT the tumor appears almost entirely fatty, with some areas of inhomogeneity. Radiographically they have been mistaken as cardiomegaly, pleural or pericardial tumors, basal atelectasis, and even pulmonary sequestration (222). Despite attaining a large size, thymolipomas do not compress or invade surrounding structures (319).

Thymic Rebound

The thymus involutes during periods of stress. The gland sustains a variable decrease in volume depending on the age of the patient and the severity and duration of the stress. The phenomenon is most marked in young children, but it has also been observed in young adults. The thymus will generally re-acquire its premorbid size several months following the stressful episode. It may exhibit "rebound" growth to a size significantly larger than its baseline status (Fig. 89). Gelfand et al. found enlargement of the thymus detected by plain chest roentgenography in five children aged 5 to 12 following recovery from burns (282). Also largely using chest roentgenography, Cohen et al. illustrated rebound thymic growth in seven children aged 3 to 11 who had received chemotherapy for 5 months to 3 years for Wilms' tumor (n = 2), malignant lymphoma (n = 2), osteosarcoma, malignant teratoma, and acute lymphatic leukemia (320). In three cases, a prominent thymus was observed in the course of chemotherapy; in the remaining four patients the changes were detected 1 to 9 months after cessation of therapy.

Since CT is more sensitive than plain chest roentgenography in detecting thymic enlargement, thymic rebound is detected with greater frequency when patients are monitored with CT (Fig. 89). Using CT, Choyke et al. made serial observations of the mediastinum in a group of patients aged 2 to 35 who were receiving chemotherapy for various malignancies including Hodgkin's disease (n = 6), osteosarcoma (n = 5), testicular

neoplasms (n = 4), Wilms' tumor (n- = 3), and rhabdomyosarcoma (n = 2) (321). An average 43% decrease in thymic volume in response to a course of chemotherapy was observed. Thymic volume was regularly observed to be restored on follow-up studies, and 25% of patients exhibited a rebound in recovery with the volume of the gland exceeding the baseline volume by 50%. Thymic rebound as visualized by CT has also been reported after treatment of Cushing's syndrome (322).

In most patients with extrathoracic malignancies, thymic rebound is unlikely to cause concern or confusion. As a practical matter, the phenomenon is most pertinent when it is observed in patients with malignant lymphoma treated with chemotherapy. When an enlarged thymus is seen in such patients, does it represent thymic rebound or recurrent lymphoma? In our experience, when a patient with lymphoma has a prominent thymus as an isolated finding with no adenopathy, it is reasonable to follow the patient conservatively with the presumption that thymic rebound is occurring (Fig. 90). In the study of Kissin et al., there was a suggestion that thymic rebound may be a favorable prognostic factor in that 13 of 14 patients with thymic enlargement after chemotherapy were free of disease after a mean follow-up of 45 months (323).

MR Evaluation of Thymic Pathology

The role of MR in the evaluation of the thymus is limited (Fig. 84). The MR appearance of the normal gland in both children and adults has been described (see Fig. 4, Chapter 11) (324–326). Characteristically, the thymus appears homogeneous, with intermediate signal intensity on T1-weighted images. The appearance of the gland is dependent to some degree on age; in patients under 30 years of age, differentiation between the thymus and adjacent mediastinal fat is somewhat easier than in older patients, where it is presumably secondary to progressive fatty replacement with age. The T2 relaxation times of the thymus are similar to fat at all ages, making visualization of the gland more difficult than on T1-weighted images (325). Occasionally the signal intensity characteristics of normal thymic tissue may be of value in identifying unusual configurations of the thymus, especially in children in whom posterior mediastinal extension between the superior vena cava and trachea is not uncommon (327). MR signal characteristics have also been reported useful in diagnosing a patient with a mediastinal thymolipoma, which not surprisingly appeared as a fatty thymic tumor (328).

The appearance of the thymus in patients with myasthenia gravis has been described and appears limited. In a study of 16 patients with myasthenia gravis studied

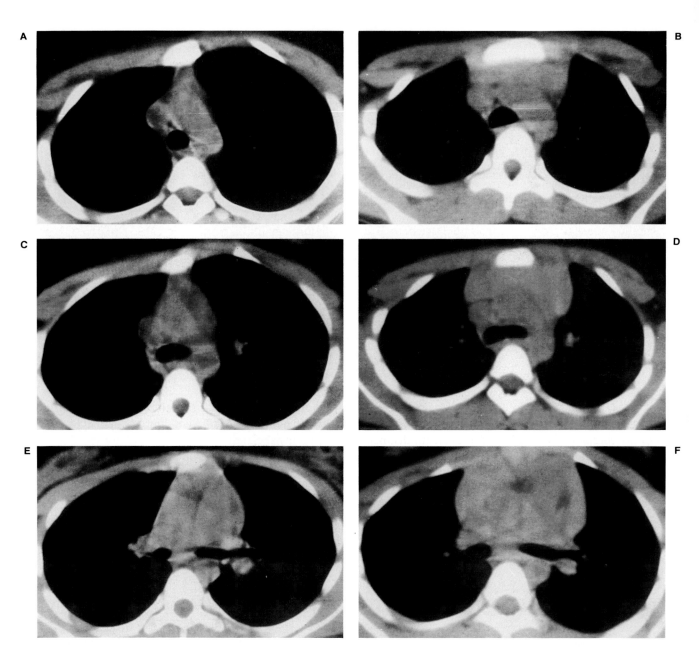

FIG. 89. Thymic rebound, osteogenic sarcoma. **A–C:** Sequential CT sections through the mediastinum in a 10-year-old girl with osteogenic sarcoma treated with chemotherapy show marked thymic involution. **D–F:** Sequential CT sections at the same levels as shown in A–C, 4 months later. Note marked thymic rebound with enlargement of both the right and left lobes of the gland.

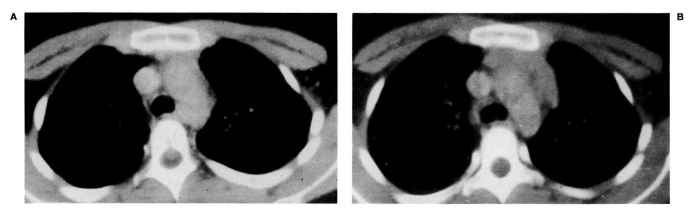

FIG. 90. Thymic rebound, lymphoma. **A:** 10-year-old girl with thymic involution following chemotherapy for malignant lymphoma. **B:** Follow-up CT obtained 8 months later shows enlargement of both lobes of the thymus without adenopathy.

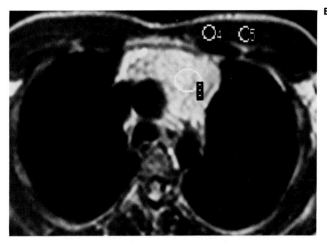

FIG. 91. Thymoma, MR assessment. **A:** T1-weighted MR image at the level of the carina shows a homogeneous soft-tissue mass of intermediate signal intensity within the anterior mediastinum (cf. Fig. 12). **B:** T2-weighted MR image at the same level as shown in A. There is considerable signal enhancement within the mass that is now more difficult to differentiate from adjacent mediastinal fat. This appearance is entirely nonspecific (compare with Fig. 55B). Biopsy proved thymoma.

with both CT and MR who subsequently underwent thymectomy, MR provided little if any distinctive information as compared with CT. Specifically, no distinctive MR features could be identified in patients with thymomas apart from morphologic identification of a mass (Fig. 12; Fig. 91) (329). In seven patients with a histologic diagnosis of thymic hyperplasia, both CT and MR displayed normal thymic morphology in five patients, and an enlarged and a small thymus in one case

each, respectively. Unfortunately, MR signal intensities were of no value in differentiating thymic hyperplasia from normal glands.

One important exception in which MR has proven valuable is in identifying vascular invasion, especially in patients for whom intravenous contrast cannot be administered (107). In these cases, MR exquisitely delineates the extent of vascular involvement, including identification of intracardiac disease extension (Fig. 92).

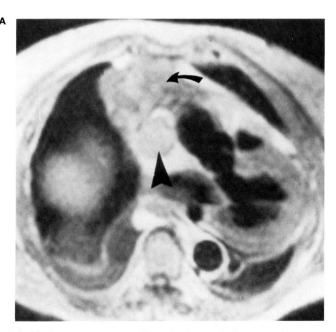
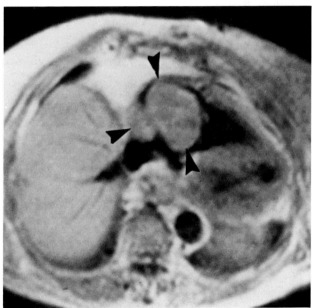

FIG. 92. Invasive thymoma, MR evaluation. **A, B:** Sequential MR images through the heart show a poorly marginated mass of intermediate signal intensity within the anterior mediastinum (*curved arrow* in A) which is directly invading the superior mediastinum (*arrowhead* in A). The mass extends into the right atrium and can be seen crossing the tricuspid valve plane to enter the right ventricle (*arrowheads* in B). A moderate-sized right pleural fluid collection is present as well. Invasive thymoma was surgically documented.

LYMPHOMA

Lymphoma is the seventh most frequent cause of cancer death in the United States, with about 40,000 cases diagnosed yearly. Lymphomas are primary neoplasms of the lymphoreticular system and are classified in two main types: Hodgkin's disease (HD) and non-Hodgkin's lymphoma (NHL). Although Hodgkin's disease is the less common of the two types, representing about 25–30% of cases, in the mediastinum it is more common than NHL. Fifty to eighty percent of patients with HD present with mediastinal adenopathy (Figs. 46 and 47) (330). The highest frequency of mediastinal involvement is in young women with nodular sclerosing HD. The mediastinum is involved in fewer than 20% of patients with NHL although up to 40% of these patients may present with some thoracic manifestation at some point in the evolution of the disease. Involvement of anterior mediastinal, paratracheal, and hilar nodes is three to four times more common with HD than with NHL. Involvement of paracardiac and posterior mediastinal nodal groups is almost exclusively seen with NHL (see Fig. 48) (331). It should be emphasized that the appearance on CT of lymphomatous nodes in itself is not distinctive; the size and appearance of the nodes span the entire spectrum, from well-defined nodes to diffuse extensive involvement (332).

Interestingly, involvement of internal mammary nodes is 10 times more common in HD than in NHL (331). Hilar adenopathy in the absence of detectable mediastinal adenopathy is unusual. Direct extension of lymphoma from the mediastinum to the lung or the chest wall is rather common with large mediastinal masses (333).

HD is believed by most to be unifocal in origin and typically spreads by contiguity to involve adjacent lymph node groups first (334). Skipped areas are therefore unlikely and if areas contiguous to the mediastinum such as the lower neck or upper abdomen are not involved by HD, it is not generally necessary to scan more distant areas such as the pelvis. In contrast, both abdomen and pelvis, as well as the neck region, must be scanned in all patients with NHL, as noncontiguous spread is common (NHL is assumed to be multi-focal in nature). Scanning in patients with mediastinal lymphoma should always be extended to the upper abdomen. Intra-abdominal periaortic adenopathy can be found in 25% of patients with HD and 49% of those with NHL (335). The spleen is involved in 37% of patients with HD and 41% of those with NHL. The liver is involved in only 8% of patients with HD and in 14% of patients with NHL at initial diagnosis. It is important to note that there is no strong correlation between liver size and liver involvement. Fewer than 30% of patients with HD with hepatic involvement at autopsy have detectable hepatomegaly at clinical examination. On the other hand, only 57% of patients with NHL and hepatomegaly demonstrate liver lymphoma at histologic examination. Thus, CT or MR demonstration of liver enlargement has no diagnostic value. Likewise, spleen size evaluation is of limited value. Lymphomatous deposits presenting as solitary or multiple abnormalities are the most reliable evidence of involvement with either CT or MR. In one series, almost two-thirds of tumor nodules involving the spleen were less than 1 cm in diameter, rendering their detection difficult on both CT and MR (336).

With the advent of CT, the detection of all thoracic manifestations of lymphomas has become significantly less of a diagnostic challenge. On the other hand, with the development of effective therapies based on the aggressive use of chemotherapeutic agents and irradiation, there has been an increasing demand for accurate means of monitoring the response of lymphoma to therapy. Indeed, a critical requirement of effective therapy is the availability of methods for assessing the disease status throughout the course of therapy. To date, CT has played a major role in the surveillance of patients undergoing therapy for lymphoma. Reduction of tumor bulk is satisfactorily monitored with CT. However, partial size regression is often observed, especially with nodular sclerosing HD. In some cases, such residual masses consist of fibrotic residual tissue with no active lymphomatous component, or so-called "sterilized" lymphoma (337). In other cases, active residual disease may still be present. This problem represents a significant clinical dilemma. Prior to the CT era, partial size regression was thought to occur in a minority of patients. More recent series indicate that this problem may occur in up to 88% of patients with HD and in up to 40% of patients with NHL (338–340).

Masses containing active tumor cannot be distinguished from "sterilized" masses by CT, since their density is identical. Biopsies are often unproductive in such cases since marked atypical cytological changes from chemotherapy or radiotherapy are the rule and prevent accurate diagnosis unless a large portion of the mass is removed. This frequent clinical problem has prompted the search for new methods capable of differentiating residual inactive masses from residual active masses.

The presence of residual mass is always of concern because over half of these patients will exhibit recurrence, most often at the site of the residual mass. Thus, close monitoring of these masses is required (341–343). A major problem in the management of lymphoma is incomplete regression of the lymphomatous mass despite presumably effective therapy (344–350). HD and up to 40% of patients with NHL (338–340,350). The clinician is limited to size monitoring when assessing these residual masses. However, size monitoring alone is not always sensitive as the rate of decrease in size is different among patients, and varies with the size of the initial mass, its site, histology, and type of treatment (351–353). CT density being identical for both active and inactive residual lymphomatous masses is of limited value. Recently promising results have been reported with gallium-67 imaging, which presumably monitors tumor cell viability (354,355). Ongoing research indicates that monitoring thymidine metabolism with positron emission tomography may also be helpful (356).

No criteria exist to predict which residual masses will eventually recur. Initial size of the mass correlates somewhat with the likelihood of recurrence. Interestingly, likelihood of recurrence has been found to be higher if the signal intensity of the initial mass is high on T2-weighted MR images (352). These masses are not always benign as resistance to treatment can occur and the relapse rate of patients presenting with residual masses approaches 50% and is more than twice that of patients without partial regression (351). In a series of patients restaged surgically following initial therapy of NHL, residual masses showed an incidence of 20%, with persistent disease and relapses occurring mainly in areas of previous involvement.

MR Evaluation of Lymphoma

As discussed in Chapter 1, the basis for the signal intensity differences exhibited by tissues in MR is fundamentally different from that of density differences in CT. Barring the presence of a high atomic number element such as calcium or iodine, CT density is directly related to physical density of tissues. Since most tissues except for fat have similar physical densities, it is not generally possible to distinguish them effectively without the use of contrast agents. In the case of lymphoma, there exists no significant difference between the CT density of fibrosis and that of active lymphoma. On the other hand, MR signal intensity is related to different properties of tissues (357,358). In simplified terms, relaxation times appear essentially dependent on the proportion of water and proteins as well as the type of proteins within a given tissue. (For a more complete discussion of these principles, see Chapter 1). Lymphomatous cells contain a larger amount of water, with a relatively lower proportion of proteins. Conversely, fibrosis contains much less water and a high proportion of highly polymerized proteins. The different compositions of lymphoma and fibrosis lead to markedly different T2 relaxation times (358). The histology of lymphoma is generally biphasic with various proportions of cells and connective tissue. For example, in nodular sclerosing HD, large amounts of sclerosis can be seen interspersed with malignant cells (Fig. 93). Conversely, in diffuse NHL, the histology may be composed almost completely of malignant cells without significant collagenous component.

Several studies have demonstrated that residual inactive masses from "sterilized" lymphoma are essentially composed of fibrosis. It is therefore reasonable to suspect that some changes in the signal intensity pattern may be perceived during the evolution of a lymphoma. This hypothesis has been the basis of research in the potential utilization of MR to monitor partially regressed lymphomatous mass (341). As demonstrated in Figure 93, differences in the histologic composition of lymphoma are paralleled by differences in the signal intensity pattern of the lesion. By systematically studying a series of patients with lymphoma, characteristic signal patterns have been defined on T2-weighted images (343). These are:

1. The homogeneous hyperintense pattern. This is characteristic of untreated lymphoma (Fig. 94). In these cases, the lymphoma demonstrates a homogeneous low signal intensity similar to that of muscle on T1-weighted images. A high signal intensity similar to that of surrounding fat is noted on T2-weighted images. This pattern is never seen in inactive residual lymphomatous masses.

2. Heterogeneous patterns with mixed hyper- and hypointensity. This pattern is characterized by a homogeneous low signal intensity on T1-weighted images and heterogeneous signal intensity on T2-weighted images characterized by interspersed areas of high and low signal. This pattern can be seen in untreated sclerosing HD where the low-signal areas are presumed to represent sclerotic regions of the tumor (Fig. 95). It is most commonly seen during the response phase of most lymphomas with the high signal areas presumably representing residual active lymphomatous masses or areas of necrosis and inflammation. The low signal areas represent presumably fibrotic tissue (Fig. 93).

An important caveat to be aware of in masses presenting a heterogeneous pattern on T2-weighted images is the possibility that mediastinal fat interspersed with residual fibrotic tissue may be responsible for this pattern. Indeed, it is commonly observed that mediastinal lymphomas may regress in a pattern that will lead to "pulling in" of surrounding mediastinal fat, leading to an appearance of "dirty" fat on CT images. Since fat has a high signal intensity on T2-weighted images, it may mimic a case of active lymphoma. However, these fibro-fatty masses are easy to recognize on T1-weighted images since the fat portions of the lesions will also exhibit high signal intensity. The important corollary is that analysis of signal intensity of lymphomas requires that both the T1-weighted and T2-weighted images of the same region be analyzed. Thus, active residual areas of lymphoma, necrosis, or inflammation can only be

A

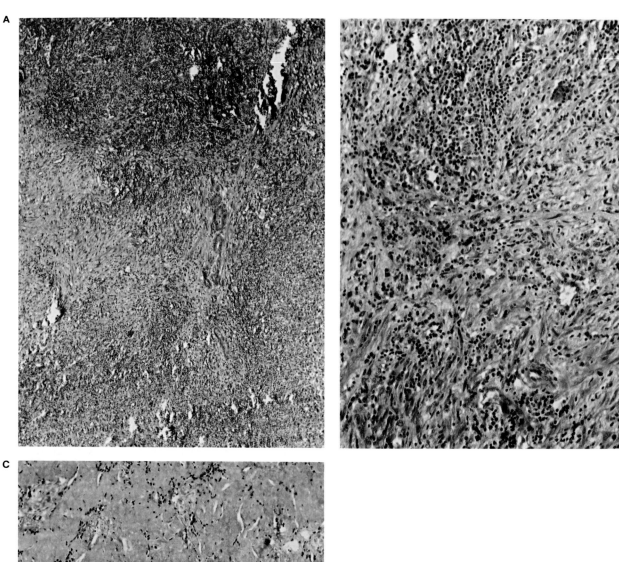

B

C

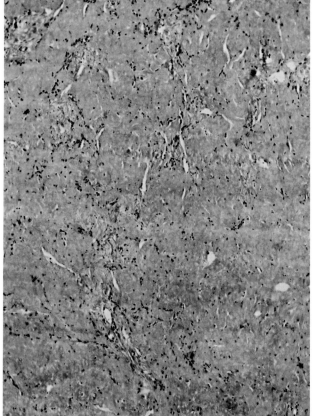

FIG. 93. Histologic changes before and after therapy of nodular sclerosing Hodgkin's lymphoma. **A:** Islands of highly cellular tissue are interspersed among more fibrotic, relatively hypocellular areas. Low-power photomicrograph of nodular sclerosing Hodgkin's lymphoma demonstrates typical biphasic histology with areas of predominant sclerosis with paucity of malignant cells and areas of malignant cell infiltrations. **B:** Higher magnification of A shows predominance of malignant cells with interspersed connective tissue components. **C:** After therapy, repeat surgical biopsy of residual mass demonstrates cell necrosis with marked hypocellularity and extensive sclerosis, presumably representing the residual fibrous component of the tumor. MR imaging of the lesion at the time of biopsy illustrated in A demonstrated a slightly heterogeneous pattern with predominantly high signal intensity on T2-weighted images. At time of biopsy in C, homogeneously low signal intensity was noted on T2-weighted images. Thus, MR appears to track, to some degree, the changes in relative proportion of cellular and fibrotic components within lymphomas because relaxation times of fibrosis and malignant cells are markedly different.

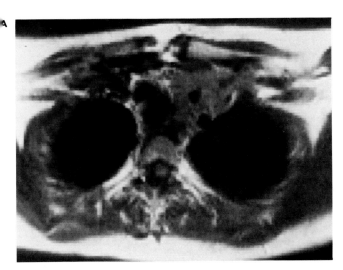

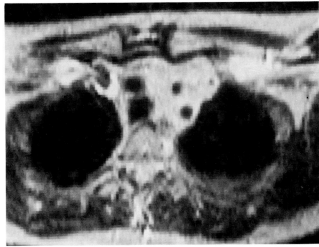

FIG. 94. Mediastinal lymphoma, MR assessment pretreatment. **A:** T1-weighted image through the mediastinum shows a mass of homogeneously low-signal intensity. **B:** T2-weighted image at the same level as A shows homogeneously high-signal intensity.

diagnosed if high signal intensity is seen on T2-weighted images, but low signal intensity is seen on T1-weighted images in the same region. A more elegant solution to this problem is the use of new pulse sequences with selective fat suppression. These new pulse sequences are now being employed and appear likely to improve the specificity of the technique.

3. Homogeneous, hypointense pattern. This pattern is characteristic of inactive residual fibrotic masses following successful therapy for lymphoma. These lesions are characterized by low signal intensity on T1-weighted images and homogeneously low signal intensity on T2-weighted images.

In our experience, monitoring the signal intensity of lymphoma by MR benefits management of the residual mass in the following ways:

1. A qualitative measure of response can be derived. In patients with a decrease in mass size and corresponding homogeneous decrease in signal intensity, favorable response can be expected.

2. Decrease in size with a persistent homogeneous hyperintense or heterogeneous hyperintense pattern suggests partial response. However, an important caveat in this group of patients is the fact that inflammation

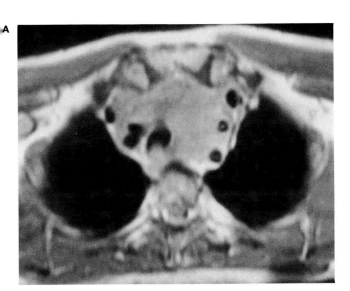

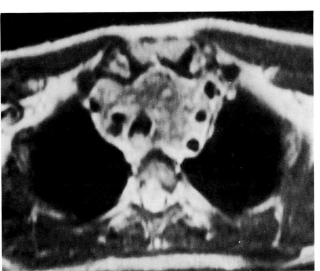

FIG. 95. 48-year-old patient with newly diagnosed Hodgkin's disease. **A:** Proton density image shows mass in superior mediastinum. **B:** T2-weighted image demonstrates a heterogeneous pattern with mixed areas of high and low signal intensity. This is typical of nodular sclerosing Hodgkin's disease with its biphasic histology comprising fibrotic areas interspersed with more cellular areas.

A

B

C

D

E

F

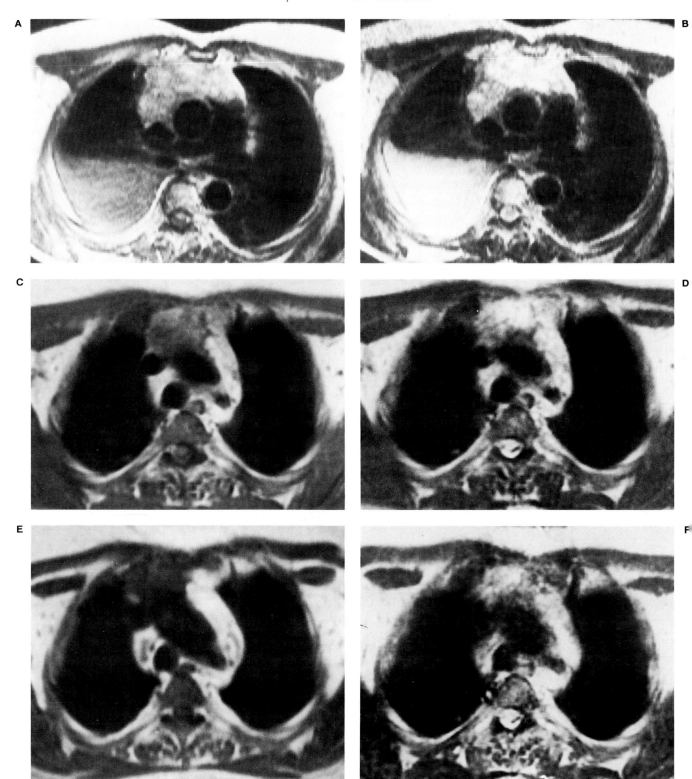

FIG. 96. 27-year-old patient with Hodgkin's lymphoma in the anterior mediastinum. **A, B:** Proton density and T2-weighted images, respectively, obtained in a patient prior to the initiation of therapy demonstrate a large mass in the anterior mediastinum with large right pleural effusion. The mass appears mostly hyperintense with a signal intensity almost equal to that of surrounding fat. Slight heterogeneity is noted within regions of the mass. **C, D:** T1- and T2-weighted images, respectively, 2 months after therapy initiation. A marked decrease in the bulk of the tumor is noted. However, a small amount of residual mass is seen immediately anterior to the arch of the aorta. Note the heterogeneous, predominantly high signal intensity seen on the T2-weighted image and the correspondingly low signal intensity on the T1-weighted scan. **E, F:** Scans obtained 5 months after start of therapy. Again there is a persistent residual mass anterior to the aorta, essentially unchanged in size from the previous examination. Note the heterogeneous high signal intensity pattern on the T2-weighted image. Even though the initial mass has regressed markedly, the lack of change in size between months 2 and 5 and the persistently "active" MR signal pattern strongly suggest residual active disease. The patient was asymptomatic at this point.

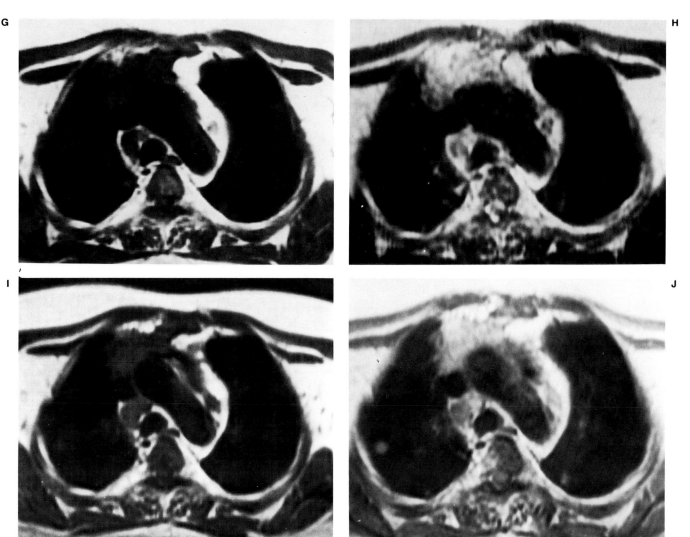

FIG. 96. *(Continued.)* **G, H:** On T1- and T2-weighted images obtained 9 months after therapy initiation, there has been a definite increase in the mass size compared to the previous examination. Note again the low homogeneous signal intensity on the T1-weighted image compared to the heterogeneous, mostly high signal intensity seen on the T2-weighted image. Additionally, an enlarged right paratracheal lymph node can now be identified. On the basis of these findings, therapy was reinitiated. **I, J:** Twelve months following the initial diagnosis, the mass has decreased somewhat in size since the previous examination. However, a pattern of high signal intensity on T2-weighted images persists, suggesting a lack of response. Note also the appearance of pulmonary lesions. The patient expired 2 months following the last study. This case represents a typical example of the dissociation between the evolution of size and that of the MR signal intensity pattern, thus demonstrating the unique information MR can provide in this category of patients.

and necrosis may appear similar to areas of active tumor in the early phase posttherapy (360). To address this issue we have studied a series of 115 patients over 3 years and all instances of false positive diagnosis due to necrosis or inflammation of the tumoral mass occurred within 4 months of therapy initiation. Thus, one should be cautious in not overinterpreting these patterns as definite evidence of lack of response within the first few months following therapy.

3. In some patients marked size regression occurs, but small residual masses with heterogeneous or homogeneous high-signal intensity are noted. A representative case of this group of patients is illustrated in Figure 96. Clearly, this is a group that may derive the most benefit from MR. Often, despite marked size regression plus

associated clinical improvement that would indicate response, a small area of the tumor is seen by MR signal intensity analysis to not respond appropriately. In these patients, the size information derived by CT as well as the clinical improvement will lead one to complacent management (361–363). MR in these cases raises the level of suspicion and justifies close monitoring. In a series of 34 patients prospectively followed by serial MRI studies over 30 months, this dissociation between decreasing size with persistently abnormal high signal intensity on MR occurred in 23% of cases (339).

4. MR signal intensity can be seen to increase in residual masses previously considered inactive. In this group of patients, "islands" of high signal intensity can be seen to reappear in residual masses previously consid-

ered inactive. This is not surprising since most recurrences in such patients occur in the location of the residual masses. The contribution of MR in these cases is the earlier detection of this sign of recurrence. In our experience, about 20% of patients will demonstrate this MR sign preceding clinical symptoms by 8–12 weeks on average.

Certain caveats should be emphasized. As mentioned above, cautious interpretation should be the rule within the first 4 to 6 months following therapy initiation. T1- and T2-weighted images should always be interpreted in parallel to exclude the possibility of fibro-fatty masses (362). Ultimately, fat suppression techniques will provide a technological solution to this problem. Motion artifacts in the phase direction of the image or flow artifacts may, on occasion, render interpretation difficult. Good technique with cardiac gating and presaturation of incoming blood is usually sufficient to resolve this problem.

Another important caveat is that MR signal intensity analysis is not valid within the pulmonary parenchyma (see Fig. 27, Chapter 4) (358). In our experience, high signal intensity can often be seen in areas of radiation fibrosis of the pulmonary parenchyma, in the absence of any tumor residual. Clearly, bronchial secretions accumulating in areas of previously irradiated lung can increase signal intensity on T2-weighted images. In areas of damaged lung, ciliated epithelium is usually damaged and the mucociliary "escalator" that is responsible for clearance of secretions from the lung is no longer functional. Secretions accumulate in damaged pulmonary areas, leading to high T2-weighted signal intensity. Thus, MR signal intensity analysis should be limited to purely mediastinal and hilar masses exclusive of their intrapulmonary manifestations.

In summary, current experience in lymphoma as well as in other disease processes such as rectal carcinoma, cervical carcinoma, and musculoskeletal tumors indicate that MR signal patterns reflect, to some extent, histologic changes within tumors. As an extension of this, it has recently been suggested that MR signal characteristics may be of value in differentiating low-grade from high-grade lymphomas (365). This property, unparalleled by other modalities, provides a unique application of MR. Since MR is more expensive and provides structural information identical to that from CT, we believe that it is most appropriate to examine patients with suspected mediastinal lymphoma first with CT.

Since in many uncomplicated cases complete regression of masses will be observed, there is no need for MR in these instances (366). For those patients in whom a residual mass is observed after one or two cycles of chemotherapy, however, MR should be used to assess whether the signal pattern is consistent with active disease. If an active pattern (homogeneous and/or hetero-geneous hyperintense) is observed, especially beyond 4 to 6 months after therapy, the remission diagnosis should be questioned.

In the majority of cases, a rapid decrease in the T2-weighted signal intensity of lymphomatous masses is the rule, with 80% of masses assuming a homogeneous hypointense pattern within 6 to 8 weeks of initiation of therapy. Thus, even though false positive diagnoses do occur in the first 4 months of therapy, a lack of rapid response may be a significant indicator of therapy effectiveness. At this time, available data are insufficient to confirm this point and assessment of signal intensities has not been reliably quantified to permit objective comparisons of disease activity status.

As demonstrated by Nyman et al., residual masses may slowly disappear over a 12- to 18-month period (360). Thus, MR should be used during that period at regular intervals to ensure resolution of this process. Indeed, in a not insignificant number of patients (20–25%), MR will reveal that the residual mass still contains areas suspicious for active disease that eventually lead to recurrence. These areas are clearly demonstrable on MR images, as illustrated in Figure 96. In other cases, even though the pattern of the residual mass is one of inactive mass (homogeneous hypointense), it is very likely that microscopic residual tumor cannot be detected by MR given the low spatial resolution and the variability of signal intensities intrinsic to the method (367). In all such cases, continued surveillance is warranted until complete resolution. Reappearance of foci of high signal intensity in such masses are strong indicators of early recurrence and are usually noted before clinical symptoms.

THYROID

Diseases of the thyroid gland generally are first evaluated with either radionuclide scintigraphy, or ultrasonography, with needle aspiration biopsy as indicated. The role of CT has generally been restricted to morphologic evaluation, especially when it is suspected that disease involves the mediastinum. Intrathoracic extension of thyroid tissue is common, in some series representing nearly 10% of mediastinal masses resected at thoracotomy (368). Usually representing direct contiguous growth of a goiter into the mediastinum, such lesions are almost always connected to the thyroid gland, even though on nuclear studies the mass may appear to be separated from the thyroid (369). Truly ectopic mediastinal thyroids are extremely rare. With progressive enlargement, the thyroid follows the path of least resistance extending into the thorax. In 80% of cases, the thyroid extends into the thyropericardiac space anterior to the recurrent laryngeal nerve and the subclavian and

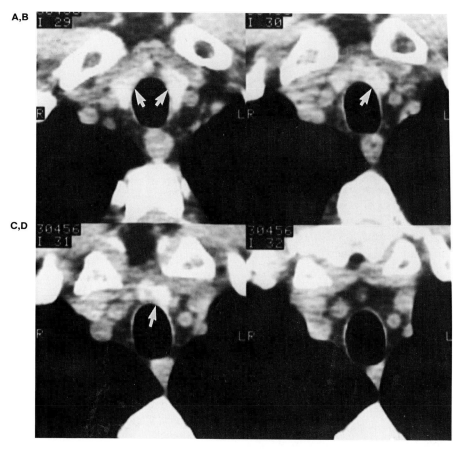

FIG. 97. Normal thyroid tissue. **A–D:** Enlargements of sequential non-enhanced CT sections through the superior mediastinum show characteristic appearance of both thyroid glands, recognizable by their increased density relative to adjacent soft tissues due to high iodine content (*arrows* in A–C). Note that the thyroid gland is closely applied to the anterolateral aspect of the trachea at all levels.

innominate vessels. Posterior mediastinal goiters constitute approximately 20% of cases. Presumably arising from the posterolateral portion of the gland, posterior goiters descend behind the brachiocephalic vessels and are most commonly found on the right side, in close proximity to the trachea, bounded inferiorly by the arch of the azygos vein. Rarely, thyroid tissue may extend either between the esophagus and trachea or even come to lie posterior to the esophagus.

The CT appearance of the thyroid gland has been a subject of investigation from the earliest use of CT (370–372). More recently, the CT appearances of both normal and abnormal thyroid glands has been extensively reviewed (368,373–381). The appearance of normal thyroid tissue is characteristic. On precontrast scans, thyroid tissue is easily identified because of its increased density relative to adjacent soft tissues due to its high iodine content (Fig. 97) (368,370,372). Follow-ing the administration of contrast, thyroid tissue markedly enhances, typically by 25 HU in at least some part of the gland (374).

Identification of substernal thyroid tissue is contingent on the following observations: (a) demonstration of a communication with the cervical portion of the thyroid gland when contiguous sections are extended to include the neck; (b) inhomogeneous densities with small, cystic-appearing areas, and curvilinear, punctate, or ringlike calcifications, and areas of high density presumably due to the iodine content of the gland [fat has not been reported in these lesions and is a differential feature from teratomas (382)]; (c) marked enhancement after contrast media injection, sometimes to the point of simulating a vascular lesion; and (d) prolonged contrast enhancement of the gland (368) due, presumably, to the thyroid actively trapping iodine contained in the contrast medium.

A,B,C

D,E,F

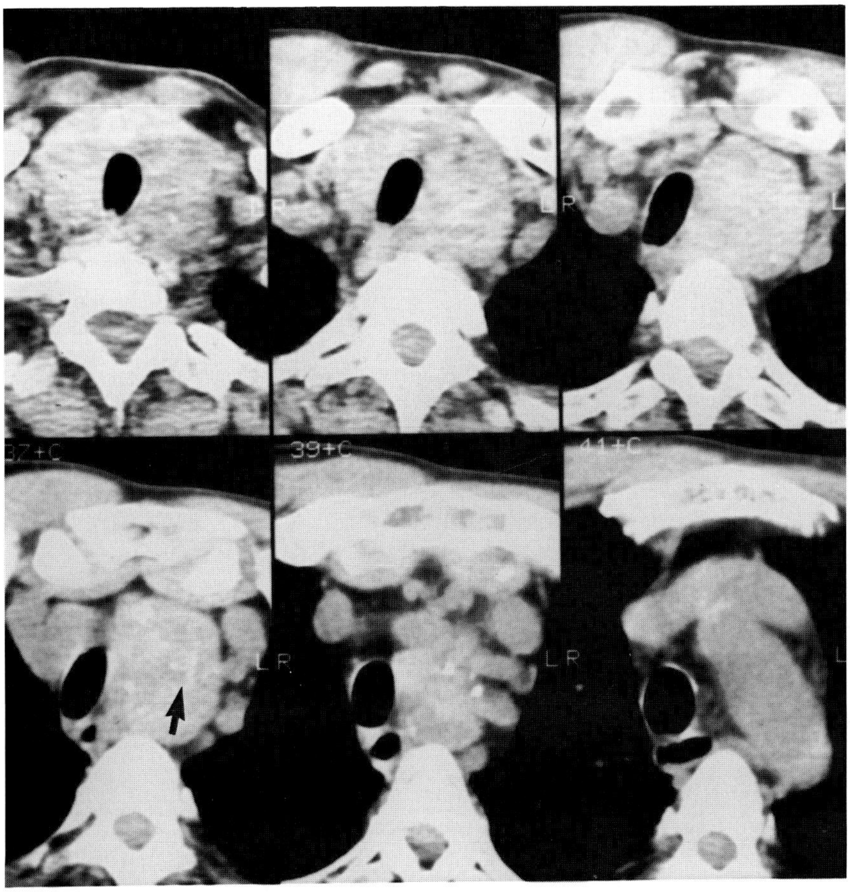

FIG. 98. Goiter: substernal extension. **A–F:** Enlargement of sequential non–contrast-enhanced CT sections through the superior mediastinum. Both the right and left lobes are markedly enlarged and slightly heterogeneous in density. Scattered foci of calcification can be identified as well (*arrow* in D).

CT is of greatest value in defining the morphologic extent of disease (Fig. 98). Marked irregularity of the gland contour, loss of distinct mediastinal fascial planes, and/or the presence of cervical or mediastinal adenopathy should signal potential malignancy (Fig. 99). Nonetheless, although correlation has been documented between areas of low density within glands identified with CT and areas of decreased tracer uptake in nuclear studies, this appearance is nonspecific. Similar limitations in histologic specificity have been noted when CT is compared to high-resolution sonography (377–381).

CT plays an especially important role in the preoperative assessment of substernal goiters (Fig. 98). It has been shown that the surgical approach to these lesions depends on precise anatomic localization. Intrathoracic goiters should be removed for symptomatic relief as well as to reduce the risk consequent to acute hemorrhage or inflammation. Although anterior substernal goiters can usually be removed through a routine cervical incision, posterior mediastinal goiters require a selective approach. In these cases, a decision as to the need for a thoracotomy or a combined cervicothoracic incision generally depends on the size of the lesion or whether or not the mass is mainly intrathoracic without a significant cervical component (369).

MR Evaluation of Thyroid Disease

The potential of MR to evaluate the thyroid gland has been long appreciated (383,384). MR has been shown to be a sensitive means for morphologically delineating the extent of disease. This includes the presence of associated abnormalities such as cervical and/or mediastinal adenopathy, displacement of mediastinal organs such as the esophagus, trachea, and great vessels, and loss of normal cervical and intrathoracic fascial planes (Fig. 99) (364,385–394). Unfortunately, MR has proven of only limited value as a means for tissue characterization.

Characteristically, on T1-weighted images signal intensity in the normal gland is equal to or slightly greater than that seen in the adjacent sternocleiodomastoid muscle; on T2-weighted scans, the signal intensity of the thyroid gland is significantly greater (Fig. 100) (389,392,394). Most focal pathologic processes, including adenomas, cysts, and cancer, are easily identified on T2-weighted sequences because of their markedly prolonged T2 values (Fig. 101). One exception appears to be functioning thyroid nodules, which have been reported to be isointense with normal thyroid tissue on both T1- and T2-weighted scans (391).

A
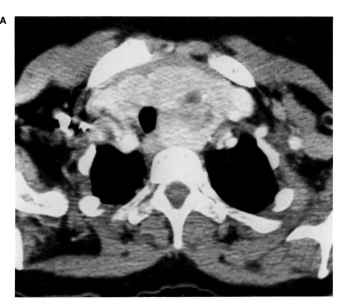

B
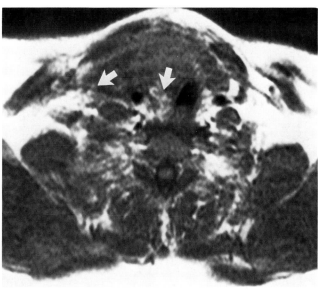

FIG. 99. Thyroid cancer. **A:** Contrast-enhanced CT section at the level of the thoracic inlet. Thyroid tissue is easily identifiable due to marked contrast enhancement which is characteristic following i.v. administration of contrast. Within the thyroid, areas of low tissue attenuation and foci of calcification can be identified. Although the thyroid is markedly enlarged, causing the trachea to deviate to the right, the outlines of the thyroid are still identifiable. Biopsy proved follicular carcinoma of the thyroid. **B:** T1-weighted MR section in a patient different than in A. The thyroid is markedly enlarged and is poorly marginated causing loss of visualization of normally discrete fascial planes (*arrows*). Note that with T1 weighting the thyroid appears relatively homogeneous. Biopsy proved follicular carcinoma of the thyroid.

Multi-nodular goiters have been shown to be relatively hypointense as compared with normal thyroid tissue on T1-weighted images, except when there are foci of either hemorrhage or cysts, in which case focal areas of high signal intensity may be visualized. On T2-weighted images, multi-nodular goiters are typically heterogeneous, with high-signal intensity noted throughout most of the gland (Fig. 101) (387–392). Although it has been suggested that benign adenomas can be differen-

tiated from follicular carcinomas based on the presence of an intact pseudocapsule surrounding adenomas, this finding has been insufficiently documented (392,393). In most series, MR has proven no more specific histologically than CT (384,387,389–391,394).

Characteristic patterns of diffuse abnormality within the thyroid have also been reported. As documented by Charkes et al., in patients with Graves' disease MR has the capability to provide physiologic insight into the

A
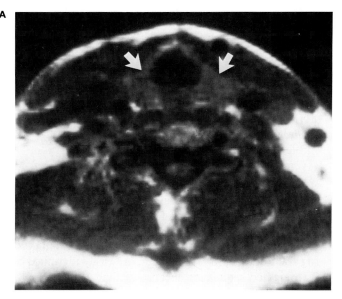

B
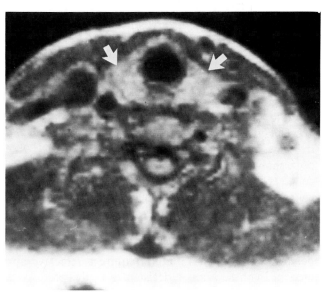

FIG. 100. Normal thyroid glands: MR assessment. **A, B:** T1- and T2-weighted MR images through a normal thyroid gland. On T1-weighted images the signal intensity in the normal gland is equal to or slightly greater than is seen in adjacent muscles (*arrows* in A). This appearance may also be seen in patients with thyroid malignancies (compare with Fig. 99). Note that the signal intensity within the thyroid is significantly greater with T2-weighting (*arrows* in B).

A

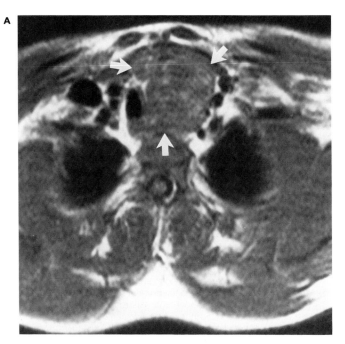

B

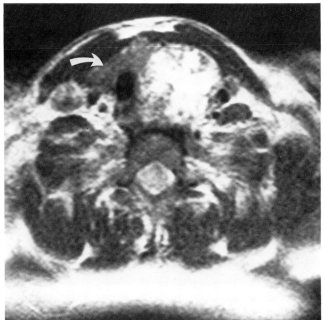

C

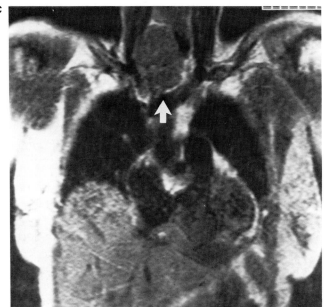

FIG. 101. Substernal goiter: MR evaluation. **A:** T1-weighted MR image through the thoracic inlet shows typical appearance of a multi-nodular substernal goiter. Note that the substernal thyroid is easily identified, separate from adjacent mediastinal fat and vessels, displacing the trachea to the right (*arrows* in A). **B:** T2-weighted MR image obtained at a slightly higher level than is shown in A. There is considerable increase in signal intensity within the goiter, which appears markedly heterogeneous. On T2-weighted images, multi-nodular goiters are typically heterogeneous, with high-signal intensity identifiable throughout the gland. Note that a portion of residual normal thyroid can be identified anterior to the trachea (*curved arrow*). **C:** Coronal T1-weighted image in another patient with a substernal goiter shows to best advantage the true extent of the thyroid. Note that inferiorly, the gland is bounded by the left brachiocephalic vein (*arrow*). Multi-planar imaging is a distinct advantage of MR, especially in presurgical assessment.

functional status of the thyroid gland (395). Typically, patients with Graves' disease have moderate to marked increased signal intensity on studies performed with both short and long TRs. Significantly, in these patients there is a linear relationship between the thyroid-muscle signal intensity contrast ratio and both the serum thyroxine (T4) level and the 24-h radioactive iodine uptake. Furthermore, these changes have been shown to normalize following therapy (395). Noma et al. have noted additional morphologic features in patients with Graves' disease, including the presence of both numerous coarse, bandlike structures traversing the thyroid gland

and dilated vascular structures within the thyroid parenchyma (392). The significance of these findings awaits further clinical investigation.

Descriptions of the thyroid gland in patients with Hashimoto's thyroiditis have also been published. Although this disorder is characterized by diffuse enlargement, no distinct pattern has been identified with MR (392).

A potential role for MR in the evaluation of patients following surgery has also been proposed (391,396–398). In one series of 24 patients with primary thyroid carcinoma evaluated postoperatively with MR reported by Auffermann et al., MR correctly diagnosed or excluded disease in 20 patients. However, MR provided a false positive diagnosis in one case, and a false negative diagnosis in three cases (396).

PARATHYROID ADENOMA

Ninety percent of normal or abnormal parathyroid glands are located near the thyroid gland. Their precise localization and number are variable. The upper pair typically are located dorsal to the superior, while the lower pair lie just below the lower poles of the thyroid gland in the region of the minor neurovascular bundle. Most parathyroid adenomas are found in the inferiorly located group of parathyroid glands, which, importantly, are also the least constant in location. Approximately 10% of parathyroid glands are ectopic. Sixty-two percent of the ectopic glands are located in the anterior mediastinum, 30% are embedded within thyroid tissue, and 8% are found in the posterior-superior mediastinum, in the region of the tracheoesophageal groove (399). Anterior mediastinal parathyroid adenomas are intimately connected with the thymus gland. Islands of parathyroid tissue carried to the anterior mediastinum by the descending thymus during embryologic development is the accepted theory that explains the presence of mediastinal parathyroid adenomas.

Primary hyperparathyroidism results from a solitary adenoma in approximately 85% of cases. Other causes include diffuse hyperplasia (10%), multiple adenomas (5%), and rarely, carcinoma (1%) (394). Various studies are available for detecting parathyroid disease. These include high-resolution ultrasonography, thallium scintigraphy, high-resolution contrast-enhanced CT, and selective venous catheterization. The CT appearance of parathyroid adenomas has been well described (401–416). With CT, normal glands cannot be identified. Parathyroid adenomas vary in size from 0.3 to 3 cm and are usually homogeneous in density, unless their vascular supply has been compromised at surgery, in which case they may appear cystic (411,412,416). Rarely, parathyroid adenomas appear calcified (413). No CT criteria reliably differentiate an adenoma from hyperplasia or carcinoma. In the anterior mediastinum they may be indistinguishable from small thymic remnants, small thymomas, or small nodes, and are found in the expected location of the thymus (Fig. 102).

The ability of CT to detect parathyroid pathology is clearly related to scan technique. Utilizing contiguous 5-mm sections from the hyoid bone to the carina, prospectively reconstructed with small fields of view, 3 sec scan time, a 512 matrix, and maximum contrast enhancement using 50 g of iodine injected through a power injector, Cates et al. documented that preoperatively CT correctly identified parathyroid adenomas prospectively in 81% of patients (416). This compares

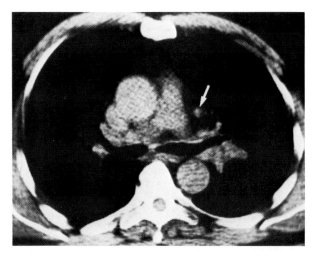

FIG. 102. Ectopic parathyroid adenoma. A 45-year-old patient with hyperparathyroidism not responding to surgical therapy. The CT scan reveals a small, 0.5-cm density in the anterior mediastinum (*arrow*). At surgery, a small parathyroid adenoma was found. Mediastinal parathyroid adenomas are found in the usual location of the thymus. They are difficult to distinguish from small nodes or residual thymic tissue.

favorably with reported sensitivities of both high-resotion ultrasonography and radionuclide imaging (414,415,417). An important potential source of error is to mistake a parathyroid adenoma for a thyroid adenoma (378,416). An association between thyroid and parathyroid disease is well known: as many as 30% of patients with parathyroid disease prove to have simultaneous thyroid abnormalities. In a recent review of 65 patients in whom parathyroid surgery was performed for primary hyperparathyroidism, Stark et al. documented that 40% of these patients had nonpalpable thyroid nodules detected either by CT or high-resolution sonography (378).

It should be emphasized that in patients with documented primary hyperparathyroidism, surgical neck exploration to remove the parathyroid tissues is curative in over 90% of cases (400). As a consequence, in most institutions no imaging procedure is obtained prior to surgery. If preoperative imaging is performed, high-resolution ultrasonography is usually the procedure of choice. In the group of patients in whom surgery fails, a higher than normal percentage of ectopic glands is seen. Ectopia is therefore a significant cause of surgical failure. Almost 50% of these patients will have mediastinal parathyroid glands; two-thirds of these glands will be located in the superior mediastinum, particularly in the posterior aspect near the tracheoesophageal groove, and one-third will be in the lower anterior mediastinum.

Reports of the accuracy of CT versus competing modalities to investigate patients postoperatively varies significantly. Miller et al. compared sonography, thallium scintigraphy, CT, and MR imaging in 53 postoperative patients, and found that no technique detected more than 50% of abnormal glands (417). Similar results have

A
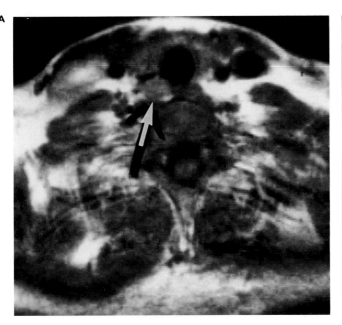
B
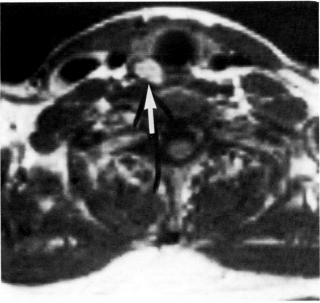

FIG. 103. Parathyroid adenoma: MR evaluation. **A, B:** T1- and T2-weighted images through the lower poles of the thyroid gland show a well-defined mass in the region of the tracheoesophageal groove (*arrows*). Note the marked signal enhancement within the mass on T2-weighted images. These findings are characteristic of parathyroid adenomas. Unfortunately, this same appearance can be seen in patients with thyroid adenomas, differentiation of which can be problematic, especially as a significant percentage of patients with hyperparathyroidism have concomitant thyroid disease.

been reported by others, including false-positive rates of nearly 20%.

MR Evaluation of Parathyroid Disease

The appearance of abnormal parathyroid glands on MR has been well documented (364,385,387, 388,394,417–424). Similar to thyroid adenomas, most parathyroid adenomas show a marked increase in signal intensity on T2-weighted images (Fig. 103). Similar findings have been documented for parathyroid hyperplasia and carcinomas. In a small but significant percentage of cases, parathyroid adenomas fail to exhibit increased signal intensity. As documented by Auffermann et al., in a study of 30 patients with recurrent hyperparathyroidism, 13% of the abnormal glands failed to display high intensity on T2-weighted images (423). Reports of the accuracy of MR, although variable, show that this modality is comparable to other noninvasive techniques for detecting parathyroid pathology (417–423). Spritzer et al., using both T1- and T2-weighted scans to evaluate 23 patients with suspected disease, reported an overall sensitivity of 78% and a specificity of 95%, with a resulting overall accuracy of 90% (421). Kneeland et al., evaluating 22 patients with hyperparathyroidism, reported a 74% and 88% sensitivity and specificity of MR imaging, respectively (419).

Given the similarities between various noninvasive modalities for imaging patients with hyperparathyroidism, each case must be individualized in order to select the most appropriate study. To some extent, availability, cost, and familiarity with these procedures will determine their usage. In our experience, following thallium scintigraphy, MR has come to replace CT in the investigation of patients with recurrent hyperparathyroidism following surgery. CT is reserved for those patients with suspected recurrent parathyroid carcinoma, especially to evaluate the lungs and the liver to rule out metastatic disease (425). Another specialized use of CT is to evaluate patients for whom angiographic ablation of mediastinal parathyroid adenomas has been performed (Fig. 104) (426).

MEDIASTINAL CYSTS

Mediastinal cysts are of congenital origin and include bronchogenic, duplication, neurenteric, and pleuropericardial cysts.

Bronchogenic Cysts

Bronchogenic cysts are one component along a continuum of developmental pulmonary anomalies usually referred to as the sequestration spectrum (427). They probably result from defective growth of the lung bud, and consequently are lined by pseudostratified ciliated columnar epithelium frequently associated with smooth muscle, mucous glands, or cartilage in the cyst wall. Two types have been described: mediastinal and intrapulmonary. Mediastinal cysts are far more frequent and

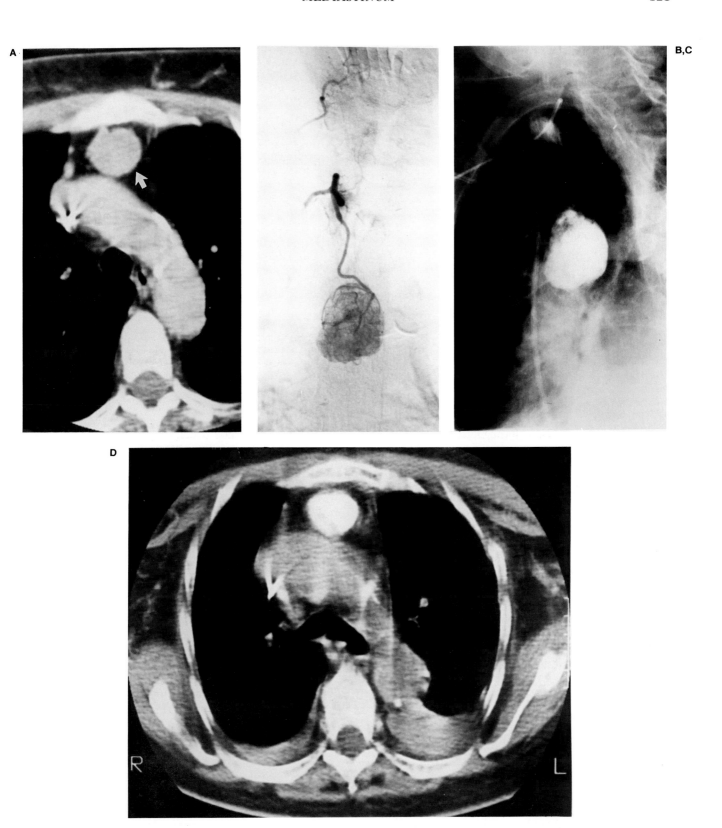

FIG. 104. Mediastinal parathyroid adenomas: angiographic ablation. **A:** Enlargement of a contrast-enhanced CT scan through the aortic arch shows a well-defined, homogeneous soft-tissue mass, otherwise indistinguishable in appearance from a thymoma (*arrow*). **B:** Subtraction angiogram demonstrates an anterior mediastinal parathyroid adenoma supplied by a descending branch of the right inferior thyroid artery. **C:** Appearance of the adenoma after selective intra-arterial injection of 180 mL of contrast material. **D:** CT section obtained 24 hr later in the same patient without additional contrast material shows dense, persistent staining of the adenoma. (From Miller et al., ref. 426, with permission.)

A

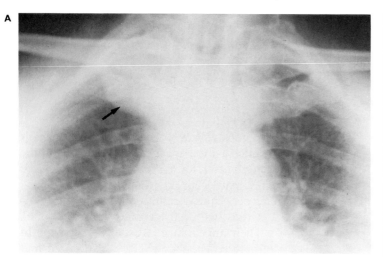

B

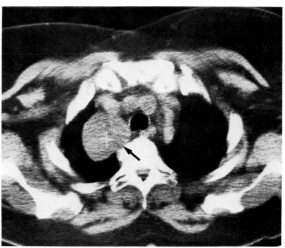

C

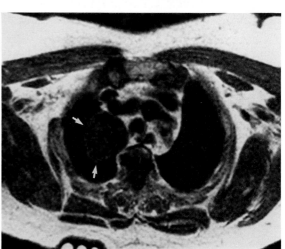

FIG. 105. Bronchogenic cyst: CT/MR correlation. A: Coned-down view from a posteroanterior radiograph of the chest shows a mass (*arrow*) of uncertain etiology, initially felt to possibly be bronchogenic carcinoma. B: Non-enhanced CT section through the superior mediastinum shows a well-demarcated mass (*arrow*) with a density measuring within the range of soft tissue. This patient could not receive i.v. contrast media because of an allergy history. C: T1-weighted MR image at the same level as in B shows the mass to be of very low signal intensity (*arrows*). The mass is clearly distinct from the adjacent vessels and mediastinal fat. D–G: Single-level, multi-echo sequence obtained at the same levels as shown in B and C, using TEs of 30, 60, 90, and 120 msec, respectively. This technique allows acquisition of heavily T2-weighted images. Note that the signal intensity of the lesion steadily increases relative to all other tissues, including fat. This combination of findings is diagnostic of a cystic mass, in this location almost certainly a bronchogenic cyst (cf. Fig. 41, Chapter 5). TE, echo time. From Naidich et al., ref. 456, with permission.

D,E

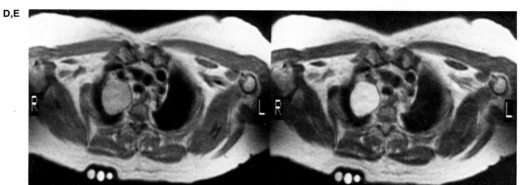

F,G

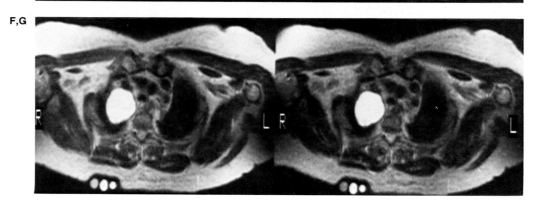

do not communicate with the bronchial tree, unlike intraparenchymal cysts in which such communications usually develop, leading to frequent recurrent infection (428). Unless infected, bronchogenic cysts contain fluid that ranges in color from clear to milky white to brown, with variable viscosity. This variable fluid composition explains the different CT densities observed in bronchogenic cysts (Fig. 105; see also Fig. 41, Chapter 5, and Figs. 18 and 19, Chapter 11) (429–434). Half of these cysts are of water density. In the other half the CT density can vary from a low soft-tissue range to higher-than-muscle density. When dense, bronchogenic cysts may be difficult to distinguish from solid lesions unless images are obtained both pre- and postcontrast enhancement. Most bronchogenic cysts are located along the right paratracheal wall or near the carina in the middle or middle-posterior mediastinum. They are sharply marginated unless infected, and are usually in contact with the carina which may be deformed. These cysts rarely can be seen in other locations such as the anterior mediastinum, the low posterior mediastinum, or in the lung itself. Although generally assumed to be asymptomatic, when strategically located and of sufficient size, bronchogenic cysts may become symptomatic due to compression of adjacent structures including the trachea and carina, mediastinal vessels, and even the left atrium (435,436).

Because of their tendency to either become infected or enlarge, surgical management has been traditional (437). Recently, considerable attention has been focused on the use of both percutaneous and transbronchial needle aspiration, not only for bronchogenic cysts, but for other benign mediastinal fluid collections, including esophageal duplication cysts and mediastinal pseudocysts (437–442). In select cases, these procedures may obviate the need for more invasive procedures such as mediastinoscopy or thoracotomy.

Duplication Cysts

Duplication cysts arise from the foregut and are sometimes grouped with bronchogenic cysts as bronchoesophageal cysts. They are lined by gastrointestinal tract mucosa and are usually located in the posterior mediastinum in a paraspinal location. They are most often connected to the esophagus, and are sometimes found within its wall. Their appearance on CT is indistinguishable from bronchogenic cysts, except for their location (see Fig. 27, Chapter 11) (443,444). Rarely, these cysts may calcify (445).

Neurenteric Cysts

These rare lesions are connected to the meninges through a midline defect in one or more vertebral bodies. They are also often connected to the esophagus. The appearance on CT of the cyst itself is the same as that of duplication cysts, but the presence of the vertebral abnormality points to the diagnosis.

Pleuropericardial Cysts

These cysts, representing defects in the embryogenesis of the coelomic cavities, are most often located in the cardiophrenic angles or lower aspect of the pericardium, although they may occur anywhere in relation to the pericardium, occasionally resulting in misdiagnosis either as a mediastinal or even an intracardiac mass (446,447). Their appearance is usually diagnostic of their cystic nature. They are sharply marginated and have low CT numbers, although pericardial cysts with high CT numbers have been reported (448,449). Pleuropericardial cysts are not always round; they may assume different shapes when studied serially (450). When small, they can sometimes be confused with enlarged cardiophrenic angle nodes.

Differential Diagnosis of Mediastinal Cysts

Differentiation of an uncomplicated congenital cyst from other cystic encapsulated lesions, such as abscesses, old hematomas, or rare cystic lymphangiomas or hemangiomas, relies on the clinical presentation, findings on correlative radiographic studies, and the location and appearance on CT of the cyst (Figs. 106 and 107).

Cystic masses of the anterior mediastinum are rarely due to congenital cysts, but are more likely related to a cystic tumor or a thymic cyst. Abscesses, hematomas, and cystic tumors commonly demonstrate thick walls, with septa on occasion, and mixed-density fluids (see Fig. 106). Cystic lymphangiomas (cystic hygromas) may be either unilocular or multilocular, and contain either serous or chylous fluid (Fig. 107). They may be associated with vascular malformations that are easily identifiable following the administration of intravenous contrast (317,429,451–453). Seventy-five percent occur within the neck and 20% in the axilla, with the remaining 5% presenting in the mediastinum and abdomen (see Fig. 62, Chapter 11) (454). Anterior meningoceles may closely resemble congenital cysts, but careful examination of adjacent sections should demonstrate the intraspinal connection of the mass through the neural foramen.

MR Evaluation of Mediastinal Cysts

The potential of MR to identify cystic or fluid-filled masses is well established (455). MR has been used successfully to diagnose a wide range of lesions, including

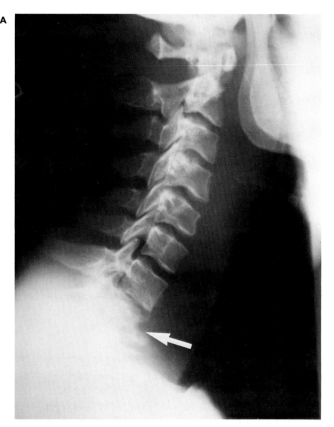

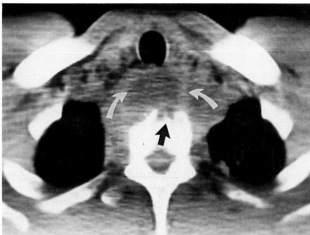

FIG. 106. Tuberculous mediastinal abscess. **A:** Lateral radiograph of the cervical spine shows destruction of the T1 vertebral body (*arrow*). **B:** Contrast-enhanced CT section confirms lytic destruction of T1 (*arrow*) associated with a large, poorly marginated posterior mediastinal fluid collection (*curved arrows*). Surgery confirmed tuberculous abscess.

bronchogenic cysts, pericardial cysts, thymic cysts, colloid cysts within goiters, cystic hygromas, and even mediastinal pseudocysts (364,385,456–460). MR is especially valuable in assessing complex cysts that do not appear fluid-filled on CT, especially when intravenous contrast cannot be administered (Fig. 105) (430–434,456). Although variable patterns of signal intensity have been noted to occur on T1-weighted sequences, presumably the result of the presence of protein and/or hemorrhage within cysts, high-signal intensity characteristically can be seen within cystic lesions on T2-weighted sequences. The ability of MR to identify cystic or fluid-filled masses in association with anomalous vessels has proven especially valuable in the diagnosis of pulmonary sequestration (see Fig. 59, Chapter 3) (456,461).

When sufficient posterior mediastinal fat is present, the esophagus can be adequately visualized with CT. The esophagus is in intimate contact anteriorly with the posterior aspect of the trachea, the left mainstem bronchus, and the left atrium. The esophagus is bordered by the aorta on the left and the azygos vein on the right. Intraluminal air is a common and normal finding with CT (see Fig. 8).

Evaluation of esophageal disease is limited if the esophagus is incompletely distended (462). This problem has been obviated to some degree by the development of a 3% barium paste that is now commercially available (Esoph-o-Cat, E-Z-EM Company, Inc., Westbury, NY) (463,464).

The manifestations on CT of esophageal disease are (a) dilatation; (b) thickening of the wall, both symmetric and asymmetric; (c) loss of periesophageal fat planes, with or without evidence of invasion of surrounding organs; and (d) periesophageal adenopathy (465).

In our experience, CT is indicated in the following settings: (a) to evaluate and stage patients with esophageal carcinoma, primarily to evaluate the mediastinum and upper abdomen, as well as to provide a means for assessing response to therapy and resultant complications; (b) to evaluate and characterize lesions that appear either intramural or especially extramural on esophagography, to identify or exclude significant mediastinal pathology; and (c) to evaluate patients with suspected esophageal perforations to assess the extent of pleural and mediastinal fluid collections. CT plays no substantial role in the evaluation of most benign esophageal disease, including benign strictures, inflammatory disease of any etiology, and disorders of esophageal motility.

ESOPHAGUS

Esophageal Carcinoma

Esophageal carcinoma represents approximately 10% of all cancers of the gastrointestinal tract. Excluding adenocarcinomas of gastric origin with secondary esophageal involvement, 90–95% of esophageal tumors are

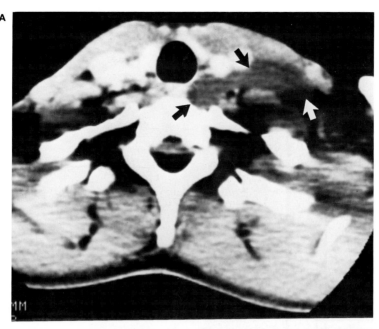

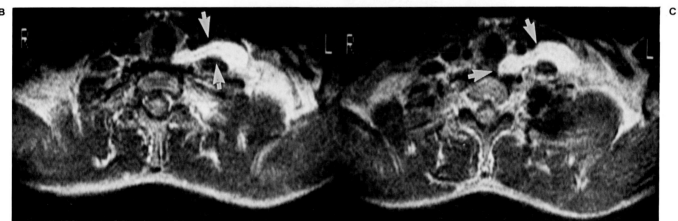

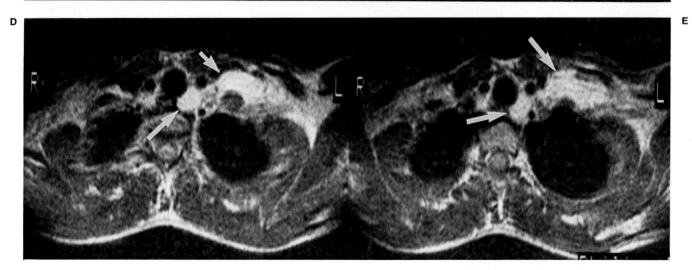

FIG. 107. Cystic hygroma. **A:** Contrast-enhanced CT section through the lower neck shows a well-defined cystic mass lying behind the carotid sheath; adjacent to the trachea, esophagus, and cervical spine; and extending laterally to lie behind the sternocleidomastoid muscle (*arrows*). This lesion also was visualized with CT extending inferiorly into the thoracic inlet and mediastinum (not shown). **B–E:** T2-weighted MR images through the lower neck and superior mediastinum in the same patient confirm the presence of an elongated cystic mass extending from the neck into the posterior mediastinum (*arrows*). Surgery confirmed cystic hygroma.

A,B

C,D

E,F

G,H

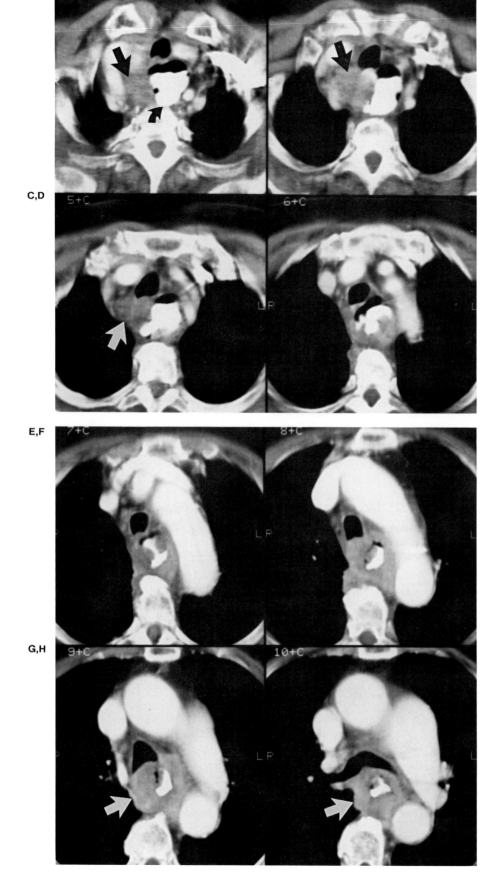

FIG. 108. Squamous cell carcinoma of the midesophagus. **A–H:** Enlargements of sequential contrast-enhanced CT sections through the mediastinum from above-downward following the oral administration of 2 tablespoons of 3% barium paste. An irregular mass is present, most easily identified as irregular thickening of the esophageal wall posterior to the distal trachea and left mainstem bronchus (*arrows* in G and H) extending at least 5 cm in length. Note that at the level of the tumor, the esophageal lumen is markedly irregular; superiorly, the esophagus is dilated due to partial obstruction (*curved arrow* in A). In addition, mediastinal adenopathy is apparent superiorly (*straight arrows* in A, B, and C). Note that the distal trachea and left mainstem bronchi are bowed forward. Although this appearance suggests direct extension of tumor into the airways, in our experience this finding is nonspecific. By CT criteria, this is at least a Stage 3 lesion.

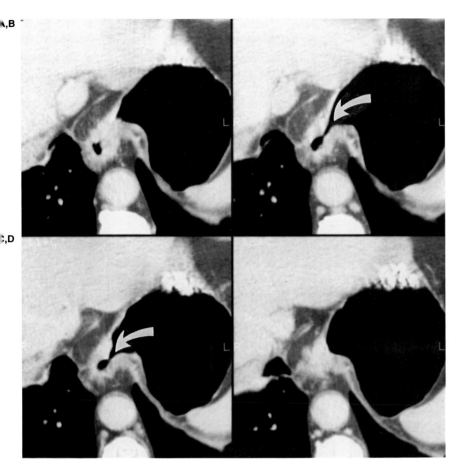

FIG. 109. Adenocarcinoma of the gastro-esophageal junction. **A–D:** Enlargements of sequential CT sections through the esophageal hiatus with the patient in a left lateral decubitus position to facilitate getting air into the distal esophagus. There is marked, irregular thickening of the distal esophageal wall (*arrows* in B and C). The immediate surrounding fat is intact. At surgery this proved to be a gastric adenocarcinoma with extension into the distal esophagus.

squamous cell carcinomas. These tumors usually present in an advanced stage, with 5-year survival rates varying between 3% and 20%. This poor prognosis results from rapid submucosal extension of tumor and early transmural invasion, facilitated by the lack of an esophageal serosa. This leads to early spread to regional and distal lymphatics as well as metastatic foci within the liver, adrenals, and lung in particular.

Accurate presurgical assessment of disease has proven elusive (466). Esophageal carcinoma has traditionally been staged according to the TNM classification of the American Joint Committee on Cancer (AJCC) (467). Moss et al. have proposed an alternative classification based on CT findings, which has been further modified by Reinig et al. to include Stage 1: intraluminal lesions or those that cause localized wall thickening of between 3 and 5 mm; Stage 2: wall thickening greater than 10 mm, either localized or circumferential; Stage 3: wall thickening associated with evidence of contiguous spread or tumor into adjacent mediastinal structures including the airways, aorta, or pericardium; and Stage 4: any locally definable disease associated with distal metastases (468,469).

The role of CT in preoperative staging of esophageal carcinoma has proven controversial (468,470–483).

Most reports suggest that CT is 80–95% accurate (Figs. 108 and 109). Thompson et al., in a series of 76 patients (12 with carcinomas of the gastroesophageal junction and 64 with esophageal carcinomas), reported that CT correctly identified 61 of 64 patients with esophageal carcinoma, 49 of whom had surgical confirmation (474). Of these 49 patients, 42 (86%) were correctly staged using the Moss et al. classification. CT was 88% accurate in evaluating regional extent of disease, correctly identifying 40 of 44 patients with mediastinal invasion and 11 of 15 patients without invasion, for a sensitivity of 90% and a specificity of 79%. CT also correctly identified 15 of 19 patients with distal metastases and 28 of 39 patients without metastatic disease for an overall accuracy of 88%.

More recently, the relationship between CT findings and prognosis in esophageal carcinoma have been investigated. In a retrospective study of 89 patients, Halvorsen et al. found significant correlation between decreased survival and CT findings of tracheal, aortic, or pericardial invasion (481). Evidence of mediastinal invasion and enlarged upper abdominal lymph nodes was especially ominous with mean survival in this group of only 90 days. These findings are consistent with recent data reported documenting parameters linked to 5- and

10-year survival in patients with esophageal carcinoma in a large series of patients in Japan (484).

Significantly different results have been reported by Quint et al., who evaluated with CT 33 patients with esophageal cancers who subsequently underwent transhiatal esophagectomies. Using a modification of the TNM system, only 13 cases (33%) were staged accurately. Thirteen of 33 cases were understaged as a result of inaccurate assessment of tumor invasion through the esophageal wall with contiguous mediastinal invasion; seven cases were overstaged due to false-positive CT diagnoses of enlarged celiac nodes. It should be noted that in this series, a significant percentage of patients proved to have adenocarcinomas of the gastroesophageal junction with secondary invasion of the esophagus. As has been documented by Freeny et al., the reliability of CT to stage this subset of esophageal tumors, in particular, is poor (477). The addition of a substantial number of adenocarcinomas, therefore, is likely to have an adverse effect on determining the efficacy of CT. This is especially important when assessing the accuracy of CT in determining unresectability such as invasion of the trachea and mainstem bronchi and the aorta, findings far more typical of squamous cell carcinomas involving the mid-thoracic esophagus (479).

The role of CT in presurgical staging must be judged against prevailing surgical opinion. This varies considerably. Recent improvements in surgical technique with a corresponding decline in operative mortality have led many to favor palliative surgery in place of more traditional curative resection (485–488). In most institutions, patients are considered unresectable a priori only if there is evidence of one of the following: (a) tumor extension into the airways; (b) invasion of the thoracic aorta, pericardium, or left atrium; and (c) metastatic disease involving the liver, adrenals, lung, or perigastric lymph nodes. Mediastinal adenopathy, CT, or even surgical evidence of transmural extension need no longer be considered contraindications to surgery (486). Using these criteria, esophagectomies have been reported with successful palliation reported in 85–95% of cases (489,490).

In our experience, CT assessment of resectability, especially in individual cases, is frequently problematic (Fig. 108). CT has been reported to be an accurate means for detecting invasion of the carina and the mainstem bronchi (480–482). However, tumor may lie

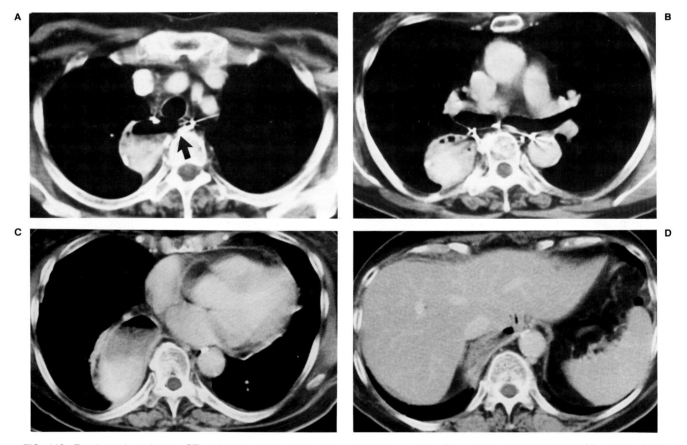

FIG. 110. Esophageal carcinoma: CT evaluation status, postesophagogastrectomy. **A–D:** Sequential contrast-enhanced CT sections from above-downward following administration of oral contrast in a patient following esophagogastrectomy. The anastomosis between the esophagus and stomach is well seen (*arrow* in A) without evidence of an anastomotic leak. Numerous surgical clips in the posterior mediastinum mark the position of the prior esophageal bed. No extraneous soft-tissue masses can be identified; there is no evidence of obstruction, mediastinal nodes, or effusions. CT is especially effective in evaluating postoperative patients due to its superior ability to visualize both luminal and extraluminal pathology.

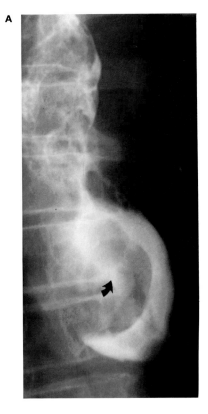

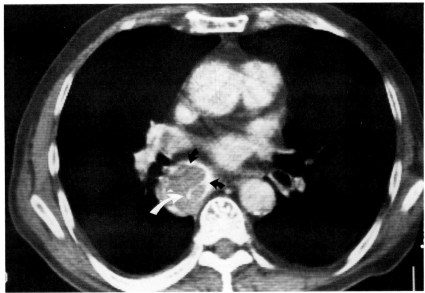

FIG. 111. Oat cell carcinoma of the esophagus. **A:** Coned-down view from an esophagram shows a lobular mass with central ulceration (*arrow*). **B:** Section through the distal esophagus shows a lobular soft-tissue mass filling most of the esophageal lumen outlined by oral contrast media (*black arrows*). Note the presence of contrast media within the mass due to central ulceration (*white arrow*). Biopsy proved oat cell carcinoma. From Naidich, ref. 444, with permission.

adjacent to the carina or mainstem bronchi, and even compress these airways, and still be resectable (470). Periesophageal invasion is usually easily identified in patients with bulky tumors. Unfortunately, definitive assessment of mediastinal invasion may be difficult in cachectic patients in whom a paucity of mediastinal fat makes visualization of the entire length of the esophagus difficult (469,471,477). Similarly, identification with CT of aortic invasion may be difficult (471,474,476,478). It has been suggested that aortic invasion may be predicted on the basis of whether or not the area of contact between the aorta and adjacent tumor is less than 45°, between 60 and 75°, or greater than 90° (478). Although these findings may have statistical significance, they are difficult to apply in individual cases, especially if the CT interpretation results in denying a patient a chance for curative surgery. CT is controversial as well in its ability to identify distant metastases. The finding of enlarged mediastinal and more particularly celiac nodes is in itself nonspecific (474,476,478). Unlike mediastinal adenopathy, CT is of proven value in detecting liver and lung metastases, as well as direct extension of tumor into the pleura, lung, or adjacent vertebral bodies (491,492). Rarely, CT may detect unusual complications of esophageal carcinoma, including the presence of fistulas between the esophagus and the spinal canal (493,494).

If the role of CT in presurgical evaluation is controversial, there is little dispute concerning the value of CT in postsurgical follow-up (Fig. 109) (495,496). As documented by Heiken et al., CT may be especially useful in detecting early postoperative complications, including anastomotic leaks with or without associated mediastinitis, parenchymal consolidation, empyema, and subphrenic abscesses (495). Equally important, CT is an accurate means for detecting early tumor recurrence. Gross et al. have reported detecting locally recurrent disease with CT in 7 of 21 patients following transhiatal esophagectomies, whereas corresponding barium studies proved positive in only four cases (496). Other unusual postoperative findings have been reported, including identifying recurrent tumor within thoracotomy incisions, as well as postoperative esophageal mucoceles (497,498).

CT has proven of little value in patients with unusual esophageal tumors, although these are occasionally encountered (Fig. 110). The esophagus may become secondarily involved by paraesophageal neoplasms that either obstruct the esophagus mechanically, or even invade the esophageal wall (499,500).

Hiatal Hernia

Thorough familiarity with the normal cross-sectional appearance of the gastroesophageal region is a necessary prerequisite for accurate identification of hiatal hernias (Fig. 111). The esophageal hiatus is formed by the decussation of muscle fibers originating from the diaphragm around the lower esophagus. The esophagus is

A

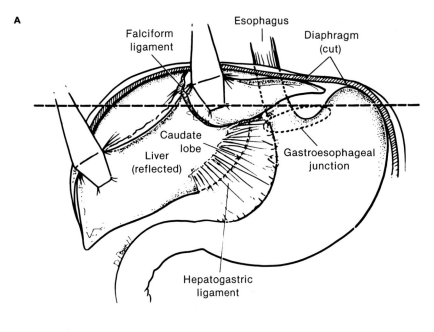

B

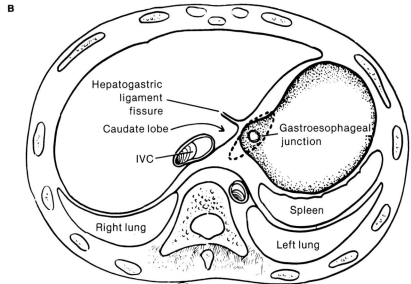

FIG. 112. Gastroesophageal junction: schematic representations of the gastroesophageal junction in the coronal and transverse planes, respectively. **A:** Note the relationship between the gastrohepatic ligament, the caudate lobe of the liver, and the medial wall of the gastroesophageal junction. **B:** A cross-section of the gastroesophageal region, corresponding to the level of the *dotted line* in A. Note that laterally the gastrohepatic ligament can be identified as a line separating the caudate lobe posteriorly from the lateral segment of the left lobe anteriorly. Adapted from Thompson et al., ref. 503.

fixed at the level of the hiatus by the phrenicoesophageal ligament, which is not routinely visible on CT scans. The esophageal hiatus is an elliptical opening just to the left of the midline, corresponding superiorly to the level of the tenth thoracic vertebral body. The margins of the hiatus are formed by the arms of the diaphragmatic crura, which are easily identified in cross-section. Variation in the normal appearance of the crura is common, especially nodular thickening that may be mistaken for either abnormally enlarged lymph nodes or rarely, crural invasion by adjacent tumor (501,502). As the esophagus passes through the upper margin of the hiatus, it assumes an oblique orientation, coursing in a posterior-to-anterior and right-to-left direction. The gastroesophageal junction itself lies just below the dia-

phragm. As it courses through the upper abdomen the distal esophagus is enveloped by the most cranial portion of the gastrohepatic ligament, which originates from a deep cleft in the liver, separating the left lobe from the caudate. This landmark serves as a convenient reference point for indentifying the esophagogastric junction (503). On cross-section the abdominal or submerged portion of the esophagus frequently appears cone-shaped with its base at the junction of the gastric fundus (504). This segment is only rarely distended by either air or barium, and hence is easily mistaken as abnormal (505). This problem may be solved by scanning patients in the left lateral decubitus position following ingestion of at least 200 ml of standard oral contrast material (Fig. 112) (506).

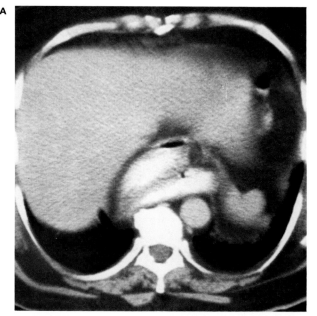

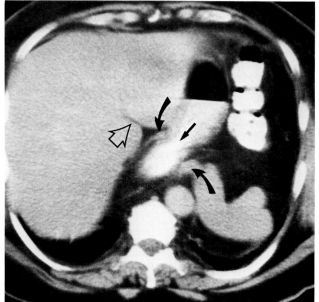

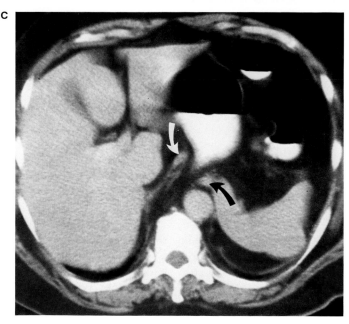

FIG. 113. Hiatal hernia. **A–C:** Sequential CT sections from above-downward following the administration of oral contrast in a patient with a moderate-sized sliding hiatal hernia. Note that the medial margins of the crura are widely separated (*curved arrows* in B and C). A portion of the contrast-filled stomach as well as peritoneal fat (*straight arrow* in B) can be identified between the widened margins of the crura. A few linear densities can be identified within the fat, presumably representing peritoneal vessels. The open arrow in B points to the fissure of the gastrohepatic ligament (cf. with Fig. 110).

In patients with sliding hiatal hernias, the most common abnormalities are dehiscence of the diaphragmatic crura and stretching of the phrenicoesophageal ligament, which ceases to exist for all practical purposes in most adults. These findings manifest as widening of the esophageal hiatus on cross-section, identifiable whenever the medial margins of the diaphragmatic crura are not tightly apposed (Fig. 113) (507). Actual measurements of the standard width of the esophageal hiatus, defined as the distance between the medial margins of the crura, have been reported. This distance measures 10.66 mm (SD ± 2.43 mm) with a maximum width of 15 mm (470). Sliding hiatal hernias are frequently associated with an apparent increase in mediastinal fat surrounding the distal esophagus, secondary to herniation of omentum through the phrenicoesophageal ligament. In the presence of massive ascites, it may be possible to actually identify fluid within herniated peritoneum anterior to the contrast-filled stomach (Fig. 114) (508).

Identification of sliding hiatal hernias rarely presents much difficulty when seen on CT (501,503,504,509). Paraesophageal herniation is easily differentiated because in these cases although the stomach is herniated, the esophagogastric junction remains in a normal position. Occasionally tumors arise in hernias; this appearance may also be mimicked by incomplete filling of the herniated stomach (510). Accurate differentiation usually requires esophagography.

A

B

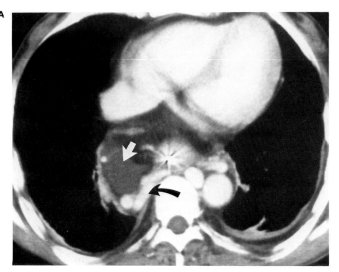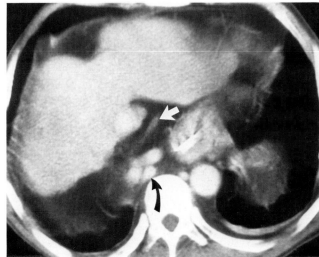

FIG. 114. Sliding hiatal hernia: esophageal varices. **A, B:** Sequential CT sections through the distal esophagus and esophageal hiatus, respectively, show a large sliding hiatal hernia. Note elevated medial margins of the right crus (*arrow* in B). In addition to the stomach, a portion of the peritoneal cavity has also herniated, within which a small quantity of ascites can be identified within the hernial sac (*arrow* in A). Posteriorly, numerous dilated vascular structures can also be identified (*curved arrows* in A, B), due to paraesophageal varices.

BENIGN ESOPHAGEAL DISEASE

The ability of CT to detect esophageal varices has been reported (511–513). CT is especially valuable in detecting paraesophageal varices (see Fig. 114). Typically these appear as either nonspecific right- or left-sided mediastinal soft-tissue masses on chest radiographs, necessitating differentiation from enlarged periesophageal lymph nodes or other posterior mediastinal masses. Although endoscopy and esophagography are able to detect esophageal varices, paraesophageal varices have previously required angiography for definite diagnosis (511). Using dynamic incremental scanning techniques following the administration of a bolus of intravenous contrast, paraesophageal varices are easily identified with CT (512). In fact, with a sufficient contrast, varices within the wall of the esophagus itself can often be seen. CT may be of value in patients following endoscopic sclerotherapy (514,515). In an assessment of nine patients evaluated by CT following otherwise uncomplicated esophageal sclerotherapy, Mauro et al. noted the following CT findings: (a) esophageal wall thickening within which areas of low density could be identified; (b) obliteration of mediastinal fat planes, often associated with a focal fluid collection; (c) thickening of the diaphragmatic crura; and (d) associated pleural effusions and subsegmental atelectasis (515). Similar findings have been reported by Saks et al. (516).

CT plays a major role in identifying extramural abnormalities that secondarily affect the esophagus. There are innumerable causes for extrinsic compression that are easily sorted out by use of CT. In the upper mediastinum CT is especially helpful in diagnosing vascular abnormalities. Detection of aortic aneurysms obviates the need for aortography. Aneurysmal dilitation of other

arteries causing compression of the esophagus also may occasionally be identified. Rarely, these may rupture into the esophagus with resultant exsanguination (see Fig. 63) (517). In addition, CT is useful in diagnosing a variety of vascular anomalies that cause compression or displacement of the esophagus, including aberrant right and left subclavian arteries, double aortic arch anomalies, and pulmonary vascular slings (47,518). CT is also helpful in diagnosing substernal thyroid glands, especially when they extend posterior to the esophagus (374–376). Throughout the length of the mediastinum the esophagus may be displaced by enlarged lymph nodes. In select cases, CT may allow a presumptive diagnosis. In particular, secondary involvement of the esophagus due to low-density tuberculous lymph nodes with resultant esophago-mediastinal fistulas has been described (519,520).

CT has proven particularly valuable in diagnosing esophageal perforation (Fig. 115). This is a potentially lethal condition that is frequently complicated by the rapid onset of severe mediastinitis, empyema, and sepsis. In addition to its association with esophageal carcinoma, perforation may occur spontaneously (Boerhaave's syndrome), or may be posttraumatic or increasingly iatrogenic in etiology, complicating endoscopy, esophageal dilatation, or attempted intubation (521). As documented by Han et al., routine radiographs may be normal in up to 12% of patients with perforations (470). Although the definitive diagnosis is generally made by an esophagram, CT may provide invaluable information concerning the extent of associated mediastinal, pleural, and parenchymal disease (523–525). Furthermore, in our experience, in select cases, CT can be used to determine which patients require immediate surgical intervention and which patients can be managed conser-

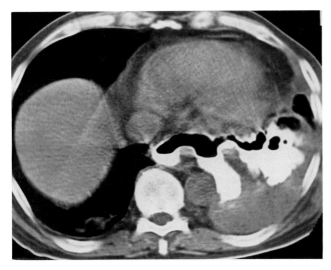

FIG. 115. Esophageal perforation: Boerhaave's syndrome. CT section through the distal esophagus following administration of oral contrast media. There is perforation of the esophagus with free extravasation of contrast into the medastinum, associated with a moderate-sized left pleural fluid collection. (Case courtesy of Robert Meisell, M.D., Booth Memorial Hospital, New York, NY.)

vatively by confirming or excluding mediastinal fluid collections.

Although the CT appearance of tracheoesophageal fistulas, esophageal foreign bodies, and even unusual entities such as idiopathic muscular hypertrophy of the esophagus have been reported, most other benign esoph-

ageal abnormalities are only infrequently seen with CT (526,528).

PARASPINAL DISEASE

Neurogenic Tumors

The richness of neural tissue in the paravertebral areas explains the frequent paraspinal location of neurogenic tumors. Tumors may involve either the peripheral nerves (neurofibromas, schwannomas, malignant peripheral nerve-sheath tumors) or the sympathetic chain (ganglioneuromas, ganglioneuroblastomas, neuroblastomas). Plexiform neurofibromas are pathognomonic of von Recklinghausen's disease, which may also be associated with abnormalities of the spine including kyphoscoliosis, scalloped vertebrae, and lateral meningoceles (529). The CT appearance of neurogenic tumors has been well described (Fig. 116; see also Figs. 25 and 26, Chapter 11) (530–538). Although neural tumors are frequently of soft-tissue density, a characteristic appearance of low density has been described by numerous authors (Fig. 116) (530,531,533,537). Kumar et al. have shown that low density areas within nerve sheath tumors are due to a number of factors, including the presence of (a) lipid-rich Schwann cells; (b) adipocytes; (c) perineural adipose tissue entrapped by plexiform neurofibromas; (d) cystic spaces caused by the coalescence of

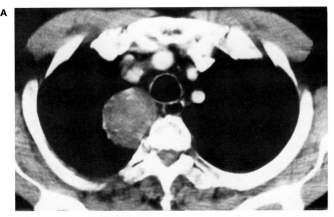

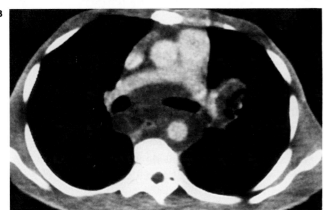

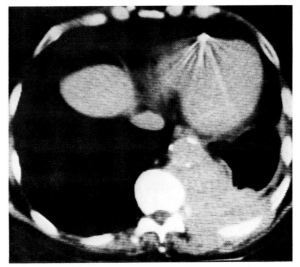

FIG. 116. Neurogenic tumors. **A:** Contrast-enhanced CT scan shows a well-defined, slightly heterogeneous posterior paravertebral mass. The appearance and location are typical. Biopsy proved neurofibroma. **B:** Contrast-enhanced CT section in a different patient with neurofibromatosis involving the vagus nerves. Note that the posterior mediastinum has been infiltrated by a mass of low tissue attenuation, causing marked anterior displacement of the right main pulmonary artery. Although the appearance of this tissue superficially mimics fat, density measurements all were consistently above zero. **C:** Malignant neurofibrosarcoma. The tumor has infiltrated the chest wall.

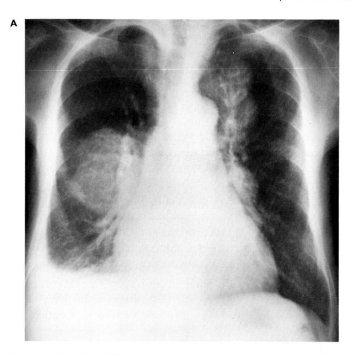

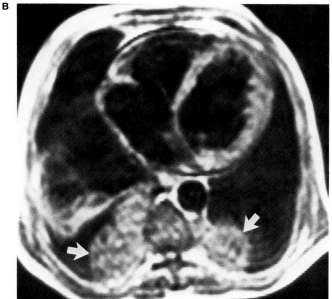

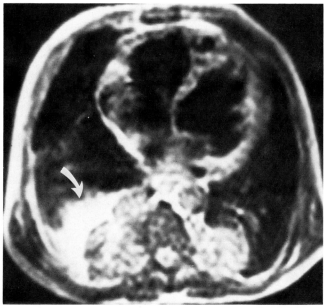

FIG. 117. Extramedullary hematopoiesis: MR evaluation. **A:** Posteroanterior chest radiograph shows massive, bilateral, paravertebral masses. **B, C:** T1- and T2-weighted MR images show typical appearance of bilateral, heterogeneous paravertebral masses (*arrows* in B). Note that there is a considerable increase in signal intensity within these lesions on the T2-weighted scan, although nowhere as near as much as in the associated right pleural fluid effusion (*curved arrow* in B). This patient had long-standing thalassemia.

interstitial fluid in schwannomas with Antoni B tissue; and (e) cystic degeneration secondary to infarction (531). Although benign tumors tend to be sharply marginated and fairly homogeneous while malignant nerve sheath tumors tend to be infiltrating and irregular, unfortunately these findings are not sufficiently reliable to obviate histologic evaluation (Fig. 116). Malignant tumors may be well defined; benign tumors may be irregular and infiltrate adjacent tissues. Both benign and malignant lesions may be symptomatic, rendering clinical differentiation of limited utility. In the rare instance of adult neuroblastoma, differentiation with lymphoma may also be problematic (538).

In addition to neurogenic tumors, a wide variety of other pathologic processes may involve the paraspinal region (539). This area is also rich in elements of the reticuloendothelial system, which explains the frequent paravertebral localization noted in patients with extramedullary hematopoesis, a phenomenon most commonly seen in conditions associated with chronic bone marrow deficiency, particularly thalassemia (Fig. 117). Lymphomas likewise may be present in these regions and simulate malignant neurogenic tumors or extramedullary hematopoesis. Infectious involvement of the spine may lead to the development of paraspinal abscesses, most commonly seen with tuberculosis (Fig. 106). Other rarer entities such as primary myelolipomas of the mediastinum, benign hemangioendotheliomas, aggressive fibromatosis, and even fibrosing mediastinitis have been reported (89,138,540,541).

The paraspinal mediastinum is also in direct communication with the retroperitoneum, especially via the esophageal hiatus. Diseases can spread between the thorax and abdomen by direct extension along this route, as demonstrated by invasive thymomas (Fig. 86). Lymphatic and neural communications through the hiatus explain the common finding of lymphomatous or neurofibromatous masses extending across it into the mediastinum. Inflammatory masses such as pancreatic pseudocysts can similarly invade the paraspinal mediastinal regions.

MR EVALUATION OF PARASPINAL PATHOLOGY

The MR appearance of both benign and malignant neural tumors has been documented (see Fig. 25,

Chapter 11) (537,542–545). Typically, these tumors have slightly greater signal intensity than muscle on T1-weighted images, and markedly increased signal intensity on T2-weighted images (Fig. 118) (542). Compared with other imaging modalities including CT, MR has several distinct advantages for imaging neurogenic tumors. In addition to identifying tumor, MR is especially helpful in assessing intraspinal extension, as well as the presence of associated spinal cord pathology (Fig. 118). The ability to obtain multi-planar images is particularly helpful as many of these tumors demonstrate longitudinal extension into structures along the axis of the spine. For these reasons, MR has largely replaced CT as an initial imaging modality in the evaluation of patients with suspected neurogenic tumors. Unfortunately, MR is no more specific than CT in differentiating benign from malignant lesions. As documented by Levine et al., in these cases, gallium scintigraphy appears to be a promising screening technique, as radiogallium uptake appears to occur only in malignant lesions (537).

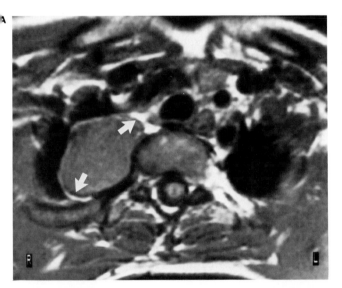
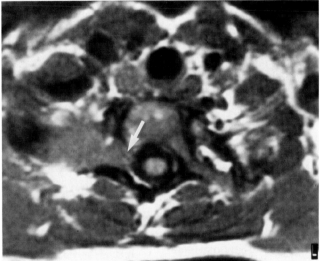
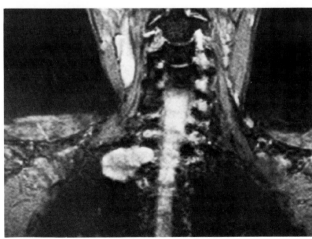

FIG. 118. Neurogenic tumor: MR evaluation. **A, B:** Sequential MR images through the lung apex from above-downward show a sharply defined, homogeneous mass in the right paravertebral space. A thin mantle of fat surrounds the lesion (*arrows* in A), confirming that this lesion arises extrapleurally. Note that the lesion clearly extends into the T1-2 foramen (*arrow* in B). **C:** Coronal MR image confirms extension of the lesion through the intervertebral foramen. This lesion has remained stable for 2 years, compatible with the clinical and morphologic diagnosis of a neurofibroma. (Case courtesy of Andrew Litt, M.D., New York University Medical Center, New York.)

SUMMARY

The potential of CT to investigate mediastinal pathology has long been recognized (4,68,73,81,86,287–289,401,466,546–548). At present, evaluation of the abnormal mediastinum is the most common indication for the use of thoracic CT. The superb density resolution of CT coupled with a lack of superimposition of densities allows a new and more precise radiographic classification of mediastinal pathology. Differentiation of benign fatty and cystic processes of the mediastinum from adenopathy, solid tumors, and vascular lesions is now routinely accomplished (2,3,45–47,429). In this regard, CT has totally replaced conventional tomography as the procedure of choice in the investigation of the mediastinum.

True fatty tumors of the mediastinum are easily differentiated from lipomatosis or herniations of abdominal fat throughout the diaphragm (69,70,72). A lesion of pure fat density with well-defined margins is almost invariably benign. Likewise, asymptomatic mediastinal cysts can be safely managed conservatively when CT confirms their fluid content and demonstrates smooth walls (98,431,439,448).

With CT, all mediastinal lymph nodes can be examined and, when found to be enlarged (>1 cm), the most appropriate method of tissue sampling can be selected (112–115,119,120). Mediastinal CT plays an important role in the staging of lung cancer, although the value of a negative CT examination of the mediastinum as a reliable indicator of resectability remains controversial.

With proper contrast enhancement, CT is reliable in distinguishing vascular from nonvascular structures (146,177). Chest roentgenographic abnormalities due to tortuous vessels are readily explained using CT. Furthermore, aneurysms and dissections of the thoracic aorta are clearly depicted (166–169,181,193–210).

CT is the most accurate noninvasive procedure used to define the extent of mediastinal neoplasms, and it is invaluable in guiding therapy (3,85,91,94,101,104,147, 260,261,263,317,336,368,531). Processes frequently missed by conventional radiography, such as thymomas in patients with myasthenia gravis (291,294, 298,307,308) or ectopic parathyroid adenomas (414–417) in patients with persistent hyperparathyroidism, are more sensitively detected with CT.

Finally, it should be emphasized that in select cases CT may be of particular value by directing transthoracic needle biopsies (549–551). The potential for CT to guide transthoracic sampling of enlarged mediastinal nodes in patients with bronchogenic carcinoma, as well as directing biopsies in patients with otherwise nondescript mediastinal masses, has been noted by numerous authors. The value of CT to direct mediastinal biopsies is dependent on a strong working relationship between radiologists, surgeons, and in particular, pathologists.

TABLE 5. *Mediastinal MR: Indications*

Vascular disease:
  Congenital arterial and venous anomalies
    (Coarctation of the aorta)
  Aortic aneursyms
  Aortic dissection
    (Marfan's syndrome)
  Postoperative assessment
  Acquired venous obstruction
    (Superior vena cava syndrome)
Neoplasia:
  Bronchogenic carcinoma
    (Pancoast tumors)
  Lymphoma (monitoring therapy)
  Neurogenic tumors
  Recurrence s/p thyroidectomy
  Parathyroid adenomas
Miscellaneous:
  Cystic masses
    (Bronchogenic cysts)
  Substernal thyroid tissue
  Fatty masses/herniations

s/p, status-post.

In diagnosed cases of esophageal carcinoma, CT is of value in assessing the extent of the disease, including the detection of distal metastases (468–478). Equally important, CT is valuable in assessing postoperative complications, including recurrent tumor as well as anastomotic leaks with associated mediastinal and pleural infection.

By comparison with CT, a potential role for MR in assessing mediastinal pathology has only developed more recently (552–556). To date, the use of MR has been limited, although indications continue to evolve (Table 5).

In our experience, the major use of MR is as a problem-solving device, especially in cases for which CT has proven equivocal or is limited, as may occur in patients with a contraindication to the administration of intravenous contrast media. MR has proven clinically efficacious in evaluating cardiovascular pathology. Virtually the entire spectrum of aortic disease can be accurately assessed, making MR a reasonable alternative to CT or angiography in most cases (53–64,221,223,229–255).

In patients with thoracic neoplasia, MR also can make significant contributions. Although most studies have evaluated small numbers of patients, MR consistently has proven more accurate than CT in assessing invasion of the chest wall and mediastinum (556). In our judgment, MR should now be considered the imaging procedure of choice to evaluate patients with suspected Pancoast tumors (556).

Additionally, MR can make a unique contribution in select patients with documented lymphoma by evaluating response to therapy, a capability previously unavailable (341–344). The ability to distinguish between residual inactive regions of fibrosis from areas of residual or recurrent tumor or inflammation represents a significant advance in the clinical management of these patients.

In patients with known or suspected intrathoracic tumors, MR can also be helpful in assessing signs of venous obstruction, especially when there is a contraindication to the use of i.v. contrast media (93,264,265). The ability to obtain multi-planar images has proven especially useful in diagnosing superior vena caval syndrome.

MR is equally as accurate as CT in assessing most benign mediastinal pathology (385). MR easily differentiates tortuous vessels from enlarged lymph nodes or masses. MR is also accurate in detecting substernal thyroid tissue, as well as mediastinal parathyroid adenomas (388–394,398,421–423). MR is especially efficacious in evaluating patients with cystic lesions, especially those with complex mediastinal cysts that are not clearly of water density (455,456).

In the assessment of most posterior mediastinal lesions, MR has also largely replaced CT as the imaging modality of choice. Because of advantages derived from multi-planar imaging in particular, MR allows precise visualization of most neurogenic lesions, including identification of dumbbell tumors extending through the neural foramina, as well as tumor extension into the chest wall and spinal canal. This has proven especially valuable in the pediatric population (537,542–545).

It is of course axiomatic to note that future indications for the use of MR can almost surely be anticipated as technological improvements continue to be made.

REFERENCES

1. de Geer G, Webb WR, Golden J. MR characteristics of benign lymph node enlargement in sarcoidosis and Castleman's disease. *Eur J Radiol* 1986;6:145–148.
2. Baron RL, Levitt RG, Sagel SS, Stanley RJ. Computed tomography in the evaluation of mediastinal widening. *Radiology* 1981;138:107–113.
3. Sones PJ, Torres WE, Colvin RS, Meier WL, Sprawls P, Rogers JR, Jr. Effectiveness of CT in evaluating intrathoracic masses. *Am J Roentgenol* 1982;139:469–475.
4. Heitzman ER. *The mediastinum: radiologic correlations with anatomy and pathology.* St. Louis: CV Mosby, 1977.
5. Lee JKT, Sagel SS, Stanley RJ. *Computed body tomography with MRI correlation,* 2nd ed. New York: Raven Press, 1989.
6. Passariello R, Salvolini U, Rossi P, Simonetti G, Pasquini U. Automatic contrast media injector for computed tomography. *J Comput Assist Tomogr* 1980;4:278.
7. Shepard JO, Dedrick CG, Spizarny DL, McLoud TC. Dynamic incremental computed tomography of the pulmonary hila using a flow-rate injector. *J Comput Assist Tomogr* 1986;10:369–371.
8. Price DB, Nardi P, Teitcher J. Venous air embolization as a complication of pressure injection of contrast media: CT findings. *J Comput Assist Tomogr* 1987;11:294–295.
9. Woodring JH, Fried AM. Nonfatal venous air embolism after contrast-enhanced CT. *Radiology* 1988;167:405–407.
10. Schnyder PA, Gamus G. CT of the pretracheal retrocaval space. *AJR* 1981;136:303–308.
11. Proto AV, Corcoran HL, Ball JB. The left paratracheal reflection. *Radiology* 1989;171:625–628.
12. McLoughlin MJ, Weisbrod G, Wise DJ, Yeung HPH. Computed tomography in congenital anomalies of the aortic arch and great vessels. *Radiology* 1981;138:399–403.
13. Reede DL, Bergeron T, McCauley DI. CT of the thyroid and of other thoracic inlet disorders. *J Otolaryngol* 1982;11:349–357.
14. Smathers RL, Buschi AJ, Pope TL, Brenbridge AN, Williamson BR. The azygos arch: normal and pathologic CT appearance. *AJR* 1982;139:477–483.
15. Friedmand AC, Chambers E, Sprayregen S. The normal and abnormal left superior intercostal vein. *AJR* 1978;131:599–602.
16. Ball JB, Proto AV. The variable appearance of the left superior intercostal vein. *Radiology* 1982;144:445–452.
17. Lane EJ, Heitzman ER, Dinn WM. The radiology of the superior intercostal veins. *Radiology* 1976;120:263–267.
18. Smathers RL, Lee JKT, Heiken JP. Clinical image: anomalous preaortic interazygous vein. *J Comput Assist Tomogr* 1983;7:732–733.
19. Takasugi JE, Godwin JD. CT appearance of the retroaortic anastomoses of the azygos system. *AJR* 1990;154:41–44.
20. Hatfield MK, Vyborny CJ, MacMahon H, Chessare JW. Case report. Congenital absence of the azygos vein: a cause for "aortic nipple" enlargement. *AJR* 1987;149:273–274.
21. Carter MM, Tarr RW, Mazer MJ, Carroll FE. The "aortic nipple" as a sign of impending superior vena caval syndrome. *Chest* 1985;87:775–777.
22. Rockoff SD, Druy EM. Tortuous azygos arch simulating a pulmonary lesion. *AJR* 1982;138:577–579.
23. Allen HA, Haney PJ. Case report: left-sided inferior vena cava with hemiazygos continuation. *J Comput Assist Tomogr* 1981;5:917–920.
24. Breckenridge JW, Kinlaw WB. Azygos continuation of the IVC. *J Comput Assist Tomogr* 1980;4:392–397.
25. Churchill RJ, Wesby G, Marsan RE, Moncada R, Reynes CJ, Love L. Case report. Computed tomographic demonstration of anomalous inferior vena cava with azygos continuation. *J Comput Assist Tomogr* 1980;4:398–402.
26. Cohen MI, Gore RM, Vogelzang RL, Rochester D, Neiman HL, Crampton AR. Case report. Accessory hemiazygos continuation of left inferior vena cava: CT demonstration. *J Comput Assist Tomogr* 1984;8:777–779.
27. Munchika H, Cohan RH, Baker ME, Cooper CJ, Dunnick NR. Case report. Hemiazygos continuation of a left inferior vena cava: CT demonstration. *J Comput Assist Tomogr* 1988;12:328–330.
28. Hayward I, Forrest JV, Sagel SS. Case report. Hemiazygos vein aneurysm: CT documentation. *J Comput Assist Tomogr* 1989;13:1072–1074.
29. Edwards J. Anomalies of derivatives of the aortic arch system. *Med Clin North Am* 1948;32:925–949.
30. Proto AV, Cuthbert NW, Raider L. Aberrant right subclavian artery: further observations. *AJR* 1987;148:253–257.
31. Salomonowitz E, Edwards JE, Hunter DW, Castaneda-Zuniga WR, Lund G, Cragg AH, Amplatz K. Pictorial essay. The three types of aortic diverticula. *AJR* 1984;142:673–679.
32. Walker TG, Geller SC. Case report. Aberrant right subclavian artery with a large diverticulum of Kommerell: a potential for misdiagnosis. *AJR* 1987;149:477–478.
33. Dominguez R, Oh KS, Dorst JP, Young LW. Left aortic arch with right descending aorta. *AJR* 1978;130:917–920.
34. Shuford WH, Sybers RG. *The aortic arch and its malformations.* Springfield, IL: Charles C Thomas, 1974.
35. Felson B, Palayew MJ. The two types of right aortic arch. *Radiology* 1963;81:745–759.
36. Stewart JR, Kincaid OW, Edwards JE. *An atlas of vascular rings and related malformations of the aortic arch system.* Springfield, IL: Charles C Thomas, 1964.
37. Taber P, Chang LWM, Campion GM. Diagnosis of retroesophageal right aortic arch by computed tomography. *J Comput Assist Tomogr* 1979;3:684–685.
38. Glanz S, Gordon DH. Right aortic arch with left descent. *J Comput Assist Tomogr* 1981;5:256–258.
39. Shufford WH, Sybers RG, Edwards FK. The three types of right aortic arch. *Am J Roentgenol R* 1970;109:67–74.
40. Eichelberger RP, Long SI, Maulsby GO. Type IIIAIB right aortic

arch: angiographic and computed tomographic evaluation. *CT* 1980;4:241–244.
41. Nath PH, Castenada-Zuniga W, Zollikofer C, et al. Isolation of a subclavian artery. *AJR* 1981;137:683–688.
42. Schlesinger AE, Leiter BE, Connors SK. Computed tomography diagnosis of right aortic arch with an aberrant left innominate artery. *CT* 1984;8:81–87.
43. Shuford WH, Sybers RG, Weens HS. The angiographic features of double aortic arches. *AJR* 1972;116:125–140.
44. Garti IJ, Aygen MM, Levy MJ. Double aortic arch anomalies: diagnosis by countercurrent right brachial arteriography. *AJR* 1979;133:251–256.
45. Webb WR, Gamsu G, Speckman JM, Kaiser JA, Federle MP, Lipton MJ. Pictorial essay. Computed tomographic demonstration of mediastinal venous anomalies. *AJR* 1982;139:157–161.
46. Baron RL, Gutierrez FR, Sagel SS, Levitt RG, McKnight RC. CT of anomalies of the mediastinal vessels. *AJR* 1981;137:571–576.
47. Webb WR, Gamsu G, Speckman JM, Kaiser JA, Federle MP, Lipton MJ. CT demonstration of mediastinal aortic arch anomalies. *J Comput Assist Tomogr* 1982;6:445–451.
48. Ketyer S, Cholankeril MV. CT detection of coarctation of the aorta. *CT* 1981;5:355–358.
49. Godwin JD, Herfkens RJ, Brundage BH, Lipton MJ. Evaluation of coarctation of the aorta by computed tomography. *J Comput Assist Tomogr* 1981;5:153–156.
50. Gaupp RJ, Fagan CJ, Davis M, Epstein NE. Case report. Pseudocoarctation of the aorta. *J Comput Assist Tomogr* 1981;5:571–573.
51. Vaid Y, Shin M, Soto B. Role of computed tomography in nonobstructive coarctation. *CT* 1987;11:95–98.
52. Kennard DR, Spigos D, Tan WS. Cervical aortic arch: CT correlation with conventional radiologic studies. *AJR* 1983;141:295–297.
53. Fletcher BD, Jacobstein MD. MRI of congenital abnormalities of the great arteries. *AJR* 1986;146:941–948.
54. Gomes AS, Lois JF, George B, Alpan G, Williams RG. Congenital abnormalities of the aortic arch: MR imaging. *Radiology* 1987;165:691–695.
55. Kersting-Sommerhoff BA, Sechten UP, Fisher MR, Higgins CB. MR imaging of congenital anomalies of the aortic arch. *AJR* 1987;149:9–13.
56. Bisset GS, Strife JL, Kirks DR, Bailey WW. Vascular rings: MR imaging. *AJR* 1987;149:251–256.
57. Fisher MR, Hricak H, Higgins CB. Magnetic resonance imaging of developmental venous anomalies. *AJR* 1985;145:705–709.
58. Park JH, Han MC, Kim CW. Pictorial essay. MR imaging of congenitally corrected transposition of the great vessels in adults. *AJR* 1989;153:491–494.
59. Amparo EG, Higgins CB, Shafton EP. Demonstration of coarctation of the aorta by magnetic resonance imaging. *AJR* 1984;143:1192–1194.
60. von Schulthess GK, Higashino SM, Higgins SS, Didier D, Fisher MR, Higgins CB. Coarctation of the aorta: MR imaging. *Radiology* 1986;158:469–474.
61. Katz ME, Glazer HS, Siegel MJ, Gutierrez F, Levitt RG, Lee JKT. Mediastinal vessels: postoperative evaluation with MR imaging. *Radiology* 1986;161:647–651.
62. Bank ER, Aisen AM, Rocchini AP, Hernandez RJ. Coarctation of the aorta in children undergoing angioplasty: pretreatment and posttreatment MR imaging. *Radiology* 1987;162:235–240.
63. Soulen RL, Kan J, Mitchell S, White RI. Evaluation of balloon angioplasty of coarctation restenosis by magnetic resonance imaging. *Am J Cardiol* 1987;60:343–345.
64. Rees S, Somerville J, Ward C, Martinez J, Mohiaddin RH, Underwood R, Longmore DB. Coarctation of the aorta: MR imaging in late postoperative assessment. *Radiology* 1989;173:499–502.
65. Lee WJ, Fatal G. Mediastinal lipomatosis in simple obesity. *Chest* 1976;70:308–309.
66. Koerner HF, Sun DIC. Mediastinal lipomatosis secondary to steroid therapy. *Am J Rad Ther* 1966;98:461–464.
67. Price JE, Rigler LG. Widening of the mediastinum resulting from fat accumulation. *Radiology* 1970;96:497–500.
68. Bein NE, Mancuso AA, Mink JH, Hansen GC. Computed tomography in the evaluation of mediastinal lipomatosis. *J Comput Assist Tomogr* 1978;2:379–383.
69. Streiter ML, Schneider HJ, Proto AV. Steroid-induced thoracic lipomatosis: paraspinal involvement. *Am J Roentgenol* 1982;139:679–681.
70. Glickstein MF, Miller WT, Dalinka MK, Lally JF. Paraspinal lipomatosis: a benign mass. *Radiology* 1987;163:79–80.
71. Homer JM, Wechsler RJ, Carter BL. Mediastinal lipomatosis. *Radiology* 1978;128:657–661.
72. Enzi G, Biondetti PR, Fiore D, Mazzoleni FD. Computed tomography of deep fat masses in multiple symmetrical lipomastosis. *Radiology* 1982;144:122–124.
73. Rohlfing BM, Korobkin N, Hall AD. Computed tomography of intrathoracic omental herniation and other mediastinal fatty masses. *J Comput Assist Tomogr* 1977;1:181–183.
74. Fagelman D, Caridi JG. CT diagnosis of hernia of Morgagni. *Gastrointest Radiol* 1984;9:153–155.
75. DeMartini WJ, House AJS. Partial Bochdalek's herniation: computed tomographic evaluation. *Chest* 1980;77:702–704.
76. Gale ME. Bochdalek hernia: prevalence and CT characteristics. *Radiology* 1985;156:449–452.
77. Ginalski JM, Schnuder P, Moss AA, Brasch RC. Incidence and significance of a widened esophageal hiatus at CT scan. *J Clin Gastroenterol* 1984;6:467–470.
78. Yeager BA, Guglielmi GE, Schiebler ML, Gefter WB, Kressel HY. Magnetic resonance imaging of Morgagni hernia. *Gastrointest Radiol* 1987;12:296–298.
79. Keely JG, Vana AJ. Lipomas of the mediastinum, 1940–1955. *Int Abst Surg* 1956;103:312–322.
80. Truwit JD, Jacobs JK, Newman JH, Dyer EL. Roentgenogram of the month. Anterior mediastinal mass following pneumonectomy. *Chest* 1988;94:173–174.
81. Cohen WN, Seidelmann FE, Bryan PJ. Computed tomography of localized adipose deposits presenting as tumor masses. *Am J Roentgenol* 1977;128:1007–1011.
82. Schweitzer DL, Aguam AS. Primary liposarcoma of the mediastinum. *J Thorac Cardiovasc Surg* 1977;741:83–97.
83. Rubin E. Case of the winter season. *Semin Roentgenol* 1978;13:5–6.
84. Yang R, Elliston L, Peterson R, Sahmel R. Roentgenogram of the month. Dysphagia and cough in a patient with a posterior mediastinal mass. *Chest* 1987;92:529–530.
85. DeSantos LA, Ginaldi S, Wallace S. Computed tomography in liposarcoma. *Cancer* 1981;47:46–54.
86. Mendez G, Isikoff MB, Isikiff SK, Sinner WN. Fatty tumors of the thorax demonstrated by CT. *Am J Roentgenol* 1979;133:207–212.
87. Quinn SF, Monson M, Paling M. Case report. Spinal lipoma presenting as a mediastinal mass: diagnosis by CT. *J Comput Assist Tomogr* 1983;7:1087–1089.
88. Kline ME, Patel BU, Agosti SJ. Noninfiltrating angiolipoma of the mediastinum. *Radiology* 1990;175:737–738.
89. Kim K, Koo BC, Davis JT, Franco-Saenz R. Primary myelolipoma of mediastinum. *CT* 1984;8:119–123.
90. Martin J, Palacio A, Petit J, Martin C. Case report. Fatty transformation of thoracic extramedullary hematopoiesis following splenectomy: CT features. *J Comput Assist Tomogr* 1990;14:477–478.
91. Suzuki M, Takashima T, Itoh H, Choutoh S, Kanwamura I, Watamabe Y. Computed tomography of mediastinal teratomas. *J Comput Assist Tomogr* 1983;7:74–76.
92. Friedman AC, Pyatt RS, Hartman DS, Downey EF Jr, Olsen WB. CT of benign cystic teratomas. *AJR* 1982;138:659–665.
93. Lewis DB, Hurt RD, Spencer-Payne W, Farrow GM, Knapp RH, Muhm JR. Benign teratoma of the mediastinum. *J Thorac Cardiovasc Surg* 1983;86:727–731.
94. Brown LR, Muhm JR, Aughenbaugh GL, Lewis BD, Hurt RD. Computed tomography of benign mature teratomas of the mediastinum. *J Thorac Imag* 1987;2:66–71.
95. Glazer HS, Siegel MJ, Sagel SS. Pictorial essay. Low-attenuation mediastinal masses on CT. *AJR* 1989;152:1173–1177.
96. Weinberg B, Rose JS, Efremidis SC, Kirshner PA, Gribetz D.

Posterior mediastinal teratoma (cystic dermoid): diagnosis by computerized tomography. *Chest* 1980;77:694–695.

97. Dobranowski J, Martin LFW, Bennett WF. Case report. CT evaluation of posterior mediastinal teratoma. *J Comput Assist Tomogr* 1987;11:156–157.

98. Seltzer SE, Herman PG, Sagel SS. Differential diagnosis of mediastinal fluid levels visualized on computed tomography. *J Comput Assist Tomogr* 1984;8:244–246.

99. Fulcher AS, Proto AV, Jolles H. Case report. Cystic teratoma of the mediastinum: demonstration of fat-fluid level. *AJR* 1990;154:259–260.

100. Yeoman LJ, Dalton HR, Adam EJ. Case report. Fat-fluid level in pleural effusion as a complication of a mediastinal dermoid: CT characteristics. *J Comput Assist Tomogr* 1990;14:307–309.

101. Shin MS, Ho KJ. Computed tomography of primary mediastinal seminomas. *J Comput Assist Tomogr* 1983;7:990–994.

102. Levitt RG, Husband JE, Glazer HS. CT of primary germ-cell tumors of the mediastinum. *AJR* 1984;142:73–78.

103. Blomlie V, Lien HH, Fossa SD, Jawbsen AB, Stenwig AE. Computed tomography in primary non-seminomatous germ cell tumors of the mediastinum. *Acta Radiol* 1988;29:289–292.

104. Lee KS, Im JG, Han CH, Kim CW, Kim WS. Pictorial essay. Malignant primary germ cell tumors of the mediastinum: CT features. *AJR* 1989;153:947–951.

105. Dooms GC, Hricak H, Sollitto RA, Higgins CB. Lipomatous tumors and tumors with fatty component: MR imaging potential and comparison of MR and CT results. *Radiology* 1985;157:479–483.

106. London J, Kim EE, Wallace S, Shirkhoda A, Coan J, Evans H. MR imaging of liposarcomas: correlation of MR features and histology. *J Comput Assist Tomogr* 1989;13:832–835.

107. Weinreb JC, Mootz A, Cohen JM. MRI evaluation of mediastinal and thoracic inlet venous obstruction. *AJR* 1986;146:679–684.

108. Beck E, Beattie EJ, Jr. The lymph nodes in the mediastinum. *J Int Coll Surgeons* 1958;29:247–251.

109. Tisi GM, Friedman PJ, Peters RM, et al. Clinical staging of primary lung cancer. American Thoracic Society node mapping scheme. *Am Rev Respir Dis* 1983;127:659–669.

110. Glazer HS, Aronberg DJ, Sagel SS, Friedman PJ. Pictorial essay. CT demonstration of calcified mediastinal lymph nodes: a guide to the new ATS classification. *AJR* 1986;147:17–25.

111. Moak GD, Cockerill EM, Farver MO, Yaw PB, Manfredi F. Computed tomography vs standard radiology in the evaluation of mediastinal adenopathy. *Chest* 1982;82:69–75.

112. Genereux GP, Howie JL. Normal mediastinal lymph node size and number: CT and anatomic study. *AJR* 1984;142:1095–1100.

113. Glazer GM, Gross BH, Quint LE, Francis IR, Bookstein FL, Orringer MB. Normal mediastinal lymph nodes: number and size according to American Thoracic Society mapping. *AJR* 1985;144:261–265.

114. Kiyono K, Sone S, Sakai F, Imai Y, Watanabe T, Izuno I, Oguchi M, Kawai T, Shigemstsu H, Watanabe M. The number and size of normal mediastinal lymph nodes: a postmortem study. *AJR* 1988;150:771–776.

115. Quint LE, Glazer GM, Orringer MB, Francis IR, Bookstein FL. Mediastinal lymph node detection and sizing at CT and autopsy. *AJR* 1986;147:469–472.

116. Glazer HS, Aronberg DJ, Sagel SS. Pictorial essay. Pitfalls in CT recognition of mediastinal lymphadenopathy. *AJR* 1985;144:267–274.

117. Mencini RA, Proto AV. The high left and main pulmonary arteries: A CT pitfall. *J Comput Assist Tomogr* 1982;6:452–459.

118. Aronberg DJ, Peterson RR, Glazer HS, Sagel SS. Superior sinus of the pericardium: CT appearance. *Radiology* 1984;153:489–492.

119. Muller NL, Webb WR, Gamsu G. Paratracheal lymphadenopathy: Radiographic findings and correlation with CT. *Radiology* 1985;156:761–765.

120. Muller NL, Webb WR, Gamsu G. Subcarinal lymph node enlargement: Radiographic findings and CT correlation. *AJR* 1985;145:15–19.

121. Rockoff SD, Rohatgi PK. Review. Unusual manifestations of thoracic sarcoidosis. *AJR* 1985;144:513–528.

122. Hamper UM, Fishman EK, Khouri NF, Johns CJ, Wang KP, Siegelman SS. Typical and atypical CT manifestations of pulmonary sarcoidosis. *J Comput Assist Tomogr* 1986;10:928–936.

123. Kuhlman JE, Fishman EK, Hamper UM, Knowles M, Siegelman SS. The computed tomographic spectrum of thoracic sarcoidosis. *Radiographics* 1989;9:449–466.

124. Vock P, Hodler J. Cardiophrenic angle adenopathy: update of causes and significance. *Radiology* 1986;159:395–399.

125. Sussman SK, Halvorsen RA, Silverman PM, Saeed M. Paracardiac adenopathy: CT evaluation. *AJR* 1987;149:29–34.

126. Frija J, Bellin MF, Laval-Jeantet M. CT mediastinum examination in recurrent nerve paralysis. *J Comput Assist Tomogr* 1984;8:901–905.

127. Aberle DR, Gamsu G, Lynch D. Thoracic manifestations of Wegener granulomatosis: diagnosis and course. *Radiology* 1990;174:703–709.

128. Andonopoulos AP, Karadanas AH, Drosis AA, Acritidis NC, Katgsiotis P, Moutsopoulous HM. CT evaluation of mediastinal lymph nodes in primary Sjogren syndrome. *J Comput Assist Tomogr* 1988;12:199–201.

129. Bergin C, Castellino RA. Mediastinal lymph node enlargement on CT scans in patients with usual interstitial pneumonitis. *AJR* 1990;154:251–254.

130. Reede DL, Bergeron RT. Cervical tuberculous adenitis: CT manifestations. *Radiology* 1985;154:701–704.

131. Im JG, Song KS, Kang HS, Park JH, Yeon KM, Han MC, Kim CW. Mediastinal tuberculous lymphadenitis: CT manifestations. *Radiology* 1987;164:115–119.

132. Scatarige JC, Fishman EK, Kuhajda FP, Taylor GA, Siegelman SS. Low attenuation nodal metastases in testicular carcinoma. *J Comput Assist Tomogr* 1983;7:682–687.

133. Yousem DM, Scatariage JC, Fishman EK, Siegelman SS. Low-attenuation thoracic metastases in testicular malignancy. *AJR* 1986;146:291–293.

134. Hopper KD, Diehl LF, Cole BA, Lynch JC, Meilstrup JW, McCauslin MA. The significance of necrotic mediastinal lymph nodes on CT in patients with newly diagnosed Hodgkin disease. *AJR* 1990;155:267–270.

135. Samuels T, Hamilton P, Shaw P. Case report. Whipple disease of the mediastinum. *AJR* 1990;154:1187–1188.

136. Goodwin RA. Disorders of the mediastinum. In: Fishman AP, ed. *Pulmonary diseases and disorders.* New York; McGraw-Hill, 1980;1482–1486.

137. Weinstein JB, Aronberg DJ, Sagel SS. CT of fibrosing mediastinitis: findings and their utility. *AJR* 1983;141:247–251.

138. Kountz PD, Molina PL, Sagel SS. Case report. Fibrosing mediastinitis in the posterior thorax. *AJR* 1989;153:489–490.

139. Goodwin RA, Nickell JA, Des Pres RM. Mediastinal fibrosis complicating healed primary histoplasmosis and tuberculosis. *Medicine* 1972;51:227–246.

140. Gross BH, Schneider HJ, Proto AV. Eggshell calcification of lymph nodes: an update. *AJR* 1980;135:1265–1268.

141. Panicek DM, Harty MP, Scicutella CJ, Carsky EW. Calcification in untreated mediastinal lymphoma. *Radiology* 1988;166:735–736.

142. Breatnach E, Myers JD, McElvein RB, Zorn GL. Roentgenogram of the month. Unusual case of a calcified anterior mediastinal mass. *Chest* 1986;89:113–115.

143. Mesisel S, Rozenman J, Yellin A, Apter S, Herczeg E, Knecht A. Castleman's disease. An uncommon computed tomographic feature. *Chest* 1988;93:1306–1307.

144. Stark P, Smith DC, Watkins GE, Chun KE. Primary intrathoracic extraosseous osteogenic sarcoma: report of three cases. *Radiology* 1990;174:725–726.

145. Groskin SA, Massi AF, Randall PA. Calcified hilar and mediastinal lymph nodes in an AIDS patient with *Pneumocystis carinii* infection. *Radiology* 1990;175:345–346.

146. Spizarny DL, Rebner M, Gross BH. CT of enhancing mediastinal masses. *J Comput Assist Tomogr* 1987;11:990–993.

147. Drucker EA, McLoud TC, Dedrick CG, Hilgenberg AD, Geller SC, Shepard JO. Case report. Mediastinal paraganglioma: radiologic evaluation of an unusual vascular tumor. *AJR* 1987;148:521–522.

148. Sheps SG, Brown ML. Localization of mediastinal paragangliomas (pheochromocytoma). *Chest* 1985;87:807–809.

149. Frances IR, Glazer GM, Shapiro B, Sisson JC, Gross BH. Complementary roles of CT and 131-I-MIBG scintigraphy in diagnosing pheochromocytoma. *AJR* 1983;141:719–725.

150. Keller AR, Hochholzer L, Castleman B. Hyaline-vascular and plasma-cell types of giant lymph node hyperplasia of the mediastinum and other locations. *Cancer* 1972;29:670–683.

151. Frizzera G. Current topics. Castleman's disease: more questions than answers. *Hum Pathol* 1985;16:202–205.

152. Gibbons CJA, Rosencrantz H, Pesey DJ, Watts CM. Angiofollicular lymphoid hyperplasia (Castleman's tumor) resembling a pericardial cyst: differentiation by computerized tomography. *Ann Thorac Surg* 1981;32:193–196.

153. Phelan MS. Castleman's giant lymph node hyperplasia. *Br J Radiol* 1982;55:158–160.

154. Fiore D, Biondetti PR, Calabro F, Rea F. Case report. CT demonstration of bilateral Castleman's tumors in the mediastinum. *J Comput Assist Tomogr* 1983;7:719–720.

155. Ferreiros J, Leon NG, Mata MI, Casanova R, Pedrosa C, Cuevas A. Computed tomography in abdominal Castleman's disease. *J Comput Assist Tomogr* 1989;13:433–436.

156. Aalbers R, Jagt E, Poppema S, Postmus PE. Roentgenogram of the month. Left paravertebral mass. *Chest* 1987;91:889–890.

157. Walter JF, Rottenberg RW, Cannon WB, Sheridan LA, Pizzimenti J, Orr JT. Giant mediastinal lymph node hyperplasia (Castleman's disease): angiographic and clinical features. *AJR* 1978;130:447–450.

158. Federle MP, Megibow AJ, Naidich DP, eds. *Radiology of AIDS.* New York; Raven Press, 1988;77–107.

159. McLoud TC, Kalisher L, Stark P. Intrathoracic lymph nodes metastases from extrathoracic neoplasms. *Am J Roentgenol* 1978;131:403–407.

160. Dooms GC, Hricak H, Crooks LE, Higgins CB. Magnetic resonance imaging of the lymph nodes: comparison with CT. *Radiology* 1984;153:719–728.

161. Dooms GC, Hricak H, Moseley ME, Bottles K, Fisher M, Higgins CB. Characterization of lymphadenopathy by magnetic resonance relaxation times: preliminary results. *Radiology* 1985;155:691–697.

162. Farmer DW, Moore E, Amparo E, Webb WR, Gamsu G, Higgins CB. Calcific fibrosing mediastinitis: demonstration of pulmonary vascular obstruction by magnetic resonance imaging. *AJR* 1984;143:1189–1191.

163. Rholl KS, Levitt RG, Glazer HS. Magnetic resonance imaging of fibrosing mediastinitis. *AJR* 1985;145:255–259.

164. Fomon JJ, Kurzweg FT, Broadaway RK. Aneurysms of the aorta: a review. *Ann Surg* 1967;165:557–563.

165. Pressler V, McNamara J. Thoracic aortic aneurysm. Natural history and treatment. *J Thorac Cardiovasc Surg* 1980;79:489–498.

166. Godwin JD, Herfkens RL, Skioldebrand CG, Federle MP, Lipton MJ. Evaluation of dissections and aneurysms of the thoracic aorta by conventional and dynamic scanning. *Radiology* 1980;136:125–133.

167. Godwin JD. Examination of the thoracic aorta by computed tomography. *Chest* 1984;85:564–567.

168. White RD, Dooms GC, Higgins CB. Advances in imaging thoracic aortic disease. *Invest Radiol* 1986;21:761–778.

169. White RD, Lipton MJ, Higgins CB, Federle MP, Pogany AC, Kerlan RK, Thaxton TS, Turley K. Noninvasive evaluation of suspected thoracic aortic disease by contrast-enhanced computed tomography. *Am J Cardiol* 1986;57:282–290.

170. Gonda RL, Gutierrez OH, Azodo MV. Mycotic aneurysms of the aorta: radiologic features. *Radiology* 1988;168:343–346.

171. Cohen BA, Efremidis SC, Dan SJ, Robinson B, Rabinowitz JG. Case report. Aneurysm of the ductus arteriosus in an adult. *J Comput Assist Tomogr* 1981;5:421–423.

172. Danza FM, Fusco A, Breda M, Bock E, Lemmo G, Colavita N. Ductus arteriosus aneurysm in an adult. *AJR* 1984;143:131–133.

173. Kurich VA, Vogelzang RL, Hartz RS, LoCicero J, Dalton D. Ruptured thoracic aneurysm: unusual manifestation and early diagnosis using CT. *Radiology* 1986;160:87–89.

174. Landtman M, Kivisaari L, Bondestam S, Taavitsainen M, Standertskjold-Nordestan CG, Somer K. Diagnostic value of ultrasound, computed tomography, and angiography in ruptured aortic aneurysms. *Eur J Radiol* 1984;4:248–253.

175. Coblentz CL, Sallee DS, Chiles C. Aortobronchopulmonary fistula complicating aortic aneurysm: diagnosis in four cases. *AJR* 1988;150:535–538.

176. Duke RA, Barrett MR, Payne SD, Salazar JE, Winer-Muram HT, Tonkin ILD. Case report. Compression of left main bronchus and left pulmonary artery by thoracic aortic aneurysm. *AJR* 1987;149:261–263.

177. Miller GA, Heaston DK, Moore AV, Korobkin M, Braun SD, Dunnick NR. CT differentiation of thoracic aortic aneurysms from pulmonary masses adjacent to the mediastinum. *J Comput Assist Tomogr* 1984;8:437–442.

178. Aronberg DJ, Glazer HS, Madsen K, Sagel SS. Normal thoracic aortic diameters by computed tomography. *J Comput Assist Tomogr* 1984;8:247–250.

179. Machida K, Tasaka A. CT patterns of mural thrombus in aortic aneurysms. *J Comput Assist Tomogr* 1980;4:840–842.

180. Torres WE, Maurer DE, Steinberg HV, Robbins S, Bernadino ME. CT of aortic aneurysms: the distinction between mural and thrombus calcification. *AJR* 1988;150:1317–1319.

181. Heiberg E, Wolverson MK, Sundaram M, Shields JB. CT characteristics of aortic atherosclerotic aneurysm versus aortic dissection. *J Comput Assist Tomogr* 1985;9:78–83.

182. Moore EH, Farmer DW, Geller SC, Golden JA, Gamsu G. Computed tomography in the diagnosis of iatrogenic false aneursyms of the ascending aorta. *AJR* 1984;142:1117–1118.

183. Thorsen MK, Goodman LR, Sagel SS. Ascending aorta complications of cardiac surgery: CT evaluation. *J Comput Assist Tomogr* 1986;10:219.

184. Chew FS, Panicek DM, Heitzman ER. Late discovery of a post-traumatic right aortic arch aneurysm. *AJR* 1985;145:1001–1002.

185. Heiberg E, Wolverson MK, Sundaram M, Shields JB. CT in aortic trauma. *AJR* 1983;140:1119–1124.

186. Mirvis SE, Kostrubiak I, Whitley NO, Goldstein LD, Rodruigez A. Role of CT in excluding major arterial injury after blunt thoracic trauma. *AJR* 1987;149:601–605.

187. Higgins WL. Infiltrated retrocrural space following thoracic aorta trauma: CT evaluation. *J Comput Assist Tomogr* 1989;13:949–951.

188. Harrington DP, Barth KH, White RI Jr, Brawley RK. Traumatic pseudoaneurysm of the thoracic aorta in close proximity to the anterior spinal artery: a therapeutic dilemma. *Surgery* 1980;87:153–156.

189. Roberts WC. Aortic dissection: anatomy, consequences, and causes. *Am Heart J* 1981;101:195–214.

190. Crawford ES, Svensson LG, Coselli JS, Safi HJ, Hess KR. Surgical treatment of aneurysm and/or dissection of the ascending aorta, transverse aortic arch, and ascending aorta and transverse arch. Factors influencing survival in 717 patients. *J Thorac Cardiovasc Surg* 1989;98:659–674.

191. Raudkivi PJ, Williams JD, Monro JL, Ross JK. Surgical treatment of the ascending aorta. Fourteen years' experience with 83 patients. *J Thorac Cardiovasc Surg* 1989;98:765–682.

192. Lytle BW, Mahfood SS, Cosgrove DM, Loop FD. Replacement of the ascending aorta. Early and late results. *J Thorac Cardiovasc Surg* 1990;99:651–658.

193. Godwin JD, Turley K, Herfkens RJ, Lipton MJ. Computed tomography for follow-up of chronic aortic dissections. *Radiology* 1981;139:655–660.

194. Stanson AW, Kazimier FJ, Lhollier LG. Penetrating atherosclerotic ulcers of the thoracic aorta: natural history and clinicopathologic correlation. *Ann Vasc Surg* 1986;1:15–23.

195. Welch TJ, Stanson AW, Sheedy PF, Johnson CM, McKusik MA. Radiologic evaluation of penetrating aortic atherosclerotic ulcer. *Radiographics* 1990;10:675–685.

196. Gross SC, Barr I, Eyler WR, Khaja F, Goldstein S. Computed tomography in dissection of the aorta. *Radiology* 1980;136:134–140.

197. Egan TJ, Neiman HL, Herman RJ, Malave SR, Sanders JH. Computed tomography in the diagnosis of aortic aneurysm dissection of traumatic injury. *Radiology* 1980;136:141–146.

198. Larde D, Belloir C, Vasile N, Frija J, Ferrane J. Computed tomography of aortic dissection. *Radiology* 1980;136:147–151.

199. Moncada R, Churchill R, Reynes C, Gunnar RM, Salinas M, Love L, Demos TC, Pifarre R. Diagnosis of dissecting aortic aneurysm by computed tomography. *Lancet* 1981;1:238–241.
200. Heiberg E, Wolverson M, Sundaram M, Connors J, Susman N. CT findings in thoracic aortic dissection. *AJR* 1981;136:13–17.
201. Pariety RA, Couffinhal JC, Wellers M, Farge C, Pradel J, Dologa M. Computed tomography versus aortography in diagnosis of aortic dissection. *Cardiovasc Intervent Radiol* 1982;5:285–291.
202. Thorsen MK, San Dretto MA, Lawson TL, Foley WD, Smith DF, Berland LL. Dissecting aortic aneurysms: accuracy of computed tomographic diagnosis. *Radiology* 1983;148:773–777.
203. Oudkerk M, Overbosch E, Dee P. CT recognition of acute aortic dissection. *AJR* 1983;141:671–676.
204. Chaudry A, Romero L, Pugatch RD. Diagnosis of aortic dissection by computed tomography. *Ann Thorac Surg* 1983;35:322.
205. Guthaner DF, Nassi M, Bradley B, Tello R. Flow determination using computed tomography: application to aortic dissection. Part 1. *Invest Radiol* 1985;20:678–681.
206. Guthaner DF, Nassi M, Bradley B, Miller C. Flow determination using computed tomography: application to aortic dissection. Part 2. *Invest Radiol* 1985;20:682–686.
207. Singh H, Fitzgerald E, Ruttley MS. Computed tomography: the investigation of choice for aortic dissection? *Br Heart J* 1987;56:171–175.
208. Yamada T, Tada S, Harada J. Aortic dissection without intimal rupture: diagnosis with MR imaging and CT. *Radiology* 1988;168:347–352.
209. Demos TC, Posniak HV, Churchill RJ. Detection of the intimal flap of aortic dissection on unenhanced CT images. *AJR* 1986;146:601–603.
210. Godwin JD, Breiman RS, Speckman JM. Problems and pitfalls in the evaluation of thoracic aortic dissection by computed tomography. *J Comput Assist Tomogr* 1982;6:750–756.
211. Meziane MA, Fishman EK, Siegelman SS. CT diagnosis of hemopericardium in acute dissecting aneurysm of the thoracic aorta. *J Comput Assist Tomogr* 1984;8:10–14.
212. Gallagher S, Dixon AK. Streak artifacts of the thoracic aorta: pseudodissection. *J Comput Assist Tomogr* 1984;8:688–693.
213. St. Amour TE, Gutierrez FR, Levitt RG, McKnight RC. CT diagnosis of type A aortic dissections not demonstrated by aortography. *J Comput Assist Tomogr* 1988;12:963–967.
214. Kastan DJ, Sharma RP, Keith F, Shetty PC, Burke MW. Case report. Intimo-intimal intussusception: an unusual presentation of aortic dissection. *AJR* 1988;151:603–604.
215. Danza FM, Fusco A, Falappa P. Letter. Re: the role of computed tomography in the evaluation of dissecting aortic aneurysms. *Radiology* 1984;152:827–829.
216. Vasile N, Mathieu D, Keita K, Lellouche D, Bloch G, Cachera JP. Computed tomography of thoracic aortic dissection: accuracy and pitfalls. *J Comput Assist Tomogr* 1986;10:211–215.
217. Turley K, Ullyot DJ, Godwin JD. Repair of dissection of the thoracic aorta: evaluation of false lumen utilizing computed tomography. *J Thorac Cardiovasc Surg* 1981;81:61–68.
218. Yamaguchi T, Naito H, Ohta M, Sugahara T, Takamiya M, Kozuka T, Nakajima N. False lumens in type III aortic dissections: progress CT study. *Radiology* 1985;156:757–760.
219. Mathieu D, Keta K, Loisance D. Post-operative CT follow-up of aortic dissection. *J Comput Assist Tomogr* 1986;10:216–218.
220. Yamaguchi T, Guthaner DF, Wexler L. Natural history of the false channel of type A aortic dissection after surgical repair: CT study. *Radiology* 1989;170:743–747.
221. Herfkins RJ, Higgins CB, Hricak H, Lipton MJ, Crooks LE, Lanzer P, et al. Nuclear magnetic resonance imaging of the cardiovascular system: normal and pathologic findings. *Radiology* 1983;147:749–759.
222. Herrera L, Oz M, Lally J, Davies A. Thymolipoma simulating pulmonary sequestration. *J Pediatr Surg* 1982;17:313–315.
223. Amparo EG, Higgins CB, Hoddick W, Hricak H, Kerlan RK, Ring EJ. et al. Magnetic resonance imaging of aortic disease: preliminary results. *AJR* 1984;143:1203–1209.
224. Dooms GC, Higgins CB. The potential of magnetic resonance imaging for the evaluation of thoracic arterial disease. *J Thorac Cardiovasc Surg* 1986;92:1088–1095.
225. O'Donovan PB, Ross JS, Sivak ED, O'Donnell JK, Meaney TF. Pictorial essay. Magnetic resonance imaging of the thorax: the advantages of coronal and sagittal planes. *AJR* 1984;143:1183–1188.
226. Webb WR, Jensen BG, Gamsu G, Sollitto R, Moore EH. Coronal magnetic resonance imaging of the chest: normal and abnormal. *Radiology* 1984;153:729–735.
227. Webb WR, Jensen BG, Gamsu G, Sollitto R, Moore EH. Sagittal MR imaging of the chest: normal and abnormal. *J Comput Assist Tomogr* 1985;9:471–479.
228. Batra P, Brown K, Steckel RJ, Collins JD, Ovenfors CO, Aberle D. MR imaging of the thorax: a comparison of axial, coronal, and sagittal imaging planes. *J Comput Assist Tomogr* 1988;12:75–81.
229. Dinsmore RE, Wedeen VJ, Miller SW, Rosen BR, Fifer M, Vlahakes GJ, Edelman RR, Brady TJ. MRI of dissection of the aorta: recognition of the intimal tear and differential flow velocities. *AJR* 1986;146:1281–1288.
230. Rumancik WM, Naidich DP, Chandra R, Kowalski HM, McCauley DI, Megibow AJ, et al. Cardiovascular disease: evaluation with MR phase imaging. *Radiology* 1986;166:63–68.
231. Sechtem U, Theissen P, Deider S, Neufang KFR, Hopp HW, Schicha H. Acute and chronic aortic dissection: demonstration of intimal tears and blood flow with MR imaging. *Radiology* 1989;173(P):321.
232. Liou J, Lee JKT, Canter C, Gutierrez F, Brown JJ. Imaging evaluation of postsurgical repair of aortic coarctation: value of cine MR imaging. *Radiology* 1989;173(P):320.
233. Dinsmore RE, Liberthson RR, Wismer GL, Miller SW, Liu P, Thompson R, et al. Magnetic resonance imaging of thoracic aortic aneurysms: comparison with other imaging modalities. *AJR* 1986;146:309–314.
234. Zeitler E, Kaiser W, Schuierer G, Wijtowycz M, Kunigk K, Oppelt A, et al. Magnetic resonance imaging of aneurysms and thrombi. *Cardiovasc Intervent Radiol* 1986;8:321–328.
235. Lois JF, Gomes AS, Brown K, Mulder DG, Laks H. Magnetic resonance imaging of the thoracic aorta. *Am J Cardiol* 1987;60:358–362.
236. Glazer HS, Gutierrez FR, Levitt RG, Lee JKT, Murphy WA. The thoracic aorta studied by MR imaging. *Radiology* 1985;157:149–155.
237. Moore EH, Webb WR, Verrier ED, Broaddus C, Gamsu G, Amparo E, Higgins CB. MRI of chronic posttraumatic false aneurysm of the thoracic aorta. *AJR* 1984;143:1195–1196.
238. Spielmann RP, Kung EE, Witte G, Heller M. Magnetic resonance imaging of ruptured aneurysm of the ascending aorta. *Br J Radiol* 1989;62:373–375.
239. Soulen RL, Fishman EK, Pyeritz RE, Zerhouni EA, Pessar ML. Marfan syndrome: evaluation with MR imaging versus CT. *Radiology* 1987;165:697–701.
240. Kersting-Sommerhoff BA, Sechtem UP, Schiller NB, Lipton MJ, Higgins CB. MR imaging of the thoracic aorta in Marfan patients. *J Comput Assist Tomogr* 1987;11:633–639.
241. Schaeffer S, Peshock RM, Malloy CR, Katz J, Parkey RW, Willerson JT. Nuclear magnetic resonance imaging in Marfan syndrome. *J Am Coll Cardiol* 1987;9:70–74.
242. Amparo EG, Higgins CB, Hricak H, Sollitto R. Aortic dissection: magnetic resonance imaging. *Radiology* 1985;155:399–406.
243. Geisinger MA, Risius B, O'Donnell JA, Zelch MG, Moodie DS, Graor RA, George CR. Thoracic aortic dissections: magnetic resonance imaging. *Radiology* 1985;155:407–412.
244. Hill JA, Lambert CR, Akins EW. Ascending aortic dissection: detection by MRI. *Am Heart J* 1985;110:894–896.
245. Barentsz JO, Ruijs JHJ, Heystraten FMJ, Buskens F. Magnetic resonance imaging of the dissected aorta. *Br J Radiol* 1987;60:499–502.
246. Kersting-Sommerhoff BA, Higgins CB, White RD, Sommerhoff CP, Lipton MJ. Aortic dissection: sensitivity and specificity of MR imaging. *Radiology* 1988;166:651–655.
247. Akins E, Hil JA, Carmichael MJ. Case report. MR imaging of blood pool signal variation with cardiac phase in aortic dissection. *J Comput Assist Tomogr* 1987;543–545.
248. Pernes JM, Grenier P, Desbleds MT, de Brix JL. MR evaluation of chronic aortic dissection. *J Comput Assist Tomogr* 1987;975–981.

249. White RD, Ullyot DJ, Higgins CB. MR imaging of the aorta after surgery for aortic dissection. *AJR* 1988;150:87–92.

250. Pucillo AL, Schechter AG, Moggio RA, Kay RH, Tenner MS, Herman MV. Postoperative evaluation of ascending aortic prosthetic conduits by magnetic resonance imaging. *Chest* 1990;97:106–110.

251. Sherry CS, Harms SE. MR imaging of pseudoaneurysms in aortocoronary bypass graft. *J Comput Assist Tomogr* 1989;13:426–429.

252. Winkler ML, Higgins CB. MRI of perivalvular infectious pseudoaneurysms. *AJR* 1986;147:253–256.

253. Lotan CS, Cranney GB, Pohost GM. Case report. Fat-shift artifact simulating aortic dissection on MR images. *AJR* 1989;152:385–386.

254. Paulin S, von Schulthess GK, Fossel E, Krayenbuehl HP. MR imaging of the aortic root and proximal coronary arteries. *AJR* 1987;148:665–670.

255. Miller DL, Reinig JW, Volkman DJ. Vascular imaging with MRI: inadequacy in Takayasu's arteritis compared with angiography. *AJR* 1986;146:949–954.

256. Borner N, Erbel R, Braun B, Henkel B, Meyer J, Rumplet J. Diagnosis of aortic dissection by transesophageal echocardiography. *Am J Cardiol* 1984;54:1157–1158.

257. Seward JB, Khandheria BK, Oh JK, Abel MD, Hughes RW, Edwards WD, et al. Transesophageal echocardiography: technique, anatomic correlations, implementation, and clinical applications. *Mayo Clin Proc* 1988;63:649–680.

258. Erbel R, Daniel W, Visser C, Engberding R, Roelandt J, Rennollet H. Echocardiography in diagnosis of aortic dissection. *Lancet* 1989;March 4:457–460.

259. Kormano MJ, Dean PB, Hamlin DJ. Upper extremity contrast medium infusion in computed tomography of upper mediastinal masses. *J Comput Assist Tomogr* 1980;4:617–620.

260. Engel IA, Auh YH, Rubenstein WA, Sniderman K, Whalen JP, Kazam E. CT diagnosis of mediastinal and thoracic inlet venous obstruction. *AJR* 1983;141:521–526.

261. Moncada R, Cardella RG, Demos TC, Churchill RJ, Cardoso M, Love L, Reynes CJ. Evaluation of superior vena cava syndrome by axial CT and CT phlebography. *AJR* 1984;143:731–736.

262. Goodman LR, Teplick SK. Computed tomography in acute cardiopulmonary disease. *Radiol Clin North Am* 1983;21:741–758.

263. Bechtold RE, Wolfman NT, Karstaedt N, Choplin RH. Superior vena caval obstruction: detection using CT. *Radiology* 1985;157:485–487.

264. McMurdo KK, de Geer G, Webb WR, Gamsu G. Normal and occluded mediastinal veins: MR imaging. *Radiology* 1986;159:33–38.

265. Templeton PA, Yang A, Tempany CMC, Zerhouni EA. MR imaging of mediastinal venous obstruction with gradient-echo and spin-echo pulse sequences. *Radiology* 1989;173(P):210.

266. Yellin A, Rosen A, Reichert N, Lieberman Y. Superior vena cava syndrome. The myths—the facts. *Am Rev Respir Dis* 1990;141:1114–1118.

267. Ishikawa T, Clark RA, Tokuda M, Ashida H. Focal contrast enhancement on hepatic CT in superior vena caval and brachiocephalic vein obstruction. *AJR* 1983;140:337–338.

268. Moncada R, Demos TC, Marsan R, Churchill RJ, Reynes C, Love L. CT diagnosis of idiopathic aneurysms of the thoracic systemic veins. *J Comput Assist Tomogr* 1985;9:305–309.

269. Zerhouni EA, Barth KW, Siegelman SS. Detection of venous thrombosis by computed tomography. *Am J Roentgenol* 1980;134:753–758.

270. Fishman EK, Pakter RL, Gayler BW, Wheeler PS, Siegelman SS. Jugular venous thrombosis: diagnosis by computed tomography. *J Comput Assist Tomogr* 1984;8:963–968.

271. Mori H, Fukuda T, Isomoto I, Maeda H, Hayashi K. CT diagnosis of catheter-induced septic thrombus of vena cava. *J Comput Assist Tomogr* 1990;14:236–238.

272. Godwin JD, Webb WR. Contrast-related flow phenomena mimicking pathology on thoracic computed tomography. *J Comput Assist Tomogr* 1982;6:460–464.

273. Baron RL, Lee JKT, Sagel SS, Peterson RR. Computed tomography of the normal thymus. *Radiology* 1982;142:121–125.

274. Heiberg E, Wolverson MK, Sundaram M, Nouri S. Normal thymus: CT characteristics in subjects under age 20. *AJR* 1982;138:491–494.

275. Moore AV, Korobkin M, Olanow W, Heaston DK, Ram PC, Dunnick NR, Silverman PM. Age-related changes in the thymus gland: CT-pathologic correlation. *AJR* 1983;141:241–246.

276. Francis IR, Glazer GM, Bookstein FL, Gross BH. The thymus: reexamination of age-related changes in size and shape. *AJR* 1985;145:249–254.

277. St. Amour TE, Siegel M, Glazer HS, Nadel SN. CT appearances of the normal and abnormal thymus in childhood. *J Comput Assist Tomogr* 1987;11:645–650.

278. Martin KW, McAlister WH. Case report. Intratracheal thymus: a rare cause of airway obstruction. *AJR* 1987;149:1217–1218.

279. Goldstein G, Mackey IR. *The human thymus*. St. Louis: Warren H Green, 1969.

280. Dixon AK, Hilton CJ, Williams GT. Computed tomography and histologic correlation of the thymic remnant. *Clin Radiol* 1981;32:255–257.

281. Perlo VP, Arnason B, Castleman B. The thymus gland in elderly patients with myasthenia gravis. *Neurology* 1975;25:294–295.

282. Gelfand DW, Goldman AS, Law EJ, MacMillan BG, Larson D, Abston S, Schreiber JT. Thymic hyperplasia in children recovering from thermal burns. *J Trauma* 1972;12:813–817.

283. Goldberg RE, Haaga JR, Yulish BS. Case report. Serial CT scans in thymic hyperplasia. *J Comput Assist Tomogr* 1987;11:539–540.

284. Chen J, Weisbrod GL, Herman SJ. Computed tomography and pathologic correlations of thymic lesions. *J Thorac Imag* 1988;3:61–65.

285. Castleman B, Norris EH. The pathology of the thymus in myasthenia gravis. A study of 35 cases. *Medicine* 1949;28:27–58.

286. LeGolvan DP, Abell MR. Thymomas. *Cancer* 1977;39:2142–2157.

287. Mink JH, Bein ME, Sukov R, Herrmann C Jr, Winter J, Sample WF, Mulder D. Computed tomography of the anterior mediastinum in patients with myasthenia gravis and suspected thymoma. *AJR* 1978;130:239–246.

288. McLoud TC, Wittenberg J, Ferrucci JT Jr. Computed tomography of the thorax and standard radiographic evaluation of the chest: A comparative study. *J Comput Assist Tomogr* 1979;3:170–180.

289. Aita JF, Wannamaker WM. Body computerized tomography and the thymus. *Arch Neurol* 1979;36:20–21.

290. Keesey J, Bein M, Mink J. Detection of thymoma in myasthenia gravis. *Neurology* 1980;30:233–239.

291. Baron RL, Lee JKT, Sagel SS, Levitt RG. Computed tomography of the abnormal thymus. *Radiology* 1982;142:127–134.

292. Fon GT, Bein ME, Mancuso AA, Keesey JC, Lupetin AR, Wong WS. Computed tomography of the anterior mediastinum in myasthenia gravis. A radiologic-pathologic correlative study. *Radiology* 1982;142:135–141.

293. Siegelman SS, Scott WW Jr, Baker RR, Fishman EK. CT of the thymus. In: Siegelman SS, ed. *Computed tomography of the chest*. New York: Churchill Livingstone, 1984:233–272.

294. Keen SJ, Libshitz HI. Thymic lesions. Experience with computed tomography in 24 patients. *Cancer* 1987;59:1520–1523.

295. Bergh N, Gatzinsky P, Larson S, Ludin P, Ridell B. Tumors of the thymus and thymic region: 1. clinicopathological studies on thymomas. *Ann Thorac Surg* 1978;25:91–98.

296. Marino M, Muller-Hermelink HK. Thymoma and thymic carcinoma. Relation of thymoma epithelial cells to the cortical and medullary differentiation of the thymus. *Virchows Arch* 1985;407:119–149.

297. Ricci C, Rendina EA, Pescarmona EO, Venuta F, Tolla RD, Ruco LP, Baroni CD. Correlations between histological type, clinical behaviour, and prognosis in thymoma. *Thorax* 1989;44:455–460.

298. Zerhouni EA, Scott WW, Baker RR, Wharam MO, Siegelman SS. Invasive thymomas: diagnosis and evaluation by computed tomography. *J Comput Assist Tomogr* 1982;6:92–100.

299. Scatariage JC, Fishman EK, Zerhouni EA, Siegelman SS. Transdiaphragmatic extension of invasive thymoma. *AJR* 1985;144:31–35.

300. Kaplan I, Swayne LC, Widmann WD, Wolff M. Case report. CT

demonstration of "ectopic" thymoma. *J Comput Assist Tomogr* 1988;12:1037–1038.

301. Korobkin M, Casano VA. Case report. Intracaval and intracardiac extension of malignant thymoma: CT diagnosis. *J Comput Assist Tomogr* 1989;13:348–350.

302. Asamura H, Morinaga S, Shimosato Y, Ono R, Naruke T. Thymoma displaying endobronchial polypoid growth. *Chest* 1988;94:647–649.

303. Maggi G, Giaccone G, Donadio M, Ciuffreda L, Dalesio O, Leria G, Trifiletti G, et al. Thymomas. A review of 169 cases, with particular reference to results of surgical treatment. *Cancer* 1986;58:756–776.

304. Fujimura S, Kondo T, Handa M, Shiraishi Y, Tamahashi N, Nakada T. Results of surgical treatment for thymoma based on 66 patients. *J Thorac Cardiovasc Surg* 1987;93:708–714.

305. Krueger JB, Sagerman RH, King GA. Stage III thymoma: results of postoperative radiation therapy. *Radiology* 1988;168:855–858.

306. Jaretzki A, Penn AS, Younger DS, Wolff M, Olarte M, Lovelace RE, Rowland LP. "Maximal" thymectomy for myasthenia gravis. *J Thorac Cardiovasc Surg* 1988;95:747–757.

307. Brown LR, Muhm JR, Sheedy PF, Unni KK, Bermatz PE, Hermann RC. The value of computed tomography in myasthenia gravis. *Am J Roentgenol* 1983;140:31–35.

308. Kaye AD, Janssen R, Arger PH, Lisak R, Coleman BG, Gefter W, Epstein D, Schatz NJ. Mediastinal computed tomography in myasthenia gravis. *J Comp Tomogr* 1983;7:273–279.

309. Heron CW, Husband JE, Williams MP. Hodgkin disease: CT of the thymus. *Radiology* 1988;167:647–651.

310. Baron RL, Sagel SS, Baglan RJ. Thymic cysts following radiation therapy for Hodgkin disease. *Radiology* 1981;141:593–597.

311. Lewis CR, Manoharan A. Benign thymic cysts in Hodgkin's disease: report of a case and review of published cases. *Thorax* 1987;42:633–634.

312. Lindfors KK, Meyer JE, Dedrick CG, Hassell LA, Harris NL. Thymic cysts in mediastinal Hodgkin disease. *Radiology* 1985;156:37–41.

313. Gouliamos A, Striggaris K, Lolas C, Deligeorgi-Politi H, Vlahos L, Pontifex G. Case report. Thymic cyst. *J Comput Assist Tomogr* 1982;6:172–174.

314. Levine C. Case report. Cervical presentation of a large thymic cyst: CT appearance. *J Comput Assist Tomogr* 1988;12:656–657.

315. Jaramillo D, Perez-Atayde A, Griscom NT. Apparent association between thymic cysts and prior thoracotomy. *Radiology* 1989;172:207–209.

316. Lagrange W, Dahm HM, Karstens J, Feichtinger J, Mittermayer C. Melanocystic neuroendocrine carcinoma of the thymus. *Cancer* 1987;59:484–488.

317. Pilla TJ, Wolverson MK, Sundaram M, Heiberg E, Shields JB. CT evaluation of cystic lymphangiomas of the mediastinum. *Radiology* 1982;144:841–842.

318. Pardes JG, LiPuma JP, Haaga JR, Petruschak MJ, Alfidi RJ. Case report. Lymphangioma of the thymus in a child. *J Comput Assist Tomogr* 1982;6:825–827.

319. Yeh HC, Gordon A, Kirshner PA, Cohen BA. Computed tomography and sonography of thymolipoma. *AJR* 1983;140:1131–1133.

320. Cohen M, Hill CA, Cangir A, Sullivan MP. Thymic rebound after treatment of childhood tumors. *AJR* 1980;135:151–156.

321. Choyke PL, Zeman RK, Gootenberg JE, Greenberg JN, Hoffer F, Frank JA. Thymic atrophy and regrowth in response to chemotherapy: CT evaluation. *AJR* 1987;149:269–272.

322. Doppman JL, Oldfield EH, Chrousos GP. Rebound thymic hyperplasia after treatment of Cushing's syndrome. *AJR* 1986;147:1145–1147.

323. Kissin CM, Husband JE, Nicholas D, Eversman W. Benign thymic enlargement in adults after chemotherapy: CT demonstration. *Radiology* 1987;163:67–70.

324. Siegel MJ, Glazer HS, Wiener JI, Molina PL. Normal and abnormal thymus in childhood: MR imaging. *Radiology* 1989;172:367–371.

325. deGeer G, Webb WR, Gamsu G. Normal thymus: assessment with MR and CT. *Radiology* 1986;158:313–317.

326. Molina PL, Siegel MJ, Glazer HS. Pictorial essay. Thymic masses on MR imaging. *AJR* 1990;155:495–500.

327. Rollins NK, Currarino G. Case report. MR imaging of posterior mediastinal thymus. *J Comput Assist Tomogr* 1988;12:518–520.

328. Shirkhoda A, Chasen MH, Eftekhari F, Goldman AM, Decaro L. MR imaging of mediastinal thymolipoma. *J Comput Assist Tomogr* 1987;11:364–365.

329. Batra P, Herrmann C Jr, Mulder D. Mediastinal imaging in myasthenia gravis: correlation of chest radiography, CT, MR, and surgical findings. *AJR* 1987;148:515–519.

330. De Vita VT, Jaffe ES, Hellman S. Hodgkin's disease and the non-Hodgkin's lymphomas. In: De Vita VT, Hellman S, Rosenberg SA, eds. *Cancer: Principles and practice of oncology.* Philadelphia: JB Lippincott, 1985.

331. Filly R, Blank M, Castellino RA. Radiographic distribution of intrathoracic disease in previously untreated patients with Hodgkin's disease and non-Hodgkin's lymphoma. *Radiology* 1976;120:277–281.

332. Burgener FA, Hamlin D. Intrathoracic histiocytic lymphoma. *Am J Roentgenol* 1981;136:499–504.

333. Schomberg TJ, Evans RG, O'Connell MJ. Prognostic significance of mediastinal mass in adult Hodgkin's disease. *Cancer* 1984;53:324–328.

334. Kaplan HS. Hodgkin's disease: unfolding concepts concerning its nature, management and prognosis. *Cancer* 1980;45:2439.

335. Kadin ME, Glatstein EJ, Dorfman RE. Clinical pathologic studies in 177 untreated patients subjected to a laparotomy for the staging of Hodgkin's disease. *Cancer* 1971;27:1277.

336. Castellino RA, Hoppe RT, Blank N. Computed tomography, lymphography and staging laparotomy: correlations with initial staging of Hodgkin's disease. *AJR* 1984;143:37.

337. Libshitz HJ, Jing BS, Walace S, Logothetis CJ. Sterilized metastases: a diagnostic and therapeutic dilemma. *Am J Roentgenol* 1983;140:14–19.

338. Radford JA, Cowan RA, Flanagan M, Dunn G, Crowtherd, Johnson RJ, Eddleston B. The significance of residual mediastinal abnormality on the chest radiograph following treatment for Hodgkin's disease. *J Clin Oncol* 1988;6:940–946.

339. Jochelson M, Mauch P, Balikian J, Rosenthal D, Canellos G. The significance of the residual mediastinal mass in treated Hodgkin's disease. *J Clin Oncol* 1988;3:637–640.

340. Surbone A, Longo DL, DeVita VT, Ihde DC, Duffey TL, Jaffe ES, Solomon D, Hubbard SM, Young RC. Residual abdominal masses in aggressive non-Hodgkin's lymphoma after combination chemotherapy: significance and management. *J Clin Oncol* 1988;6:1832–1837.

341. Zerhouni EA, Fishman EK, Jones R, Siegelman SS, Soulen RL. (Abstr) MR imaging of sterilized lymphoma. *Radiology* 1986;161(P):207.

342. Zerhouni EA. MRI in the management of lymphoma. In: Margulis AR, Gooding CA, eds. *Diagnostic radiology 1987.* San Francisco: Radiology Research and Education Foundation, University of California, 1987;375–384.

343. Rahmouni AD, Zerhouni EA. Role of MRI in the management of thoracic lymphoma. In: Zerhouni EA, ed. *CT and MRI of the thorax.* New York: Churchill-Livingstone, 1990;23–35.

344. Katz M, Piekarski JD, Bay-Wesberger C, Laval-Jeantet M, Teillet F. Masses mediastinales residuelles post-radiotherapiques au cours de al maladie de Hodgkin. *Ann Radiol* 1977;20:667–672.

345. Durkin W, Durant J. Benign mass lesions after therapy for Hodgkin's disease. *Arch Intern Med* 1979;139:333–336.

346. Marman M. Mediastinal fibrosis simulating residual Hodgkin's disease. *Am J Med Sci* 1984;187:40–42.

347. Stewart FM, Williamson BR, Innes DJ, Hess CE. Residual tumor masses following treatment for advanced histiocytic lymphoma. *Cancer* 1985;55:620–623.

348. Chen JL, Osborne EM, Butler JJ. Residual fibrous masses in treated Hodgkin's disease. *Cancer* 1987;60:407–413.

349. Lewis E, Bernardino ME, Salvador PG, Cabanillas FF, Barnes PA, Thomas JL. Post therapy CT detected mass in lymphoma patients: is it viable tissue? *J Comput Assist Tomogr* 1982;6:792–795.

350. Fuks JZ, Aisner J, Wiernik PH. Restaging laparotomy in the management of the non-Hodgkin lymphomas. *Med Pediatr Oncol* 1982;10:429–438.

351. North LB, Fuller LM, Sullivan-Halley JA, Hagemeister FB. Re-

gression of mediastinal Hodgkin disease after therapy: evaluation of time interval. *Radiology* 1987;164:599–602.

352. Nyman RS, Rehn SM, Glimelius BLG, Hagber ME, Hemmingsson AL, Sundstrom CJ. Residual mediastinal masses in Hodgkin disease: prediction of size with MR imaging. *Radiology* 1989;170:435–440.

353. Oliver TW, Bernardino ME, Sones PJ. Monitoring the response of lymphoma patients to therapy: correlation of abdominal CT findings with clinical course and histologic cell type. *Radiology* 1983;149:219–224.

354. Israel O, Front D, Lam M, Ben-Haim S, Kleinhaus U, Ben-Schachar M, Robinson E, Kolodny G. Gallium 67 imaging in monitoring lymphoma response to treatment. *Cancer* 1988;61:2439–2443.

355. Tumeh SS, Rosenthal DS, Kaplan WD, English RJ, Holman BL. Lymphoma: evaluation with Ga-67 SPECT. *Radiology* 1987;164:111–114.

356. Martiat P, Ferrant A, Labar D, Cogneau M, Bol A, Michel C, Michaux JL, Soukal G. In vivo measurement of carbon-11 thymidine uptake in non-Hodgkin's lymphoma using positron emission tomography. *J Nucl Med* 1988;29:1633–1637.

357. Dooms GC, Hricak H, Moseley ME, Bottles K, Fisher M, Higgins CB. Characterization of lymphadenopathy by magnetic resonance relaxation times: preliminary results. *Radiology* 1985;155:691–697.

358. Glazer HS, Lee JKT, Levitt RG, Heiken JP, Ling D, Totty WG, Balf DM, Emani B, Wasseman TH, Murphy WA. Radiation fibrosis: differentiation from recurrent tumor by MR imaging. *Radiology* 1985;156:721–726.

359. Rahmouni A, Tempany C, Jones R, Mann R, Zerhouni EA. Relative value of size versus signal intensity changes by MRI in the management of lymphoma. [In preparation].

360. Nyman R, Rehn S, Glimelius B, Hagberg H, Hemmingson A, Jung B. Magnetic resonance imaging for assessment of treatment effects in mediastinal Hodgkin's disease. *Acta Radiol* 1987;28:145–151.

361. Schein PS, Chabner BA, Canellos GP, Young RC, de Vita VT. Non-Hodgkin's lymphoma: patterns of relapse from complete remission after combination chemotherapy. *Cancer* 1975;35:334–357.

362. Rostock RA, Giangreco A, Wharam MD, Lenhard R, Siegelmann SS, Order SE. CT scan modification in the treatment of mediastinal Hodgkin's disease. *Cancer* 1982;49:2267–2275.

363. Weller SA, Glatstein E, Kaplan HS, Rosenberg SA. Initial relapses in previously treated Hodgkin's disease: results of second treatment. *Cancer* 1976;37:2840–2846.

364. von Schulthess GK, McMurdo K, Tscholakopff, de Geer G, Gamsu G, Higgins CB. Mediastinal masses: MR imaging. *Radiology* 1986;158:289–296.

365. Rehn SM, Nyman RS, Glimelius BL, Hagberg HE, Sundström JC. Non-Hodgkin lymphoma: predicting prognostic grade with MR imaging. *Radiology* 1990;176:249–253.

366. Webb WR. MR imaging of treated mediastinal Hodgkin disease [editorial]. *Radiology* 1989;170:315–316.

367. Head GM, Mackintosh FR, Burke SS, Rosenberg SA. Late relapse from complete remission in nodular and diffuse histiocytic lymphoma. *Cancer* 1983;52:1356–1359.

368. Glazer GM, Axel L, Moss AA. CT diagnosis of mediastinal thyroid. *Am J Roentgenol* 1982;138:495–498.

369. Shahian DM, Rossi R. Posterior mediastinal goiter. *Chest* 1988;94:599–602.

370. Wolf BS, Nakagawa H, Yeh HS. Visualization of the thyroid gland with computed tomography. *Radiology* 1977;1223:368.

371. Sekiya T, Tada S, Kawakami K, Kino M, Fukuda K, Watanabe H. Clinical application of computed tomography to thyroid disease. *Comput Tomogr* 1979;3:185–193.

372. Machida K, Yoshikawa K. Case report. Aberrant thyroid gland demonstrated by computed tomography. *J Comput Assist Tomogr* 1979;3:689–690.

373. Silverman PM, Newman GE, Korobkin M, Moore AV, Coleman RE. Computed tomography in the evaluation of thyroid disease. *AJR* 1984;141:897–902.

374. Bashist B, Ellis K, Gold RP. Computed tomography of intrathoracic goiters. *AJR* 1983;140:455–460.

375. Binder RE, Pugatch RD, Faling LJ, Kanter RA, Sawin CT. Case

376. Morris UL, Colletti PM, Ralls PW, Boswell WD, Lapin SA, Quinn M, Halls JM. Case report. CT demonstration of intrathoracic thyroid tissue. *J Comput Assist Tomogr* 1982;6:821–824.

377. Radecki PD, Arger PH, Arenson RL, Jennings AS, Coleman RG, Mintz MC, Kressel HY. Thyroid imaging: comparison of high-resolution real-time ultrasound and computed tomography. *Radiology* 1984;153:145–147.

378. Stark DD, Clark OH, Gooding GAW, Moss AA. High-resolution ultrasonography and computed tomography of thyroid lesions in patients with hyperparathyroidism. *Surgery* 1983;94:863–868.

379. Katz JF, Kane RA, Reyes J, Clarke MP, Hill TC. Thyroid nodules: sonographic-pathologic correlation. *Radiology* 1984;151:741–745.

380. Takashima S, Ikezoe J, Morimoto S, Arisawa J, Hamada S, Ikeda H, et al. Primary thyroid lymphoma: evaluation with CT. *Radiology* 1988;168:765–768.

381. Takashima S, Morimoto S, Ikezoe J, Arisawa J, Hamada S, Ikeda H, et al. Primary thyroid lymphoma: comparison of CT and US assessment. *Radiology* 1989;171:439–443.

382. Kier R, Silverman PM, Korobkin M, Wain S, Leight G, Burch W Jr. Case report. Malignant teratoma of the thyroid in an adult: CT appearance. *J Comput Assist Tomogr* 1985;9:174–176.

383. deCertaines J, Herry JY, Lancien G, Benoist L, Bernard AM, LeClech G. Evaluation of human thyroid tumors by proton nuclear magnetic resonance. *J Nucl Med* 1982;23:48–51.

384. Tennvall J, Biorklund A, Moller T, Olsen N, Persson B, Akerman M. Studies of NMR-relaxation-times in malignant tumours and normal tissues of the human thyroid gland. *Prog Nucl Med* 1984;8:142–148.

385. Gamsu G, Stark DD, Webb WR, Moore EH, Sheldon PE. Magnetic resonance imaging of benign mediastinal masses. *Radiology* 1984;151:709–713.

386. Stark DD, Moss AA, Gamsu G, Clark OH, Gooding GAW, Webb WR. Magnetic resonance imaging of the neck, part 1: normal anatomy. *Radiology* 1984;150:447–454.

387. Stark DD, Moss AA, Gamsu G, Clark OH, Gooding GAW, Webb WR. Magnetic resonance imaging of the neck, part 2: pathologic findings. *Radiology* 1984;150:455–461.

388. Stark DD, Clark OH, Moss AA. Magnetic resonance imaging of the thyroid, thymus, and parathyroid glands. *Surgery* 1984;96:1083–1091.

389. Higgins CB, McNamara MT, Fisher MR, Clark OH. MR imaging of the thyroid. *AJR* 1986;147:1255–1261.

390. Mountz JM, Glazer GM, Dmuchowski C, Sisson JC. MR imaging of the thyroid: comparison with scintigraphy in the normal and diseased gland. *J Comput Assist Tomogr* 1987;11:612–619.

391. Gefter WB, Spritzer CE, Eisenberg B, LiVolsi VA, Axel L, Velchik M, et al. Thyroid imaging with high-field strength surface-coil MR. *Radiology* 1987;164:483–490.

392. Noma S, Nishimura K, Togashi K, Itoh K, Fujisawa I, Nakano Y, et al. Thyroid gland: MR imaging. *Radiology* 1987;164:495–499.

393. Noma S, Kanaoka M, Minami S, Sagoh T, Yamashita K, Nishimura K, et al. Thyroid masses: MR imaging and pathologic correlation. *Radiology* 1988;168:759–764.

394. Higgins CB, Auffermann W. MR imaging of thyroid and parathyroid glands: a review of current status. *AJR* 1988;151:1095–1106.

395. Charkes ND, Maurer AH, Siegel JA, Radecki PD, Malmud LS. MR imaging in thyroid disorders: correlation of signal intensity with Graves disease activity. *Radiology* 1987;164:491–494.

396. Auffermann W, Clark OH, Thurnher S, Galante M, Higgins CB. Recurrent thyroid carcinoma: characteristics on MR images. *Radiology* 1988;168:753–757.

397. Barakos JA, DeMarco RD, Higgins CB. MR imaging of recurrent medullary thyroid carcinoma. *Radiology* 1989;173(P):252.

398. Holliday RA, Weinreb J. Utility of MR imaging in postthyroidectomy patients. *Radiology* 1989;173(P):253.

399. Norris EH. The parathyroid adenoma: a study of 322 cases. *Int Abst Surg* 1947;84:1–41.

400. Satava RM, Beahrs OH, Scholz DA. Success rate of cervical

exploration for hyperparathyroidism. *Arch Surg* 1975;110:625–627.

401. Doppman JL, Brennan MF, Koehler JO, Marx SJ. Computed tomography for parathyroid localization. *J Comput Assist Tomogr* 1977;1:30–36.
402. Shimshak RR, Sundaram M, Eddelston B, Prendergast J. Diagnosis of parathyroid adenoma by computed tomography. *J Comput Assist Tomogr* 1979;3:117–119.
403. Whitley NO, Bohlman M, Connor TB, McCrea ES, Mason GR, Whitley JE. Computed tomography for localization of parathyroid adenomas. *J Comput Assist Tomogr* 1981;5:812–817.
404. Wolverson MK, Sundaram M, Eddelston B, Prendergast J. Diagnosis of parathyroid adenoma by computed tomography. *J Comput Assist Tomogr* 1981;5:818–821.
405. Krudy AG, Doppman JL, Brennan MF, Marx SJ, Spiegel AM, Stock JL, Aurbach GD. The detection of mediastinal parathyroid glands by computed tomography, selective arteriography, and venous sampling. *Radiology* 1981;140:739–744.
406. Adams JE, Adams PH, Mantora H. Computed tomography in localization of parathyroid tumors. *Clin Radiol* 1981;32:251–254.
407. Ovenfors CO, Stark D, Moss A, Goldberg H, Clark O, Galante M. Localization of parathyroid adenoma by computed tomography. *J Comput Assist Tomogr* 1982;6:1094–1098.
408. Sommer B, Welter HF, Spelsberg F, Scherer U, Lissner J. Computed tomography for localizing enlarged parathyroid glands in primary hyperparathyroidism. *J Comput Assist Tomogr* 1982;6:521–526.
409. Doppman JL, Krudy AG, Brennan MF, Schneider P, Lasker RD, Marx SJ. CT appearance of enlarged parathyroid glands in the posterior superior mediastinum. *J Comput Assist Tomogr* 1982;6:1099–1102.
410. Takagi H, Tominaga Y, Uchida K, Yamada N, Ishii T, Morimoto T, Yasue M. Preoperative diagnosis of secondary hyperparathyroidism using computed tomography. *J Comput Assist Tomogr* 1982;6:527–528.
411. Krudy AG, Doppman JL, Shawker TH, Spiegel AM, Marx SJ, Norton J, et al. Hyperfunctioning cystic parathyroid glands: CT and sonographic findings. *AJR* 1984;142:175–178.
412. College D, Rohatgi PK. Mediastinal parathyroid cyst. *J Comput Assist Tomogr* 1983;7:140–142.
413. Lineaweaver W, Clore F, Mancuso A, Hill S, Rumley T. Calcified parathyroid glands detected by computed tomography. *J Comput Assist Tomogr* 1984;8:975–977.
414. Krubsack AJ, Wilson SD, Lawson TL, Collier BD, Hellman RS, Isitman AT. Prospective comparison of radionuclide, computed tomographic, and sonographic localization of parathyroid tumors. *World J Surg* 1986;10:579–585.
415. Stark DD, Gooding GAW, Moss AA, Clark OH, Ovenfors CO. Parathyroid imaging: comparison of high-resolution CT and high-resolution sonography. *AJR* 1983;141:633–638.
416. Cates JD, Thorsen K, Lawson TL, Middleton WD, Foley WD, Wilson SD, Krubsack AJ. CT evaluation of parathyroid adenomas: diagnostic criteria and pitfalls. *J Comput Assist Tomogr* 1988;12:626–629.
417. Miller DL, Doppman JL, Shawker TH, Krudy AG, Norton JA, Vucich JJ, et al. Localization of parathyroid adenomas in patients who have undergone surgery. Part 1. Noninvasive imaging methods. *Radiology* 1987;162:133–137.
418. Levin KE, Gooding GAW, Okerlund MD. Localizing studies in patients with persistent or recurrent hyperparathyroidism. *Surgery* 1987;102:917–925.
419. Kneeland JB, Krubsack AJ, Lawson TL, Wilson SD, Collier BD, Froncisz W, Jesmanowicz A, Hyde JS. Enlarged parathyroid glands: high-resolution local coil MR imaging. *Radiology* 1987;162:143–146.
420. Peck WW, Higgins CB, Fisher MR, Ling M, Okerlund MD, Clark OH. Hyperparathyroidism: comparison of MR imaging with radionuclide scanning. *Radiology* 1987;163:415–420.
421. Spritzer CE, Gefter WB, Hamilton R, Greenberg BM, Axel L. Kressel HY. Abnormal parathyroid glands: high-resolution MR imaging. *Radiology* 1987;162:487–491.
422. Kier R, Blinder RA, Herfkins RJ, Leight GS, Spritzer CE, Carroll BA. MR imaging with surface coils in primary hyperparathyroidism. *J Comput Assist Tomogr* 1987;11:863–868.
423. Auffermann W, Gooding GAW, Okerlund MD, Clark OH, Thrurnher S, Levin KE, Higgins CB. Diagnosis of recurrent hyperparathyroidism: comparison of MR imaging and other imaging techniques. *AJR* 1988;150:1027–1033.
424. Kang EH, Schiebler ML, Gefter WB, Kressel HY. Case report. MR demonstration of bilateral intrathyroidal parathyroid glands. *J Comput Assist Tomogr* 1988;12:349–350.
425. Krudy AG, Doppman JL, Marx SJ, Brennan MF, Spiegel A, Aurback GD. Radiographic findings in recurrent parathyroid carcinoma. *Radiology* 1982;142:625–629.
426. Miller DL, Doppman JL, Chang R, Simmons JT, O'Leary TJ, Norton JA, et al. Angiographic ablation of parathyroid adenomas: lessons from a 10-year experience. *Radiology* 1987;165:601–607.
427. Panicek DM, Heitzman ER, Randall PA, Groskin SA, Chew FD, et al. The continuum of pulmonary developmental anomalies. *Radiographics* 1987;7:747–772.
428. Dahmash NS, Chen JTT, Ravin CE, Reed JC, Pratt PC. Unusual radiologic manifestations of bronchogenic cyst. *South Med J* 1984;77:762–764.
429. Pugatch RD, Faling LJ, Spira R. CT diagnosis of benign mediastinal abnormalities. *AJR* 1980;134:685–694.
430. Marvasti MA, Mitchell GE, Burke WA, Meyer JA. Misleading density of mediastinal cysts on computerized tomography. *Ann Thorac Surg* 1981;31:167–170.
431. Nakata H, Nakayama C, Kimoto T, Nakayama T, Tsukamoto Y, Nobe T, Suzuki H. Computed tomography of mediastinal bronchogenic cysts. *J Comput Assist Tomogr* 1982;6:733–738.
432. Mendelson DS, Rose JS, Efremidis SC, Kirschner PA, Cohen BA. Bronchogenic cysts with high CT numbers. *AJR* 1983;140:463–465.
433. Nakata H, Sato Y, Nakayama T, Yoshimatsu H, Kobayashi T. Bronchogenic cyst with high CT number: analysis of contents. *J Comput Assist Tomogr* 1986;10:360–362.
434. Yemault JC, Kuhn G, Dumortier P, Rocmans P, Ketelbant P, Vuyst PD. "Solid" mediastinal bronchogenic cyst: mineralogic analysis. *J Comput Assist Tomogr* 1986;146:73–74.
435. Bankoff MS, Daly BDT, Johnson HA, Carter BL. Case report. Bronchogenic cyst causing superior vena cava obstruction: CT appearance. *J Comput Assist Tomogr* 1985;9:951–952.
436. Volpi A, Cavalli A, Maggioni AP, Pieri-Nerli F. Left atrial compression by a mediastinal bronchogenic cyst presenting with paroxysmal atrial fibrillation. *Thorax* 1988;43:216–217.
437. Haller JA, Golladay ES, Pickard LR, Tepas JJ, Shorter NA, Shermeta DW. Surgical management of lung bud anomalies: lobar emphysema, bronchogenic cyst, cystic adenomatoid malformation, and intralobar pulmonary sequestration. *Ann Thorac Surg* 1979;28:33–43.
438. Schwartz DB, Beals TF, Wimbish KJ, Hammersley JR. Transbronchial fine needle aspiration of bronchogenic cysts. *Chest* 1985;88:573–575.
439. Zimmer WD, Kamida CB, McGough PF, Rosenow EC. Mediastinal duplication cyst. Percutaneous aspiration and cystography for diagnosis and treatment. *Chest* 1986;90:772–773.
440. Kuhlman JE, Fishman EK, Wang KP, Zerhouni EA, Siegelman SS. Mediastinal cysts: diagnosis by CT and needle aspiration. *AJR* 1988;150:75–78.
441. Kuhlman JE, Fishman EK, Wang KP, Siegelman SS. Esophageal duplication cysts: CT and transesophageal aspiration. *AJR* 1985;145:531–532.
442. Wittich GR, Karnel F, Schurawitzki H, Jantsch H. Percutaneous drainage of mediastinal pseudocysts. *Radiology* 1988;167:51–53.
443. Weiss LM, Fagelman D, Warhit JM. CT demonstration of an esophageal duplication cyst. *J Comput Assist Tomogr* 1983;7:716–718.
444. Naidich DP. Esophagus. In: Megibow AJ, Balthazar EJ, eds. *Computed tomography of the gastrointestinal tract.* St. Louis: CV Mosby, 1986;33–98.
445. Maroko I, Hirsch M, Sharon N, Benharroch D. Calcified mediastinal enterogenous cyst. *Gastrointest Radiol* 1984;9:105–106.
446. Rogers CI, Seymour Q, Brock JG. Case report. Atypical pericardial cyst location: the value of computed tomography. *J Comput Assist Tomogr* 1980;4:683–684.
447. Patel BK, Markivee CR, George EA. Pericardial cyst simulating intracardiac mass. *AJR* 1983;141:292–294.

448. Pugatch RD, Braver JH, Robbins AH, Faling J. CT diagnosis of pericardial cysts. *AJR* 1978;131:515–516.
449. Brunner DR, Whitley NO. A pericardial cyst with high CT numbers. *AJR* 1984;142:279–280.
450. Parienty RA, Fontaine Y, Guillemette D. Transformation of a pericardial cyst observed on long-term follow-up. *CT* 1984;8:125–128.
451. Angtuaco EJC, Jiminez JF, Burrows P, Ferris E. Case report. Lymphatic-venous malformation (lymphangiohemangioma) of the mediastinum. *J Comput Assist Tomogr* 1983;7:895–897.
452. Shaked A, Raz I, Gottehrer A, Romanoff H. Aymptomatic, highly vascularized superior mediastinal mass. *Chest* 1984;86:621–622.
453. Joseph AE, Donaldson JS, Reynolds M. Neck and thorax venous aneurysm: association with cystic hygroma. *Radiology* 1989;170:109–112.
454. Murayama S. Retrocrural cystic lymphangioma. *Chest* 1985;88:930–931.
455. Terrier F, Revel D, Pajannen H, Richardson M, Hricak H, Higgins CB. MR imaging of body fluid collections. *J Comput Assist Tomogr* 1986;10:953–962.
456. Naidich DP, Rumancik WM, Ettenger NA, Feiner HD, Harnaz-Schulman M, Spatz EM, et al. Congenital anomalies of the lungs in adults: MR diagnosis. *AJR* 1988;151:13–19.
457. Stark DD, Higgins CB, Lanzer P, Lipton MJ, Schiller N, Crooks LE, et al. Magnetic resonance imaging of the pericardium: normal and pathologic findings. *Radiology* 1984;150:469–474.
458. Barakos JA, Brown JJ, Brescia RJ, Higgins CB. High signal intensity lesions of the chest in MR imaging. *J Comput Assist Tomogr* 1989;13:797–802.
459. Siegel MJ, Nadel SN, Glazer HS, Sagel SS. Mediastinal lesions in children: Comparison of CT and MR. *Radiology* 1986;160:241–244.
460. Winsett MZ, Amparo EG, Fagan CJ, Bedi DG, Gallagher P, Nealon WH. Case report. MR imaging of mediastinal pseudocyst. *J Comput Assist Tomogr* 1988;12:320–322.
461. Oliphant L, McFadden RG, Carr TJ, Mackenzie DA. Magnetic resonance imaging to diagnose intralobar pulmonary sequestration. *Chest* 1987;91:500–502.
462. Halber MD, Daffner RH, Thompson WM. CT of the esophagus: normal appearance. *AJR* 1979;133:1047–1050.
463. Cayea PD, Seltzer SE. A new barium paste for computed tomography of the esophagus. *J Comput Assist Tomogr* 1985;9:214–216.
464. Conces DJ, Tarver RD, Lappas JC. The value of opacification of the esophagus by low density barium paste in computer tomography of the thorax. *J Comput Assist Tomogr* 1988;12:202–205.
465. Kressel HY, Callen PW, Montagne JP, Korobkin M, Goldberg HI, Moss AA, et al. Computed tomographic evaluation of disorders affecting the alimentary tract. *Radiology* 1978;129:451–455.
466. Mori S, Kasai M, Watanabe T. Preoperative assessment of resectability for carcinoma of the thoracic esophagus. *Ann Surg* 1979;190:100–105.
467. Beahrs OH, Meyers MH, eds. *Manual for staging of cancer,* 2nd ed. Philadelphia: JB Lippincott, 1983.
468. Moss AA, Schnyder P, Thoeni RF, Margulis AR. Esophageal carcinoma: pretherapy staging by computed tomography. *AJR* 1981;136:1051–1056.
469. Reinig JW, Stanley JH, Schabel SI. CT evaluation of thickened esophageal walls. *AJR* 1983;140:951–958.
470. Schneekloth G, Terrier F, Fuchs WA. Computed tomography in carcinoma of esophagus and cardia. *Gastrointest Radiol* 1983;8:193–206.
471. Samuelson L, Hambraeus GM, Mercke EC. CT staging of esophageal carcinoma. *Acta Radiol Diag* 1984;25:7–11.
472. Terrier F, Schapira CL, Fuchs WA. CT assessment of operability in carcinoma of the esophagogastric junction. *Eur J Radiol* 1984;4:114–117.
473. Daffner RH, Halber MD, Postlethwait RW, Korobkin M, Thompson WM. CT of the esophagus. Part 2. Carcinoma. *AJR* 1979;133:1051–1055.
474. Thompson WM, Halvorsen RA, Foster WL, Williford ME, Postlethwait RW, Korobkin M. Computed tomography for staging esophageal and gastroesophageal cancer: reevaluation. *AJR* 1983;141:951–958.
475. Kron IL, Cantrell RW, Johns ME, Joob A, Minor G. Computerized axial tomography of the esophagus to determine the suitability for blunt esophagectomy. *Ann Surg* 1984;49:173–174.
476. Quint LE, Glazer GM, Orringer MB, Gross BH. Esophageal carcinoma: CT findings. *Radiology* 1985;155:171–175.
477. Freeny PC, Marks WM. Adenocarcinoma of the gastroesophageal junction: barium and CT examination. *AJR* 1982;138:1077–1084.
478. Picus D, Balfe DM, Koehler RE, Roper CL, Owen JW. Computed tomography in the staging of esophageal carcinoma. *Radiology* 1983;146:433–438.
479. Moss AA. Critical reviews. Esophageal carcinoma: CT findings. *Invest Radiol* 1987;22:84–87.
480. Quint LE, Glazer GM, Orringer MB, Gross BH. Esophageal imaging by MR and CT: study of normal anatomy and neoplasms. *Radiology* 1985;156:727–731.
481. Halvorsen RA, Magruder-Habib K, Foster WL, Roberts L, Potlethwait RW, Thompson WM. Esophageal cancer staging by CT: long-term follow-up study. *Radiology* 1986;161:147–151.
482. Halvorsen RA, Thompson WM. Computed tomographic staging of gastrointestinal tract malignancies. Part 1. Esophagus and stomach. *Invest Radiol* 1987;22:2–16.
483. Vilgrain V, Mompoint D, Palazzo L, Menu Y, Gayet B, Ollier P. Staging of esophageal carcinoma: comparison of results with endoscopic sonography and CT. *AJR* 1990;155:277–281.
484. Iizuka T, Isono K, Kakegawa T, Watanabe H. Parameters linked to ten-year survival in Japan of resected esophageal carcinoma. Report of the Japanese Committee for Registration of Esophageal Carcinoma Cases. *Chest* 1989;96:1005–1011.
485. Drucker MH, Mansour KA, Hatcher CR. Esophageal carcinoma: an aggressive approach. *Ann Thorac Surg* 1979;28:133–138.
486. Gatzinsky P, Berglin E, Dernevik L. Resectional operations and long-term results in carcinoma of the esophagus. *J Thorac Cardiovasc Surg* 1985;89:71–76.
487. Orringer MB. Transhiatal esophagectomy without thoracotomy for carcinoma of the thoracic esophagus. *Ann Surg* 1984;200:282–288.
488. Beatty JD, Beboer G, Rider WD. Carcinoma of the esophagus: pretreatment assessment, correlation or radiation treatment parameters with survival, and identification and management of radiation treatment failure. *Cancer* 1979;43:2254–2267.
489. Piccone VA, LeVeen HH, Ahmed N. Reappraisal of esophagogastrectomy for esophageal malignancy. *Am J Surg* 1979;137:32–38.
490. Ellis FH, Gibb SP, Watkins E. Esophagogastrectomy. *Ann Surg* 1983;198:531–540.
491. Wippold FJ, Scnapf D, Bennet LL. Case report. Esophagosubarachnoid fistula: an unusual complication of esophageal carcinoma. *J Comput Assist Tomogr* 1982;6:147–149.
492. Reddy SC. Esophagopleural fistula. *J Comput Assist Tomogr* 1983;7:376–378.
493. Wippold FJ, Schnapf D, Bennet LL, Friedman AC. Case report. Esophago-subarachnoidal fistula: an unusual complication of esophageal carcinoma. *J Comput Assist Tomogr* 1982;6:147–149.
494. Cornwell J, Walden C, Ghahremani GG. Case report. CT demonstration of fistula between esophageal carcinoma and spinal canal. *J Comput Assist Tomogr* 1986;10:871–873.
495. Heiken JP, Balfe DM, Roper CL. CT evaluation after esophagogastrectomy. *AJR* 1984;143:555–560.
496. Gross BH, Agha FP, Glazer GM, Orringer MB. Gastric interposition following transhiatal esophagectomy: CT evaluation. *Radiology* 1985;155:177–179.
497. Recht MP, Coleman BG, Barbot DJ, Rosato EF, Aronchick JM, Epstein DM, Gefter WB, Miller WT. Recurrent esophageal carcinoma at thoracotomy incisions: diagnostic contributions of CT. *J Comput Assist Tomogr* 1989;13:58–60.
498. Glickstein MF, Gefter WB, Low D, Stephenson LW. Case report. Esophageal mucocele after surgical isolation of the esophagus. *AJR* 1987;149:729–730.

499. Pakter RL, Fishman EK. Metastatic osteosarcoma to the heart and mediastinum presenting as esophageal obstruction. *J Comput Assist Tomogr* 1983;7:1114–1115.

500. Gale ME, Birnbaum SB, Gale DR, Vincent ME. Esophageal invasion by lung cancer: CT diagnosis. *J Comput Assist Tomogr* 1984;8:694–698.

501. Callen PWQ, Filly RA, Korobkin M. Computed tomographic evaluation of the diaphragmatic crura. *Radiology* 1978;126:413–416.

502. Naidich DP, Megibow AJ, Ross CR. CT of the diaphragm: Normal anatomy and variants. *J Comput Assist Tomogr* 1983;7:633–640.

503. Thompson WM, Halvorsen RA, Williford ME, Foster WL, Korobkin M. Computed tomography of the gastroesophageal junction. *Radiographics* 1982;2:179–193.

504. Govoni AF, Whalen JP, Kazam E. Hiatal hernia: a relook. *Radiographics* 1983;3:612–644.

505. Marks WM, Callen PW, Moss AA. Gastroesophageal region: Source of confusion on CT. *AJR* 1981;136:359–362.

506. Thompson WM, Halvorsen RA, Foster W, Roberts L, Korobkin M. Computed tomography of the gastroesophageal junction: value of the left lateral decubitus view. *J Comput Assist Tomogr* 1984;8:346–349.

507. Ginalski JM, Schnyder P, Moss AA. Incidence and significance of a widened esophageal hiatus at CT scan. *J Clin Gastroenterol* 1984;6:467–470.

508. Godwin JD, MacGregor JM. Case report. Extension of ascites into the chest with hiatal hernia: visualization on CT. *AJR* 1987;148:31–32.

509. Lindell MM, Bernadino ME. Diagnosis of hiatus hernia by computed tomography. *Comput Radiol* 1981;5:16–19.

510. Pupols A, Ruzicka FF. Hiatal hernia causing a cardia pseudomass on computed tomography. *J Comput Assist Tomogr* 1984;8:699–700.

511. Clark KE, Foley WD, Lawson TL, Berland LL, Maddison FE. CT evaluation of esophageal and upper abdominal varices. *J Comput Assist Tomogr* 1980;4:510–515.

512. Balthazar EJ, Naidich DP, Megibow AJ, Lefleur RS. CT evaluation of esophageal varices. *AJR* 1987;148:131–135.

513. Hirose WJ, Takashima T, Suzuki M, Matsui O. Case report. "Downhill" varices demonstrated by dynamic computed tomography. *J Comput Assist Tomogr* 1984;8:1007–1009.

514. Halden WJ, Harnsberger HR, Mancuso AA. Computed tomography of esophageal varices after sclerotherapy. *AJR* 1983;140:1195–1196.

515. Mauro MA, Jaques PF, Swantkowski TM, Staab EV, Bozymski EM. CT after uncomplicated esophageal sclerotherapy. *AJR* 1986;147:57–60.

516. Saks BJ, Kilby AE, Dietrich PA. Pleural and mediastinal changes following endoscopic injection sclerotherapy of esophageal varices. *Radiology* 1983;149:639–642.

517. Shaer AH, Bashist B. Case report. Computed tomography of bronchial artery aneurysm with erosion into the esophagus. *J Comput Assist Tomogr* 1989;13:1069–1071.

518. Day DL. Aortic arch in neonates with esophageal atresia: preoperative assessment using CT. *Radiology* 1985;155:99–100.

519. Williford ME, Thompson WM, Hamilton JD, Postlethwait RW. Esophageal tuberculosis: findings on barium swallow and computed tomography. *Gastrointest Radiol* 1983;8:119–122.

520. Im KG, Kim JH, Han MC, Kim CW. Computed tomography of esophagomediastinal fistula in tuberculous mediastinal lymphadenitis. *J Comput Assist Tomogr* 1990;14:89–92.

521. Wechsler RJ, Steiner RM, Goodman LR, Teplick SK, Mapp E, Laufer I. Iatrogenic esophageal-pleural fistula: subtlety of diagnosis in the absence of mediastinitis. *Radiology* 1982;144:239–243.

522. Han SY, McElvein RB, Aldrete JS. Perforation of the esophagus: correlation of site and cause with plain film findings. *AJR* 1985;145:537–540.

523. Glenny RW, Fulkerson WJ, Ravin CE. Occult spontaneous esophageal perforation. Unusual clinical and radiographic presentation. *Chest* 1987;92:562–565.

524. Pezzulli FA, Aronson D, Goldberg N. Case report. Computed tomography of mediastinal hematoma secondary to unusual

525. Brown BM. Case report. Computed tomography of mediastinal abscess secondary to posttraumatic esophageal laceration. *J Comput Assist Tomogr* 1984;8:765–767.

526. Berkmen YM, Auh YH. CT diagnosis of acquired tracheoesophageal fistula in adults. *J Comput Assist Tomogr* 1985;9:302–304.

527. Gamba JL, Heaston DK, Ling D, Korobkin M. CT diagnosis of an esophageal foreign body. *AJR* 1983;140:289–290.

528. Agostini S, Salducci J, Clement JP. Case report. Idiopathic muscular hypertrophy of the esophagus: CT features. *J Comput Assist Tomogr* 1988;12:1041–1043.

529. Healy JF, Wells MV, Carlstom T, Rosenkrantz H. Lateral thoracic meningocele demonstrated by computerized tomography. *Comput Tomogr* 1980;4:159–163.

530. Ross CR, McCauley DI, Naidich DP. Intrathoracic neurofibroma of the vagus nerve associated with bronchial obstruction. *J Comput Assist Tomogr* 1982;6:406–412.

531. Kumar AJ, Kuhajda FP, Martinez CR, Fishman EK, Jezic DV, Siegelman SS. CT of extracranial nerve sheath tumors. *J Comput Assist Tomogr* 1983;7:857–865.

532. Biondetti PR, Vigo M, Fiore D, De Faveri D, Ravasini R, Benedetti L. CT appearance of generalized von Recklinghausen neurofibromatosis. *J Comput Assist Tomogr* 1983;7:866–869.

533. Bourgouin PM, Shepard JO, Moore EH, McLoud TC. Plexiform neurofibromatosis of the mediastinum: CT appearance. *AJR* 1988;151:461–463.

534. Joseph SG, Tellis CJ. Posterior mediastinal mass with intraspinous extension. *Chest* 1988;93:1101–1103.

535. Aughenbaugh GL. Thoracic manifestations of neurocutaneous diseases. *Radiol Clin North Am* 1984;22:741–756.

536. Coleman BG, Arger PH, Dalinka MK, Obringer AL, Raney BR, Meadows AT. CT of sarcomatous degeneration in neurofibromatosis. *AJR* 1983;140:383–387.

537. Levine E, Huntrakoon M, Wetzel LH. Malignant nerve-sheath neoplasms in neurofibromatosis: distinction from benign tumors by using imaging techniques. *AJR* 1987;149:1059–1064.

538. Feinstein RS, Gatewood OMB, Fishman EK, Goldman SM, Siegelman SS. Computed tomography of adult neuroblastoma. *J Comput Assist Tomogr* 1984;8:720–726.

539. Efremidis SC, Dan SJ, Cohen BA, Mitty HA, Rabinowitz JG. Displaced paraspinal line: role of CT and lymphography. *AJR* 1981;136:505–509.

540. Black WC, Armstrong P, Daniel TM, Cooper PH. Case report. Computed tomography of aggressive fibromatosis in the posterior mediastinum. *J Comput Assist Tomogr* 1987;11:153–155.

541. Tarr RW, Glick AG, Shaff MI. Case report. Benign hemangioendothelioma involving posterior mediastinum: CT findings. *J Comput Assist Tomogr* 1986;10:865–867.

542. Burk DL, Brunberg JA, Kanal E, Latchaw RE, Wolf GL. Spinal and paraspinal neurofibromatosis: surface coil MR imaging at 1.5T. *Radiology* 1987;162:797–801.

543. Dietrich RB, Kangarloo H, Lenarsky C, Feig SA. Neuroblastoma: the role of MR imaging. *AJR* 1987;148:927–942.

544. Cohen MD, Weetman R, Provisor A. Magnetic resonance imaging of neuroblastoma with 0.15-T magnet. *AJR* 1984;143:1241–1248.

545. Siegel MJ, Jamroz GA, Glazer HS, Abramson CL. MR imaging of intraspinal extension of neuroblastoma. *J Comput Assist Tomogr* 1986;10:593–595.

546. Mintzer RA, Malave SR, Neiman HL, Michaelis LL, Vanecko RM, Sanders JH. Computed vs conventional tomography in evaluation of primary and secondary pulmonary neoplasms. *Radiology* 1979;132:659–663.

547. Jost RG, Sagel SS, Stanley RJ, Levitt RG. Computed tomography of the thorax. *Radiology* 1978;126:125–136.

548. Crowe JK, Brown LR, Muhm JR. Computed tomography of the mediastinum. *Radiology* 1978;128:75–87.

549. van Sonnenberg E, Casola G, Ho M, et al. Difficult thoracic lesions: CT-guided biopsy experience in 150 cases. *Radiology* 1988;167:457–461.

550. Westcott JL. Percutaneous transthoracic needle biopsy. *Radiology* 1988;169:593–601.

esophageal laceration: a Boerhaave variant. *J Comput Assist Tomogr* 1989;13:129–131.

551. Perlmutt LM, Johnston WW, Dunnick NR. Percutaneous transthoracic needle aspiration: a review. *AJR* 1989;152:451–455.

552. Kundel HL, Kressel HY, Epstein D. The potential role of NMR imaging in thoracic disease. *Radiol Clin North Am* 1983;21:801–808.

553. Newhouse JH. Nuclear magnetic resonance studies of the chest. *Clin Chest Med* 1984;5:307–312.

554. Berquist TH, Brown LR, May GR, Jett JR, Bernatz PE. Magnetic resonance imaging of the chest: a diagnostic comparison with computed tomography and hilar tomography. *Magn Reson Imaging* 1984;2:315–327.

555. Ross JS, O'Donovan PB, Nonoa R, Mehta A, Buonocore E, MacIntyre WJ, Golish JA, Ahmad M. Magnetic resonance of the chest: initial experience with imaging and in vivo T1 and T2 calculations. *Radiology* 1984;152:95–101.

556. RDOG imaging study. (Abst). *Radiology* 1989;173(P):69.

Chapter 3

Airways

The central airways include the trachea, the carina, the main-stem bronchi, and the lobar, segmental, and subsegmental bronchi. Because of the clarity of anatomic detail that can be obtained with cross-sectional imaging, these structures are easily definable with computed tomography (CT) (1,2). Evaluation of the central airways is important for the following reasons: (a) The bronchi are important sites of disease, both neoplastic and inflammatory. The ability to detect and potentially differentiate between various forms of bronchial pathology is of obvious clinical significance. (b) The bronchi, as seen in cross-section, provide a road map into the pulmonary parenchyma. This is important for both localization and characterization of pulmonary parenchymal disease. (c) The bronchi serve as a lattice on which the pulmonary arteries and veins are draped in characteristic fashion and, therefore, serve as the point of orientation for interpreting the pulmonary hila (3–6). The purpose of this chapter will be, first, to review CT technique as well as CT anatomy of the airways and, second, define clinical indications for the use of CT, with special emphasis on correlation with fiberoptic bronchoscopy (FOB).

GENERAL PRINCIPLES AND METHODOLOGY

Accurate evaluation of the airways necessitates both detailed knowledge of normal anatomy and variants, as well as careful attention to technique. In a classic study of 50 patients with normal chest radiographs evaluated with contiguous 10-mm thick sections, Osborne et al. (7) documented that only 70% of segmental bronchi could be identified reliably. Similar results have been reported

by Jardin and Remy (6). These limitations point up the necessity for developing clearly defined methodologies for adequately scanning the airways.

Following detailed evaluation of all relevant plain radiographic studies, the following strategies may be applied.

Routine Studies

This approach is a modification of routine chest scans as performed in most institutions, and is most appropriate when indications for studying the airways are vague or nonspecific. An initial sequence of contiguous 8–10-mm sections is obtained from the thoracic inlet to the hemidiaphragms. Based on the appearance of the airways and parenchyma on these baseline scans, a limited number of additional thin sections is then obtained: either to more convincingly visualize a focal abnormality (especially in patients with some suspicion of endobronchial disease), or to identify airways not visualized initially (for example, in patients with a vague history of hemoptysis and a nonlocalizing chest radiograph).

In our experience, this approach is least sensitive for evaluating the airways: additional sections are almost always necessary in order to avoid inadequate or misleading interpretation of airway pathology, especially due to partial volume averaging artifacts. As shown in Fig. 1, given the small size of lobar and segmental bronchi, 8–10-mm thick sections can easily distort otherwise normal airways, creating a false impression of abnormality. The number of additional slices acquired should reflect the length and size of the airways in question. For lobar bronchi, a few contiguous 5-mm thick sections are

A

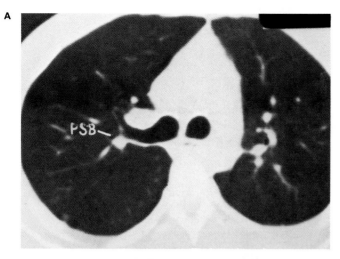

B

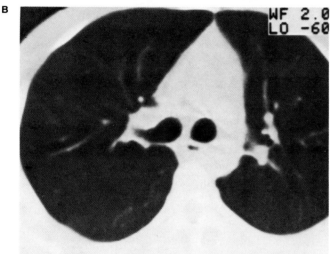

FIG. 1. Technique: normal variant. **A,B:** Sections through the center of the right upper lobe bronchus and 10 mm below the center of the right upper lobe bronchus, respectively. It is easy to simulate bronchial pathology by scanning below or above the center of the right upper lobe bronchus. The appearance could be misinterpreted as showing narrowing from tumor. PSB, posterior segmental bronchus.

generally sufficient, whereas thinner (1.5–2 mm) sections are best reserved for smaller (subsegmental) airways or bronchi within the lung parenchyma. Although oblique CT scans with the gantry angled cranially 20° may be advantageous, especially for visualizing the course of the lingular and middle lobe bronchi, angling the gantry is usually not indicated provided care is taken to obtain appropriate axial thin sections (8).

Tailored Studies

In patients for whom bronchial pathology is to be ruled out specifically, a reasonable modification of rou-

tine scan technique is as follows. An initial sequence of contiguous 8–10-mm sections is acquired from the thoracic inlet to the level of the carina. Following this, contiguous 5-mm sections are obtained through the hila to approximately the level of the inferior pulmonary veins. Contiguous 8–10-mm sections are then obtained inferiorly to the level of the hemidiaphragms. While this technique results in between eight to ten additional scans, the increased exposure is more than offset by the resultant marked improvement in visualization of the central segmental and subsegmental bronchi (Fig. 2). Acquisition of these additional images is especially valuable in patients in whom central airways disease in particular is suspected, as for example, patients with chronic parenchymal infiltrates, or segmental or subsegmental atelectasis. As a practical matter, newer scanners allow acquisition in one predetermined sequence of sections of varying thickness: obtaining 5-mm thick sections through the airways, therefore, does not require that each part of the study be programmed separately.

As a further modification of this technique, utilizing the same spacing outlined above, 1.5–2-mm thick sections can be used in place of 8–10-mm thick sections from the outset. This would result in a sequence of 1.5–2-mm thick sections every 10 mm from the thoracic inlet to the distal trachea, followed by 5-mm thick sections every 5 mm through the central airways, followed again by another sequence of 1.5–2-mm thick sections to the hemidiaphragms (Fig. 2). As discussed in the section on bronchiectasis, optimal identification of bronchiectatic airways requires high resolution, 1.5–2-mm thick sections should be obtained. The approach outlined above, therefore, emphasizing thin-section evaluation of both the central airways and the distal parenchyma, represents the most sensitive methodology for detecting radiographically occult causes of hemoptysis, and is most applicable to patients with hemoptysis in whom chest radiographs are either nonspecific or normal.

Whenever possible, the strategies outlined above can be modified to incorporate the use of intravenous (i.v.) contrast administration. In select cases, especially when the extent of peribronchial disease needs to be established (e.g., in patients with airway lesions who are potential candidates for transbronchial needle aspiration or biopsy, or laser therapy for obstructed airways) sections obtained following a bolus of i.v. contrast material may prove invaluable. Whenever possible, dynamic scanning should be utilized, either with multiple images at a single preselected level (dynamic static scanning), or through multiple levels (dynamic incremental scanning) as indicated. As previously noted, iodine content should be sufficient to cause dense vascular opacification (see Chapter 1).

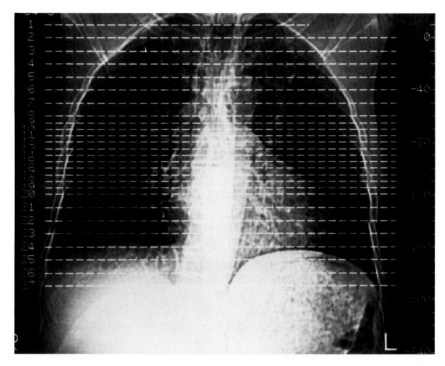

FIG. 2. CT evaluation of the airways: Technique. Annotated AP scanogram. Optimal evaluation of the central segmental and subsegmental airways requires obtaining 5-mm thick sections from the distal trachea through the basilar bronchi, corresponding to sections numbered 8 to 20. While 8–10-mm thick sections are adequate in most cases for all other sections illustrated, corresponding to sections numbered 1 to 7, and 21–27, respectively, in patients suspected of bronchiectasis, these may be replaced by 1.5–2-mm thick sections.

TRACHEA

Anatomically, the trachea is a cartilaginous and membranous tube that extends from the larynx superiorly (at the level of the sixth cervical vertebra) to the carina (at the level of the fifth thoracic vertebra). There is marked variability in the cross-sectional appearance of the trachea, which normally may appear rounded, oval, or horseshoe-shaped with a flattened posterior wall (9,10). Despite variability, the tracheal wall is almost always a thin, delicate structure, well defined internally by the central air column, and frequently as well delineated externally by the presence of mediastinal fat (Fig. 3). The position of the trachea will vary, depending on what level sections are obtained through the superior mediastinum. As the trachea courses with a slight anteroposterior obliquity, progressively caudal sections will show the trachea to lie more posteriorly. At all levels, the trachea lies anterior to the esophagus, which usually lies slightly to the left (Fig. 3).

Along most of its length, the right wall of the trachea is in contact with the mediastinal pleural reflections of the

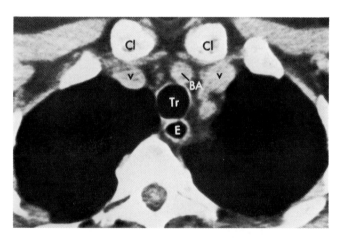

FIG. 3. Normal tracheal anatomy. Section at the level of the great vessels through the trachea (Tr). The full thickness of the tracheal wall is exquisitely well defined internally by the central air column and externally by mediastinal fat, except for that portion of the posterior wall which lies immediately adjacent to the esophagus (E). The left subclavian artery is clearly separate from the trachea. On the right side lung outlines the lateral wall; some lung also extends just posterior to the trachea, approximating the right lateral wall of the esophagus. This space has been called the retrotracheal recess and gives rise on lateral radiograph to the posterior tracheal band. BA, brachiocephalic artery; v, brachiocephalic veins; Cl, clavicles.

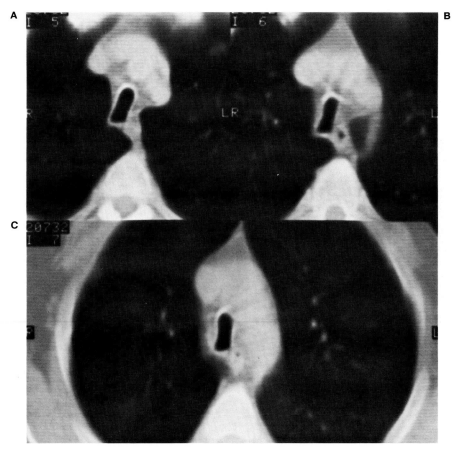

FIG. 4. Saber-sheath trachea. **A–C:** Sequential images from above downward show the typical configuration of a saber-sheath trachea. As shown in B, the trachea measures 2.16 cm in length in the sagittal plane and 0.67 cm in width in the coronal plane.

right upper lobe (Fig. 3). This gives rise to the right paratracheal stripe seen on routine posterior-anterior (PA) radiographs. Additionally, a potential space exists between the posterior right half of the trachea anteriorly and the right lateral wall of the esophagus medially. This has been called the retrotracheal recess and is frequently occupied by lung. These relationships give rise on lateral radiographs to the posterior tracheal band (11).

Abnormal variations in the configuration of the trachea are easily defined with CT. Figure 4 is a section at the level of the great vessels in a patient with a saber-sheath trachea. Although described classically as a static deformity consisting of marked coronal narrowing associated with sagittal widening of the trachea, abnormal narrowing of the tracheal lumen during expiration can be documented when patients are examined using CT during a Valsalva maneuver and during forced expiration (10). This may be significant, since these patients invariably have chronic obstructive pulmonary disease (12).

CT is most efficacious in analyzing tracheal neoplasia, both primary and secondary (9,10,13). Despite the pres-

ence of air within the tracheal lumen, visualization and definition of tracheal tumors are difficult with routine radiographs, including tomography. This point is illustrated in Fig. 5 (a patient with adenoid-cystic carcinoma). Among primary tracheal neoplasms, adenoid-cystic carcinomas are second only to squamous cell carcinoma in frequency (14). These tumors arise from the tracheobronchial mucous glands, most frequently on the posterolateral wall of the trachea, and they show a marked propensity for local invasion (Fig. 6). Although endoscopic biopsy can reliably establish the diagnosis, proper preoperative evaluation requires definition of the presence and extent of extraluminal involvement. This is especially important since recent advances in tracheal surgery have made resection of long tracheal segments possible (Figs. 6 and 7) (15–17). In addition to adenoid-cystic carcinomas, the CT appearance of other lesions, including granular cell tumors and benign leiomyomas, has been reported (18–20).

Secondary neoplastic involvement of the trachea usually results from direct invasion, frequently from esophageal carcinoma. Metastases to the trachea are rel-

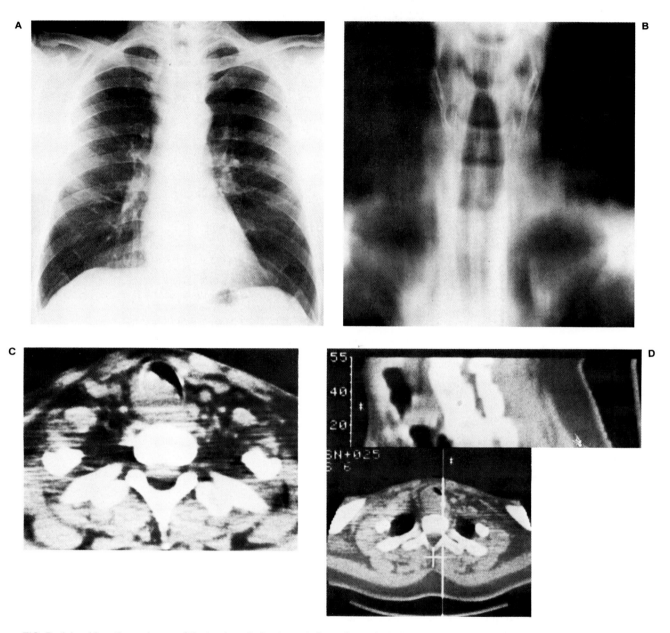

FIG. 5. Adenoid-cystic carcinoma of the trachea. **A:** Posteroanterior radiograph. **B:** Anteroposterior tomogram. A mass in the trachea can be defined inferiorly. **C:** Section through the midtrachea. The tracheal lumen is narrowed by tumor, which extends posteriorly into the prevertebral fascia. Proper therapy of these tumors is contingent on defining the true extent of disease, both intra- and extraluminally. **D:** Sagittal reconstruction demonstrates, to good advantage, the true extent of tumor.

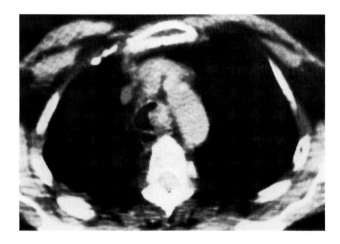

FIG. 6. Adenoid-cystic carcinoma of the trachea. Section at the level of the aortic arch shows a focal, well-defined soft-tissue mass arising from the left lateral wall of the trachea. Note that although the mass extends outside the wall into the mediastinum, there is a clear plane of separation between the mass and adjacent mediastinal structures, indicating potential resectability, later confirmed surgically (compare with Fig. 5).

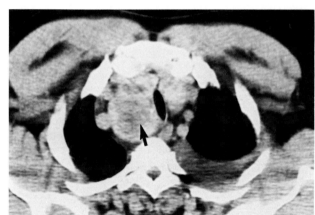

FIG. 7. Squamous cell carcinoma of the trachea. Section through the trachea at the level of the great vessels. The trachea wall is thickened, and the lumen appears circumferentially and irregularly narrowed. A soft-tissue mass can be identified infiltrating deeply into the mediastinum, obliterating the normal fascial planes surrounding the brachiocephalic artery and medial wall of the right brachiocephalic vein. As compared with the appearance of the trachea shown in Fig. 6, this tumor proved unresectable.

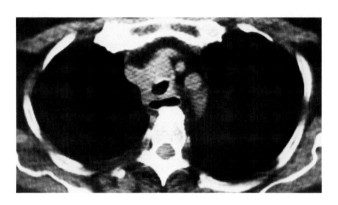

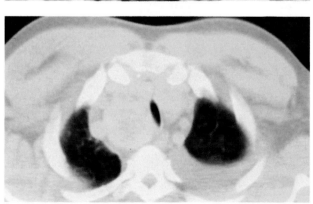

FIG. 8. Extrinsic compression of the trachea-substernal thyroid. **A,B:** Section through the superior mediastinum, imaged with (A) narrow and (B) wide windows, respectively. There is a soft-tissue mass both to the right and left of the trachea causing marked narrowing of the lumen. Irregular low density is definable within the mass, especially to the right (*arrow*). These findings are typical of substernal extension of the thyroid. Further characterization requires histologic evaluation.

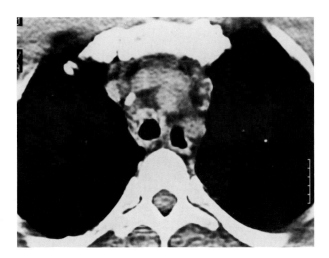

FIG. 9. Tracheal sarcoid. Section through the aortic arch. The trachea is circumferentially thickened; the tracheal lumen is narrowed. Enlarged mediastinal nodes are present as well. Biopsy confirmed tracheal sarcoid. This appearance may be indistinguishable from other infiltrative-inflammatory diseases of the tracheal wall.

atively uncommon and are usually seen in association with bronchogenic carcinoma.

Mediastinal masses, both benign and malignant, cause displacement or narrowing of the trachea (Fig. 8). The trachea is a relatively flexible structure, allowing for significant deviation without necessarily causing symptoms. A mass adjacent to the trachea per se is not good evidence of tracheal involvement; tumor invasion can be diagnosed reliably only when there is marked irregularity of the tracheal wall and/or lumen.

Tracheal stenosis may also be defined with CT. However, due to inaccuracies resulting from limitations inherent in imaging in the transaxial plane only, CT may overestimate both the degree and the length of the stenosis, as compared with tomograms, tracheograms, or endoscopy (10). Short stenotic segments (i.e., <0.5 cm) in particular may prove difficult to define with routine transaxial imaging.

A wide variety of inflammatory diseases, both primary and mediastinal, may also directly affect the tracheal wall (21). In these cases, CT may disclose circumferential, uniform thickening of the entire tracheal wall, as in a patient with biopsy-proven tracheal sarcoidosis (Fig. 9). A similar appearance has been documented to occur in other inflammatory diseases, including tuberculosis, amyloidosis, Wegener's granulomatosis, and relapsing polychondritis (Fig. 10) (22–25). In patients with tracheobronchopathia osteochondroplastica, multiple, characteristically calcified nodules irregularly projecting into the tracheal lumen are more easily documented than with routine tomography (26). The CT diagnosis of congenital and acquired tracheoesophageal fistulae has also been reported (27,28).

As compared with CT, magnetic resonance (MR) offers the unique advantage of sectioning the trachea in both coronal and sagittal planes (17,29,30). Diffuse involvement may be more easily evaluated when the trachea can be identified along its entire length (Fig. 11). As with CT, MR allows simultaneous evaluation not only of the dimensions of the tracheal lumen, but measurements of the true thickness of the tracheal wall, as well as the extent of extraluminal disease. In patients with tracheal tumors, both primary and secondary, MR appears comparable to CT in identification of the extent of disease (Fig. 12).

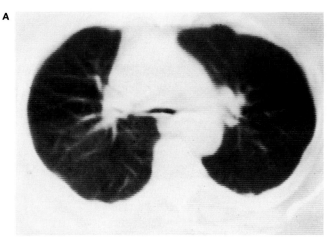

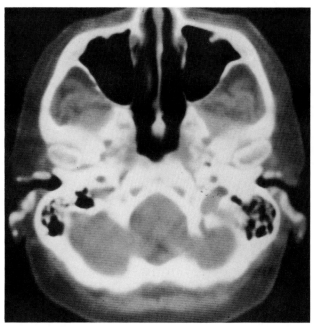

FIG. 10. Relapsing polychondritis. A: Section through the carina shows marked narrowing of the right and left main-stem bronchi, as well as the right upper lobe bronchus. The lung fields appear normal. B: Scan through the base of the skull shows diffuse calcifications of the pinnae of both ears. This combination of findings is pathognomonic of relapsing polychondritis. (Case courtesy of Burton Cohen, M.D., Mt. Sinai Hospital, New York, NY.)

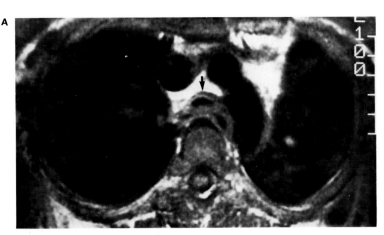

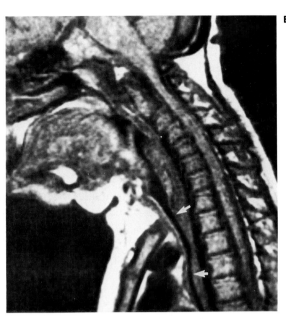

FIG. 11. Benign narrowing of the trachea: MR evaluation. **A:** Transaxial, cardiac gated, T1-weighted section at the level of the origin of the brachiocephalic artery. There is marked thickening of the tracheal wall and significant narrowing of the tracheal lumen easily identified as an area of abnormal, intermediate signal intensity, clearly distinguishable from the brighter signal originating from adjacent mediastinal fat (*arrow*). Although the wall of the esophagus also appears thickened, this is less specific, possibly due to partial collapse. **B:** Sagittal midline section through the midtrachea, obtained with the same technique as in A. Abnormal thickening of the wall is easily identified along the entire length of the trachea (*arrows*). Despite clear delineation of diffuse tracheal disease, the findings are nonspecific. In this case, these abnormalities occurred in a patient with a documented mucopolysaccharidosis. (From Naidich, ref. 114.)

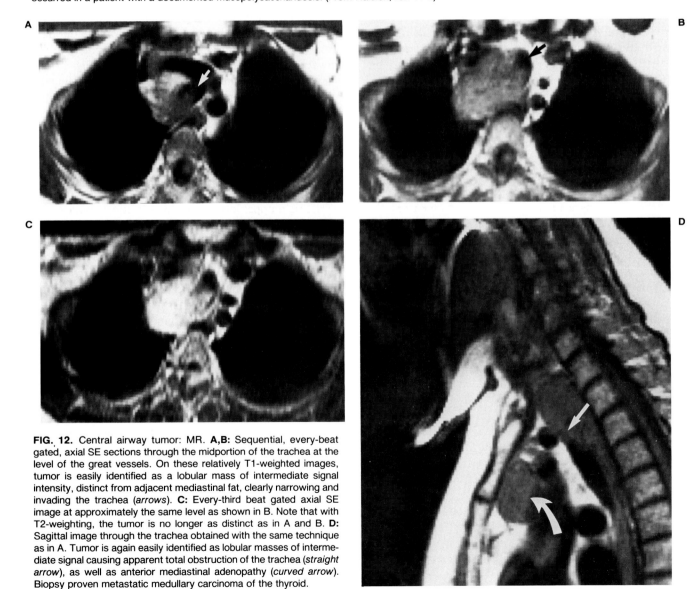

FIG. 12. Central airway tumor: MR. **A,B:** Sequential, every-beat gated, axial SE sections through the midportion of the trachea at the level of the great vessels. On these relatively T1-weighted images, tumor is easily identified as a lobular mass of intermediate signal intensity, distinct from adjacent mediastinal fat, clearly narrowing and invading the trachea (*arrows*). **C:** Every-third beat gated axial SE image at approximately the same level as shown in B. Note that with T2-weighting, the tumor is no longer as distinct as in A and B. **D:** Sagittal image through the trachea obtained with the same technique as in A. Tumor is again easily identified as lobular masses of intermediate signal causing apparent total obstruction of the trachea (*straight arrow*), as well as anterior mediastinal adenopathy (*curved arrow*). Biopsy proven metastatic medullary carcinoma of the thyroid.

Despite the advantages inherent in imaging the trachea with both CT and MR, a significant role for both fluoroscopy and even routine tomography still remains (16). Fluoroscopy allows functional evaluation of the trachea (e.g., in patients with tracheomalacia), which cannot be obtained with routine CT scanners, although the potential for physiologic evaluation with ultrafast CT scanning has been documented, especially in the pediatric age group (see Chapter 11) (31–33). Routine tomography, by virtue of its greater spatial resolution, may remain an important adjunct to CT (or MR) specifically for the preoperative assessment of patients with focal tracheal and main-stem bronchial lesions for whom plastic surgical reconstruction is planned (17).

BRONCHIAL ANATOMY

The ability to visualize a given bronchus on CT depends on the size and orientation of that bronchus. The origin and proximal portion of every major bronchus that courses horizontally can be identified regularly on CT, provided meticulous scanning technique is employed (see above). These include the right upper lobe bronchus (including both the anterior and posterior segmental bronchi), the left upper lobe bronchus (including the anterior segmental bronchus), the middle lobe bronchus (generally including some portion of both the medial and lateral segmental bronchi), and the superior segmental bronchi of both lower lobes.

Bronchi having a vertical course will be seen only in cross-section and will then appear as circular lucencies. These include the apical segmental bronchus of the right upper lobe, the apical-posterior segmental bronchus of the left upper lobe, the bronchus intermedius, and the proximal portions of both lower lobe bronchi (below the takeoff of the superior segmental bronchi).

The most difficult bronchi to visualize are those that run obliquely. This is especially true of the lingular bronchus, including the superior and inferior lingular divisions; the lateral and medial segmental bronchi of the middle lobe also course with a shallow obliquity. Such bronchi appear oval or elliptical when viewed in cross-section.

Only the proximal portions of the bronchial tree, specifically the proximal portions of the segmental bronchi, can be visualized and identified on CT. Reduced size as well as variable anatomic course limit interpretation distal to the proximal portions of fourth-order, subsegmental bronchi. As will be discussed later, visualization of bronchi in the periphery of the lung, especially on 10-mm thick sections is abnormal, suggesting either thickening of the bronchial walls and/or parenchymal disease.

The right and left bronchial trees will be considered independently. For simplicity, standard nomenclature and letter-number codes will be consistently used (Table 1) (34–38). Emphasis will be placed on recognition of characteristic sections, as illustrated in Figs. 13, 14, and 21 (see pages 159 and 164).

Right Lung Segmental Anatomy

As shown in Fig. 13, the right bronchial tree may be viewed as a sequence of five characteristic sections: the distal trachea-carina, the right upper lobe bronchus, the bronchus intermedius, the middle lobe bronchus, and the lower lobe bronchus.

Figure 15 shows a series of 5-mm thick sections through the right upper lobe bronchus and its segmental divisions. At the level of the distal trachea, the apical segmental bronchus of the right upper lobe can be seen in cross-section, appearing as a circular lucency in close proximity to accompanying branches of the right upper lobe pulmonary artery and right superior pulmonary vein (Fig. 15). The right upper lobe bronchus itself is always found at or just below the carina. In Fig. 15, the carina is easily identified as a thin septum separating the right from the left main-stem bronchi. The right upper lobe bronchus originates more cephalad than the left upper lobe bronchus, above the level of the right main pulmonary artery. The right upper lobe bronchus courses horizontally; the origins and proximal portions of the anterior and posterior segmental bronchi are visualized routinely. Characteristically, the posterior wall of the right upper lobe bronchus is in direct contact with air either in the posterior segment of the right upper lobe or the superior segment of the right lower lobe. Differentiation between the posterior segment of the right upper lobe and the superior segment of the right lower lobe is facilitated by identification of the upper portion of the oblique fissure (Fig. 15).

The origin of the apical segment of the right upper lobe bronchus can be visualized routinely with careful scanning technique. The origin appears as a rounded area of decreased density "superimposed" on the distal portion of the right upper lobe bronchus (Fig. 15).

Although some variability in the cross-sectional appearance of the airways is to be anticipated, this is more often the result of variations in the plane of the scan than true anatomic variants (Figs. 16 and 17). As has already been discussed, accurate visualization of bronchi requires meticulous technique. As shown in Fig. 1, it is easy to "distort" the normal appearance of a bronchus if sections are not obtained through the center of the bronchus.

MacGregor et al. (39) have noted on scans obtained through both the anterior and posterior segmental bronchi and their subsegmental divisions that in ~15%

TABLE 1. *Segmental and subsegmental bronchi: nomenclature and variants*

Bronchial segments	Subsegments	Most common variants/comments
Right lung		
Right upper lobe		
B1, apical	a, apical	Widely distributed in apex (35%)
	b, anterior	
B2, anterior	a, lateral	
	b, anterior	
B3, posterior	a, apical	
	b, posterior	
Axillary		Subsegment formed by B2a and B3b (or both)
Middle lobe		
B4, lateral	a, lateral	B4 and B5 equivalent in size (44%); B5 > B4 (27%). Trifurcation
	b, medial	(B4a, B4b, B5a + b) (13%)
B5, medial	a, superior	
	b, inferior	
Right lower lobe		
B6, superior segmental bronchus	a, medial	B6c, B6a + b bifurcation (60%)
	b, superior	
	c, lateral	
B*, subsuperior bronchus		Variable, arises posteriorly between B6 and B7 (30%)
Truncus basalis		Segment extending between B6 and B7
B7, medial basilar bronchus	a, anterior	B7a + b course anterior to the right inferior pulmonary vein (60%)
	b, medial	
B8, anterior	a, lateral	B8, B9–10 bifurcation (60%); B8, B9, B10
	b, basilar	
B9, lateral	a, lateral	Trifurcation (15%); rudimentary B8 (10%)
	b, basilar	
B10, posterior basilar bronchi	a, posterior	
	b, lateral	
	c, basilar	
Left lung		
Left upper lobe		
B1 + 2, apicoposterior	a, apical	
	b, posterior	
	c, lateral	
B3, anterior	a, lateral	B3 may arise anywhere between B1 + 2 and B4 + 5; B3 poorly
	b, medial	defined (25%)
	c, superior	
B4, superior lingular bronchus	a, lateral	Anatomic extent varies with size and distribution of B3. Well-
	b, anterior	developed B4a (40%)
B5, inferior lingular bronchus	a, superior	
	b, inferior	
B6+, superior bronchus	a, medial	B6a, B6b + c bifurcation (45%)
	b, superior	
	c, lateral	
B*, subsuperior bronchus		Variable, arises as single stem (30%)
Truncus basalis		Segment extending between B6 and B7 (9 mm wide and 13 mm
		long)
B7 + 8, anteromedial bronchus	B7a, medial	B7 + 8, B9–10B bifurcation (45%); B7 + 8, 9, 10 trifurcation
	B7b, lateral	(15%); separate origin of B7 (<5%)
	B8a, lateral	
	B8b, basilar	
B9, lateral basilar bronchus	a, lateral	
	b, basilar	
B10, posterior basilar bronchus	a, lateral	
	b, basilar	

Percentages in parentheses represent general approximations.
Modified from Jackson and Huber, ref. 34; Boyden, ref. 35; and Yamashita, ref. 38.

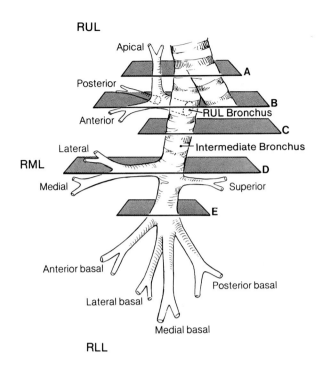

FIG. 13. Diagrammatic representation of the right bronchial tree in a steep oblique projection. Levels A–E represent key levels. RUL, right upper lobe; RML, right middle lobe; RLL, right lower lobe.

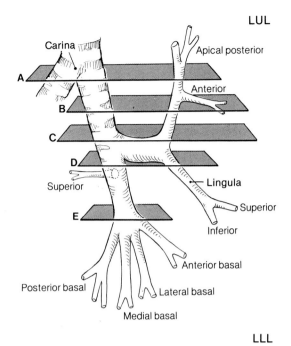

FIG. 14. Diagrammatic representation of the left bronchial tree in 45° oblique projection. LUL, left upper lobe; LLL, left lower lobe. Note that in both these diagrams, anatomic detail corresponding to the basilar segmental bronchi in particular is extremely sketchy (compare with Fig. 21).

of normal patients an independent ramus of the posterior segmental bronchus of the right upper lobe can be recognized, supplying a discrete axillary subsegment. More often, this actually represents a prominent posterior subsegmental division, easily identified in cross-section (Fig. 15).

The posterior wall of the right upper lobe bronchus is an important anatomic landmark. In general, this stripe is uniform in caliber. Although there is some variability in the overall thickness, the upper limits of normal should be <0.5 cm. This posterior stripe should have a uniform configuration; nodularity or irregularity is abnormal, generally signifying tumor infiltration and/or adenopathy. One significant exception is the finding of a prominent azygos vein (40). This appearance should not cause confusion; analysis of sections just above and below should establish the presence of a prominent azygos vein. If doubt persists, scans taken following a Valsalva maneuver should show marked decrease in the size of the azygos vein.

True anatomic variants are unusually encountered. Most frequent is the finding of a tracheal bronchus (Fig. 17). This anomalous airway usually arises at or within 2 cm of the tracheal bifurcation and typically supplies a variable extent of the medial-apical portion of the right upper lobe (41–43). Although often supernumerary, tracheal bronchi may also represent a replaced segment or subsegment of the right upper lobe bronchus proper. Though usually asymptomatic, recurrent infection and/or bronchiectasis may result from partial obstruction;

associated vascular and tracheobronchial anomalies have also been reported.

Figure 18 is a section through the bronchus intermedius. The bronchus intermedius extends from the point at which the right upper lobe bronchus originates to the point of origin of the middle lobe bronchus. The bronchus intermedius lies directly posterior to the right main pulmonary artery and, at a slightly lower level, just medial to the right intralobar pulmonary artery. The entire posterior wall of this bronchus is in contact with air in the superior segment of the right lower lobe. Pulmonary parenchyma also extends posteromedial to the bronchus intermedius, in the aptly named "azygoesophageal recess," the medial border of which is formed by the azygos vein. Except for the pediatric population, lung in this recess is normally convex medially. This convexity is obliterated when there are enlarged subcarinal lymph nodes. The region of the minor fissure separating the right upper and middle lobes is generally manifested as a hypovascular zone lateral to the right interlobar pulmonary artery frequently seen at this level (Fig. 18).

Figure 19 shows sequential 5-mm thick sections through the origin of the middle lobe bronchus and medial and lateral segmental bronchi, respectively. The middle lobe bronchus extends anteriorly at a slightly oblique angle. The origin of the middle lobe bronchus also marks the point of origin of the right lower lobe bronchus. Although a thin septum of tissue or spur may be identified separating the orifices of two airways, more

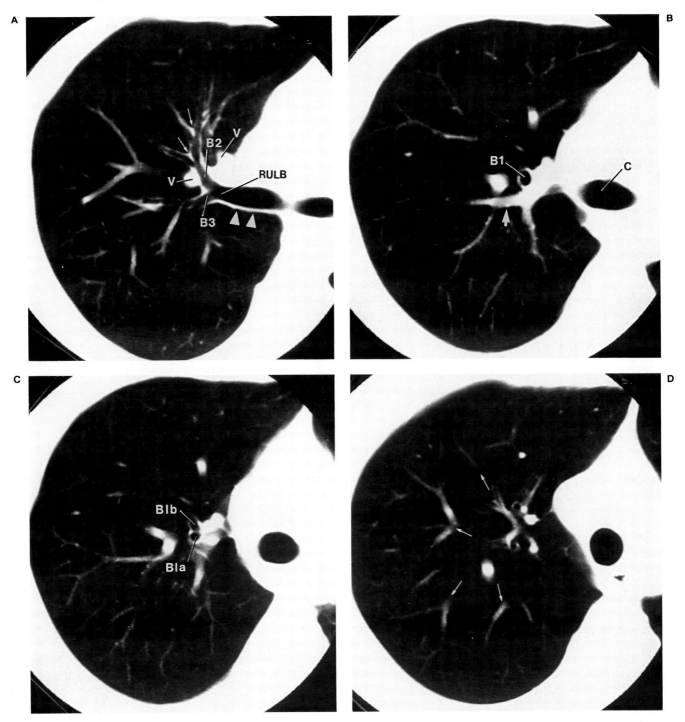

FIG. 15. RUL lobar and segmental bronchi. Sequential 5-mm thick sections beginning at the level of the right upper lobe bronchus (RULB) and proceeding upward at 5-mm intervals. **A:** The RULB originates from the lateral aspect of the right main-stem bronchus at or just below the carina (corresponding to level B in Fig. 13). The RULB courses horizontally. Posteriorly, air within either the posterior segment of the RUL or the superior segment of the RLL normally comes in contact with the posterior wall of the RULB, which is uniformly smooth (*arrowheads*); occasionally, a prominent azygos vein will be identifiable posteromedially. The anterior (B2) and posterior (B3) segmental bronchi also have a horizontal configuration in most cases, making their identification particularly easy. As a rule, sections through the anterior segmental bronchus allow identification of both third- and often fourth-order subsegmental divisions. As elsewhere within the bronchial tree, the origins of particular airways are marked by the presence of spurs. These are soft-tissue divisions between contiguous airways, easily identified as thin lines or, when sectioned obliquely, triangular densities. Prominent spurs can be identified in A, separating the origins of B2 from B3, as well as the origins of two third-order subdivisions of B2 (*small arrows*). **B–D:** Sequential 5-mm thick sections show the proximal portion of the apical segmental bronchus (B1) arising from the superior aspect of the RULB (corresponding to level A in Fig. 13) and quickly subdividing into anterior and posterior subsegments. As a general rule, branches of the pulmonary artery to the RUL, the truncus anterior, lie medial to B1, although in this case a large horizontally oriented upper lobe vein can be seen crossing behind the apical segmental bronchus in B (*arrow*). Note that the arteries and veins of the apical segment have a vertical orientation, whereas vessels to the anterior and posterior segments course more horizontally. This distinction can be easily seen in D (*small arrows*).

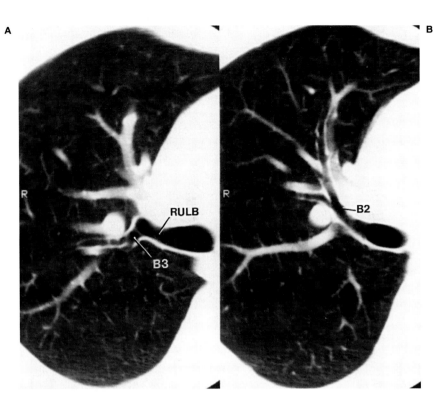

FIG. 16. RULB: normal variant. **A,B:** Sequential 5-mm thick sections obtained 5-mm apart through the RULB. The anterior (B2) and posterior (B3) segmental bronchi both course horizontally but originate at slightly different levels (compare with Fig. 15).

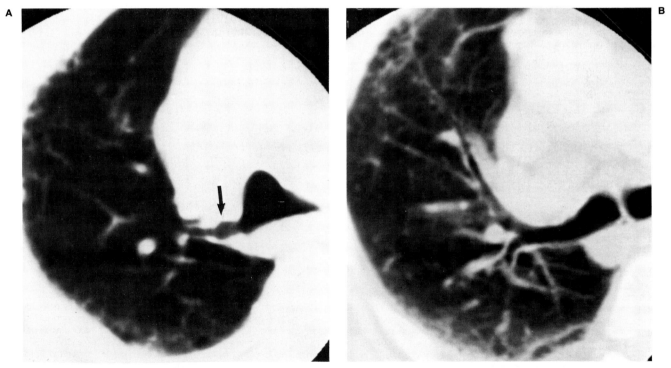

FIG. 17. Tracheal bronchus. **A,B:** Enlargements of sections through the distal trachea (A) and right upper lobe bronchus (B), respectively. An accessory bronchus arises from the lateral wall of the distal trachea to supply a part of the apical segment of the RUL (*arrow* in A). Note the otherwise normal appearance of the RULB in B.

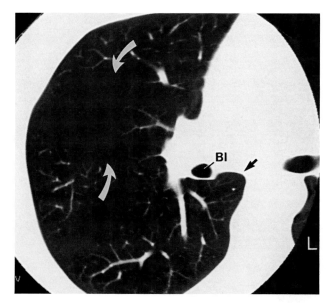

FIG. 18. Bronchus intermedius (BI). The BI lies immediately posterior and medial to the right main and interlobar pulmonary arteries (corresponding to level C in Fig. 13). Typically, a portion of the superior segment of the RLL extends medially to form a convexity—the azygoesophageal recess (*arrow*). The circular hypovascular region on the right is caused by the minor fissure, the so-called right midlung window (*curved arrows*).

frequently only the lateral aspect of the spur can be seen. Typically, this can be identified as a triangular wedge of tissue just lateral to the bronchial bifurcation (Figs. 15 and 19). In either case, identification of spurs is important: first, because they are convenient landmarks marking the point of origin of any airway and, second, because they are frequent sites of bronchial pathology, including bronchogenic carcinoma.

In 60% of cases, the middle lobe bronchus divides into equally prominent medial and lateral segmental bronchi (44). The medial segmental bronchus has a more oblique orientation than does the lateral segmental bronchus, which courses horizontally. In a small percentage of cases, a large medial segmental bronchus is associated with a small lateral segmental bronchus. Even more rarely, the two segmental bronchi appear to arise independently from a very truncated middle lobe bronchus. None of these variations should cause confusion when scans are viewed sequentially.

As may be noted in Figure 19, the middle lobe bronchus courses inferiorly as well as anteriorly. If the origin of the middle bronchus is visualized, the medial and lateral segmental bronchi may be located in a slightly inferior plane. In select cases, bronchi that course in an oblique plane may be visualized to better advantage when the gantry is tilted 20° cranially (Fig. 20) (8).

The basilar bronchi and their subdivisions are listed in Table 1 and are illustrated schematically in Fig. 21. As with the lobar bronchi, the basilar segmental bronchi are best conceptualized through a series of characteristic sections.

The superior segmental bronchus of the right lower lobe may arise at the same level as the point of origin of the middle lobe bronchus or, frequently, at a slightly lower level. The superior segmental bronchus courses posteriorly and runs in a horizontal plane (Fig. 22). Typically, the superior segmental bronchus bifurcates, al-

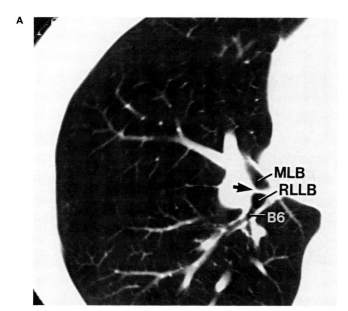

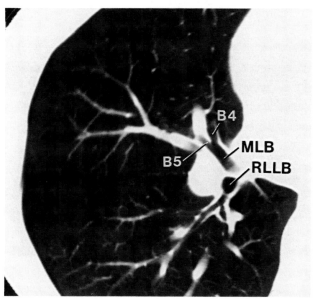

FIG. 19. Middle lobe bronchus (MLB). **A:** CT section shows the origin of the MLB coursing anteriorly on an oblique angle (corresponding to level D in Fig. 13). There is a thin line, or septum, separating the MLB anteriorly from the right lower lobe bronchus (RLLB); this represents the middle lobe spur (*arrow*). B6, superior segmental bronchus of the right lower lobe. **B:** Section just caudal to that shown in A, through the main portion of the MLB as well as the origins of the medial (B4) and lateral (B5) segmental bronchi.

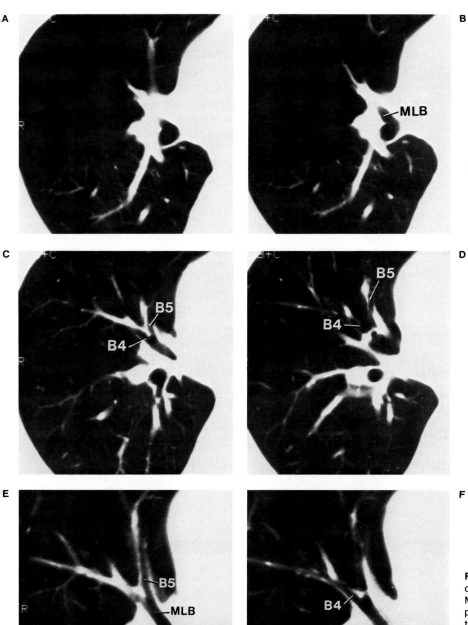

FIG. 20. MLB: 20° angulation. **A–D:** Sequential 5-mm thick sections through the MLB and its subdivisions, B4 and B5 (compare with Fig. 19). **E,F:** Sequential 5-mm thick sections through the MLB in the same patient as A–D, obtained with 20° cephalic angulation of the gantry. Due to its oblique orientation, the MLB is seen along its entire length, as are the lateral (B4) and medial (B5) segmental bronchi, when the gantry is tilted 20°. In select cases, this may allow easier interpretation.

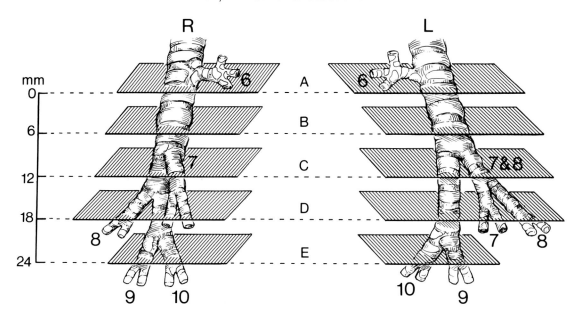

FIG. 21. Schematic oblique representations of the right and left basilar segmental bronchi. A, B, C, D, and E represent characteristic levels through the origins of the superior segmental bronchi (B6) (level A); the truncus basalis (level B); the medial basilar segmental bronchus (B7) on the right, and the anteromedial basilar segmental bronchus (B7 & 8) on the left (level C); the anterior basilar segmental bronchus (B8) on the right, and the medial (B7) and anterior (B8) basilar segmental bronchi on the left (level D); and the origins of the lateral (B9) and posterior (B10) basilar segmental bronchi from their common trunks (level E), respectively. The scale on the right indicates approximate distances between these levels, given a wide range of variations encountered. (From Naidich et al., ref. 46.)

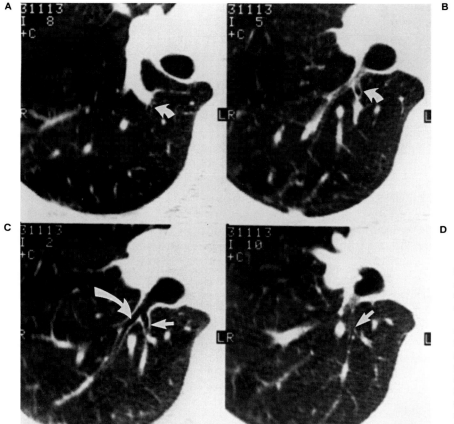

FIG. 22. Superior segmental bronchus: B6. **A–D:** Enlargements of sequential 1.5-mm thick sections through the superior segmental bronchus, obtained every 3 mm (see level A in Fig. 15). The origin of the superior segmental bronchus is clearly seen originating from the posterolateral wall of the distal bronchus intermedius. The superior segmental bronchus on the right typically bifurcates into a prominent lateral subsegment (B6c) (*curved arrow* in C) and a common trunk for the medial (B6a) (*small arrows* in C and D) and superior (B6b) (*small curved arrows* in A and B) subsegmental bronchi. Note how far superiorly the superior subsegmental bronchus can be traced.

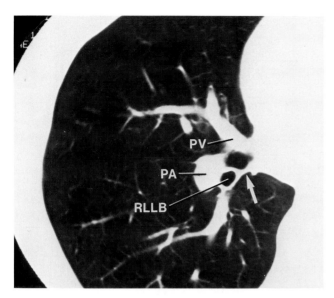

FIG. 23. Truncus basalis. CT section through the proximal portion of the RLLB (corresponding to level E in Fig. 13 and level B in Fig. 21) at a level just below the origin of the superior segmental bronchus. An *arrow* points to the superior portion of the inferior pulmonary ligament. PA, interlobar pulmonary artery; PV, right superior pulmonary vein.

though trifurcation into medial, superior, and lateral subsegments is not unusual.

Below the origin of the superior segmental bronchus, the lower lobe bronchus continues for ~7–10 mm as the truncus basalis (Fig. 23). The lower lobe bronchus, at this level, is vertically oriented and, hence, is visualized as a circular lucency. The lower lobe bronchi always lie medial and anterior to the corresponding lower lobe pulmonary arteries, which also course vertically. The lower lobe bronchi characteristically appear "suspended" in the lung by the superior portions of the inferior pulmonary ligaments.

Despite considerable variability in the cross-sectional appearance of the basilar segmental bronchi, each can be identified routinely, provided that 1.5–5-mm thick sections are obtained (Fig. 24) (45,46). As with other airways, anatomical identification of individual basilar segmental and subsegmental bronchi is facilitated by reference to characteristic sections (Fig. 21). Typically, the medial basilar segmental bronchus arises first, characteristically lying just anterior to the inferior pulmonary vein. Subsequently, although variable in appearance, the remaining basilar segmental bronchi always course in the direction of their respective basilar pulmonary segments. This is the key to their identification. The anterior, lateral, and posterior basilar bronchi may all be identified individually because of their positions

relative to one another and because of their general configuration coursing toward the anticipated positions of their respective pulmonary segments. This makes identification of normal variants and anomalies relatively easy (Figs. 25 and 26).

As shown in Fig. 27, utilizing thin sections, the central airways generally can be identified only within the central portions of the lung parenchyma. More peripheral identification is strong evidence of either intrinsic bronchial or pulmonary parenchymal abnormality.

Left Lung Segmental Anatomy

Sequential sections through the lower trachea and carina are shown in Fig. 28, corresponding to levels A and B in Fig. 14. These two levels are grouped together because they both represent sections through the apical-posterior segmental bronchus of the left upper lobe. The left upper lobe bronchus originates at a level lower than the right upper lobe bronchus and forms a "sling" over which the main left pulmonary artery passes. In Fig. 28, the apical-posterior segmental bronchus is seen as a circular lucency surrounded medially and laterally by main branches of the left upper lobe pulmonary artery and vein.

The key to understanding the anatomy of the left upper lobe bronchus and its branches is to realize that the left upper lobe bronchus is large, and it is therefore possible to obtain sections through both the upper and lower portions of this bronchus. Each has a characteristic appearance (Fig. 29).

In a section through the "upper" portion of the left upper lobe bronchus, the posterior wall of the left upper lobe bronchus is smooth and slightly concave; this concavity is caused by the left pulmonary artery as it passes above and then posterior to the left upper lobe bronchus. At this level, the origin of the apical-posterior segmental bronchus can be recognized as a rounded area of increased lucency "superimposed" on the distal portion of the left upper lobe bronchus (Fig. 29). Just posterior to the medial portion of the left upper lobe bronchus, air in the superior segment of the left lower lobe abuts the posteromedial wall of the bronchus. This invagination of lung between the descending aorta and the left interlobar pulmonary artery has been referred to as the left "retrobronchial stripe" (47). Adenopathy and/or a hilar mass will efface this segment of lung, similar to the effacement of the azygoesophageal recess on the right side caused by subcarinal adenopathy.

The most important anatomic landmark identifying a scan as being through the lower portion of the left upper lobe bronchus is the left upper lobe spur. This spur marks the point of origin of the left lower lobe bronchus

(*Text continues on page 171.*)

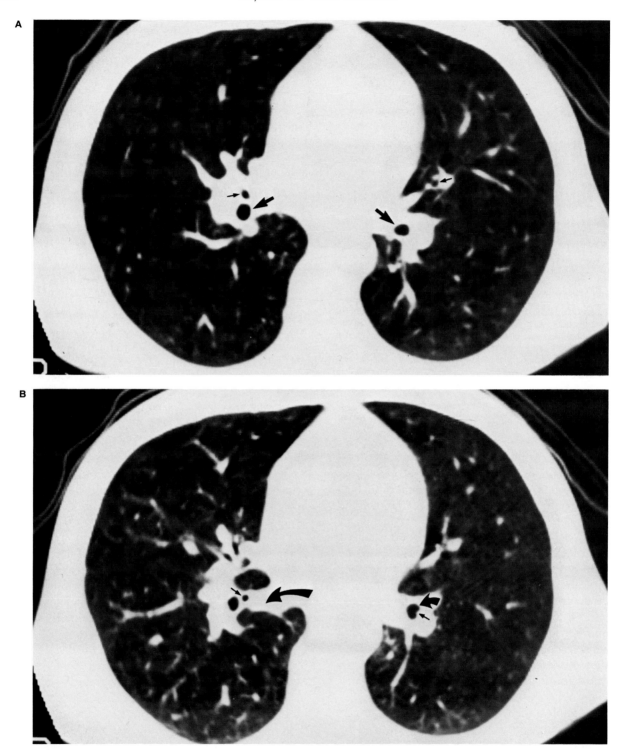

FIG. 24. B7, 8, 9, and 10: basilar segmental bronchi. Sequential 1.5-mm thick sections obtained every 3 mm, beginning at the level of the distal lower lobe bronchi (truncus basalis), bilaterally. **A:** Section through the truncus basalis on the right and left sides, respectively (level B in Fig. 21). The truncus basalis represents a continuation of the lower lobe bronchus below the origin of the superior segmental bronchus. It is considerably longer on the left side. This bronchus typically appears circular or ovoid, as it is oriented in a vertical plane (*arrows* in A). The MLB is easily identified on the right (*small arrow* on right), as is the lingular bronchus (*small arrow* on the left). **B:** Section through the medial basilar segmental bronchus on the right and the origin of the anteromedial segmental bronchus on the left (level C in Fig. 21). The medial basilar bronchus on the right is the first branch of the truncus basalis and typically lies anteromedially (*short arrow* on right) in close proximity to the right inferior pulmonary vein (*curved arrow*). On the left, the origin of the anteromedial segmental bronchus can be identified (*curved arrow* on left) originating anteromedially from the truncus basalis, clearly demarcated by the presence of a well-defined spur laterally (*short arrow* on left). The MLB has bifurcated anteriorly into well-defined medial and lateral subdivisions. **C:** Section through the origin of the anterior basilar segmental bronchus on the right and the proximal common trunks of the anteromedial and posterolateral segmental bronchi on the left (level D on the right and level C on the left in Fig. 21). The origin of the anterior basilar segmental bronchus on the right is easily defined, extending anteriorly and laterally (*short arrow* on right), separating

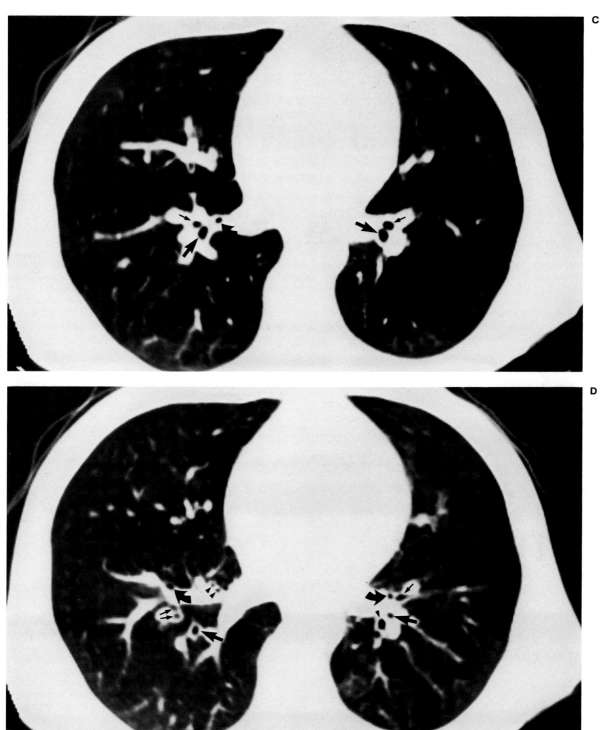

from the right lower lobe bronchus, which in this case continues as a common posterolateral basilar trunk (*large straight arrow* on right). The medial basilar segmental bronchus is still identifiable (*curved arrow*), anterior to the right inferior pulmonary vein. On the left, two large bronchi can be identified. These represent the anteromedial basilar bronchus, anterolaterally (*small arrow* on left) and the continuation of the lower lobe bronchus as a common posterolateral trunk (*large arrow* on left). Note the similarity in size of these two airways. **D:** Section through all four segmental bronchi, bilaterally (level E in Fig. 21). On the right side, the posterior basilar segmental bronchus continues inferiorly as the largest of the basilar segmental airways (*large arrow* on right). In this case, subsegmental divisions of the medial (*double arrowheads* on right) and lateral (*small double arrows* on right) are apparent. The anterior basilar segmental bronchus is easily definable as a continuation of the airway identified at its origin in C (*large curved arrow* on the right). On the left, the anteromedial segmental bronchus has divided into a smaller medial basilar branch (*small black arrow* on left) and a larger anterior segmental bronchus (*curved white arrow* on left). The posterior segmental bronchus can be identified easily as a continuation of the lower lobe bronchus (*straight white arrow* on left), analogous to its counterpart on the right. The lateral segmental bronchus can be identified just lateral to the posterior segmental bronchus (*straight black arrow*). Note the overall symmetry of the basilar segmental bronchi at this level, as well as the fact that outside of these main trunks, more peripheral airways cannot be defined at any level (see A–D). (From Naidich et al., ref. 46.)

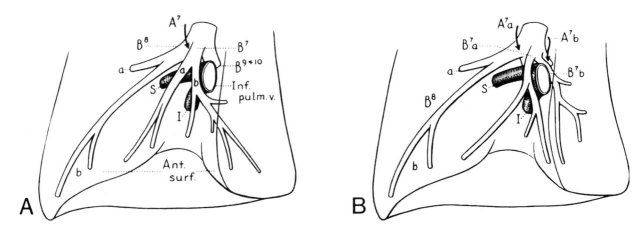

FIG. 25. Schematic representations of the two commonest variations in the subdivisions of the medial basilar bronchus. **A:** The medial basilar segmental bronchus (B7) generally subdivides into an anterior (B7a) and a medial (B7b) ramus. Characteristically, these two subsegmental bronchi lie anterior to the right inferior pulmonary vein (Inf. pulm. v.). In approximately one-third of cases, B7b extends solely to the anterior surface of the right lower lobe (Ant. surf.), whereas in approximately one-fifth of cases a subdivision extends to the paravertebral surface of the medial basilar segment inferiorly. A7, medial basilar segmental artery; S, superior; I, inferior rami of the right inferior pulmonary vein; B8 (a and b), subdivisions of the anterior basilar segmental bronchus. **B:** Diagrammatic representation of the most common variation in the subdivision of the medial basilar segmental bronchus. In approximately one-fourth of cases, the medial ramus (B7b) courses posterior to the right inferior pulmonary vein, unlike the anterior ramus (B7a), which remains anteriorly oriented. Knowledge of this variation is significant, especially to surgeons attempting medial basilar segmental resections. A7a and b, corresponding arterial rami supplying the medial basilar segment. (From Naidich et al., ref. 46.)

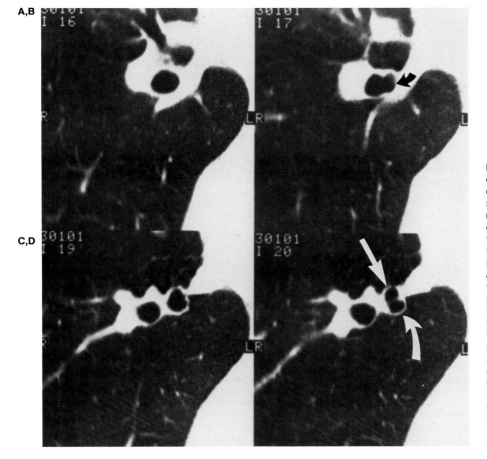

FIG. 26. B7-variant/B*-subsuperior bronchus. **A–H:** Sequential 1.5-mm thick sections obtained through the origin of the medial segmental bronchus (B7) and its anterior (B7a) and medial (B7b) subdivisions. The origin of B7 is easily identified, arising characteristically from the anteromedial surface of the truncus basalis (*curved black arrow* in B). B7a (*white arrow* in D) and B7b (*curved white arrow* in D) originate as equivalent sized trunks, which then split around the inferior pulmonary vein (v in E). B7a and its subdivisions are easily defined, coursing anterior to the vein (*single white arrows* in E and F), whereas B7b courses posteriorly (*curved white arrows* in E and F). Note the position and origin of the anterior segmental bronchus (*white arrowhead* in E), the point of origin of the lateral (B9) and posterior (B10) segmental bronchi from a common trunk (B9–10) (*black arrow* in F) as well as the subsuperior segmental bronchus (B*) (*double white arrows* in E and F). (From Naidich et al., ref. 46.)

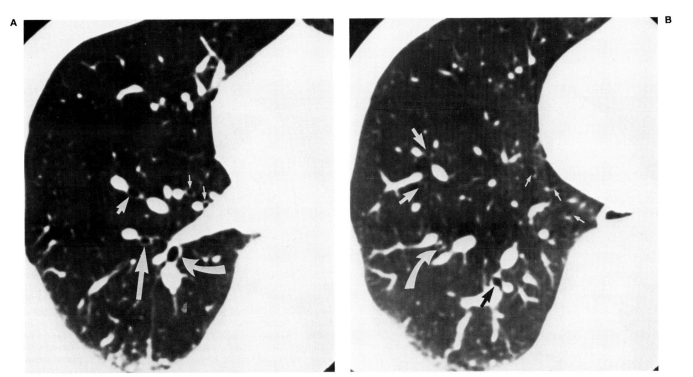

FIG. 27. Normal basilar airways: peripheral distribution. **A:** Enlargement of a 1.5-mm thick section obtained through the right lower lobe, through all four basilar segmental airways, respectively. Proximally, it is easy to identify individual segmental airways, largely due to their characteristic location and configuration. Note that B7a and b have both subdivided into fourth-order bronchi (*small arrows* in A), whereas B8 (*small arrow* in A), B9 (*large arrow* in A), and B10 (*curved arrow* in A) remain undivided in close proximity to their respective adjacent pulmonary arteries. **B:** Enlargement of a 1.5-mm thick section obtained 1.5 cm below that shown in A. This represents the most peripheral level at which subdivisions of all four segmental bronchi can still be discerned. B10 (*black arrow* in B), still the largest of the basilar airways, is especially easy to identify. B9 (*curved white arrow* in B) and several small subdivisions of B8 (*large white arrows* in B) are also identifiable. More difficult to decipher are branches of B7, although some can be faintly identified (*small white arrows* in B). Note that identification of these airways is contingent on extrapolation from scans obtained more proximally and that the number of identifiable airways at this level is few. (From Naidich et al., ref. 46.)

E,F

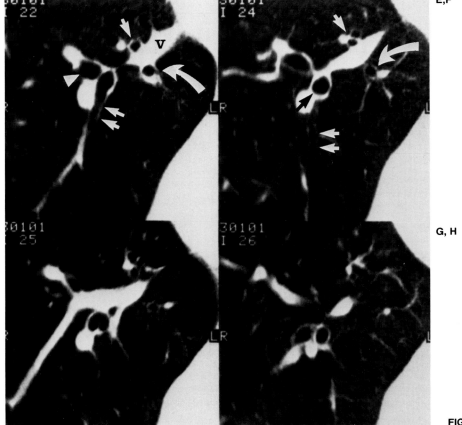

G, H

FIG. 26. (*Continued*)

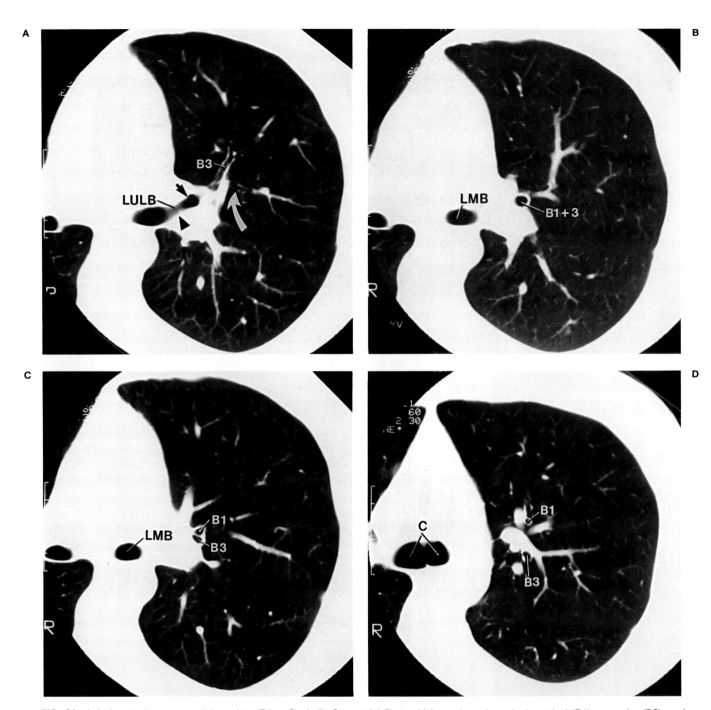

FIG. 28. Apical-posterior segmental bronchus (B1 + 3). **A–D:** Sequential 5-mm thick sections through the apical (B1), posterior (B3), and apical-posterior segmental bronchus (B1 + 3), from below up (corresponding to levels A and B in Fig. 14). The apical-posterior segmental bronchus arises as a common trunk from the superior surface of the left upper lobe bronchus (LULB). The posterior wall of the LULB is slightly concave (*arrowhead*) due to extrinsic compression from the left interlobar pulmonary artery, which courses posteriorly. The origin of the apical-posterior segmental bronchus can be identified as a circular lucency superimposed on the distal portion of the LULB (*arrow*). After briefly coursing superiorly, this bronchus divides into anterior (B1) and posterior (B3) divisions. LMB, left main-stem bronchus; C, carina. Note that the anterior segmental bronchus of the left upper lobe (B3) is easily identifiable coursing anteriorly on a horizontal axis. The *curved arrow* in A points to a prominent axillary subdivision. (From Naidich et al., ref. 46.)

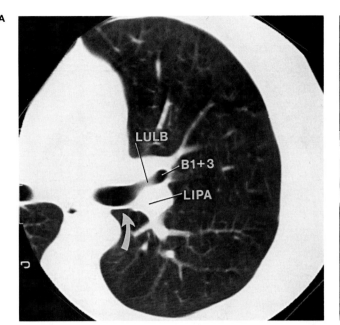

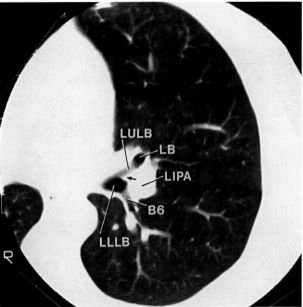

FIG. 29. LULB: secondary carina. **A:** Section through the upper portion of the LULB (corresponding to level C in Fig. 14). At this level, the LULB is angulated slightly anterior. There is a smooth convexity along the posterior border of the LULB caused by the left interlobar pulmonary artery. Note that there is a slight increase in density in the midportion of the LULB; this is due to partial volume averaging of the left main pulmonary artery as it crosses over the LULB. The origin of the apical-posterior segmental bronchus (B1 + 3) can be identified as a circular lucency "superimposed" over the distal end of the LULB. A portion of the superior segment of the LLL abuts the posteromedial wall of the LULB at this level, the left "retrobronchial stripe" (*curved arrow*). **B:** Section through the lower portion of the LULB (corresponding to D in Fig. 14). At this level, the lower portion of the LULB is separated from the origin of the LLLB by a triangular spur—the secondary carina (*arrow*). The origin of the lingular bronchus (LB) can be identified as a circular lucency "superimposed" on the distal end of the left upper lobe bronchus.

and is also referred to as the "secondary carina." This spur can be recognized as a triangular density separating the lower portion of the left upper from the left lower lobe bronchus and is visually analogous to the middle lobe spur of the right side (compare with Fig. 19).

The lingular bronchus arises from the undersurface of the distal portion of the left upper lobe bronchus and has an oblique course inferiorly (Figs. 29 and 30). The origin of the lingular bronchus can be identified as a circular area of increased lucency "superimposed" on the distal portion of the left upper lobe bronchus, in much the same manner in which the origin of the apical-posterior segmental bronchus can be identified. The key to differentiating the origin of the apical-posterior segmental bronchus from the origin of the lingular bronchus is identification of the left upper lobe spur (Fig. 29) and confirming that the section showing the origin of the lingular bronchus is through the lower portion of the left upper lobe bronchus.

The lingular bronchus runs inferiorly on an oblique path. In cross-section, the lingular bronchus has an oval or elliptical shape. If sections are obtained just below the left upper lobe bronchus, the lingular bronchus will appear as a discrete oval lucency separated spatially from the left lower lobe bronchus (Fig. 30). Sequential sections obtained below the origin of the lingular bronchus will show progressively wider separation between the lingular bronchus anteriorly and the left lower lobar bronchus posteriorly.

The superior and, especially, the inferior divisions of

the lingular bronchus are seen on CT only infrequently, utilizing standard 8–10-mm thick sections. These segmental bronchi tend to originate at a considerable distance from the origin of the lingular bronchus and may be too small and peripheral to be visualized with standard technique. Identification, however, is significantly enhanced with use of 1.5–5-mm thick sections (Fig. 30). As noted previously, in select cases, 20° angulation of the beam may be beneficial (8).

The anterior segmental bronchus of the left upper lobe has been omitted from discussion so far because it is highly variable. In ~75% of individuals, the left upper lobe bronchus divides into superior and lingular divisions (48). In this instance, the anterior segmental bronchus originates as a branch of the apical-posterior segmental bronchus (Fig. 31).

In 25% of cases, the left upper lobe trifurcates. The anterior segmental bronchus then arises between a modified superior division bronchus (apical-posterior segmental bronchus) superiorly and the lingular bronchus inferiorly. When the left upper lobe bronchus trifurcates in this manner, the anterior segmental bronchus will arise in close proximity to the apical-posterior segmental bronchus (Fig. 31) or, occasionally, close to the origin of the lingular bronchus.

Identification of the anterior segmental bronchus is facilitated by recognizing that it is the only bronchus arising from the left upper lobe bronchus that courses anteriorly in a horizontal plane.

The superior segmental bronchus of the left lower

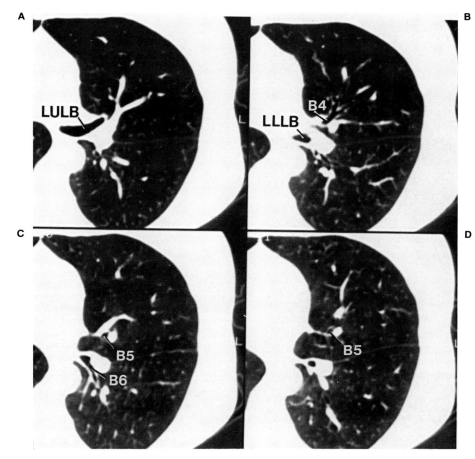

FIG. 30. LB. **A–D:** Sequential 5-mm thick sections starting at the level of the LULB and continuing inferiorly through the LB. The LB originates from the inferior surface of the LULB and courses obliquely, both inferiorly and anteriorly. Note progressively wider separation between the lingular bronchi and the LLLB as scans proceed caudally. The superior lingular bronchus (B4) runs horizontally and usually can be identified along its course when thin sections are obtained. Below B4, the inferior LB (B5) can be identified as an oblong lucency coursing with its adjacent pulmonary artery.

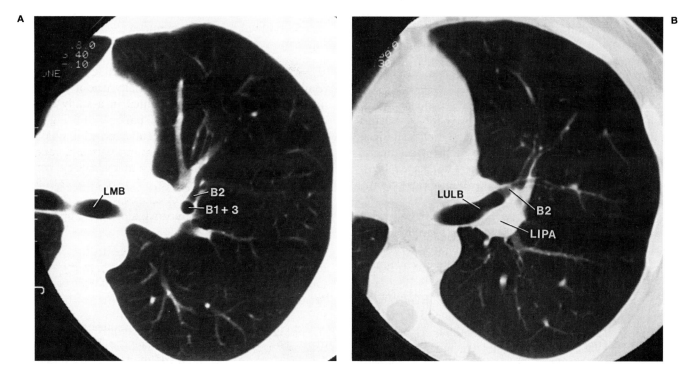

FIG. 31. Anterior segmental bronchus, LUL: normal variants. **A:** Section through the apical-posterior segmental bronchus of the LUL (B1 + 3). The anterior segmental bronchus (B2) originates from the anterior aspect of B1 + 3 (compare with Fig. 29). **B:** Section through the upper portion of the LULB, in a different patient than shown in A. The anterior segmental bronchus (B2) is easily identified, originating at the same level as the origin of the apical-posterior segmental bronchus (B1 + 3). Despite variations in origin, the anterior segmental bronchus is always identifiable as coursing anteriorly in a horizontal plane.

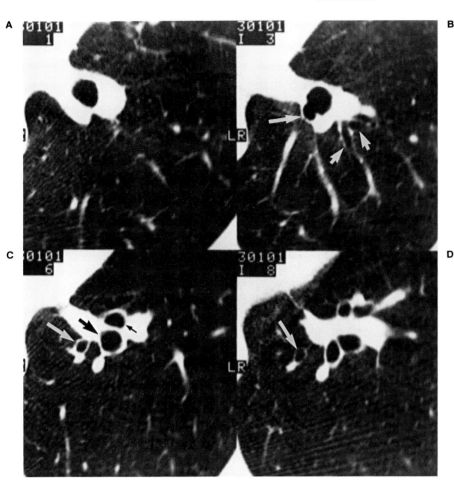

FIG. 32. B*-subsuperior segmental bronchus: LLL. **A–D:** Sequential 1.5-mm thick sections obtained through the proximal divisions of the LLL basilar segmental bronchi. An anomalous bronchus can be defined originating off the posteromedial aspect of the truncus basalis (*white arrow* in B), which then extends inferomedially (*white arrows* in C and D). This subsuperior bronchus is easily differentiated from the anteromedial segmental bronchus (B7 + 8) (*small black arrow* in C), as well as a common trunk of the lateral and posterior segmental bronchi (B9 and 10) (*large black arrow* in C). Note that superiorly, inferior branches of the superior segmental bronchus (B6) can be identified (*short white arrows* in B), distinct from the subsuperior bronchus.

lobe is analogous in shape and configuration to the same bronchus on the right side (Fig. 21).

The left lower lobe bronchus usually conforms to the same general pattern as the right lower lobe bronchus (Figs. 23 and 24). The proximal portion of the left lower bronchus, below the origin of the superior segmental bronchus, the truncus basalis, appears at this level suspended in the lung by the upper portion of the left inferior pulmonary ligament.

The basilar segmental bronchi are essentially mirror images of the patterns shown for the right lower lobe basilar bronchi, except that on the left side the medial and anterior basilar bronchi characteristically originate together as a common trunk (Fig. 24). Again, the key to their identification is to note the general configuration and position of these bronchi as they course to their corresponding basilar lung segments.

As noted repeatedly, segmental and even subsegmental bronchi have characteristic cross-sectional appearances that are easily identified when images are obtained and analyzed sequentially. Familiarity with these char-acteristic sections allows easy identification of other less common variations. This is especially true if thin sections are obtained. As documented in a study of the basilar segmental bronchi of 31 patients utilizing thin sections, in each case all segmental bronchi could be identified, regardless of variations in origin and course; in a majority of cases, most subsegmental airways could be identified as well (Figs. 25, 26, and 32) (46). The implications of this degree of accuracy for the potential use of CT in evaluating abnormal airways is apparent.

CORRELATION WITH FIBEROPTIC BRONCHOSCOPY: GENERAL PRINCIPLES

The clinical utility of CT in the management of patients with airway disease can only be determined by comparison with FOB. This is made necessary due to the widespread availability of FOB, as well as the obvious advantages that derive both diagnostically and ther-

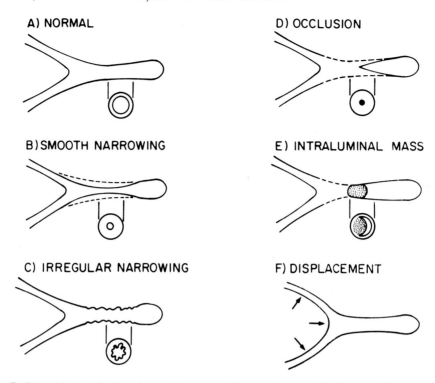

FIG. 33. Radiographic classification of bronchial abnormalities detectable by CT. (From Naidich et al., ref. 50.)

apeutically from direct visualization of the airway lumen. Although, in most cases, the role of CT will be complementary, the precise clinical contexts in which CT is indicated are still evolving (49–52).

Meaningful correlation between CT and FOB requires the use of standardized definitions. Specifically, analysis of the airways on CT scans requires a radiologic classification (Fig. 33). Attempts to describe abnormalities identified on CT scans utilizing bronchoscopic terminology, such as mucosal or submucosal, in particular, are invalid.

Numerous reports comparing CT and FOB have documented that CT is an extremely accurate modality for detecting pathologic changes within the airways (50–54). In a retrospective report utilizing scans with both thin (1.5- or 5-mm) and thick (10-mm) sections, CT accurately identified 59 (92%) of 64 cases in which lesions were detected endoscopically (50). Analyzed individually, CT successfully identified 88 (90%) of 98 lesions. False-negative studies often resulted from too low a clinical index of suspicion of bronchial disease (Fig. 34). In this same series, CT correctly excluded dis-

A

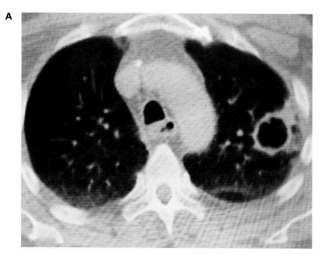

B

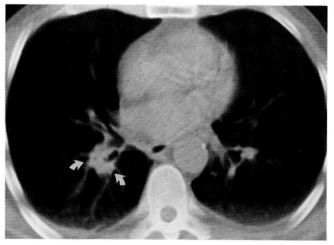

FIG. 34. CT localization: false-negative study. **A:** Section obtained at the level of the aortic arch shows a thin-walled cavity in the LUL diagnosed subsequently as adenocarcinoma. **B:** Section through the RLLB, on the right at the level of the origin of the medial basilar segmental bronchus. Compared with the left side, a soft-tissue mass can be identified deforming the basilar bronchi on the right (*curved arrows*). In this case, contralateral metastases went undiagnosed at CT due to a low clinical index of suspicion that the cavity was neoplastic. (From Naidich et al., ref. 50.)

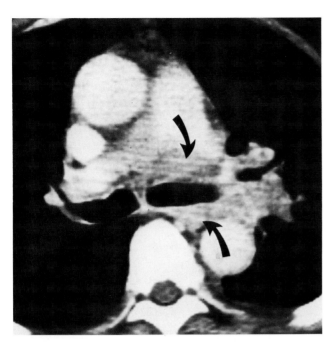

FIG. 35. Submucosal extension, left main-stem bronchus. Section through portions of both the left main-stem and apical-posterior bronchus after a bolus of intravenous contrast medium. There is extensive tumor throughout the left hilum extending into the mediastinum lying adjacent to the left main-stem bronchus both anteriorly and posteriorly (*arrows*). This is the only finding to suggest submucosal involvement, which was subsequently confirmed bronchoscopically. Note that the overall configuration of the left main-stem bronchus is grossly normal, also true when viewed with wide windows (not illustrated). (From Naidich et al., ref. 50.)

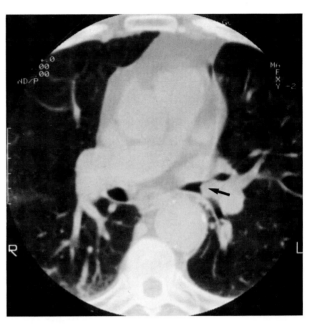

FIG. 36. Endobronchial tumor: squamous cell carcinoma. Section through the left main-stem bronchus shows a curvilinear soft-tissue density within the bronchial lumen (*arrow*). This appearance is consistent with endobronchial disease as visualized bronchoscopically. Endobronchial biopsy proven bronchogenic carcinoma. (Case courtesy of Burton Cohen, M.D., Mt. Sinai Hospital, New York, NY.)

ease in 35 (92%) of 38 cases that were subsequently verified to be normal by FOB. CT accurately identified all cases in which malignancy was verified.

More recently, Mayr et al. used CT to evaluate 142 patients thought to have endobronchial lesions, in whom 121 patients had documented endobronchial masses confirmed either at bronchoscopy or surgery (54). Evaluating each individual bronchus from the level of the trachea to the segmental bronchi independently, the sensitivity of CT was found to be 100% and 99%, respectively, for identification of abnormal bronchi, with a corresponding specificity of 97% and 96%, respectively, for CT identification of normal airways (54). Importantly, when only 8-mm thick sections were analyzed, the sensitivity of CT proved to be 94% and 91%, respectively; however, when contiguous 4-mm thick sections were obtained (n = 23 patients: 71 abnormal bronchi; 189 normal bronchi), there were no false positive or false negative CT interpretations. Improved visualization of airway abnormalities using thinner sections was reported.

Unfortunately, when abnormalities identified on CT scans are analyzed using a radiographic classification and compared with the results of FOB, it has been shown that CT is imprecise in predicting whether a given abnormality will be primarily endobronchial, sub-

mucosal, or extrinsic as seen endoscopically (Fig. 35) (50). Smooth narrowing, for example, which is the most commonly identified finding, may be associated with either endobronchial, submucosal, or peribronchial disease. Exceptions in which CT findings have high specificity include cases in which a discrete filling defect can be identified (Figs. 36 and 37) or an abnormal intraluminal density can be defined (see Figs. 38 and 39).

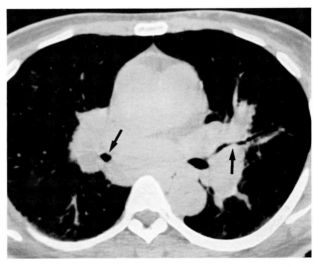

FIG. 37. Endobronchial sarcoidosis. CT section through the bronchus intermedius and left upper lobe bronchus in a patient with endoscopically confirmed endobronchial sarcoid. There is marked narrowing of the airways, which appear nodular and markedly irregular (*arrows*). Note presence of significantly enlarged hilar and subcarinal lymph nodes.

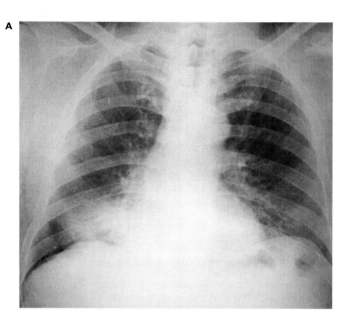

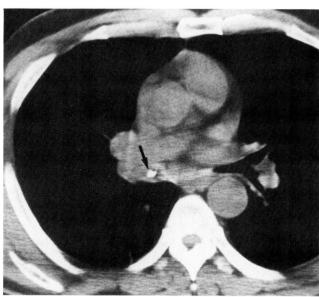

FIG. 38. CT localization: endobronchial foreign body. **A:** PA radiograph shows consolidation in the RLL. **B:** 5-mm thick section through the proximal RLLB, imaged with narrow windows, shows a well-defined ring-like shadow within the lumen of the airway (*arrow*). This proved to be a chicken bone at bronchoscopy. The ring-like shadow is caused by sectioning the bone orthogonally, allowing identification of both cortex and medulla. Accurate differentiation of a calcified broncholith from peribronchial calcified lymph nodes may require use of thin sections. (From Naidich et al., ref. 114.)

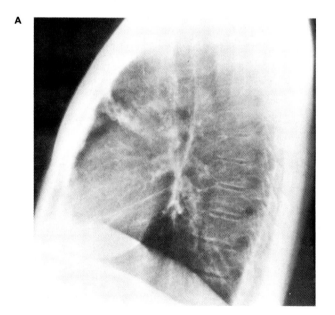

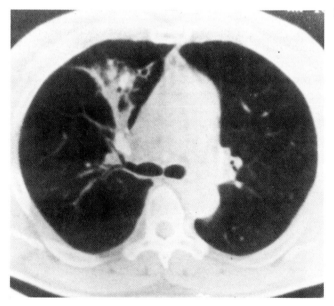

FIG. 39. Tuberculosis (calcified broncholith). Section at the level of the RULB. The anterior segmental bronchus is patent. At the level of first bifurcation, the medial subsegmental bronchus is obliterated by an adjacent calcified lymph node. At bronchoscopy, this had eroded into the bronchus, causing obstruction. (From Naidich et al., ref. 13.)

A 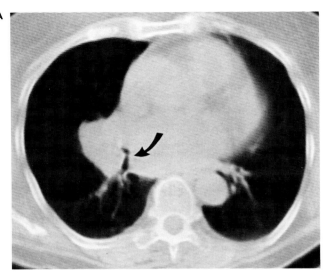 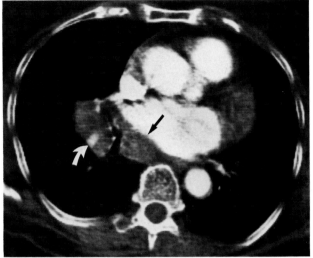 B

FIG. 40. CT localization: peribronchial disease. **A,B:** Sections at the level of the origin of the MLB, imaged with wide and narrow windows, respectively, following a bolus of i.v. contrast. The airways are narrowed (*curved arrow* in A). There is a large soft-tissue mass in the right hilum, displacing the right interlobar pulmonary artery laterally (*curved arrow* in B) and deforming the lateral border of the left atrium (*straight arrow* in B). At bronchoscopy, the MLB and LLB appeared extrinsically narrowed; no other abnormalities were appreciated. In this case, CT is complementary to bronchoscopy by accurately delineating the extent of peribronchial disease. Transbronchial biopsy proved small cell carcinoma. (From Naidich et al., ref. 114.)

Fortunately, although the appearance of the airways themselves is often a nonspecific predictor of findings at FOB, CT is extremely accurate in delineating the extent of peribronchial abnormalities, especially in cases in which a bolus of i.v. contrast media has been given (Fig. 40). These findings indicate that CT can be complementary to FOB in both the staging and therapy of lung cancer (see Chapter 6). As graphically illustrated in Fig. 41, by defining the precise location of peribronchial disease, CT can be used to localize and guide transbronchial needle aspiration and biopsy, as well as play a critical role in selecting patients for endobronchial laser therapy (55–57). As documented by Lam et al. (57), CT can be utilized to predict which patients will benefit from photodynamic therapy by delineating the extent of peribronchial tumor.

In addition to delineating central airway disease, CT may also play a complementary role to FOB in the delineation and evaluation of parenchymal disease. In select cases, CT may define the location and precise extent of parenchymal infiltrates otherwise poorly seen or localized on plain chest radiographs (Fig. 42). In addition to patients with parenchymal consolidation and/or collapse, CT may also play a complementary role with FOB in evaluating localized parenchymal masses or nodules. In a retrospective evaluation of 65 patients with solitary pulmonary nodules or masses evaluated with CT, when a bronchus was found in association with a lesion on

cross-section (a positive bronchus sign) the yield from FOB was twice that of a similar number of patients in whom this sign was absent (60% versus 30%, respectively) (Fig. 43) (58). Most significantly, in those cases in which thin (1.5-mm) sections were obtained, a negative bronchus sign was associated with a positive endoscopic biopsy in only one of seven cases (14%).

For those cases in which it has been determined that a lesion is most easily approached transthoracically, CT can also have several potentially useful roles. First, CT can be used to plan the best approach for percutaneous biopsy (CT-assisted, transthoracic needle biopsy). Small subpleural blebs are frequently seen with CT, for example, that were unsuspected on plain films; their presence frequently necessitates a change in the direction of biopsy. More significantly, it is well documented that CT-guided transthoracic needle biopsies are of value, despite a somewhat higher complication rate than reported for fluoroscopically guided needle biopsies, especially for cases in which peripheral lesions are difficult to identify accurately with biplanar fluoroscopy (59–61). Even in those cases in which the lesion is easily seen and localized fluoroscopically, CT may be useful in determining the exact site at which a biopsy should be performed, especially in larger lesions, by disclosing areas of viable tumor tissue distinct from areas of necrosis, following a bolus of i.v. contrast media, thus establishing the best location for biopsy (62).

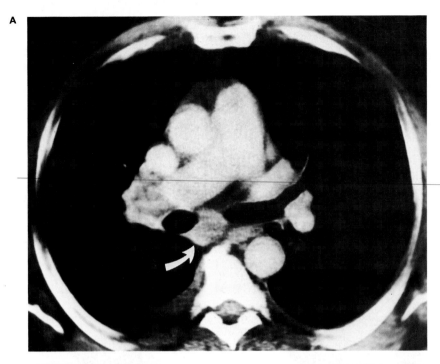

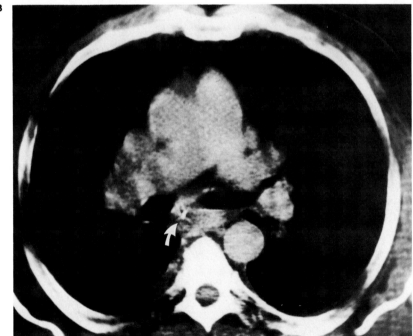

FIG. 41. CT-guided transcarinal needle aspiration. **A:** Section just below the carina in a patient with a widened mediastinum and no apparent parenchymal lesion. Despite extensive subcarinal (*curved arrow*) and right hilar adenopathy, the adjacent airways appear entirely normal. A small pleural effusion is present on the right side. **B:** Repeat CT section following passage of a transcarinal aspirating needle confirming that the tip is within the subcarinal nodes seen in A (*arrow*). Evaluation of the aspirate in this case showed only nonspecific inflammatory cells. (From Naidich et al., ref. 114.)

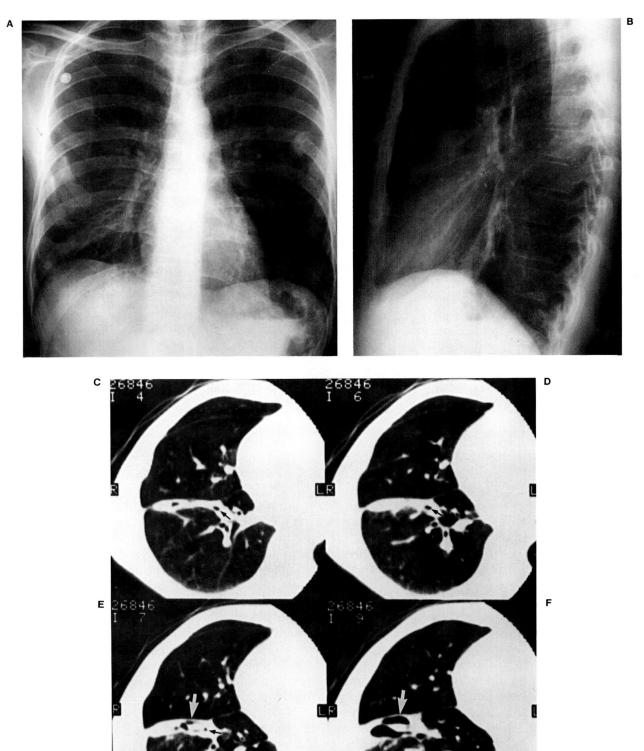

FIG. 42. Pulmonary infarction: segmental localization. **A,B:** Posteroanterior and lateral radiographs, respectively, in an intravenous drug addict with documented endocarditis show an ill-defined infiltrate in the RLL, best seen on the lateral radiograph, just posterior to the oblique fissure. **C–F:** Enlargements of sequential 1.5-mm thick sections through the proximal basilar bronchi of the RLL. A dense infiltrate can be identified in the anterior basilar segment, within which cavitation can be seen (*white arrows* in E and F). Soft-tissue density is present within the cavity, possibly due to necrotic debris resulting from pulmonary infarction. Note that the anterior segmental bronchus is well-defined and clearly patent (*black arrows* in C–E). Precise localization and characterization of the parenchymal abnormalities seen in A and B are clearly enhanced in this case by precise delineation of segmental anatomy. (From Naidich et al., ref. 114.)

A,B

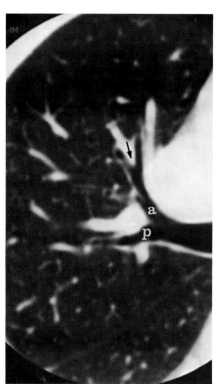 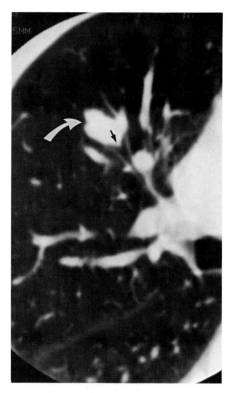

FIG. 43. CT/bronchoscopic correlation: the positive bronchus sign. **A,B:** Sequential, magnified 1.5-mm thick sections through the anterior (a) and posterior (p) segmental bronchi of the right upper lobe, and their distal subdivisions, respectively. Spurs dividing both third and fourth order bronchi can be identified (*black arrow* in A). The tumor is easily identified (*curved arrow* in B), infiltrating the spur dividing a fourth order division of the right upper lobe bronchus (*black arrow* in B). Endoscopically biopsy-proved adenocarcinoma. (From Naidich et al., ref. 56.)

BRONCHIAL NEOPLASIA: CARCINOIDS

The CT appearance of carcinoid tumors serves as a useful model for all bronchial neoplasia (see Chapter 7 for further reference to CT in the evaluation of carcinoid tumors). Previously categorized as one of a subset of tumors labeled "bronchial adenomas," carcinoid tumors are presently classified as part of the spectrum of neuroendocrine lung neoplasms (63–67). This classification includes both typical and atypical carcinoids, as well as small-cell lung carcinomas (SCLC) (66). These tumors have in common features of neuroendocrine differentiation, including the ability to produce neurosecretory granules, as well as peptide hormones and biogenic amines. Histologically, they constitute a spectrum of cytologically malignant forms, ranging from the relatively indolent typical carcinoid on one end of the spectrum, through clinically and histologically intermediate atypical carcinoids, to aggressively malignant SCLC.

Precise terminological classification of these tumors is controversial. Initially thought to be derived from migrating amine precursor uptake and decarboxylation (APUD) cells of neural crest origin, specifically from bronchopulmonary Kulchitzky cells, it has been suggested that these tumors be called "Kulchitzky cell carcinomas" (KCC-1, KCC-2, and KCC-3, respectively) (65). However, there is evidence to suggest that both typical and atypical carcinoids, as well as SCLC, differentiate from pluripotential bronchial epithelial cells instead (66).

Bronchial carcinoids, both typical and atypical, tend to exhibit variable growth patterns (68,69). They may grow primarily intraluminally, or, alternatively, they may have a small intraluminal component and extend deeply into the adjacent peribronchial soft tissues. As compared with typical carcinoids, atypical carcinoids show a marked propensity to metastasize, especially to regional lymph nodes. Although ~5% of typical carcinoids metastasize (and nearly all SCLC metastasize), ~40–50% of atypical carcinoids will have metastasized at the time of presentation (63–67). Proper preoperative evaluation requires accurate definition of both the intra- and extraluminal components of these tumors (Fig. 44) (67,68,70–72).

The diagnosis of a typical carcinoid tumor should be suspected in any patient with a central, well-defined tumor, which is either narrowing, deforming, or obstructing an adjacent airway, especially when associated either with diffuse or punctate calcifications, or significant homogeneous enhancement following a bolus of i.v. contrast media (Fig. 45) (13,68,73,74). In a study of 12 pulmonary carcinoid tumors, all surgically proved, Magid et al. showed that five were central, defined by CT evidence of involvement of central airways, while

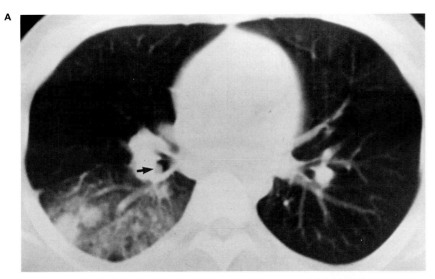

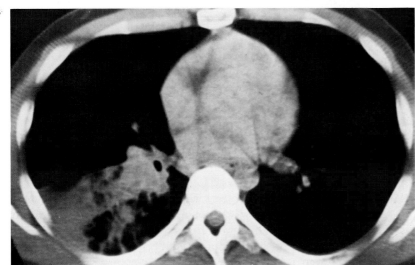

FIG. 44. Typical carcinoid-endobronchial disease. A: CT section through the origin of the RLLB imaged with lung windows shows a curvilinear soft-tissue density within the bronchial lumen, characteristic of an endobronchial lesion (*arrow*). The right hilum has a distinctly lobular configuration, compatible with enlarged lymph nodes. B: CT section obtained ~1.5 cm below A, imaged with mediastinal windows, following a drip infusion of i.v. contrast, shows that the presence of extensive consolidation within the RLL limits precise delineation of the tumor mass.

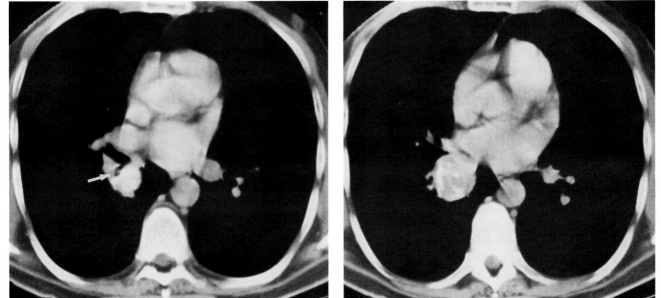

FIG. 45. Typical central carcinoid, calcified. A,B: Sequential scans through the inferior portion of the right hilum, imaged with narrow windows. A well-defined mass can be identified, compressing adjacent lower lobe basilar bronchi (*arrow* in A), within which foci of tumoral calcification are easily identified.

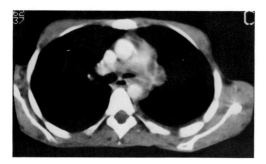

FIG. 46. Atypical carcinoid-nodal disease. CT section at the level of the carina following a bolus of i.v. contrast media shows extensive left hilar and mediastinal adenopathy encasing the left main pulmonary artery.

TABLE 2. Bronchiectasis: differential diagnosis

Congenital
  Congenital cystic bronchiectasis
  Selective immunoglobulin A (IgA) deficiency
  Primary hypogammaglobulinemia
  Cystic fibrosis
  Congenital deficiency of bronchial cartilage
  Immotile cilia syndrome (Kartagener's syndrome)
  Bronchopulmonary sequestration

Acquired
  Infection (bacterial or viral)
  Bronchial obstruction
    Intrinsic: neoplasm, foreign body, mucous plug
    Extrinsic: enlarged lymph nodes
  "Middle lobe syndrome"
  Traction bronchiectasis
  Acquired hypogammaglobulinemia

Modified from Barker and Bardana, ref. 73.

seven were peripheral (surrounded by parenchyma). Four tumors (three central; one peripheral) proved calcified by CT criteria: typically, these calcifications were punctate and peripheral. Nine lesions appeared smooth and round while two were irregular and lobulated (67). Similarly, in a review of 21 cases of both typical and atypical carcinoid tumors evaluated with CT, some combination of these findings was present in 11 of 14 patients with typical carcinoids and six of seven patients with atypical carcinoids (Meary E, Naidich DP, Huang RM, unpublished data).

The diagnosis of an atypical carcinoid is suggested by (a) an irregular or spiculated lesion, especially when associated with (b) markedly heterogeneous enhancement following administration of i.v. contrast, presumably secondary to tumor necrosis adenopathy, and/or (c) either hilar or mediastinal adenopathy (Fig. 46). The presence of adenopathy, in particular, should arouse suspicion. As documented by Forster et al., in a study of 31 patients with neuroendocrine carcinomas of the lung, only one of 10 patients with KCC-1 tumors had adenopathy, while four of 10 patients with KCC-2, and 10 of 11 patients with KCC-3 tumors, proved to have enlarged hilar and/or mediastinal lymph nodes (65).

BRONCHIECTASIS

Bronchiectasis is defined as generally localized, irreversible dilatation of the bronchial tree. Although the etiology of bronchiectasis is usually infectious, secondary either to airway obstruction due to tumor or, more rarely, due to impacted foreign bodies or mucus, inherited abnormalities clearly also play a significant role (see Table 2) (75–81). More recently, a form of central bronchiectasis has also been identified in patients following heart–lung transplantation (82).

The radiographic manifestations of bronchiectasis have been described (83). Typically, there is crowding and loss of definition of vascular markings in specific

segments of lung, changes reflecting peribronchial fibrosis, and loss of volume. With more extensive disease, discrete cystic spaces can be defined, occasionally containing air-fluid levels. In its most severe form, bronchiectasis causes a "honeycomb" pattern. The honeycombing is caused by fibrosis and resultant emphysema, not by dilated bronchi. Bronchiectasis rarely is associated with a normal chest radiograph (83).

Bronchiectasis has been classified by Reid (84) into three groups, depending on the severity of bronchial dilatation—all cylindrical, in which the bronchi have "ballooned" and are progressively more dilated toward the periphery.

Each type of bronchiectasis has a characteristic appearance on CT; however, the differentiation among various forms of bronchiectasis is less important than the simple identification of the disease process per se

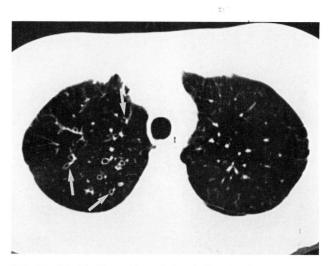

FIG. 47. Cylindrical bronchiectasis (cystic fibrosis). Cylindrical bronchiectasis involving a vertically oriented bronchus results in the "signet-ring" sign (arrows). This appearance is due to dilated bronchi lying adjacent to an accompanying pulmonary artery.

(85). Dilated bronchi with thickened walls and air-filled distended lumens are distinguishable in cross-section from normal lung parenchyma. The key to the CT diagnosis of bronchiectasis is the recognition of distinct and characteristic patterns of abnormalities within the pulmonary parenchyma.

Cylindrical bronchiectasis may be recognized by the finding of dilated, thick-walled bronchi extending to-ward the lung periphery (Fig. 47). Using both 10- and/or 1.5-mm thick sections, bronchi are normally visualized only in the medial or proximal portions of the lung parenchyma (Fig. 27). Peribronchial fibrosis, with resultant thickening of the bronchial wall and dilatation of the bronchial lumen, allows visualization of bronchi in more peripheral locations.

The appearance of cylindrically dilated bronchi will

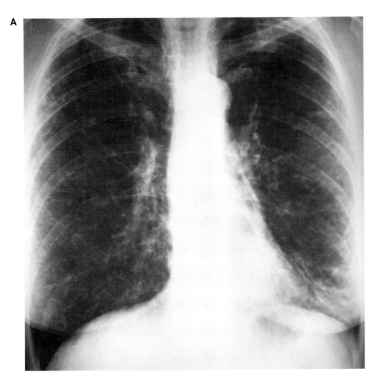

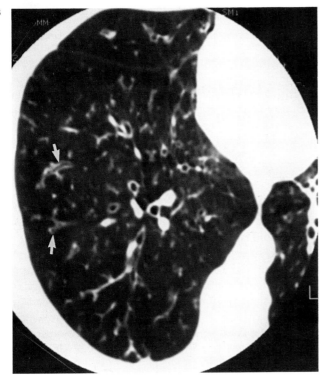

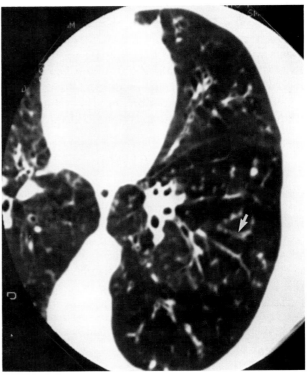

FIG. 48. Cylindrical bronchiectasis. **A:** PA radiograph shows extensive tram-tracking throughout both lower lobes medially, associated with apparent significant volume loss in the LLL, changes compatible with the clinical diagnosis of bronchiectasis. **B,C:** Enlargements of 1.5-mm thick sections obtained through the RLL and LLL, respectively. Note the presence of innumerable peripheral airways identifiable throughout both lower lobes in areas where otherwise normal caliber airways should not be definable. Many of these dilated peripheral airways would be difficult to define as such and might even have gone unrecognized without the use of thin sections (*arrows* in B and C).

vary depending on whether the bronchi have a horizontal or vertical course. When horizontal, the bronchi are visualized along their length; they are recognizable as "tramlines." When cylindrically dilated, bronchi course in a vertical direction; they are cut in cross-section and appear as thick-walled, circular lucencies (Fig. 48). Distended bronchi can be differentiated from emphysematous blebs in two ways. First, blebs generally have no definable wall thickness. Second, and more characteristically, bronchi, even in the lung periphery, are accompanied by branches of the pulmonary artery. When cut in cross-section, the result is a "signet ring" pattern (Fig. 47).

Varicose bronchiectasis is essentially similar in appearance to cylindrical bronchiectasis, the chief difference being that with varicose bronchiectasis the walls of the bronchi assume a beaded appearance (Fig. 49). Varicose bronchiectasis is easiest to identify when the involved bronchi course horizontally.

Cystic bronchiectasis may be most reliably recognized by the following pattern: (a) air-fluid levels (retained secretions in the dependent portions of dilated bronchi are a very specific sign of cystic bronchiectasis); (b) strings of cysts (the presence of a patent bronchus with consecutive areas of cystic dilatation leads to the production of a linear array or string of cysts if the bronchus

courses horizontally within the scanning plane; the greater the length of bronchus visualized on one section, the longer is the string of cysts, although these need not be lengthy to be diagnostic of cystic bronchiectasis); and (c) cluster of cysts (in more severe cases, dilated bronchi can be found grouped together; the appearance suggests a cluster of grapes). Recognition of some combination of dilated bronchi, air-fluid levels, and strings and clusters of cysts should be diagnostic of cystic bronchiectasis (Fig. 50). More than one pattern may be present, often on a single section. It should be emphasized that the findings on CT of bronchiectasis may be quite focal and exceedingly subtle. Reliance on the patterns described above should lead to accurate diagnosis.

It should also be emphasized that certain patterns of bronchiectasis are sufficiently characteristic to suggest a specific diagnosis. For example, central bronchiectasis is a frequent finding in patients with allergic bronchopulmonary aspergillosis (Fig. 51).

If the role of CT in the detection and characterization of bronchiectasis has proven controversial, this is due to delayed recognition of the significance of the use of proper technique in evaluation. The results of early reports, utilizing only 10-mm thick sections, proved surprisingly consistent, with sensitivities ranging between 60% and 80%, and specificities between 90% and 100% (86–89). This has led several investigators to conclude that CT was of only limited value in the diagnosis of bronchiectasis, especially as a potential screening modality. Significant improvement in diagnostic sensitivity, however, can be achieved by the use of 1.5–5-mm thick sections (Figs. 52 and 53) (90–93). Grenier et al. (90), utilizing 1.5-mm thick sections obtained every 10 mm, retrospectively compared CT and bronchography in 44 lungs in 36 patients and found that CT confirmed the diagnosis of bronchiectasis with a sensitivity of 97% and a specificity of 93%. In two lungs, CT underestimated the extent of disease, although in only one case with proven lower lobe disease was the CT scan interpreted as normal. Significantly, in one case CT detected bronchiectasis when bronchography was equivocal due to incomplete opacification of mucus-filled airways. Similar results have been reported by Joharjy et al. (91). Utilizing 4-mm thick sections obtained every 5 mm, CT correctly identified bronchiectasis in 98 (97%) of 101 segmental bronchi identified as abnormal with bronchography.

It should be emphasized that not all investigators have reported such good results (93). Munro et al. compared the accuracy of 3-mm thick sections and bronchography in 27 patients evaluated for chronic sputum production. Overall, the sensitivity of CT was 84% and the specificity was 82% compared with bronchography. Interestingly, in five cases the diagnosis of bronchiectasis was made by CT only in five cases, including two cases in which bronchial segments were underfilled at bronchography, sug-

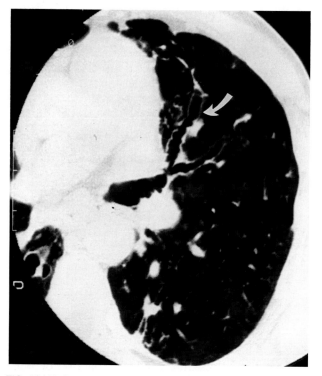

FIG. 49. Varicose bronchiectasis. Section through the anterior segmental bronchus of the LUL. This airway has a distinctly accordion or pleated appearance, compatible with varicose bronchiectasis (*arrow*). In this case, bronchiectasis is the result of long-standing tuberculosis, resulting in significant traction bronchiectasis.

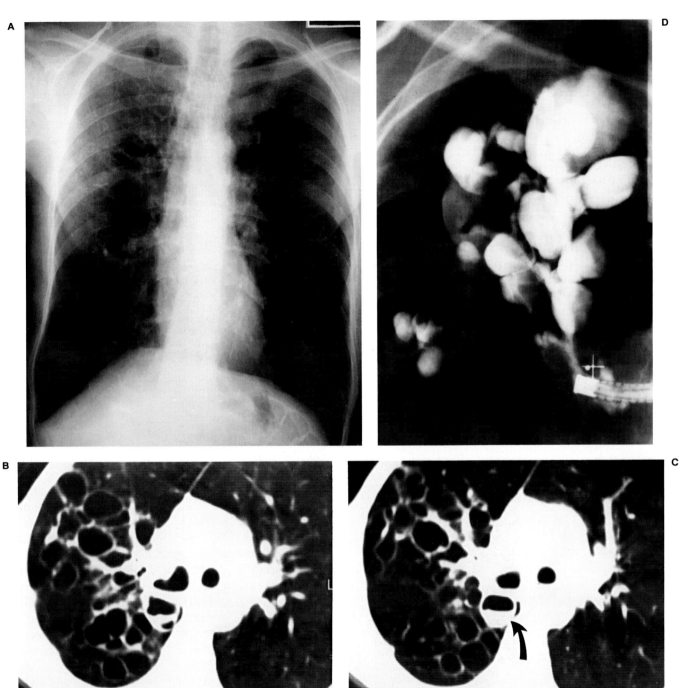

FIG. 50. Cystic bronchiectasis. **A:** PA radiograph shows numerous cystic spaces identifiable in the RUL. **B,C:** Enlargements of sections through the RUL. Numerous dilated bronchi can be identified having the configuration of a cluster of grapes; a few discrete air-fluid levels can be identified within dilated bronchi (*arrow* in C). **D:** Coned-down fluoroscopic spot film following selective injection of oily contrast medium into the apical segmental bronchus of the RUL following bronchoscopy.

gesting that bronchography may not be an absolute standard for identification of bronchiectasis.

On the basis of these findings, CT is recommended as the imaging procedure of choice following plain chest radiography in the diagnosis of bronchiectasis (94). As suggested by Phillips et al. (88), given the high specificity of CT findings in patients with documented bronchiectasis and the unpleasantness and potential risks of bronchography, CT is best utilized to confirm clinically or radiographically suspected disease. CT is especially valuable in cases in which there is unequivocal evidence of bilateral disease as it eliminates unnecessary surgery.

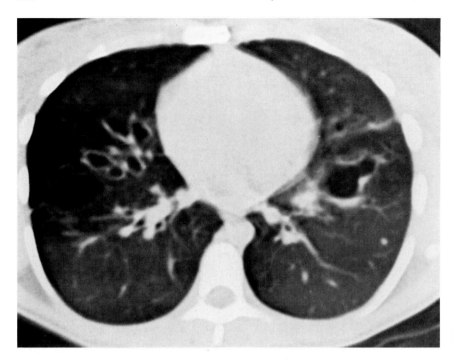

FIG. 51. Allergic bronchopulmonary aspergillosis. Section through the origin of the right middle lobe bronchus (RMLB) shows characteristic findings of central cystic bronchiectasis.

Bronchography should be reserved only for select surgical candidates in whom CT has documented segmental or unilateral involvement (95). Although the role of CT as a screening test is somewhat more controversial, due to a small but definite incidence of false-negative examinations, in our practice CT has proven frequently invaluable, especially in cases in patients who present with a history of hemoptysis (52,96,97).

In our experience, most cases are referred because of subtle abnormalities identified on routine radiographs in patients with clinically suspected disease. Symptomatic patients with entirely normal radiographs are the exception. As a consequence, the following technique is recommended: in cases in which there are no specific clinical or radiographic signs to help localize disease, 1.5-mm thick sections initially should be obtained every

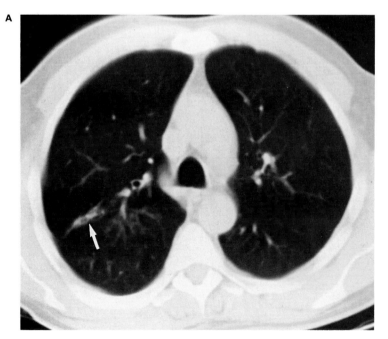
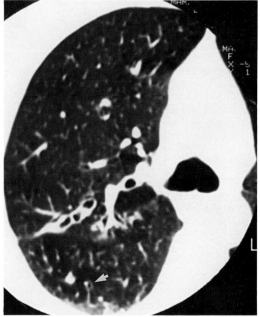

FIG. 52. Bronchiectasis: thin-section evaluation. A: 10-mm thick section through the carina shows ill-defined linear densities in the posterior segment of the RUL (arrow). The appearance is nonspecific. B: Enlargement of a 1.5-mm thick section at the same level as shown in A, reconstructed utilizing an edge-enhancing (bone) algorithm. Dilated bronchi are now easily identifiable, allowing a confidant diagnosis of bronchiectasis to be made. Note isolated small bronchiectatic airway in superior segment with characteristic ring shadow (arrow).

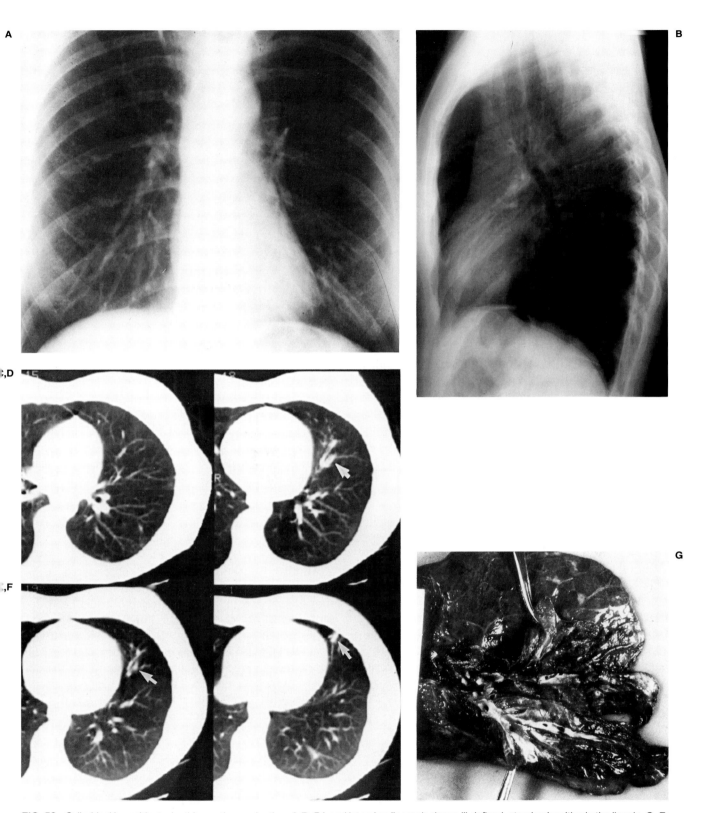

FIG. 53. Cylindrical bronchiectasis: thin-section evaluation. **A,B:** PA and lateral radiograph shows ill-defined, streaky densities in the lingula. **C–F:** Enlargements of select, sequential, 5-mm thick sections through the lingula. There is subtle tram-tracking along the entire length of the lingular bronchus, which can be traced almost to the pleural surface (*arrows*). **G:** Resected specimen, following sectioning, documenting the presence of cylindrical bronchiectasis in the lingula.

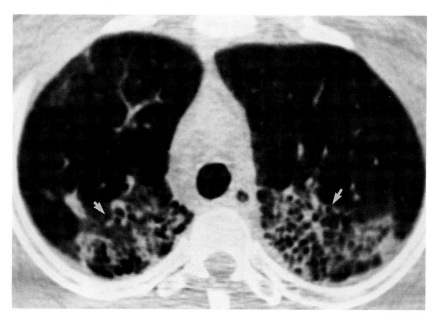

FIG. 54. Interstitial fibrosis, traction bronchiectasis, sarcoid. Section through the upper lobes shows focal interstitial fibrosis in a patient with known sarcoidosis. Dilated bronchi are easily identified (*arrows*), presumably reflecting traction bronchiectasis. The finding of dilated airways in the periphery of the lung may be the consequence of parenchymal disease, not bronchiectasis.

10 mm; if there is no suspicion of mediastinal or hilar disease, these may be reconstructed from the outset using an edge-enhancing or bone algorithm to enhance resolution. By markedly enhancing visualization of parenchymal anatomy, this approach allows more than adequate evaluation of the lungs, despite the lack of contiguous sections.

If localizing signs are present radiographically, this approach can be modified to obtain more sections as needed through specific regions of interest.

Recognition of potential pitfalls in the diagnosis of bronchiectasis can obviate misdiagnoses (see Table 3) (98). Diagnosis is especially difficult in patients with concurrent foci of parenchymal consolidation. In these cases, CT frequently discloses dilated peripheral airways that nonetheless revert to normal following adequate therapy, so-called reversible bronchiectasis. In this setting, follow-up scans are recommended pending radiographic resolution. Interstitial fibrosis also limits the diagnosis of bronchiectasis, as peribronchial fibrosis causes visualization of peripheral airways in cases in which true inflammatory destruction of bronchi is absent pathologically (Fig. 54) (99).

TABLE 3. *Bronchiectasis: potential pitfalls on CT*

Poor technique
   Inadequate collimation
   Respiratory/cardiac motion
Parenchymal consolidation (reversible bronchiectasis)
Interstitial fibrosis
Mucoid impaction of the airways
Pseudobronchiectasis (alveolar cell carcinomatosis)
Histiocytosis X

Another limitation frequently encountered is the presence of mucus-filled airways. The typical cross-section appearance of mucoid impaction has been described (Fig. 55) (100). Uncommonly, subtle focal involvement of peripheral airways may simulate otherwise nondescript pulmonary masses or nodules (Fig. 56). The appearance of cavitary nodules in patients with widespread bronchoalveolar cell carcinoma has given rise to the diagnosis "pseudobronchiectasis." In fact, this appearance is rare, only superficially resembles bronchiec-

→

FIG. 55. Mucoid impaction/bronchial atresia. CT/MR correlation. **A:** PA radiograph shows branching soft-tissue densities emanating from the left hilum (*arrow*) characteristic of mucoid impacted airways. **B,C:** CT sections obtained pre- and postadministration of a bolus of i.v. contrast material. Note the lack of contrast enhancement due to fluid within dilated, blind-ending airways (*arrows* in B and C), distinct from the marked enhancement apparent within the left interlobar pulmonary artery. **D:** Every-beat gated axial MR section through the left hilum at the same level as shown in B and C. Intermediate signal is present within dilated, branching airways on this relatively T1-weighted sequence, presumably due to the mucoid nature of the fluid (*arrow*) (compare with B and C). **E–H:** Sections at the same level as shown in B–D, obtained with a single level, multi-echo, heavily weighted T2 (every-third beat gated) sequence. With progressive T2-weighting persistent bright signal is apparent within these abnormal branching airways (*arrow* in G and H), findings diagnostic of mucoid filled airways.

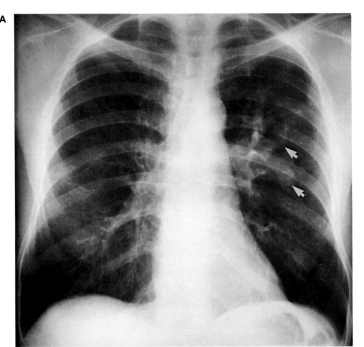

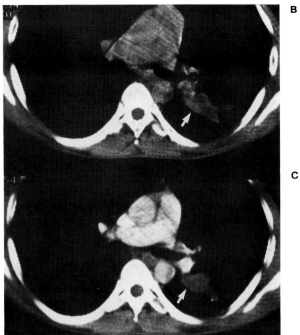

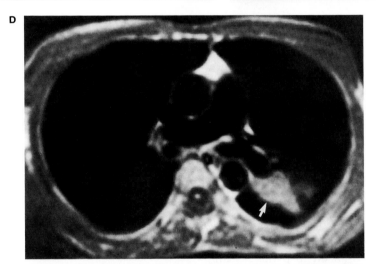

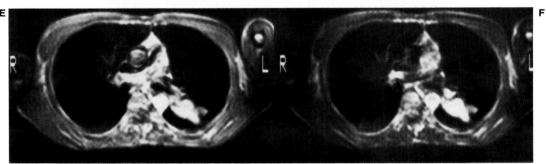

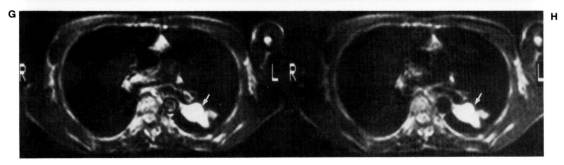

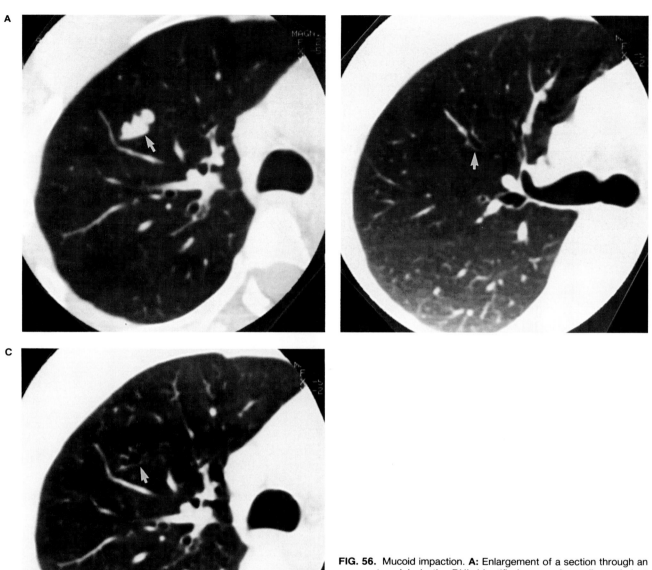

FIG. 56. Mucoid impaction. **A:** Enlargement of a section through an apparent nodule in the RUL identified on a prior radiograph (not shown). A density with an unusual configuration can be identified, with a straight border posteriorly (*arrow*). **B,C:** Sequential 1.5-mm thick sections obtained at the same level as A, following expectoration of a mucous plug on conservative antibiotic therapy. Note that the cystic space in B is a ghost of the density identified in A (*arrow*) and that a dilated bronchus leading to this region can be identified as well (*arrow* in C).

tasis, and should not be cause for confusion (Fig. 57). Uncommonly, central tumor may obstruct and then fill peripheral airways (Fig. 58). In cases of mucoid or tumor-filled airways, in addition to the use of thin sections, contrast-enhanced bolus CT or MR may prove invaluable (Figs. 55, 58, and 59) (102–104). Finally, the appearance of multiple odd-shaped cysts has been described in patients with histiocytosis X (105). In addition to careful evaluation of sequential sections, detailed clinical correlation usually suffices to avoid misdiagnosis (see chapter 8, Figs. 49 and 50).

CT/FOB CORRELATION: EVALUATION OF HEMOPTYSIS

Although CT is of proven value for delineating abnormalities of both the central and peripheral airways, the role of CT to evaluate patients with hemoptysis is controversial (52,96,97). Millar et al., evaluating 22 consecutive patients presenting with hemoptysis and normal chest radiographs, found that CT disclosed previously unsuspected abnormalities in 15 (68%) individuals, three of whom had bronchiectasis (97). These authors

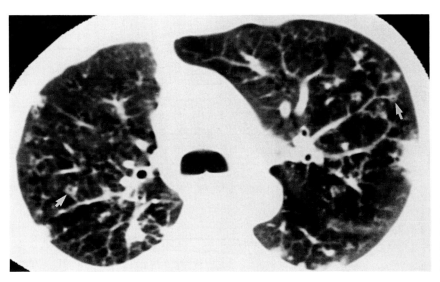

FIG. 57. Pseudobronchiectasis. Section through the carina shows multiple, scattered cavitary nodules that superficially resemble cylindrical bronchiectasis. Note that some lie adjacent to vessels, mimicking a signet ring appearance (*arrows*). Biopsy proved diffuse bronchoalveolar cell carcinoma.

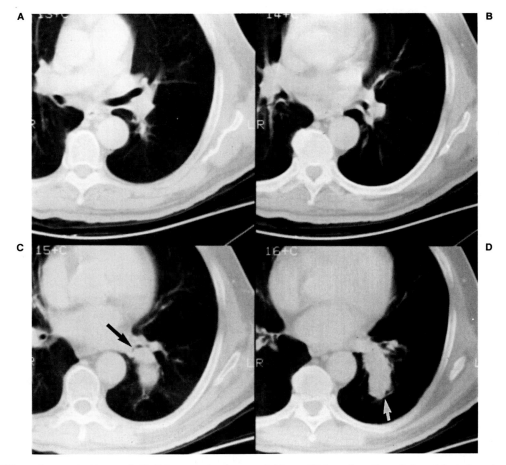

FIG. 58. Mucoid impaction, central tumor. **A–D:** Enlargements of sequential 5-mm thick sections through the origin and proximal portions of the LLLB, respectively, following a bolus of contrast medium show that there is marked narrowing and irregularity of the origins of the basilar segmental bronchi (*arrow* in C), as well as a somewhat unusual lobular, branching density just inferiorly (*arrow* in D).

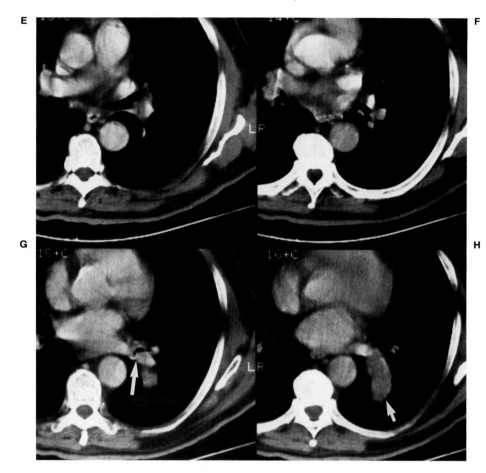

E   F

G   H

FIG. 58. (*Continued*) E–H: Identical images as shown in A–D, imaged with narrow windows. Note that there is no enhancement of the branching density illustrated in E, in conjunction with abnormal airways, a finding highly suggestive of mucoid impaction (*arrow* in H). Slight increased soft-tissue density can be seen adjacent to basilar bronchi (*arrow* in G). At surgery, portions of the segmental airways were filled with tumor growing distally from a central endobronchial focus. In this case, the key to diagnosing tumor instead of simple mucoid impaction is in identifying an abnormal configuration of a central airway. (Case courtesy of Ira Tyler, M.D., Albert Einstein Medical Center, Bronx, NY.)

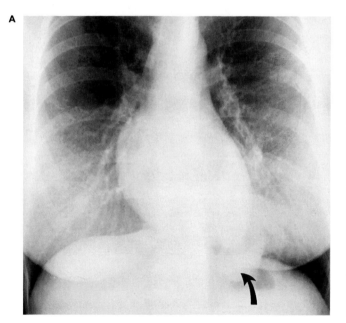

A

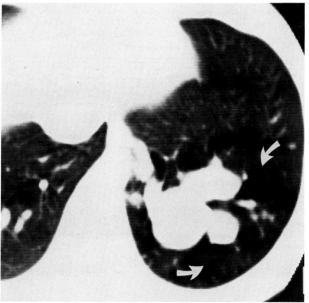

B

FIG. 59. Intralobar pulmonary sequestration. A: PA radiograph shows serpiginous densities at the left lung base, suggestive of pulmonary sequestration (*curved arrow*). B: CT scan through the left lung base, imaged with lung windows, shows characteristic appearance of dilated, branching densities surrounded by hyperaerated, emphysematous pulmonary parenchyma (*arrows*). C: Section through the lung bases following a bolus of i.v. contrast media. An anomalous vessel can be identified (*curved arrow*) coursing within the LLL, showing the same degree of opacification as the descending aorta confirming this as arterial. Note the lack of enhancement within fluid-filled, dilated airways (*small arrows*).

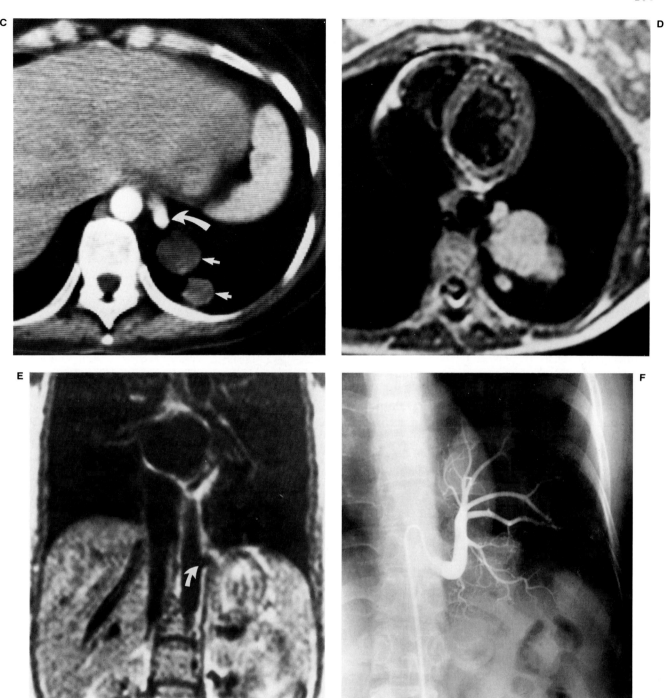

FIG. 59. (*Continued*) **D:** Every-beat gated, axial MR section through the LLL shows dilated, mucoid impacted bronchi, easily identified due to their characteristic, branching configuration (compare with B and C). Considerable signal is present within these airways, even on this relatively T1-weighted sequence, presumably due to the high protein content of the bronchial secretions. Note that unlike the corresponding CT scan, emphysematous changes within the LLL cannot be identified (compare with B). **E:** ECG-gated coronal section through the descending aorta shows an anomalous artery arising from the distal descending aorta, clearly originating above the diaphragm (*curved arrow*). **F:** Coned-down view following selective catheterization of the anomalous vessel.

concluded that CT should be considered an essential examination in all cases in which both chest radiography and bronchoscopy prove nondiagnostic. Haponik et al. correlated CT findings with chest radiographs and bronchoscopic findings in 32 patients (96). In 23 of 26 cases (88%), CT accurately showed the source of bleeding when the site was identified bronchoscopically. Furthermore, in 15 cases (47%), CT provided new diagnostic information, including identifying a previously unsuspected carcinoma in one case. Despite these findings, however, the authors concluded that CT offered little aid in the management of patients, and did not obviate the need for bronchoscopy. It should be emphasized that although 14 of 32 cases (44%) reported by Haponik et al. had documented lung cancers, these authors made no mention of any contribution CT may have made in staging these patients. Additionally, there were no cases of bronchiectasis.

It should be noted that the role of FOB in evaluating patients with hemoptysis is itself controversial, especially in cases with nonlocalizing chest radiographs (106–111). Jackson et al. (106) in a review of 48 consecutive patients presenting with hemoptysis with normal or nonlocalizing chest radiographs found that FOB resulted in a diagnosis other than endobronchial inflammation in only four patients, of whom only two proved to have bronchogenic carcinoma. Similarly, Poe et al. examined 196 patients with nonlocalizing chest radiographs and found that only 12 (6%) proved to have lung cancer (108). Applying univariate and discriminant analyses using age (older than 50 years), sex (male) and severity of hemoptysis (>30 mL/d), it was concluded that use of these criteria could have reduced the need for bronchoscopy by as much as 28% (108).

The use of CT to evaluate patients presenting with hemoptysis both with and without localizing chest radiographs has been documented (52). In a comparative retrospective study of 58 patients evaluated both by CT and FOB, abnormalities involving the airways were identified by CT in a total of 28 cases (48%). In 18 cases, CT identified focal abnormalities involving the central airways, 17 of which were subsequently proven to be malignant; in 10 cases, CT showed bronchiectasis. In all cases in which FOB depicted focal airway pathology, CT proved abnormal; CT abnormalities were identified in all cases of malignancy. Furthermore, in the same study, in 10 of 21 cases (48%) of non-small cell lung cancer, CT allowed definitive staging by documenting either direct mediastinal invasion or metastatic disease. Although the results of this study are preliminary, there appears to be a definite role for CT in evaluating patients with hemoptysis, especially for those in whom there is a low clinical index of suspicion for underlying malignancy.

MR OF AIRWAYS

The potential role of MR specifically to evaluate the airways has received relatively little attention (102,103,112). As documented by Mayr et al. (112) in a retrospective evaluation of 79 pathological and 319 normal bronchi confirmed bronchoscopically, only ~70% of the pathological and 45% of the normal bronchi, respectively, were visualized, compared to an overall accuracy of ~98% for CT. The superiority of CT over MR in visualizing the airways is the result of higher spatial resolution. Although this is a significant limiting factor in the evaluation of smaller bronchi, larger airways, such as

the trachea and main-stem bronchi, may be comparably imaged (Figs. 11 and 12). As already illustrated, due to the sensitivity of MR in identifying and delineating fluid, MR can also be utilized to evaluate mucus-filled airways (Figs. 55 and 59). In select cases, this may obviate the need for more invasive procedures, especially in the pediatric age group.

As discussed in more detail in Chapter 5, MR may also play a role in the evaluation of patients with lobar or segmental collapse (103,104). Although small endobronchial lesions may be difficult to define because of intrinsically high-contrast resolution, in select cases MR can be used to differentiate central obstructing tumor from peripheral lung collapse.

REFERENCES

1. Naidich DP, Terry PB, Stitik FP, Siegelman SS. Computed tomography of the bronchi: 1. Normal anatomy. *J Comput Assist Tomogr* 1980;4:746–753.
2. Proto AV. Evaluation of the bronchi with CT. *Semin Roentgenol* 1984;19:199–210.
3. Naidich DP, Stitik FP, Khouri NF, Terry PB, Siegelman SS. Computed tomography of the bronchi. Part 2. Pathology. *J Comput Assist Tomogr* 1980;4:754–762.
4. Naidich DP, Khouri NF, Scott WW, Wang KP, Siegelman SS. Computed tomography of the pulmonary hila. 1. Normal anatomy. *J Comput Assist Tomogr* 1981;5:459–467.
5. Naidich DP, Khouri NF, Stitik FP, McCauley DI, Siegelman SS. Computed tomography of the hila. 2. Abnormal anatomy. *J Comput Assist Tomogr* 1981;5:468–475.
6. Jardin M, Remy J. Segmental bronchovascular anatomy of the lower lobes: CT analysis. *AJR* 1986;147:457–468.
7. Osborne D, Vock P, Godwin JD, Silverman PM. CT identification of bronchopulmonary segments: 50 normal subjects. *AJR* 1984;142:47–52.
8. Jardin MR, Remy J. Comparison of vertical and oblique CT in evaluation of the bronchial tree. *J Comput Assist Tomogr* 1988;12:956–962.
9. Kittredge RD. Computed tomography of the trachea: a review. *Computed Tomography* 1981;5:44–49.
10. Gamsu G, Webb WR. Computed tomography of the trachea: normal and abnormal. *AJR* 1982;139:321–326.
11. Kittredge RD. The right posterolateral tracheal band. *J Comput Assist Tomogr* 1979;3:348–354.
12. Greene R. "Saber sheath" trachea: relation to chronic obstructive pulmonary disease. *AJR* 1978;130:441–445.
13. Naidich DP, McCauley DI, Siegelman SS. Computed tomography of bronchial adenomas. *J Comput Assist Tomogr* 1982;6:725–732.
14. Houston HE, Payne WS, Harrison EG, Olsen AM. Primary cancers of the trachea. *Arch Surg* 1969;99:132–140.
15. Jensik RJ, Faber LP, Brown CM, Kittle CF. Bronchoplastic and conservative resectional procedures for bronchial adenoma. *J Thorac Cardiovasc Surg* 1974;68:556–565.
16. Ross JAT. Techniques in the surgical repair of tracheal stenosis. *Otolaryngol Clin North Am* 1979;12:893–899.
17. Moore EH, Templeton PA, Grillo HC, Shepard J, McCloud TC. Bronchoplastic and lung preservation surgery: indications, imaging, complications, and the impact of the new TNM classification. *Radiology* 1988;169:62.
18. Thaller S, Fried MP, Goodman ML. Symptomatic solitary granular cell tumor of the trachea. *Chest* 1985;88:925–928.
19. Allen HA, Angell F, Hankins J, Whitley NO. Leiomyoma of the trachea. *AJR* 1983;141:683–684.
20. Swain ME, Coblentz CL. Clinical images. Tracheal chondroma: CT appearance. *J Comput Assist Tomogr* 1988;12:1085–1086.

21. Choplin RH, Wehunt WD, Theros EG. Diffuse lesions of the trachea. *Semin Roentgenol* 1983;18:38–50.

22. Cohen MI, Gore RM, August CZ, Ossoff RH. Case report. Tracheal and bronchial stenosis associated with mediastinal adenopathy in Wegener granulomatosis: CT findings. *J Comput Assist Tomogr* 1984;8:327–329.

23. Stein MG, Gamsu G, Webb WR, Stulbarg MS. Case report. Computed tomography of diffuse tracheal stenosis in Wegener granulomatosis. *J Comput Assist Tomogr* 1986;10:868–870.

24. Mendelson DS, Som PM, Crane R, Cohen BA, Spier H. Relapsing polychondritis studied by computed tomography. *Radiology* 1985;157:489–490.

25. Shepard JO. Radiology of the bronchial tree. In: Taveras JM, Ferrucci JT, eds. *Radiology: diagnosis—imaging—intervention.* Philadelphia: J. B. Lippincott, 1987.

26. Bottles K, Nyberg DA, Clark M, Hinchcliffe WA. Case report. CT diagnosis of tracheobronchopathia osteochondroplastica. *J Comput Assist Tomogr* 1983;7:324–327.

27. Berkmen YM, Auh YH. CT diagnosis of acquired tracheoesophageal fistula in adults. *J Comput Assist Tomogr* 1985;9:302–304.

28. Liu P, Daneman A. Computed tomography of intrinsic laryngeal and tracheal abnormalities in children. *J Comput Assist Tomogr* 1984;8:662–669.

29. Hoffman EA, Gefter WB, Schnall M, Nordberg J, Listerud J, Lenkinski RE. Work in progress. Upper airway evaluation: a multidimensional-multiparameter approach. *Radiology* 1988;169:374.

30. Okada K, Lee MO, Hitmi S, Nagayama Y, Noma S. Case report. Sinus histiocytosis with massive lymphadenopathy and tracheobronchial lesions: CT and MR findings. *J Comput Assist Tomogr* 1988;12:1039–1040.

31. Ell SR, Jolles H, Keyes WD, Galvin JR. Cine CT technique for dynamic airway studies. *AJR* 1985;145:35–36.

32. Stein MG, Gamsu G, de Geer G, Golden JA, Crumley RL, Webb WR. Cine CT in obstructive sleep apnea. *AJR* 1987;148:1069–1074.

33. Frey EE, Smith WL, Grandgeorge S, McCray P, Wagener J, Franken EA, Sato Y. Chronic airway obstruction in children: Evaluation with cine-CT. *AJR* 1987;148:347–352.

34. Jackson CL, Huber JF. Correlated applied anatomy of the bronchial tree and lungs with a system of nomenclature. *Dis Chest* 1943;9:319–326.

35. Boyden EA. The nomenclature of the bronchopulmonary segments and their blood supply. *Dis Chest* 1961;39:1–6.

36. Ferry RM, Boyden EA. Variations in the bronchovascular patterns of the right lower lobe of fifty lungs. *J Thorac Cardiovasc Surg* 1951;22:188–201.

37. Pitel M, Boyden EA. Variations in the bronchovascular patterns of the left lower lobe in fifty lungs. *J Thorac Cardiovasc Surg* 1953;26:633–653.

38. Yamashita H. *Roentgenologic anatomy of the lung.* Stuttgart: Thieme Medical Publishers, 1978.

39. MacGregor JH, Chiles C, Godwin JD, Ravin CE. Imaging of the axillary subsegment of the right upper lobe. *Chest* 1986;90:763–765.

40. Landay M. Azygos vein abutting the posterior wall of the right main and upper lobe bronchi: a normal CT variant. *AJR* 1983;140:461–462.

41. Siegel MJ, Shakelford GD, Francis RS, McAlister WH. Tracheal bronchus. *Radiology* 1979;130:353–355.

42. Shipley RT, McCloud TC, Dedrick CG, Shepard JO. Computed tomography of the tracheal bronchus. *J Comput Assist Tomogr* 1985;9:53–55.

43. Morrison SC. Case report. Demonstration of a tracheal bronchus by computed tomography. *Clin Radiol* 1988;39:208–209.

44. Felson B. *Chest roentgenology.* Philadelphia: W.B. Saunders, 1973.

45. Jardin M, Remy J. Segmental bronchovascular anatomy of the lower lobes: CT analysis. *AJR* 1986;147:457–468.

46. Naidich DP, Zinn WL, Ettenger NA, McCauley DI, Garay SM. Basilar segmental bronchi: thin-section CT evaluation. *Radiology* 1988;169:11–16.

47. Webb WR, Gamsu G. Computed tomography of the left retrobronchial stripe. *J Comput Assist Tomogr* 1983;7:65–69.

48. Borman N. Broncho-pulmonary segmental anatomy and bronchography. *Minn Med* 1958;41:820–830.

49. Colice GL, Chappel GJ, Frenchman SM, Solomon DA. Comparison of computerized tomography with fiberoptic bronchoscopy in identifying endobronchial abnormalities in patients with suspected lung cancer. *Am Rev Respir Dis* 1985;131:397–400.

50. Naidich DP, Lee JJ, Garay SM, McCauley DI, Aranda CP, Boyd AD. Comparison of CT and fiberoptic bronchoscopy in the evaluation of bronchial disease. *AJR* 1987;148:1–7.

51. Henschke CI, Davis SD, Auh PR, Westcott J, Berkman YM, Kazam E. Detection of bronchial abnormalities: comparison of CT and bronchoscopy. *J Comput Assist Tomogr* 1987;11:432–435.

52. Naidich DP, Funt S, Ettenger NA, Arranda C. Hemoptysis: CT-bronchoscopic correlations in 58 cases. *Radiology* 1990;177:357–362.

53. Woodring JH. Determining the cause of pulmonary atelectasis: a comparison of plain radiography and CT. *AJR* 1988;150:757–763.

54. Mayr B, Ingrisch H, Haussinger K, Huber RM, Sunder-Plassmann L. Tumors of the bronchi: role of evaluation with CT. *Radiology* 1989;172:647–652.

55. Wang KP. Flexible transbronchial needle aspiration biopsy for histological specimens. *Chest* 1985;88:860–864.

56. Shure D, Fedillo PF. Transbronchial needle aspiration in the diagnosis of submucosal and peribronchial bronchogenic carcinoma. *Chest* 1985;88:49–51.

57. Lam S, Muller NL, Miller RR, Kostashuk EC, Szasz IJ, LeRiche JC, Lee-Chuy E. Predicting the response of obstructive endobronchial tumors to photodynamic therapy. *Cancer* 1986;58:2298–2306.

58. Naidich DP, Sussman R, Kutcher WL, Aranda CP, Garay SM, Ettenger NA. Solitary pulmonary nodules: CT–bronchoscopic correlation. *Chest* 1988;93:595–598.

59. Fink I, Gamsu G, Harter L. CT-guided aspiration biopsy of the thorax. *J Comput Assist Tomogr* 1982;6:958–962.

60. van Sonnenberg E, Casola G, Ho M, Neff CC, Varney RR, Wittich GR, Christensen R, Friedman PJ. Difficult thoracic lesions: CT-guided biopsy experience in 150 cases. *Radiology* 1988;167:457–461.

61. Tolly TL, Feldmeier JE, Czarnecki D. Case report. Air embolism complicating percutaneous lung biopsy. *AJR* 1988;150:555–556.

62. Pinstein ML, Scott RL, Salazaar J. Avoidance of negative percutaneous lung biopsy using contrast-enhanced CT. *AJR* 1983;140:265–267.

63. Arrigoni MG, Woolner LB, Bernatz PE. Atypical carcinoid tumors of the lung. *J Thorac Cardiovasc Surg* 1972;64:413–421.

64. Mills SE, Walker AN, Cooper PH, Kron IL. Atypical carcinoid tumor of the lung. A clinicopathologic study of 17 cases. *Am J Surg Pathol* 1982;6:643–654.

65. Paladugu RR, Benfield JR, Pak HY, Ross RK, Teplitz RL. Bronchopulmonary Kulchitzky cell carcinomas. A new classification scheme for typical and atypical carcinoids. *Cancer* 1985;55:1303–1311.

66. Churg A. Tumors of the lung. In: Thurlbeck WM, ed. *Pathology of the lung.* Stuttgart: Thieme Medical Publishers, 1988.

67. Magid D, Siegelman SS, Eggleston JC, Fishman EK, Zerhouni EA. Pulmonary carcinoid tumors: CT assessment. *J Comput Assist Tomogr* 1989;13:244–247.

68. Forster BB, Muller NL, Miller RR, Nelems B, Evans KG. Neuroendocrine carcinomas of the lung: clinical, pathologic, and radiologic correlation. *Radiology* 1988;169:63.

69. Choplin RH, Kawamoto EH, Dyer RB, Geisinger KR, Mills SE, Pope TL. Atypical carcinoid of the lung: radiographic features. *AJR* 1986;146:665–668.

70. Boyd AD, Spencer FC, Lind AL. Why has bronchial resection and anastomosis been reported infrequently for treatment of bronchial adenoma? *J Thorac Cardiovasc Surg* 1970;59:359–365.

71. Jensik RJ, Faber LP, Brown CM, Kittle CF. Bronchial adenoma. *J Thorac Cardiovasc Surg* 1974;68:556–565.

72. Grote TH, Macon WR, Davis B, Greco FA, Johnson DH. Atypi-

cal carcinoid of the lung: a distinct clinicopathologic entity. *Chest* 1988;93:370–375.

73. Aronchick JM, Wexler JA, Christen B, Miller W, Epstein D, Gefter WB. Computed tomography of bronchial carcinoid. *J Comput Assist Tomogr* 1986;10:71–74.

74. Webb WR, Gamsu G, Birnberg FA. CT appearance of bronchial carcinoid with recurrent pneumonia and hyperplastic hilar lymphadenopathy. *J Comput Assist Tomogr* 1983;7:707–709.

75. Barker AF, Bardana EJ. State of the art. Bronchiectasis: update of an orphan disease. *Am Rev Respir Dis* 1988;137:969–978.

76. Davis PB, di Sant'Agnese PA. Diagnosis and treatment of cystic fibrosis: an update. *Chest* 1984;85:802–809.

77. Annest LS, Kratz JM, Crawford FA. Current results of treatment of bronchiectasis. *J Thorac Cardiovasc Surg* 1982;83:546–550.

78. Lewiston NJ. Bronchiectasis in childhood. *Pediatr Clin North Am* 1984;31:865–876.

79. Watanabe Y, Nishiyama Y, Kanayama H, Enomoto K, Kato K, Takeichi M. Case report. Congenital bronchiectasis due to carti-lage deficiency: CT demonstration. *J Comput Assist Tomogr* 1987;11:701–703.

80. Dunne MG, Reiner B. CT features of tracheobronchomegaly. *J Comput Assist Tomogr* 1988;12:388–391.

81. Shin MS, Jackson RM, Ho KJ. Case report. Tracheobroncho-megaly (Mounier-Kuhn syndrome): CT diagnosis. *AJR* 1988;150:777–779.

82. Skeens JL, Fuhrman CR, Yousem SA. Bronchiolitis obliterans in heart-lung transplantation patients: radiologic findings in 11 pa-tients. *AJR* 1989;153:253–256.

83. Gudjberg CE. Roentgenologic diagnosis of bronchiectasis. An analysis of 112 cases. *Acta Radiol* 1955;43:209–226.

84. Reid LM. Reduction in bronchial subdivision in bronchiectasis. *Thorax* 1950;5:233–236.

85. Naidich DP, McCauley DI, Khouri NF, Stitik FP, Siegelman SS. Computed tomography of bronchiectasis. *J Comput Assist To-mogr* 1982;6:437–444.

86. Muller NL, Bergin CJ, Ostrow DN, Nichols DM. Role of com-puted tomography in the recognition of bronchiectasis. *AJR* 1984;143:971–976.

87. Silverman PM, Godwin JD. CT/bronchographic correlations in bronchiectasis. *J Comput Assist Tomogr* 1987;11:52–56.

88. Phillips MS, Williams MP, Flower CDR. How useful is com-puted tomography in the diagnosis and assessment of bronchiec-tasis? *Clin Radiol* 1986;37:321–325.

89. Cooke JC, Currie DC, Morgan AD, Kerr IH, Delany D, Strick-land B, Cole PJ. Role of computed tomography in diagnosis of bronchiectasis. *Thorax* 1987;42:272–277.

90. Grenier P, Maurice F, Musset D, Menu Y, Nahum H. Bron-chiectasis: assessment by thin-section CT. *Radiology* 1986;161:95–99.

91. Joharjy IA, Bashi SA, Abdullah AK. Value of medium-thickness CT in the diagnosis of bronchiectasis. *AJR* 1987;1133–1137.

92. Mootoosamy IM, Reznek RH, Osman J. Assessment of bron-chiectasis by computed tomography. *Thorax* 1985;40:920–924.

93. Munro NC, Cooke JC, Currie D, Stickland B, Cole PJ. Compari-son of thin section computed tomography with bronchography for identifying bronchiectatic segments in patients with chronic sputum production. *Thorax* 1990;45:135–139.

94. Stanford W, Galvin JR. The diagnosis of bronchiectasis. *Clin Chest Med* 1988;9:691–699.

95. Breatnach ES, Nath PH, McElvein RB. Case report. Preoperative evaluation of bronchiectasis by computed tomography. *J Com-put Assist Tomogr* 1985;9:949–950.

96. Haponik EF, Britt EJ, Smith PL, Bleecker ER. Computed chest tomography in the evaluation of hemoptysis. *Chest* 1987;91:80–85.

97. Millar AB, Boothroyd A, Edwards D, Hetzel MR. Abstract. Value of computed tomography in unexplained haemoptysis. *Thorax* 1988;43:811.

98. Tarver RD, Conces DJ, Godwin JD. Technical note. Motion artifacts on CT simulate bronchiectasis. *AJR* 1988;151:1117–1119.

99. Westcott JL, Cole SR. Traction bronchiectasis in end-stage pul-monary fibrosis. *Radiology* 1986;161:665–669.

100. Pugatch RD, Gale ME. Obscure pulmonary masses: bronchial impaction revealed by CT. *AJR* 1983;141:909–914.

101. Chasen MH, McCarthy MJ, Gilliland JD, Floyd JL. Concepts in computed tomography of the thorax. *Radiographics* 1986;6:793–832.

102. Gooding CA, Lallemand DP, Brasch RC, Wesbey GE, Davis B. Magnetic resonance imaging in cystic fibrosis. *J Pediatr* 1984;105:384–388.

103. Naidich DP, Rumancik WM, Ettenger NA, Feiner HD, Har-nanz-Schulman M, Spatz EM, Toder ST, Genieser NB. Congeni-tal anomalies of the lungs in adults: MR diagnosis. *AJR* 1988;151:13–19.

104. Naidich DP, Rumancik WM, LeFleur RS, Estioko MR, Brown S. Case report. Intralobar pulmonary sequestration. MR evalua-tion. *J Comput Assist Tomogr* 1987;11:531–533.

105. Moore AD, Godwin JD, Muller NL, Naidich DP, Hammar SP, Buschman DL, et al. Pulmonary histiocytosis X (eosinophilic granuloma): CT findings. *Radiology* 1989;172:249–254.

106. Jackson CV, Savage PJ, Quinn DL. Role of fiberoptic bronchos-copy in patients with hemoptysis and a normal chest roentgeno-gram. *Chest* 1985;87:142–144.

107. Adelman M, Haponik EF, Bleeker ER, Britt EJ. Cryptogenic hemoptysis. Clinical features, bronchoscopic findings, and natu-ral history in 67 patients. *Ann Int Med* 1985;102:829–834.

108. Poe RH, Israel RH, Marin MG, et al. Utility of fiberoptic bron-choscopy in patients with hemoptysis and a nonlocalizing chest roentgenogram. *Chest* 1988;92:70–75.

109. Lederle FA, Nichol KL, Parenti CM. Bronchoscopy to evaluate hemoptysis in older men with nonsuspicious chest roentgeno-grams. *Chest* 1989;95:1043–1047.

110. Rohwedder JJ. [Editorial.] Enticements for fruitless bronchos-copy. *Chest* 1989;96:708–710.

111. Sen RP, Walsh TE. [Editorial.] Bronchoscopy. Enough or too much? *Chest* 1989;96:710–712.

112. Mayr B, Heywang SH, Ingrisch H, Huber RM, Haussinger K, Lissner J. Comparison of CT with MR imaging of endobronchial tumors. *J Comput Assist Tomogr* 1987;11:43–48.

113. Naidich DP. CT/MR correlation in the evaluation of tracheo-bronchial neoplasia. *Rad Clin N Amer* 1990;28:555–571.

114. Naidich DP. CT and MRI of the airways. In: *CT and MRI of the Thorax.* Zerhouni EA, ed. New York: Churchill-Livingstone, 1990.

115. Tobler J, Levitt RG, Glazer HS, Moran J, Crouch E, Evens RG. Differentiation of proximal bronchogenic carcinoma from postobstructive lobar collapse by magnetic resonance imaging: comparison with computed tomography. *Invest Radiol* 1987;22:538–543.

116. Shioya S, Haida M, Ono Y, Fukuzaki M, Yamabayashi H. Lung cancer: differentiation of tumor, necrosis, and atelectasis by means of T1 and T2 values measured *in vitro*. *Radiology* 1988;167:105–109.

Chapter 4

Lobar Collapse

The radiographic patterns of lobar collapse have been extensively reviewed (1–9). A wide range of abnormalities has been described, characterizing the appearance of the collapsed lobe as well as secondary, compensatory changes, including shifts or changes of position of mediastinal structures, the hila, the hemidiaphragms, and the fissures.

Computed tomography (CT) is a useful adjunct to routine radiography in the evaluation of lobar collapse (10–16). This is because CT allows unobstructed cross-sectional visualization of thoracic anatomy. Not only can the affected lobe and involved airways be evaluated, but changes involving the mediastinum, chest wall, hilum, pleura, and adjacent lung can be appreciated as well.

The purpose of this chapter is to review the basic patterns of lobar collapse, with specific emphasis on the underlying pathophysiology. It is only through an understanding of the mechanics of collapse that cross-sectional images can be interpreted properly.

GENERAL PRINCIPLES AND METHODOLOGY

Obviously, accurate interpretation of the cross-sectional appearance of lobar collapse necessitates thorough knowledge of normal CT anatomy, especially bronchial anatomy (see Chapter 3). CT can accurately identify and localize the presence of an obstructing bronchial lesion (17–22). Even in the absence of bronchial obstruction, alterations in the normal appearance of the bronchi are to be expected consequent to volume loss in the affected lobe and resultant changes in the position of normal bronchi. Although these changes

may be appreciated on routine radiographs, they are far more apparent with CT.

Proper technique for evaluating the airways has been described in detail previously (see Chapter 3). When evaluating patients with pulmonary atelectasis, specific modifications need to be applied. This is because adequate evaluation requires not only precise visualization of the airways but detailed examination of the collapsed lung itself, as well as evaluation of the mediastinum, hilum, and pleura. Correlation with appropriate radiographs is mandatory to define which lobar, or segmental bronchi need to be most closely evaluated. This is most easily accomplished with an initial series of contiguous 8–10-mm sections. Additional, thinly collimated (1.5–5 mm) sections can be obtained through the regions of greatest interest, as necessary. As discussed in detail previously (see Chapter 3), this approach ensures accurate delineation of the presence or confirmation of the absence of bronchial pathology.

Following detailed airway evaluation, especially in cases in which endobronchial tumor is suspected, additional sections should be obtained following the administration of intravenous contrast. This should be in the form of a bolus, either hand delivered, or preferentially, if available, by means of a power injector (22). As will be discussed and illustrated in greater detail below, intravenous contrast serves a critically important role in defining the presence and extent of central masses, as well as differentiating tumor from adjacent collapsed lung and associated mediastinal and pleural disease (10–12,14,15,21,23).

Although it is generally accepted that intravenous contrast should be administered as a bolus, some uncertainty persists concerning the most appropriate imaging sequence to be followed. Two options are available: *dynamic-incremental* scanning and *dynamic-static* scanning. The first technique, dynamic-incremental scanning, requires rapid acquisition of images with table incrementation through a preselected region of interest, usually through the hila in patients with either lobar or segmental collapse (24). The alternative method, dynamic-static scanning, involves acquisition of images in the dynamic mode at one level only. In the case of pulmonary atelectasis, this involves obtaining a minimum of six to eight sections, usually at the level of an abnormal lobar or segmental bronchus, ideally identified on an initial, precontrast enhanced series of scans. Either method will generate acceptable images; as will be discussed, however, preliminary work suggests a significant advantage to utilizing the dynamic-static approach (23). Although less critical, intravenous contrast should also be administered to evaluate causes of pulmonary atelectasis other than endobronchial obstruction (11,21).

Lobar collapse may be caused by one of four mechanisms: endobronchial obstruction; passive atelectasis (collapse caused by extrinsic pressure, either from air, fluid, or both in the pleural space); cicatrization; and, more rarely, adhesions, such as may be caused by radiation with resultant loss of surfactant (25). Each of these mechanisms results in a distinctive radiographic pattern and is easily assessed with CT.

ENDOBRONCHIAL OBSTRUCTION

Endobronchial obstruction causes a spectrum of radiographic changes, reflecting both the nature and extent of the disease process within the affected lobe, as well as compensatory changes involving the adjacent lung, the mediastinum, the diaphragm, and the chest wall. Lobar collapse due to endobronchial occlusion should thus be viewed as a dynamic process accounting for a wide variability of radiographic appearances.

Bronchial obstruction usually causes increased density within the affected lobe, secondary to the presence of intra-alveolar fluid. How much fluid is present within the obstructed lung is generally a function of both the degree of obstruction and time.

Occasionally, in the presence of endobronchial obstruction, the affected lobe may contain air and appear relatively normal in density. In this situation, obstruction may be difficult to detect (Fig. 1). In the presence of total bronchial obstruction, distal lung may appear normally aerated if there is sufficient collateral air-drift. This may occur between various portions of a single lobe or, as illustrated in Fig. 1, between lobes, presumably as a function of incompletely formed fissures.

Despite great variability, lobar collapse secondary to endobronchial obstruction forms a discrete and easily

TABLE 1. *CT of lobar collapse: primary changes*

Segmental bronchi are variable in appearance. Endobronchial tumor causes irregular narrowing and/or occlusion; patent bronchi may be established with other forms of lobar collapse.

With collapse, the involved lobe becomes pie-shaped rather than hemispherical in cross section.

The proximal portion of the lobe assumes a V-shape, with the apex situated at the origin of the affected bronchus.

There is an overall increase in the density of the lobe. Endobronchial obstruction, over time, produces an airless lobe with soft-tissue density. Lucency within collapsed lobes is generally secondary to extensive bronchiectasis, such as is seen with cicatrization atelectasis.

Large tumor masses produce a bulge in the contour of the collapsed lobe (S-sign of Golden) and may be identified separately from the remainder of the collapsed lobe following a bolus of i.v. contrast medium.

Lose of volume results in a reduced zone of contact between the pleural surface of the lobe and the chest wall.

Partial fixation of the lobe by prior pleural adhesions may affect the pattern of collapse, as will fluid and/or air in the pleural space, in which case the affected lobe may be displaced from the chest wall or mediastinum.

An entire lobe may be replaced by tumor; this gives a lobular rather than wedge-shaped appearance to the collapsed lobe in the absence of endobronchial occlusion.

definable subset, the characteristic appearance of which is described in Table 1.

Right Upper Lobe Collapse

The right upper lobe is bordered medially by the mediastinum, superiorly by the chest wall, inferiorly by the minor fissure, and posteroinferiorly by the superior portion of the oblique fissure. When collapsed, the right upper lobe progressively pancakes against the mediastinum, maintaining its connection to the hilum by a tongue of tissue referred to as the "mediastinal wedge" (Figs. 2 and 3).

The lower and middle lobes both become hyperaerated in compensation; this results in upward displacement of the minor fissure and anterior displacement of the upper portion of the oblique fissure. As the right upper lobe collapses toward the midline, the middle lobe (especially the lateral segment) insinuates itself laterally between the chest wall and the lateral portion of the collapsing right upper lobe. With hyperaeration and expansion, the pulmonary vessels within the middle and lower lobes will appear abnormally spaced. Compensatory hyperexpansion of the right lower lobe, especially the superior segment, may lead to visualization of a sliver of lung invaginating between the mediastinum

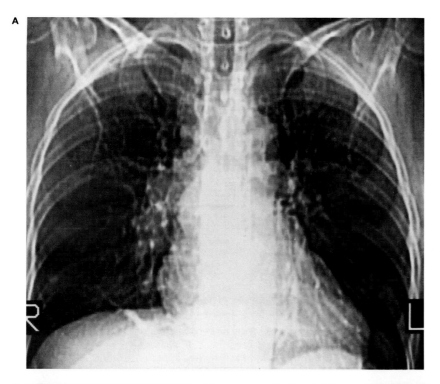

FIG. 1. Endobronchial obstruction: metastatic renal cell carcinoma. **A:** Scanogram. A nodular density is present in the right lower lobe. A subcarinal mass is present as well. There is no evidence of volume loss on the right side. **B–E:** Sequential images through the right upper lobe bronchus, bronchus intermedius, right lower lobe bronchus, and right lower lobe, respectively. A small density can be seen within the lumen of the right upper lobe bronchus. The bronchus intermedius is obliterated. Despite this, there is normal aeration of the middle and right lower lobes. Total obstruction was confirmed bronchoscopically.

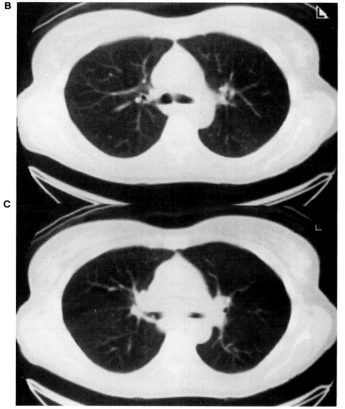

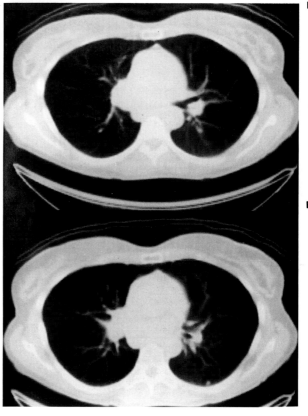

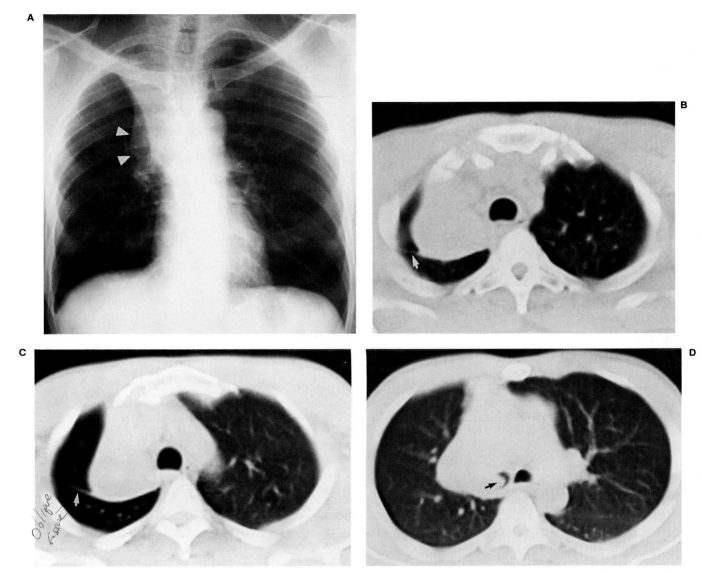

FIG. 2. Right upper lobe collapse: adenocarcinoma. **A:** PA radiograph shows right upper lobe collapse. The line that is convex medially represents the elevated middle lobe fissure; the line that is convex laterally represents tumor mass (*arrowheads*). **B–D:** Sequential images through the mid and lower trachea and the right upper lobe bronchus. The collapsed right upper lobe can be identified as a wedge of uniform density extending along the mediastinum to the anterior chest wall. There is hyperinflation of the middle and lower lobes, which can be clearly separated by identification of the lateral margin of the oblique fissure (*arrows* in B and C). The middle lobe is insinuated between the collapsed upper lobe medially and the lateral chest wall. A large polypoid lesion obstructs the origin of the right upper lobe bronchus (*arrow* in D). Notice that there is convex bulging of the contour of the collapsed upper lobe laterally, which becomes more pronounced as sections are taken closer to the right upper lobe bronchus. This bulge is caused by central tumor mass and accounts for the S-shaped configuration of the collapsed right upper lobe scan on the PA radiograph.

medially and the posterior aspect of the collapsed right upper lobe laterally. This phenomenon has been referred to as "Luftsichel" on plain radiographs and results in a triangular configuration of the posterior-inferior portion of the collapsed right upper lobe (Fig. 3) (15). As will be illustrated, Luftsichel is far more commonly seen with left upper lobe collapse. Ancillary changes, such as shift to the right of the trachea and mediastinum and elevation of the right hemidiaphragm, may occur but are more variable.

This sequence of events is readily identifiable with CT. As illustrated in Fig. 2, the collapsed right upper

lobe appears as a wedge of soft-tissue density extending alongside the mediastinum to the anterior chest wall. Hyperaerated middle and lower lobes can be differentiated by identification of the oblique fissure, which marginates the posterior border of the collapsed right upper lobe. Separation of vessels within the hyperaerated middle and lower lobes is easy to appreciate by comparison with the normal, contralateral lung. As the right upper lobe retracts from the lateral chest wall, the apex of the lobe remains affixed to the hilum.

Endobronchial obstruction is readily identifiable with CT. In the case illustrated in Fig. 2, a polypoid mass

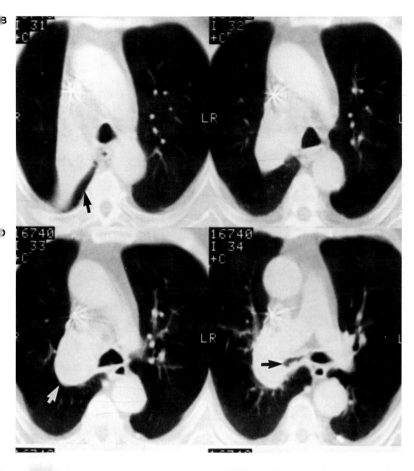

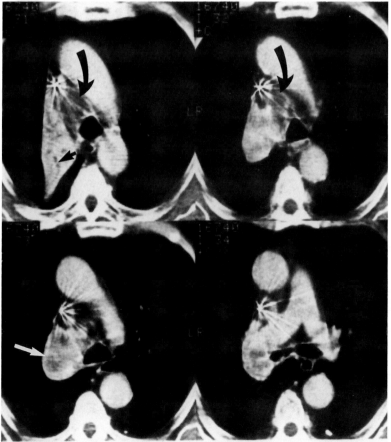

FIG. 3. Right upper lobe collapse: bronchogenic carcinoma. **A–D:** Sequential sections through the distal trachea and carina in a patient with an obstructing bronchogenic carcinoma, imaged with lung windows. There is complete obstruction of the right upper lobe bronchus and marked narrowing of the proximal bronchus intermedius by tumor (*arrow* in D). Central tumor causes a convexity in the margin of the collapsed lobe (*arrow* in C). The middle lobe is hyperaerated and lies lateral to the collapsed right upper lobe. Note that a portion of the superior segment of the right lower lobe has become invaginated medial to the collapsed right upper lobe (*arrow* in A), so-called Luftsichel. **E–H:** Identical sections corresponding with A–D, only imaged with narrow, mediastinal windows, following a bolus of i.v. contrast material. Central tumor is easily identified as an irregular mass of low attenuation (*arrow* in G) causing convexity in the contour of the collapsed right upper lobe. Collapsed lung enhances uniformly, except for obviously identifiable fluid-filled bronchi (*arrow* in E). Not the presence of enlarged, low-density, pretracheal mediastinal lymph nodes (*curved arrows* in E and F).

occludes the origin of the right upper lobe bronchus and prolapses into the right main-stem bronchus and proximal portion of the bronchus intermedius, causing partial occlusion. Unfortunately, there is little specificity in the appearance of most endobronchial lesions. Primary bronchogenic carcinoma, bronchial adenomas, endobronchial metastases, and even lymphoma may be indistinguishable. Accurate histologic diagnosis requires biopsy (26).

In the absence of a large, proximally obstructing lesion, the collapsed right upper lobe should taper relatively smoothly into the hilum. When central tumor mass is present, the lateral border of the collapsed lobe widens centrally, having a convex border directed laterally, as shown in Figs. 2 and 3. This is the CT counterpart of the radiologic "S-sign of Golden" and may be seen on CT with collapse of any lobe that is caused by central tumor (27). With right upper lobe collapse, the concave line seen on posteroanterior (PA) films is caused by upward displacement of the minor fissure; the convex line is caused by tumor (Fig. 2). Identification of central tumor mass necessitates the use of a bolus of intravenous (i.v.) contrast medium. As shown in Fig. 3, following contrast medium administration the borders of a central tumor can be distinguished from the remainder of the collapsed lobe: the presence of mediastinal lymphadenopathy may be delineated as well.

In addition to the changes already mentioned, right upper lobe collapse may result in a rearrangement of bronchial anatomy. Such changes may be difficult to detect with routine films. Rotation of the carina, such as may occur in right upper lobe collapse, probably reflects the fact that, unlike the left upper lobe bronchus, which

TABLE 2. *CT of lobar collapse: specific findings*

Right upper lobe
  Posterior margin of the collapsed lobe (the major fissure) is displaced anteromedially
  Medial margin of collapsed lobe abuts the mediastinum
  Anterior margin of collapsed lobe consists of a reduced zone of pleural contact

Left upper lobe
  Posterior margin of collapsed lobe (the major fissure) is displaced anteromedially
  Medial margin of collapsed lobe approaches the mediastinum but frequently makes incomplete contact because of intrusion of overexpanded superior segment of left lower lobe

Middle lobe collapse
  Medial margin of lobe abuts the right heart border
  Posterior margin of collapsed lobe is displaced anteromedially
  Compensatory changes are less marked because of small volume of middle lobe

Lower lobe collapse
  Medial margin makes contact with the mediastinum inferiorly
  The anterior margin (the major fissure) is displaced posteromedially
  Contact between the collapsed lobe and the medial portion of the diaphragm is maintained, probably as a result of the inferior pulmonary ligament.

is anchored superiorly by the left main pulmonary artery, the right upper lobe bronchus is more freely able to change position.

The findings on CT in right upper lobe collapse are summarized in Tables 1 and 2, and shown pictorially in Fig. 4.

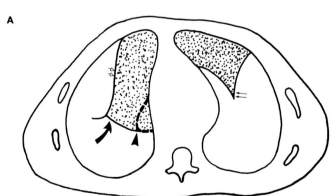
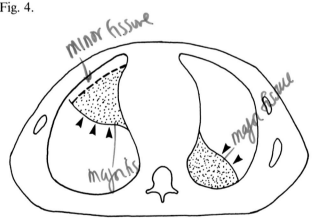

FIG. 4. Schematic representations of collapse. **A:** Cross-sectional appearance of idealized collapse of the right and left upper lobes secondary to central obstructing tumors. The right upper lobe (*stippled area* on the left side of the image) typically collapses anteromedially against the mediastinum. The middle lobe fissure rotates anteromedially as the hyperinflated middle lobe insinuates between the collapsed lobe medially and the lateral chest wall (*open arrows*). The major fissure is shifted slightly anteriorly (*curved arrow*). Rarely, a small portion of the superior segment invaginates between the collapsed lung laterally and the mediastinum, so-called Luftsichel (*dashed lines*), giving a triangular appearance to the posterior aspect of the collapsed right upper lobe (*arrowhead*). Unlike right upper lobe collapse, left upper lobe collapse (*stippled area* on the right side of the image) typically is anterosuperior, and the posterior portion of the collapsed lobe is more characteristically V-shaped (*double arrows*). This appearance is caused by pronounced medial insinuation of the hyperaerated superior segment of the left lower lobe. (Modified from Khoury et al., ref. 15.) **B:** Cross-sectional appearance of idealized collapse of the middle lobe and left lower lobe, secondary to central obstructing tumors. The middle lobe characteristically collapses anteromedially against the right heart border (*stippled area* on the left side of the image). The major fissure rotates anteriorly (*triple arrowheads*) and is typically sharply defined. The minor fissure is deviated inferiorly (*dotted lines*) and is usually indistinct due to its oblique orientation. The lower lobes collapse posteromedially against the spine. As a consequence, the major fissure is displaced posteriorly (*double arrowhead*).

Left Upper Lobe Collapse

The left upper lobe is bounded medially by the mediastinum and more inferiorly by the left heart border, superiorly and laterally by the chest wall, and posteriorly by the major fissure. With collapse, the left upper lobe moves anterosuperiorly. Unlike the right upper lobe, which collapses against the mediastinum along its entire length, the left upper lobe generally retains more contact with the anterior and lateral chest wall as it collapses. Superiorly, the left upper lobe may be displaced from the mediastinum by hyperaeration of the superior segment of the left lower lobe. This accounts for the frequent finding of periaortic lucency or Luftsichel on PA radiographs following left upper lobe collapse (Figs. 4 and 5). Inferiorly, the left upper lobe, like the right upper lobe, marginates the mediastinum and is connected to the left hilum by a wedge of collapsed tissue.

Superiorly, the collapsed upper lobe has a wedge-shaped, triangular configuration, with the apex pointing posteriorly. This configuration is caused by the general anterosuperior direction of collapse; the broad base of the triangular collapsed lobe retains its connection to the anterior chest wall. Posteriorly, this V-shaped contour is caused by anterior displacement of the superior segment of the left lower lobe along both the medial and lateral limbs of the V (15). Hyperinflation of the left lower lobe and right lung (which crosses the midline) is somewhat greater than that seen in right upper lobe collapse, probably because the left upper lobe has a much greater volume. Superiorly, hyperaerated left lower lobe insinuates between the aorta and mediastinum medially and the collapsed upper lobe laterally.

Depending on the degree of collapse, the left hilum will become elevated. The degree of elevation of the left hilum, and subsequent rotation of the left bronchial tree, is of less magnitude on the left side, compared with changes accompanying right upper lobe collapse, because the left upper lobe bronchus is "anchored" by the left pulmonary artery superiorly. As shown in Fig. 5, despite considerable volume loss in the left upper lobe, the left upper lobe bronchus has undergone little elevation or rotation.

Endobronchial obstruction is easily defined with CT. Tumor infiltration frequently results in irregular tapering of the distal portion of the left upper lobe bronchus. Care must be taken to confirm this appearance as abnormal with sequential, thin sections. The left upper lobe bronchus normally may have a tapered appearance if sections are obtained at the level at which the left main pulmonary artery courses over the left upper lobe bronchus (see Chapter 3).

The triangular, wedge-shaped configuration of the collapsed left upper lobe is generally a result of considerable volume loss. Acutely, the degree of volume loss within the left upper lobe may be minimal, in which case the posterior margin of the collapsed lobe may appear convex posteriorly.

Collapse may be associated with a large hilar mass, as well as with extensive mediastinal disease. With the use of a bolus of intravenous contrast, separation of these components is generally possible (Fig. 5). Differentiation between the collapsed lung and masses in the hilum and mediastinum depends on identification of the characteristic triangular configuration of the collapsed left upper lobe.

Although lesions involving the left upper lobe bronchus generally cause collapse of the whole lobe, occasionally collapse is more pronounced in one of the segments of the left upper lobe. As illustrated in Fig. 6, despite total occlusion of the left upper lobe bronchus, volume loss is most marked in the lingula. This portion of the left upper lobe collapses against the left heart border, causing marked anteromedial displacement of the major fissure. Presumably, volume differential to this degree between different segments of a lobe implies prior segmental obstruction.

The findings of CT in left upper lobe collapse are reviewed in Tables 1 and 2, and illustrated pictorially in Fig. 4.

Middle Lobe Collapse

The middle lobe is bounded medially by the right heart border, anteriorly and laterally by the chest wall, posteriorly by the major fissure, and superiorly by the minor fissure. As the middle lobe collapses, the two fissures begin to approximate one another; that is, there is downward shift of the minor fissure and forward displacement of the oblique fissure. The major fissure is clearly seen with CT because the axis of this fissure is perpendicular to the plane of the scan. The minor fissure, parallel to the plane of the scan, is never as sharply defined. As the middle lobe loses volume, it collapses medially against the right heart border. This accounts for the silhouette sign on PA radiographs. The middle lobe normally has a triangular or wedge-shaped configuration; this becomes accentuated as the lobe collapses, with the apex of the triangle directed toward the hilum. Because of the relatively smaller volume of the middle lobe, compared with the other lobes, compensatory changes, such as shift of the mediastinum and hyperaeration of the remainder of the lung, tend to be less pronounced (Fig. 7).

The typical configuration of middle lobe collapse, as in any other form of lobar collapse, will be altered if adhesions form between the pleural surfaces. This may cause confusion, especially when seen on routine chest radiographs; in this setting, CT may prove invaluable. The findings on CT of middle lobe collapse are summarized in Tables 1 and 2.

A

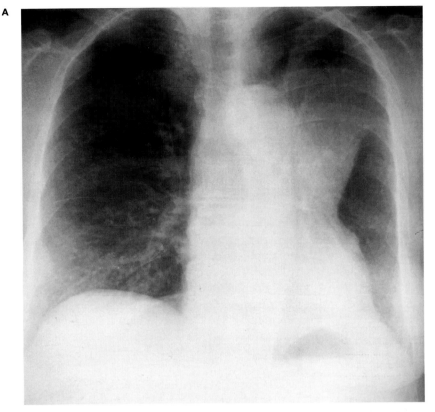

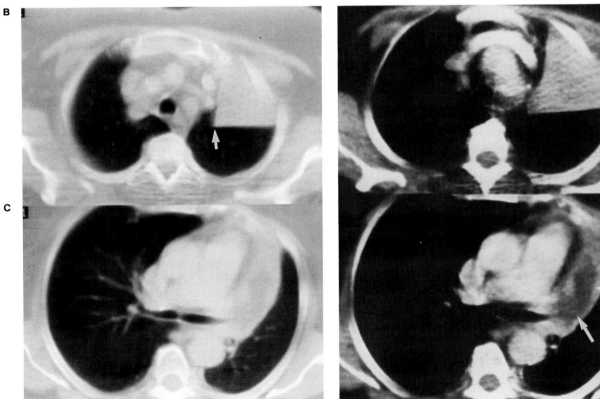

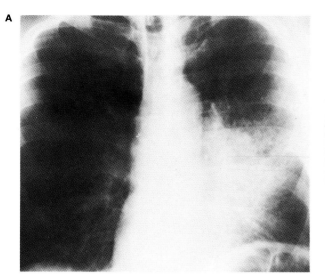

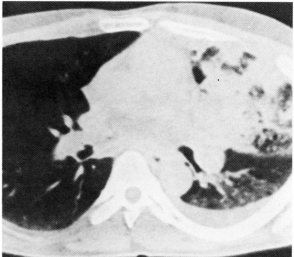

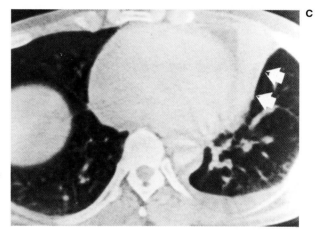

FIG. 6. Left upper lobe collapse: large cell carcinoma. **A:** PA radiograph shows left upper lobe collapse. Increased density in the left lung is more apparent inferiorly. **B:** Section at the level of the left upper lobe spur. The left upper lobe bronchus is obliterated by tumor. Mass and infiltrate are present in the left upper lobe, sharply marginated posteriorly by the major fissure. At this level, volume loss is slight. **C:** Section through the lower thorax. The lingula is totally collapsed, identifiable as a wedge of uniformly increased density, marginating the left heart border and extending to the anterior chest wall. The major fissure has rotated anteromedially (*arrow*). In this case, obstruction of the lingular bronchus must have antedated obstruction of the left upper lobe bronchus.

FIG. 5. Left upper lobe collapse: squamous cell carcinoma. **A:** PA radiograph. Characteristic appearance of left upper lobe collapse. **B,C:** Sections at the level of the great vessels and left upper lobe bronchus, respectively, imaged with lung windows. The appearance is classic of left upper lobe atelectasis. The collapsed left upper lobe forms a sharply defined triangular density, with the apex pointing posteriorly (*arrow* in B). The hyperinflated left lower lobe lies between the collapsed upper lobe and the mediastinum. There is shift of the carina and great vessels to the left, and hyperaeration of the right upper lobe that crosses the midline anteriorly. Note that the left upper lobe bronchus is obstructed laterally and is slightly elevated superiorly, lying at the same level as the right upper lobe bronchus. **D,E:** Identical sections as shown in B and C, imaged with narrow, mediastinal windows. Images obtained following a bolus of i.v. material show an irregular, necrotic tumor mass centrally (*arrows* in E) causing obstruction of the left upper lobe bronchus. Peripherally, there is strikingly uniform enhancement of the collapsed lung. Note the absence of any significant mediastinal adenopathy.

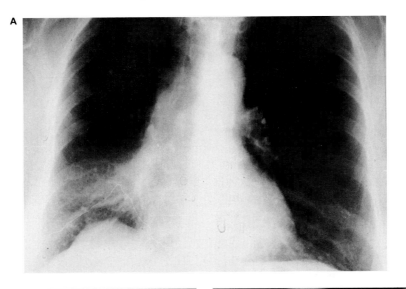

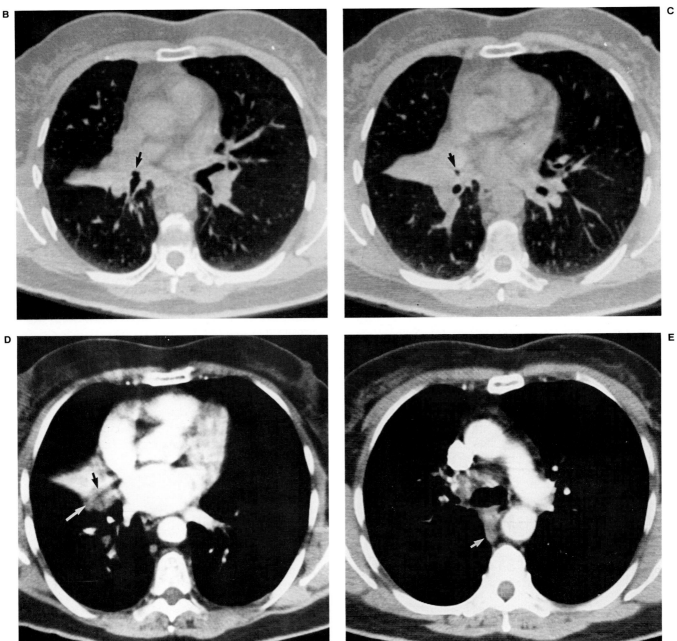

Lower Lobe Collapse

The lower lobes should be considered together, since anatomically they appear identical in the collapsed state. The lower lobes are bordered inferiorly by the hemidiaphragms, posteriorly and laterally by the chest wall, medially by the heart and mediastinum, and anteriorly by the major fissure. The lower lobes collapse medially toward the mediastinum, generally maintaining contact with the hemidiaphragms. These changes reflect the attachments of the inferior pulmonary ligaments. Occasionally, the attachments between the lower lobes and the pulmonary ligaments are incomplete. In this case, collapse of the lower lobes may assume an unusual or rounded configuration. The major fissure, especially the lateral portion, moves posteriorly. This accounts for the usually sharp line of the lateral portion of the collapsed lobe on PA radiographs (Fig. 8).

Right lower lobe collapse mimics the appearance of left lower lobe collapse. Collapse is generally posteromedial against the posterior mediastinum and spine. The lateral contour of the collapsed lobe is convex laterally when collapse is secondary to central tumor. Occasionally, a central tumor will cause atelectasis of the superior segment alone. Isolated from the remainder of the basilar segmental bronchi, a strategically placed tumor can obstruct the superior segmental orifice without compromising the main portion of the right lower lobe bronchus. Although this appearance may cause confusion on plain radiographs, identification of isolated superior segmental collapse is greatly simplified when seen in cross-section (Fig. 9).

The findings on CT of lower lobe collapse are reviewed in Tables 1 and 2.

BENIGN VERSUS MALIGNANT BRONCHIAL OBSTRUCTION

CT can be used to differentiate between benign and malignant causes of pulmonary atelectasis. Recognition of malignancy is based on the following triad: abnormal or obstructed airways, a central mass causing distinct bulging of the proximal contour of the collapsed lobe or segment, and differential enhancement of tumor versus collapsed peripheral lung following administration of intravenous contrast (Figs. 3, 5, and 7–9).

In a retrospective analysis of 50 patients with segmental or lobar atelectasis, Woodring (21) compared the accuracy of chest radiographs with CT in identifying patients with central obstructing tumors. Utilizing the findings of bronchial obstruction and a central mass causing a contour abnormality, unlike chest radiographs, which identified 24 (89%) of 27 patients, CT proved 100% sensitive, correctly identifying all 27 obstructing carcinomas. In three cases (10%), CT findings led to false-positive diagnoses; in each, benign causes of bronchial obstruction led to the false assumption of central tumor. Significantly, in no case in which the airways were shown to be patent was tumor ultimately found. A similar degree of accuracy utilizing CT to detect central tumor has been documented by others (10,18,19).

It should be emphasized that central airway patency should be distinguished from the finding on CT of airbronchograms within collapsed lobes. These latter may be seen within consolidated or collapsed segments, even when not apparent on routine chest radiographs. Their presence should not be assumed to be evidence of central airway patency, either because central obstruction may be of recent onset, central obstruction may not be complete, or the effects of central obstruction may be mitigated by collateral air-drift. It is for this reason that careful scanning with thin sections through the origin and proximal portions of potentially abnormal airways is mandatory. As documented by Woodring (21), in 32 cases in which air-bronchograms could be identified with CT, in 11 (34%) a central obstructing tumor was present.

Although the findings of bronchial pathology and central masses causing contour abnormalities have proven reliable signs of malignant collapse, there is less certainty concerning the role of intravenous contrast in delineating the presence of tumor (10,12,15,23). In a retrospective study of 25 cases of obstructive lobar collapse, Khoury et al. (15), administering first an intravenous bolus and then a rapid drip of contrast material, and utilizing contiguous 1 cm sections, found that differential enhancement separated tumor from collapsed lung in only two of eight patients (15). Tobler et al. (23), however, in their evaluation of 18 patients with proximal bronchogenic carcinoma and postobstructive lobar collapse, found that in eight (80%) of ten patients evaluated with a bolus of intravenous contrast, differentiation

FIG. 7. Middle lobe collapse: squamous cell carcinoma. **A:** PA radiograph showing increased density inferiorly on the right, suggestive of collapse of the middle lobe. **B,C:** Sections through and just below the origin of the middle lobe bronchus, imaged with wide windows. The middle lobe bronchus is patent at its origin (*arrow* in B); just below, however, the distal portion of the middle lobe bronchus is significantly narrowed (*arrow* in C). The apex of the middle lobe can be defined as a small airless wedge extending laterally from the hilum towards the lateral chest wall, defined posteriorly by the right lower lobe and anteriorly by the hyperinflated upper lobe. **D:** Section at almost the same level as B, imaged with narrow windows, following administration of a bolus of i.v. contrast medium via a power injector, imaged with narrow windows. Central tumor can be identified as an area of low attenuation, easily differentiated from the uniformly enhancing collapsed middle lobe (*arrows*). **E:** Section through the carina shows extensive precarinal lymphadenopathy, as well as extensive posterior lymph nodes (*arrow*), which on more inferior scans proved to be continuous with markedly enlarged subcarinal lymph nodes (not shown).

A,B

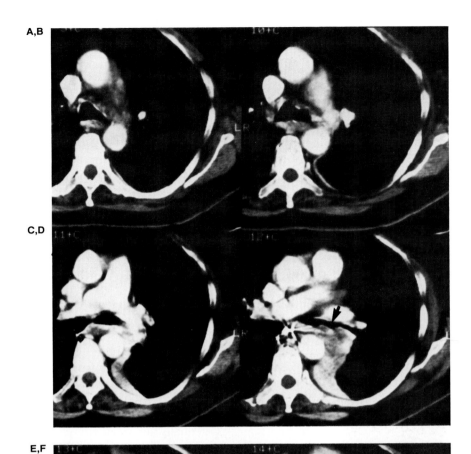

C,D

E,F

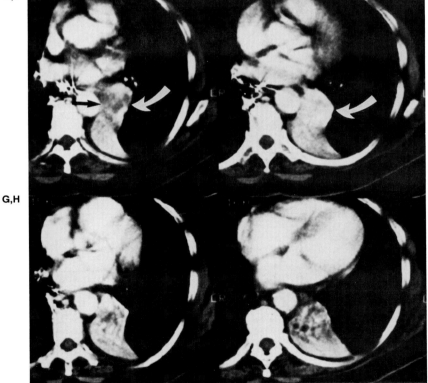

G,H

FIG. 8(A–T). Left lower lobe collapse: squamous cell carcinoma. CT/MR correlation. **A–H:** Sequential images beginning at the level of the aorticopulmonary window and extending caudally through the collapsed left lower lobe, imaged with narrow, mediastinal windows. Following a bolus on i.v. contrast, central tumor is identifiable as a mass of low density, causing convexity of the lateral border of the collapsed lobe (*curved arrows* in E and F). Note that the left lower lobe bronchus is obliterated and that there is significant nodular narrowing of visualized portions of the left upper lobe bronchus (*small arrow* in D). Numerous small mediastinal nodes are present in the aorticopulmonary window. The left lower lobe is airless and collapsed against the posterior mediastinum. Uniform enhancement of the collapsed lobe allows confident identification of the left hilar mass causing obstruction (*straight arrow* in E). Note the presence of fluid-filled airways within the collapsed lung. Equally significant, no pleural fluid can be identified, an observation difficult to determine from the plain radiograph.

,J

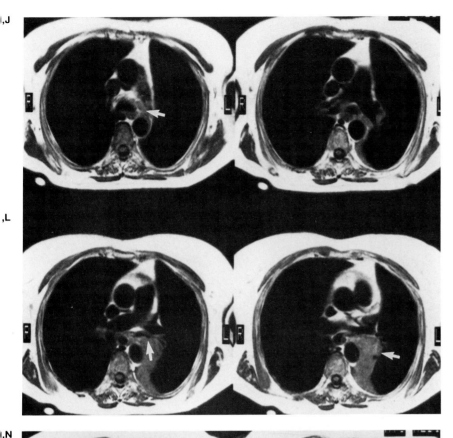

,L

,N

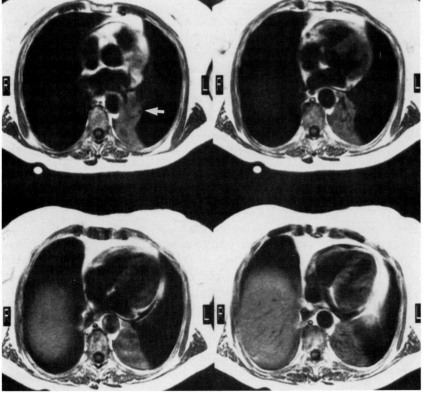

,P

FIG. 8. (*Continued*) **I–P:** Sequential, T1-weighted images corresponding precisely to the same levels shown in A–H. Anatomic correspondence is strikingly similar, including the presence of enlarged nodes in the aorticopulmonary window (*arrow* in I), obstruction of the left lower lobe bronchus, and nodular narrowing of the left upper lobe bronchus (*arrow* in K), as well as a convex bulge along the lateral margin of the collapsed lobe (*arrows* in L and M). Note that on this T1-weighted sequence it is not possible to differentiate tumor from collapsed lung.

Q,R

S,T

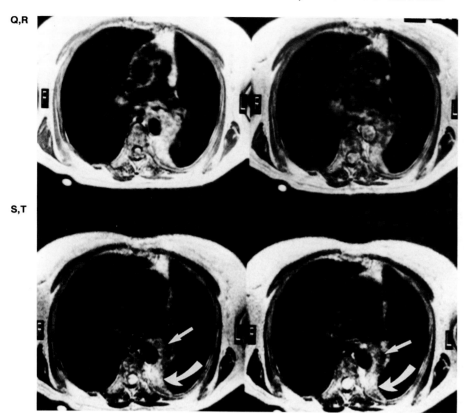

FIG. 8. (*Continued*) **Q–T:** T2-weighted images all obtained at the level of the left upper lobe spur, with echo-times (TE's) of 30, 60, 90, and 120 msecs, respectively. Note that with progressively longer TE's, considerable signal can be identified within the collapsed lung (*curved arrows* in S and T), allowing easy differentiation from central tumor (*arrows* in S and T).

of tumor from adjacent lung was possible. Significantly, as compared with previous reports, Tobler et al. (23) utilized a dynamic-static sequence, in which six 3-sec scans were obtained with a 2-sec interscan delay, providing six sequential images all at the same level with variable degrees of contrast enhancement. Interestingly, in the two cases in this study evaluated with a dynamic-incremental technique following first a bolus and then a rapid drip infusion of contrast, central tumor could not be differentiated from peripheral collapse with either technique.

That variable findings should be reported utilizing intravenous contrast to differentiate tumor from collapse is not surprising. Differentiation is based on numerous factors, most significantly including the degree of vascularity of the tumor, the presence and extent of tumor necrosis, and the state of the collapsed lung. Significantly, no attempt has yet been made to correlate the CT appearance of collapse following intravenous contrast administration with actual tissue histology. As will be discussed in greater detail later in this chapter, in addition to differences in tumor behavior and histology, there is a wide range of pathological changes that occur over time within collapsed lobes themselves (28). It is to be anticipated that with so many variables determining the role of both CT and magnetic resonance (MR) in evaluating lobar atelectasis will be complex. Nonetheless, despite limitations, in our experience, the use of

dynamic scanning following a bolus of intravenous contrast material has proven invaluable. Not only can tumors be identified, but, with few reservations, changes within the collapsed lung can be identified as well, including the findings of both micro- and macro-abscesses, as well as bronchiectasis (Fig. 10). Tumor typically is identifiable as a poorly marginated area of low density (Figs. 3, 5, and 7–11). This is strikingly different from the appearance of otherwise uncomplicated pulmonary collapse, which can be identified as an area of uniformly increased attenuation, frequently with "mucous" bronchograms within, or a lung abscess, which characteristically can be sharply delineated from adjacent lung or tumor (Fig. 10).

An important caveat is that sometimes residual aerated lung behind an endobronchial obstructing lesion may assume bizarre configurations, mimicking parenchymal infection or necrosis (Fig. 12 A–H). Follow-up CT scans, however, easily confirm that this appearance is transitory. It should also be emphasized that despite optimal technique, well-vascularized, nonnecrotic tumors may not be differentiable from adjacent collapsed lung with CT (Fig. 12 H–I).

Bronchial obstruction with resultant collapse may be caused by a variety of benign conditions, including bronchostenosis, congenital bronchial atresia, and trauma with bronchial laceration, among others. The findings on CT of obstruction secondary to an aspirated

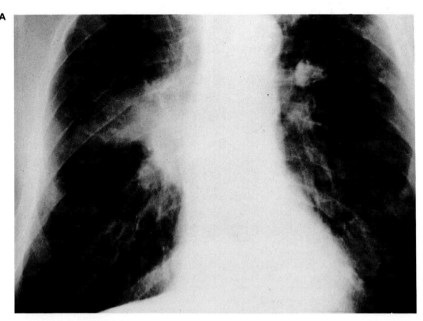

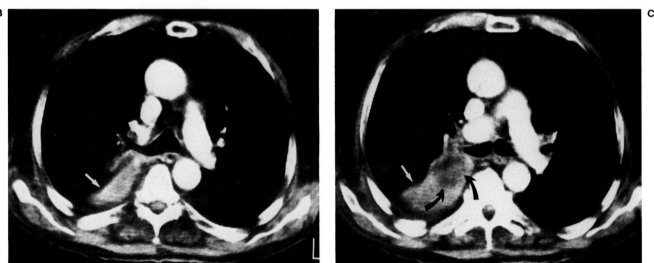

FIG. 9. Superior segmental collapse: bronchogenic carcinoma. **A:** PA radiograph shows increased density in the region of the right hilum. **B,C:** Sections through the right upper lobe bronchus and 1 cm below, respectively, imaged with narrow, mediastinal windows following a bolus of i.v. contrast. The superior segment is collapsed medially against the spine (*arrows* in B and C). A necrotic tumor can be seen within the apical portions of the superior segment, identifiable as an ill-defined area of low attenuation (*curved arrows* in C), distinct from the otherwise uniform enhancement present in the remainder of the atelectatic lobe uninvolved by tumor.

A 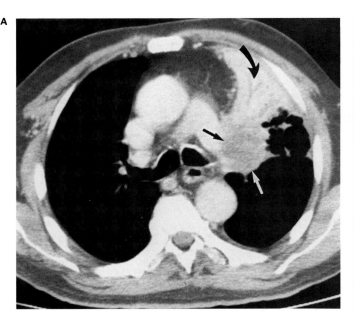 B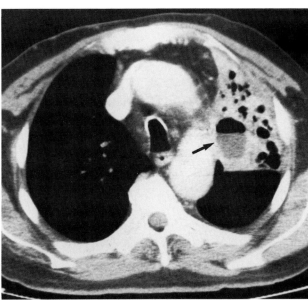

FIG. 10. Central tumor versus peripheral collapse with infection. **A:** Enlargement of a CT section obtained through the carina in a patient with tumor obstructing the left upper lobe bronchus, confirmed bronchoscopically. Following a bolus of i.v. contrast, central tumor is easily identified as an irregular area of low attentuation adjacent to the left pulmonary artery (*arrows*). Note that peripherally there is uniform enhancement of the collapsed left upper lobe, within which dilated, fluid-filled bronchi can be identified (*curved arrow*). **B:** Enlargement of a section obtained 2 cm above A. A large cavity is present medially with an air-fluid level within (*arrow*). Smaller cavities, some with fluid can also be identified. As compared with tumor, abscesses within obstructed, collapsed lung are characteristically sharply circumscribed (compare with A), allowing easy differentiation. (From Naidich, ref. 74.)

A 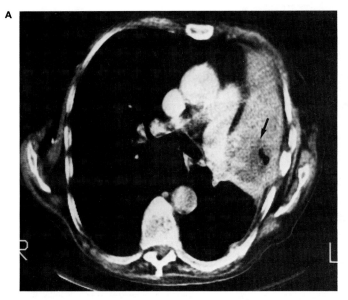 B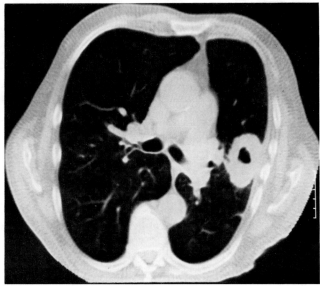

FIG. 11. Bronchogenic carcinoma: appearance following i.v. contrast. **A:** Enlargement of a CT section through the left main pulmonary artery in a patient with left upper lobe collapse due to central tumor. Following a bolus of i.v. contrast, the collapsed left upper lobe is easily identified, within which there is an ill-defined mass with low attenuation (*arrow*). A small quantity of air can be defined within this mass, which nonetheless does not appear like a typical lung abscess (compare with Fig. 10B). Note the marked shift of the mediastinum to the left secondary to left upper lobe collapse. **B:** Enlargement of a section obtained through the left upper lobe several weeks prior to A. A large, partially necrotic mass can be identified within the left upper lobe. This corresponds in position to the mass identified within the collapsed lobe seen in A. Collapse in this case was due to an endobronchial metastasis.

A,B

C,D

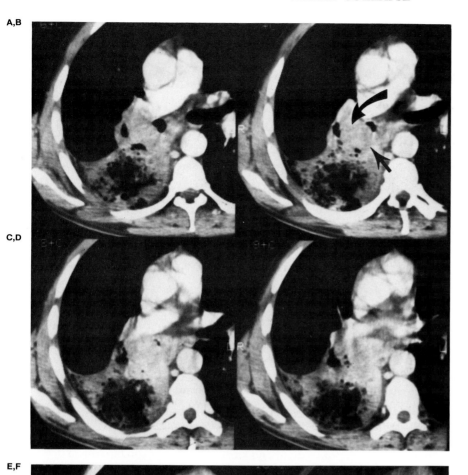

E,F

G,H

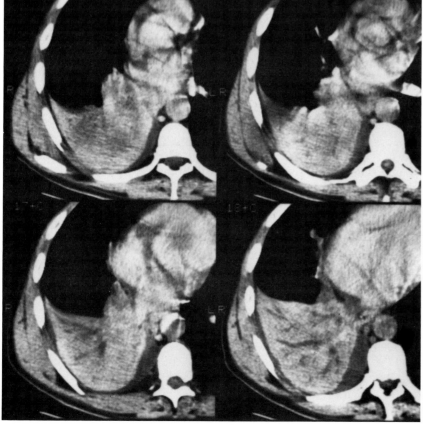

FIG. 12 (A–J). Right lower lobe collapse. (A–H) Pseudo-necrosis. **A–D:** Enlargements of sequential CT sections through the bronchus intermedius and lower lobe bronchi, respectively, following a bolus of i.v. contrast media. A large mass can be identified partially obstructing the bronchus intermedius (*arrows* in B). Mottled areas of low density and air can be seen within the collapsed right lower lobe, an appearance suggestive of post-obstructive infection and necrosis. Clinical signs of infection, however, were notably absent. **E–H:** Enlargements of CT sections obtained following a bolus of i.v. contrast media, at approximately the same levels as shown in A–D, acquired four days later. Note that except for some well-defined fluid bronchograms, there is now uniform consolidation of the right lower lobe. This rapid change in appearance is secondary to resorption of residual air within the collapsed lobe. (From Naidich, ref. 74.)

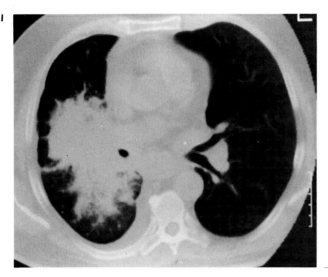
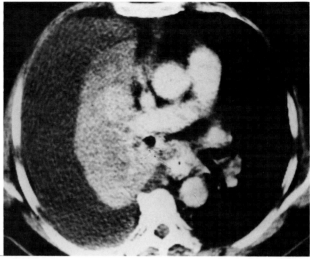

FIG. 12. (Continued.) Right lung collapse: small cell carcinoma. I: Section through the bronchus intermedius in a patient with documented small cell carcinoma. J: Section at the same level as shown in I, several weeks later, following development of a large right-sided pleural effusion. Following a bolus of i.v. contrast, the collapsed right lung has an overall uniform density. Differentiation between tumor and collapsed lung cannot be confidently identified, despite adequate opacification.

foreign body, as well as a broncholith, have been reported (29–32). Perhaps the most important and most common benign cause of endobronchial obstruction is mucous plugs. These frequently form when there is some interruption in the normal mechanism for clearing bronchial secretions, such as, for example, in the immediate postoperative period. A mucus-filled bronchus can mimic an endobronchial lesion (Fig. 13). Mucus may also collect in bronchi distal to an occluding tumor, giving rise to the CT finding of "mucous" bronchograms (21). These are especially easy to identify following administration of a bolus of intravenous contrast (Fig. 13).

PASSIVE ATELECTASIS

"Passive atelectasis" denotes loss of volume within a lobe or lobes secondary to interference with the normal balance that exists between the lung, which tends to retract toward the hilum, and the chest wall, which tends to expand the lung and keep it aerated. This most frequently occurs because of pleural disease, i.e., the presence of air, fluid, or both within the pleural space. Of all forms of collapse, in our experience, this is the most common. Fluid within the pleural space is easily defined, even when the underlying lung is collapsed. This differentiation may be made simpler by use of i.v. contrast medium because of the difference in density between pleural fluid and consolidated, collapsed pulmonary parenchyma (Figs. 12 and 14). Pleural fluid, when sufficiently massive, will distort the "usual" configuration of collapsed lobes. The configuration of collapse caused by endobronchial obstruction is typified by

characteristic relationships between the collapsed lobes and the chest wall; these are distorted in the presence of fluid (Fig. 14).

Once a lobe has collapsed, it is frequently difficult to exclude the presence of tumor (21). If the lobar bronchi are patent and air-bronchograms can be defined in every portion of the collapsed lobe, tumor is unlikely. Unfortunately, this is not often the case. However, if tumor within the collapsed lobe is difficult to exclude, the presence of tumor within the pleural space is generally easy to recognize. If collapse is passive, secondary to a large accumulation of fluid in the pleural space, characterization of the nature of the pleural disease process is clearly of primary concern. The value of CT in differentiating benign from malignant pleural effusions is illustrated in Figs. 15 and 16. The diagnosis of malignant pleural disease is dependent on recognition of the presence of soft-tissue densities within the pleural space. These will appear either as nodular foci of soft-tissue density or as an enveloping rind of thickened nodular pleura, usually in association with loculated areas of pleural fluid (11). Of course, in cases in which microscopic seeding only is present, malignant pleural disease will be nondescript in appearance on CT (see Chapter 9).

As already noted, unusual configurations of collapse may result when fluid or air is present in the pleural space. The magnitude of pressure exerted on lung by adjacent pleural fluid or, especially, by air may be great; the result may be initially confusing radiographically. Of particular interest is the phenomenon of lung torsion (33–36). Torsion has been noted to occur spontaneously, usually in association with some other pulmonary abnormality, such as pneumonia or tumor, following traumatic pneumothorax, and especially as a complica-

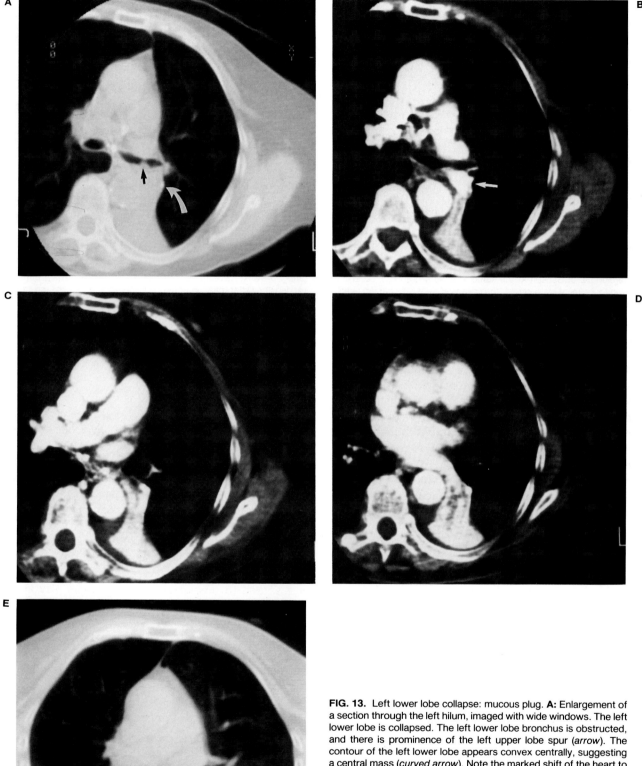

FIG. 13. Left lower lobe collapse: mucous plug. **A:** Enlargement of a section through the left hilum, imaged with wide windows. The left lower lobe is collapsed. The left lower lobe bronchus is obstructed, and there is prominence of the left upper lobe spur (*arrow*). The contour of the left lower lobe appears convex centrally, suggesting a central mass (*curved arrow*). Note the marked shift of the heart to the left, and hyperaeration of the right lung. **B–D:** Enlargements of sequential sections through the left lower lobe, following a bolus of i.v. contrast. Note uniform enhancement of the entire left lower lobe. Fluid-filled airways can be identified, but there is no evidence of a central, low-density tumor mass. The convex contour noted in A is in fact caused by prominence of the left interlobar pulmonary artery (*arrow* in B). Note the small quantity of pleural fluid present, loculated posteromedially behind the collapsed lower lobe (*curved arrow* in C). **E:** Section through the left lower lobe bronchus following removal of a mucous plug at bronchoscopy. Both the left upper and left lower lobe bronchi are normal; collapse has entirely resolved.

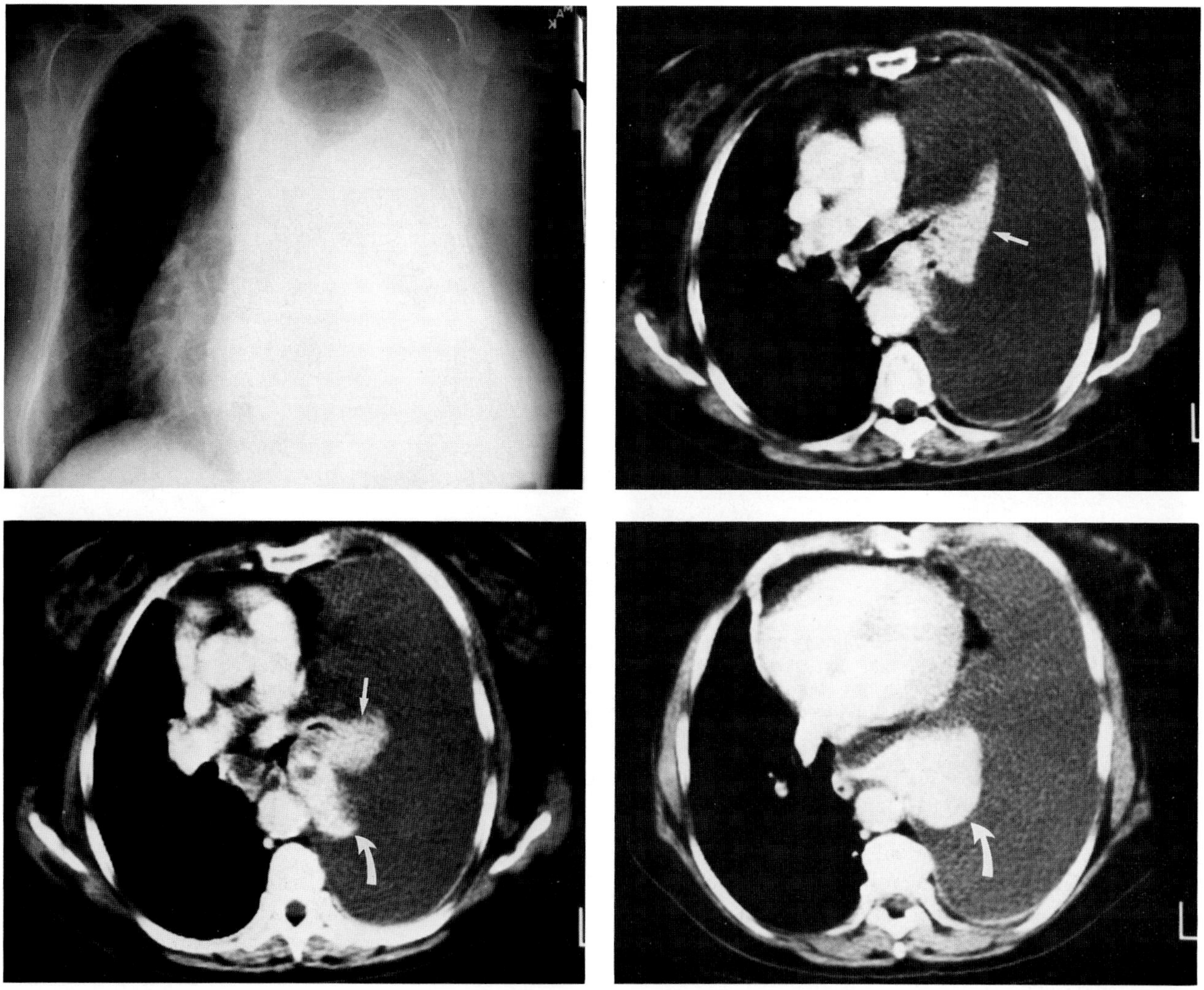

FIG. 14. Passive atelectasis: left pleural effusion. **A:** PA radiograph shows large left-sided pleural fluid collection associated with contralateral shift of the heart and mediastinum. **B–D:** Sequential images through the left upper and lower lobes. There is a massive left-sided pleural fluid collection causing collapse of the left upper lobe (*arrow* in B), lingula (*arrow* in C), and left lower lobes (*curved arrow* in C and D), respectively. The pattern of collapse is different from that seen in endobronchial occlusion, in that the collapsed lobes have been displaced away from the chest wall by the pleural fluid. There is no evidence of a central endobronchial tumor.

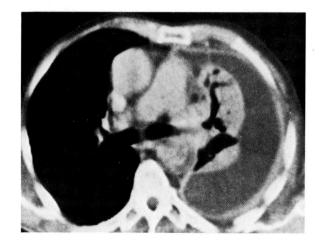

FIG. 15. Passive atelectasis. A large pleural fluid collection has collapsed the left lung. Air-bronchograms can be defined in both the left upper and lower lobes. Note that the pleural margins are slightly thickened in a uniform manner. Despite the nondescript appearance of the pleural space, pleural biopsy was compatible with metastic pleural disease.

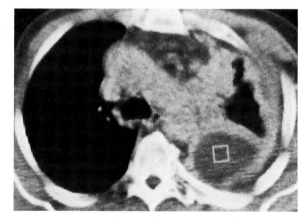

FIG. 16. Passive atelectasis: malignant pleural disease. Section through the aortic arch shows considerable volume loss in the left upper lobe, within which discrete air-bronchograms can be defined (better seen with wide windows). A loculated pleural fluid collection is present posteriorly (*cursor*). Note that the pleural surface is markedly irregular and that anterior mediastinal adenopathy is present. These changes are characteristic of malignant pleural disease. Biopsy revealed poorly differentiated adenocarcinoma.

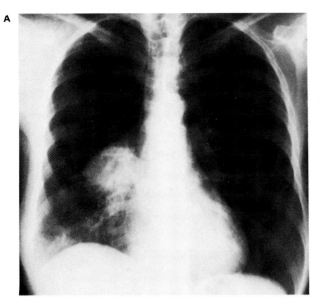
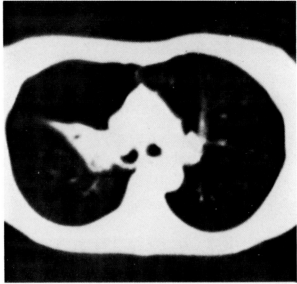

FIG. 17. Pulmonary torsion: right upper lobe. **A:** PA radiograph shows a right apical pneumothorax. A right hilar density is present, of uncertain significance. **B:** Section through the right upper lobe bronchus. The right upper lobe is collapsed, identifiable as a triangular wedge of uniform density, with the apex pointing toward the hilum. A focal anterior pneumothorax can be seen. The right upper lobe bronchus appears to be obstructed. This appearance is a result of torsion of the right upper lobe secondary to the pneumothorax. Following chest tube placement and re-expansion of the right upper lobe, bronchoscopy was negative.

tion of surgery. Radiographically, the hallmark of this entity is the finding of a collapsed lobe, almost always either the right or left upper lobes, or the middle lobe, rarely the lower lobes, occupying an unusual position (Fig. 17). Marked change in position of the collapsed lobe on sequential radiographs is considered characteristic (33). Although rare, the diagnosis is significant, especially in postoperative patients, as unrecognized torsion is associated with a high mortality due to resultant pulmonary infarction.

CICATRIZATION ATELECTASIS

Cicatrization atelectasis is lobar collapse consequent to scarring and fibrosis from inflammatory disease. This form of collapse is a frequent sequela of tuberculosis and is best typified by the chronic middle lobe syndrome (Fig. 18).

Cicatrization atelectasis may be differentiated from other forms of lobar collapse by the following criteria.

(a) Endobronchial obstruction is absent. With careful scan technique, patency of the bronchial tree subtending the involved lobe can be confirmed (Figs. 18–21).

(b) The degree of volume loss, in general, is more marked in cicatrization atelectasis than in other forms of collapse, particularly collapse from endo-

bronchial obstruction. Any question of central obstruction, of course, is easily resolved by scanning through the appropriate lobar bronchus (Fig. 19).

(c) Collapse is frequently accompanied by bronchiectatic changes within the involved lobe.

(d) Collapse is present in the absence of demonstrable pleural or chest wall pathology.

There has been some controversy about whether the chronic middle lobe syndrome is due to bronchostenosis or to cicatrization from inflammatory parenchymal disease. In our and others' experience, in all cases of chronic middle lobe syndrome examined with CT, the middle lobe bronchus has been patent, excluding bronchostenosis (i.e., fibrous narrowing of the middle lobe bronchus) as etiologic (37). The syndrome appears to be most common in middle-aged women with histories of chronic cough and chest pain, and usually involves the middle lobe or the inferior lingular segment. Although the precise etiology of this syndrome is unknown, it is generally held that the middle lobe and inferior lingular segments are characteristically involved, at least, in part, due to a lack of normal collateral ventilation that may occur due to intact pleural investments surrounding these otherwise isolated lung segments (37,38). The result is that inflammation and secretions in the peripheral airways of these segments produce varying degrees of atelectasis that cannot be offset by collateral ventilation.

A

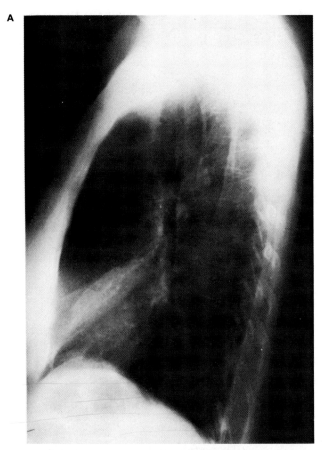

FIG. 18. Cicatrization atelectasis: chronic middle lobe syndrome.
A: Lateral radiograph shows marked volume loss in the middle lobe.
B: Section through the middle lobe bronchus. The middle lobe
bronchus is patent. Adjacent to the origins of the medial and lateral
segmental bronchi, punctate calcification can be identified (*arrows*).
C: Section through the middle lobe bronchi. Dilated, irregular bronchi can be identified within the collapsed lobe. The lateral border of
the collapsed middle lobe is sharply defined by the major fissure,
which is displaced anteromedially (*arrowheads*). The anterior border
of the collapsed middle lobe is less well defined. This is because the
minor fissure is roughly parallel to the plane of the CT scan. Despite
the appearance of retraction of the middle lobe from the anterior
chest wall, some contact may persist, usually at a more inferior level
(not shown).

B

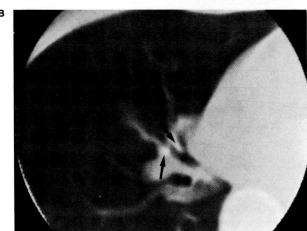

C

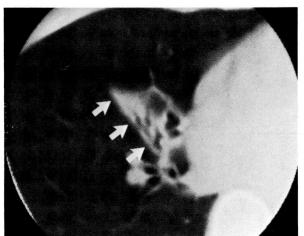

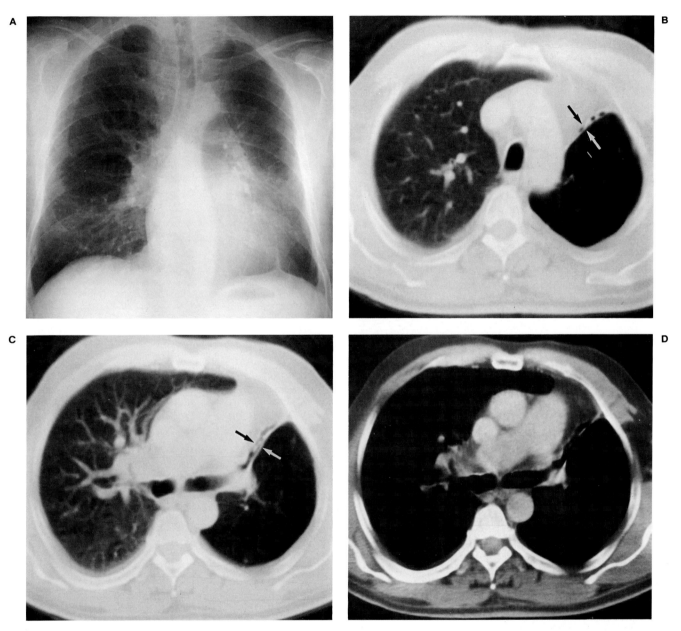

FIG. 19. Cicatrization atelectasis (left upper lobe). **A:** PA radiograph. **B–D:** Sequential images through the left upper lobe bronchus, and the great vessels, imaged with wide (B,C) and narrow (D) mediastinal windows, respectively. There is profound volume loss within the left upper lobe that can be identified as only a thin sliver of tissue marginated posteriorly by a markedly displaced major fissure and anteriorly by anterior mediastinal fat (*arrows* in B and C). The left upper lobe bronchus can be identified and is patent, confirming the benign nature of the collapse. The etiology in this case was presumed to be secondary to tuberculosis.

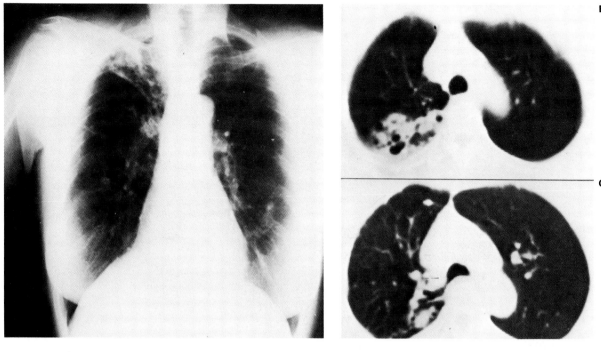

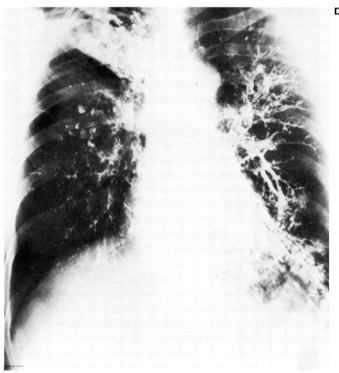

FIG. 20. Cicatrization atelectasis (right upper lobe). Tuberculosis. **A:** PA radiograph. The right upper lobe is collapsed; there is increased lucency in this lobe. **B,C:** Sequential images through the right upper lobe. There are extensive bronchiectatic changes throughout the right upper lobe, which has collapsed posteriorly against the chest wall. There is marked posterior rotation of the right upper lobe bronchus. **D:** PA radiograph following bronchography. Extensive bronchiectasis in the right upper lobe is apparent.

Bronchiectasis within scarred and shrunken lobes is common. This may occur even in the absence of bronchial occlusion. Although the pathogenesis of this form of bronchiectasis is disputed, it probably results from stasis of secretions with subsequent infection (37–41). In the absence of endobronchial occlusion, bronchi within a collapsed lobe may appear dilated on CT. If the degree of collapse is marked and bronchiectasis is extensive, the overall result may be hyperlucency of a shrunken lobe on routine radiography (Fig. 20).

Occasionally, cicatrization atelectasis may result in the compromise of respiratory function as a result of compensatory spatial rearrangements affecting otherwise uninvolved portions of the lung. This detrimental

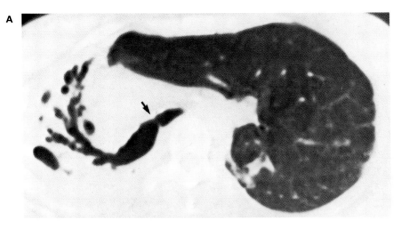

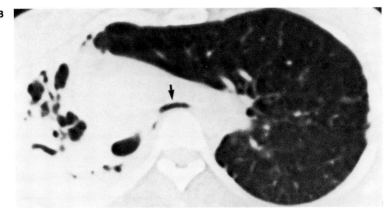

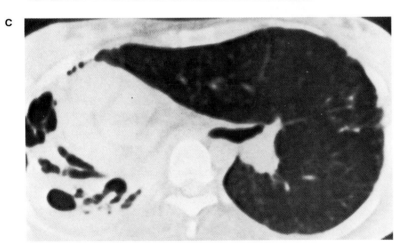

FIG. 21. Cicatrization atelectasis: bronchiectasis (right upper lobe). **A–C:** Sequential images show right upper lobe collapse, with evidence of extensive bronchiectasis. The carina (*arrow* in A) is displaced to the right. The left main-stem bronchus is stretched across the spine (*arrow* in B), with resultant narrowing. The left upper lobe bronchus (in C) is of normal caliber. In this case, respiratory distress resulted not from pathology in the right upper lobe but was secondary to compression of the left main-stem bronchus, caused by its displacement.

effect on other portions of the airways and lung may not be apparent on routine radiographs (Fig. 21).

When collapse is as marked as that shown in Figs. 19–21, the etiology can safely be considered to be inflammatory, provided a central endobronchial lesion has been ruled out. Especially characteristic is the appearance of cicatrization atelectasis of the right upper lobe. As shown in Figs. 20 and 21, unlike collapse associated with endobronchial obstruction where the vector of collapse is anteromedial, with cicatrization, the vector of retraction is posteromedial. This results in characteristic posterior displacement of the right upper lobe bronchus, as well as the bronchus intermedius. These airways frequently come to lie in close proximity or even posterior to the upper thoracic vertebral bodies, an appearance never seen in cases with collapse due to endobronchial obstruction (Fig. 21). Even in this setting, however, care must be taken, as previously suggested, to

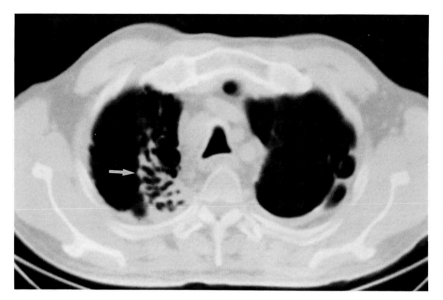

FIG. 22. Adhesive atelectasis: radiation. Section through the upper lung fields. A sharp line demarcates normal pulmonary parenchyma laterally from irradiated parenchyma that is paramediastinal in location (*arrow*). Numerous dilated airways can be identified within the atelectatic lung. A large bulla is present on the left side, accounting for the lack of any obvious paramediastinal parenchymal changes.

A

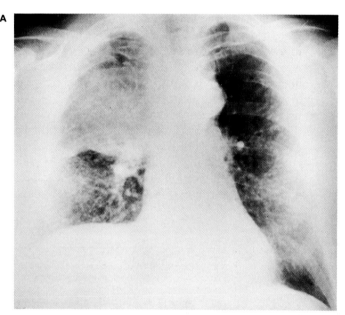

FIG. 23. Replacement atelectasis: small cell carcinoma. **A:** PA radiograph shows uniform density in the right upper lobe. There is slight elevation of the middle lobe fissure and the right hemidiaphragm. **B:** Section through the right upper lobe bronchus. The proximal portion of the bronchus is patent. There is uniform density throughout the right upper lobe, which superficially mimics consolidation. **C:** Section through the right upper lobe. Uniform density is present; however, this does not conform to the shape of the right upper lobe. Tumor has replaced the lobe and infiltrated into the chest wall anteriorly (*arrows*).

B

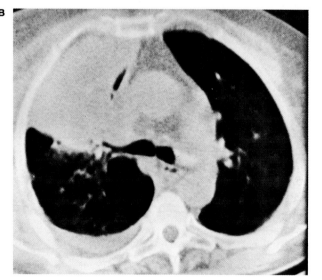

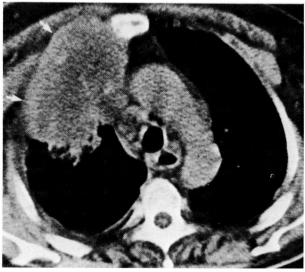

C

define dilated, bronchiectatic airways in each portion of the collapsed lung in order to survey for a peripheral rather than a central malignancy in the involved lobe.

ADHESIVE ATELECTASIS

Adhesive atelectasis is a somewhat controversial subject. Presumably, this form of atelectasis occurs as a result of an absence or lack of production of surfactant and may be thought of as a form of resorption atelectasis occurring without bronchial obstruction. The prototype for this form of collapse is radiation pneumonitis. The spectrum of changes seen in the thorax consequent to radiation have been described (42–44). The hallmark of this type of atelectasis is that involved lung is sharply demarcated from normal lung, usually conforming to known radiation ports (Fig. 22). The finding of dilated bronchi within known radiation ports is commonplace and may be the primary abnormality visualized on cross-section.

REPLACEMENT ATELECTASIS

Rarely, volume loss may occur as a consequence of obliteration of pulmonary parenchyma by unchecked tumor growth. Endobronchial obstruction is generally absent. We have termed this "replacement atelectasis" (Fig. 23). The key to identifying this type of collapse is to note that the margins of the "collapsed" lobe do not conform to lobar or segmental anatomy. In the case illustrated in Fig. 23, there is uniform density through-out the right upper lobe. Superficially, this mimics parenchymal consolidation. However, the contours of this density do not conform to the shape of the right upper lobe. Unchecked tumor growth has resulted in replacement of the right upper lobe, with extension into the chest wall. More frequently, tumor is restricted to the involved lobe; in this setting, the diagnosis can be made by noting that the magins of the collapsed lobe are exceedingly nodular and irregular.

POSTLOBECTOMY CHEST

In addition to the types of atelectasis already described, it is frequently necessary to analyze radiographs and CT scans in patients postlobectomy. With some exceptions, alterations caused by the surgical resection of pulmonary segments may mimic findings observed in cases of extreme lobar collapse resulting from endobronchial obstruction. These changes have been well described by Holbert et al. (45). Briefly, left-sided lobectomies result in a reorientation of the remaining lobe, which can be characterized by new pleuromediastinal/lung interfaces (Fig. 24). On the right side, each type of lobectomy results in the realignment of the remaining two lobes, with creation of a postlobectomy neofissure (Fig. 25). Although these rearrangements may cause confusion radiographically, they are readily apparent in cross-section (45,46). Another concern in these patients is the early identification of recurrent tumor, especially at the site of resection (Fig. 25), for which CT may also be of value.

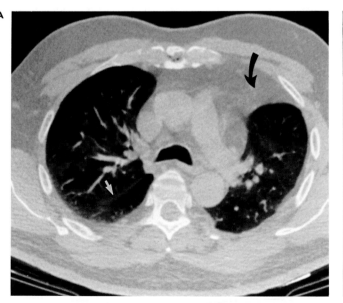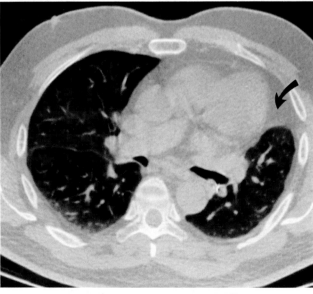

FIG. 24. Post left upper lobectomy. **A,B:** Sequential images through the carina and left hilum, respectively. Volume loss is apparent on the left side. The left oblique fissure cannot be identified [compare with the appearance of the major fissure on the right side (*arrow* in A)]. There is a marked increase in the amount of mediastinal fat present immediately anterior to the hyperinflated left lower lobe (*curved arrows* in A and B), accounting for the frequent similarity in radiographic appearances between patients with collapsed left upper lobes and patients with left upper lobectomies. Note surgical clips present in the left hilum, at this level posterior to the left main-stem bronchus.

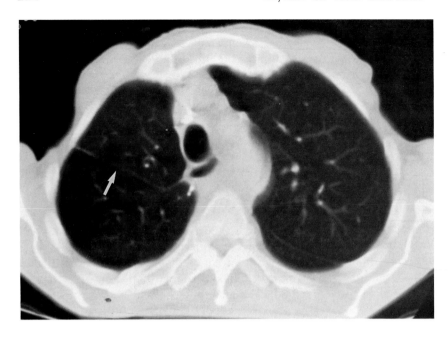

FIG. 25. Post right upper lobectomy. Section through the right upper lung field in a patient following right upper lobectomy. A neofissure between the middle and lower lobes has formed (*arrow*). Note the normal position and configuration of the superior portion of the left major fissure, by comparison.

LOBAR ATELECTASIS: MR EVALUATION

Considerable interest has been directed towards the potential of MR to evaluate pulmonary atelectasis (47–54). Although early descriptions emphasized the use of T1-weighted sequences, most reports have documented the need for relatively T2-weighted sequences to adequately differentiate central, obstructing tumor from peripheral collapsed lung (Fig. 8; Fig. 39, p. 263) (49–54,74). In a retrospective study of 18 patients with proximal bronchogenic carcinomas and postobstructive lobar collapse evaluated both with postintravenous contrast dynamic CT and MR, Tobler et al. (53) reported that, utilizing T2-weighted sequences, MR showed different signal intensities of tumor and collapsed lung in only five (50%) of ten patients, whereas dynamic CT differentiated tumor from collapsed lung in eight (80%) of ten patients. Of 18 patients evaluated with T1-weighted sequences, MR accurately differentiated tumor from collapse in only one patient (5%). Despite these differences, the authors concluded that there was no significant statistical difference between the two modalities. Of particular interest was the finding that CT and MR were apparently complementary in that, in two cases in which differentiation was not possible with dynamic CT scanning, MR was successful (Fig. 26).

Experimental verification of improved delineation of tumor versus collapsed lung utilizing T2-weighted sequences in both animal and human tissue samples has been reported, and has been presumed, at least in part, to be due to differences in total water content of tumor and lung (52,54) (see Chapter 1, Figs. 24 and 25).

In fact, as documented by Burke and Fraser (28) in their evaluation of 50 consecutive patients undergoing pulmonary resection of bronchogenic carcinomas, a wide spectrum of histologic changes can be identified within collapsed lung. Initially, eosinophilic proteinaceous material accumulates within airspaces, representing, at least in part, retained surfactant. Subsequently, aggregates of lipid-laden macrophages accumulate, and there is progressive lymphocytic infiltration and collagen deposition within the pulmonary interstitium (so-called lipid pneumonia). Finally, with sufficient time, interstitial fibrosis supervenes. Surprisingly, in their series, infection per se proved relatively rare and, when present, appeared either as focal bronchitis or bronchiolitis, with only minimal or absent parenchymal involvement.

These factors clearly have implications for the potential role of both contrast-enhanced CT and, especially, MR for evaluating patients with pulmonary atelectasis. Significantly, when tumor to fat and collapsed lung to fat MR signal intensity ratios are calculated utilizing T2-weighted sequences, at least in one study, tumor could be differentiated from collapsed lung only in patients with collapsed lung to fat ratios >1. These preliminary findings suggest that MR may be most useful in the subacute stage of collapse, in which lipid-laden macrophages are most conspicuous (53).

Another form of collapse that has been evaluated preliminarily with MR is adhesive atelectasis secondary to pulmonary irradiation (55). On the assumption that, with time, radiated lung becomes fibrotic, it has been suggested that T2-weighted sequences may be of value in differentiating fibrosis from residual or recurrent tumor, or areas of radiation-induced pneumonitis. Unfortunately, at least in our experience, considerable signal is almost always present within areas of irradiated lung, even when these areas have been stable radiographically over a prolonged time interval (Fig. 27). This

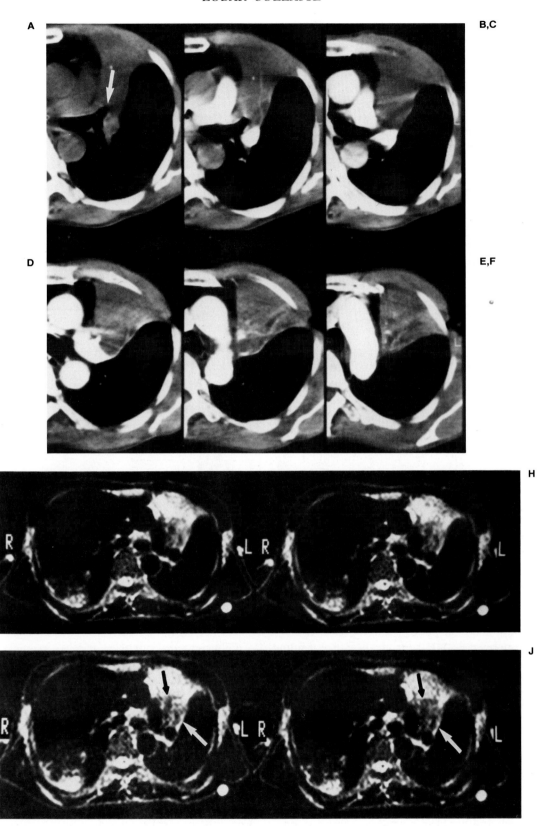

FIG. 26. Left upper lobe collapse: CT/MR correlation. **A–F:** Dynamic incremental CT sections through the left upper lobe obtained following a bolus of 60 cc of 60% iodinated contrast media injected at a rate of 2 cc/sec using a power injector. Note that the left upper lobe bronchus is obstructed (*arrow* in A). Despite good opacification of vessels, differentiation of tumor from collapsed lung is impossible. **G–J:** MR images obtained at the level of the left main pulmonary artery (compare with C), utilizing a single level, multiecho technique. Note that with progressively longer TE's (150, 180, 210, and 240 msec, respectively), central tumor is easily differentiable from peripheral collapse as an area of relatively lower signal intensity (*arrows* in I and J). Abnormal signal is also present in the right lower lobe corresponding to a documented aspiration pneumonia. (From Naidich, ref. 74.)

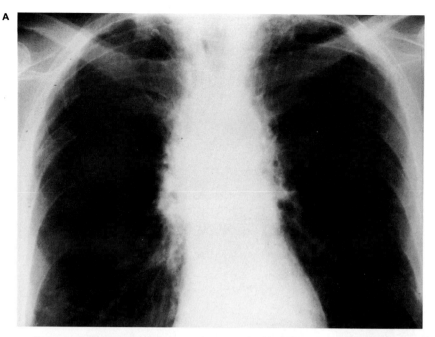

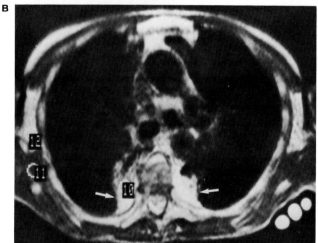

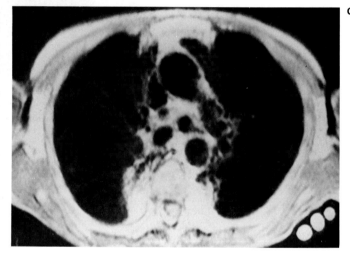

FIG. 27. Adhesive atelectasis: radiation. MR evaluation. **A:** PA radiograph shows characteristic paramediastinal changes following thoracic irradiation. **B:** T1-weighted scan shows prominent signal originating from paramediastinal lung bilaterally (*arrows*). **C:** T2-weighted scan obtained at the same level as B shows an increase in the signal originating from the irradiated lung (compare with B). This appearance is nonspecific and may be due either to radiation pneumonitis, recurrent tumor, superimposed infection, or retained bronchial secretions. In this case, radiographic changes had been stable for over a year.

signal presumably reflects either some degree of residual pneumonitis or may be related to the presence of retained secretions within dilated, damaged airways, due to decreased mucociliary clearance.

Clearly, the ability of both CT and MR to differentiate and potentially characterize both tumor and collapsed lung is dependent on multiple variables, the relative significances of which will require further elucidation (see Chapter 1, Figs. 24 and 25). Of considerable interest is the potential role of MR contrast agents to delineate lung tumors. As shown in Fig. 28, the use of gadolinium (Gd) diethylenetriaminepentaacetic acid (DTPA) may obviate the need for T2-weighted sequences. Following the intravenous injection of 0.1 mmol/kg, it has been shown that Gd-DTPA causes an immediate increase in the signal intensity of vascularized tumors, emphasizing their inhomogeneous structure (Fig. 28) (56). Although

collapsed lung also demonstrates signal enhancement, this is usually delayed by several minutes compared with tumor enhancement. These preliminary findings suggest that Gd-DTPA may ultimately prove to be the most efficacious manner to study collapse in patients with central, obstructing tumors.

CONCLUSION

Lobar collapse is a significant indicator of a variety of pulmonary abnormalities. Commonly associated with central endobronchial tumor, collapse may also denote, among other disease processes, long-standing infection, pleural disease (both benign and malignant), or evidence of radiation. The sorting out of these various etiologies is a frequently difficult and perplexing problem encountered by all radiologists.

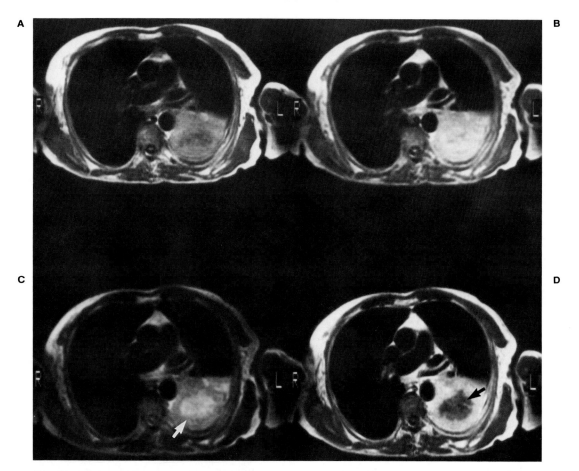

FIG. 28. Left lower lobe collapse: contrast-enhanced MRI. **A:** T1-weighted image through the left upper lobe spur in a patient with atelectasis of the left lower lobe due to central tumor. Slightly heterogeneous signal can be identified within the collapsed lobe. **B:** image acquired at the same level as A. **C:** T2-weighted image obtained at the same level as A and B. With T2-weighting, a central mass can be identified within which considerable signal is present, consistent with tumor necrosis (*arrow*). **D:** T1-weighted obtained at the same levels as A–C, immediately following i.v. administration of Gd-DTPA. An irregular shaped, necrotic mass is easily identifiable within the collapsed left lower lobe (*arrow*).

In the preceding sections, representative examples of "typical" forms and patterns of collapse have been reviewed. As has been stressed repeatedly, collapse, in all its forms, represents a pathophysiologic spectrum; images obtained at any given time, therefore, represent only one point on a continuum of changes (Fig. 1). Nonetheless, certain patterns are characteristic and are important models. It is in this sense that the examples illustrated have been chosen to be representative.

In our judgment, CT is indicated in the evaluation of all patients suspected of or known to have lobar or segmental obstruction secondary to central endobronchial tumor.

Diagnostically, in patients in whom the cause of collapse is unknown, CT may play a critical role by differentiating endobronchial obstruction from other forms of collapse. In select cases in which no bronchial pathology is identified, CT may obviate the need for bronchoscopy (Figs. 18–21). In those cases in which endobronchial tumor is found, CT serves several useful diagnostic roles. By allowing routine visualization of the mediastinum, pleura, chest wall, and adrenals, CT provides detailed information critical to accurate tumor staging (Figs. 3, 5, 7, 8, 16, and 23). Additionally, by defining the presence and extent of peribronchial tumor, CT may serve as a road map for transbronchial needle biopsies (Fig. 29) (57–59).

In cases not amenable to resection, CT may play a critical therapeutic role. Precise delineation of the extent of tumor has important implications in the planning of adequate radiotherapy ports (60–64). Babcock (65) has compared the efficacy of CT to that of routine radio-

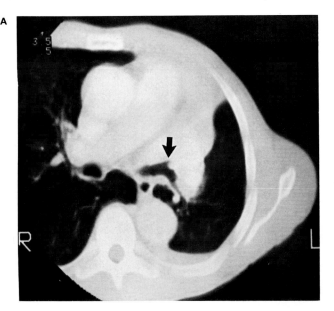
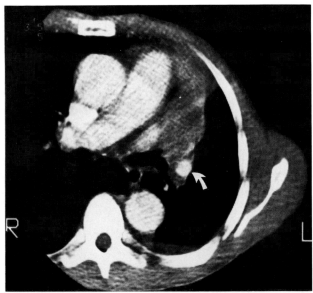

FIG. 29. Left upper lobe collapse: bronchogenic carcinoma. **A,B:** Enlargements of a section through the secondary carina imaged with wide and narrow windows, respectively, following a bolus of i.v. contrast material. The left upper lobe is collapsed due to endobronchial obstruction (*arrow* in A). In addition, tumor has infiltrated into the left hilum, causing thickening of the left upper lobe spur and lateral displacement of the left interlobar artery (*arrow* in B). In this case, CT served as a road map for bronchoscopy by documenting the extent of tumor and its relation to adjacent hilar vessels.

graphs in determining tumor location, volume, and expected radiation doses in 59 patients with primary unresectable bronchial tumors. Fifty-nine percent of the patients required alterations in their radiation treatment plans because of additional information supplied by CT.

CT may also be of vital importance to patients with both benign and malignant central endobronchial tumors who are candidates for photodynamic therapy. The role of laser therapy in the palliation of otherwise unresectable tumors has been established (66–68). By demonstrating the extent of peribronchial tumor and, in particular, by delineating the precise location of major hilar vessels, CT may provide the bronchoscopist a detailed road map, decreasing or eliminating the incidence of accidental penetration of the tracheobronchial wall with subsequent damage to adjacent major arteries and veins (Fig. 29) (69). CT may also play a role in predicting the response of individual patients to photodynamic therapy. In an evaluation of the usefulness of CT and bronchoscopy in assessing which patients would most likely benefit from photodynamic therapy, in a series of 24 patients, Lam et al. (70) showed that a main determinant of response was the extent of submucosal and peribronchial spread—information easily assessed with CT but frequently underestimated by bronchoscopy alone.

It is clear that CT can complement routine radiographs in the evaluation of patients with lobar collapse. This is especially important in patients with radiographically atypical forms of collapse (Fig. 30) (71–73). Pulmonary atelectasis associated with pleural effusions should be evaluated further with CT whenever

possible in order to detect pleural malignancy. The hallmarks of pleural malignancy are thickened, irregular, nodular pleural surfaces associated with loculated fluid. Despite limitations, CT represents a marked improvement over plain radiographs in the assessment of pleural malignancy because of its ability to differentiate more precisely among various tissue densities (Figs. 14–16). Differentiation between pleural fluid and collapsed lung also is usually possible, and, furthermore, endobronchial obstruction can be excluded with confidence, in select cases, obviating the need for bronchoscopy.

In addition to atelectasis associated with endobronchial obstruction and pleural disease, discrete etiological subsets may also be easily identified in cross-section, frequently obviating the need for any further diagnostic evaluation. Cicatrization atelectasis in particular has a characteristic appearance on CT (Figs. 18–21). Endobronchial obstruction is absent, affected lobes tend to be markedly shrunken, and there is frequent evidence of diffuse bronchiectasis. CT is especially efficacious in the evaluation of this group of patients because collapse so frequently tends to be "atypical" radiographically. Although tumor may be superimposed on chronically inflamed, fibrotic lobes, identification of this complication may be possible if care is taken to examine individually each segment of the collapsed lobe. Clearly, recognition of tumor is dependent on the size of the lesion; it may be anticipated that small lesions may be overlooked.

Other forms of collapse are equally characteristic, including collapse secondary to radiation and collapse caused by unchecked tumor growth (Figs. 22 and 23).

A

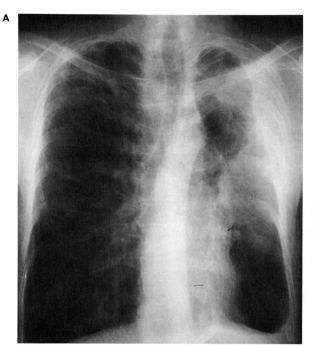

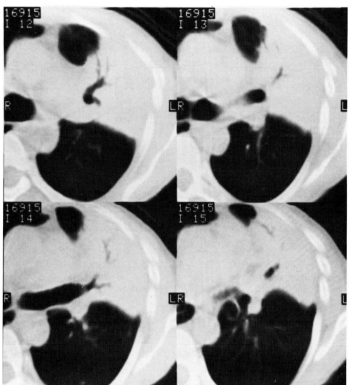

B,C

D,E

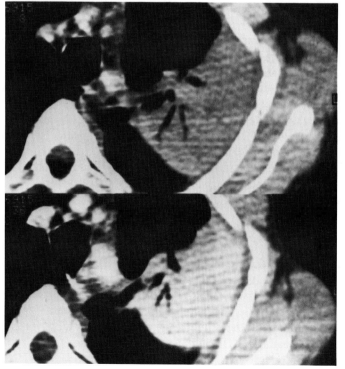

F

G

FIG. 30(A–G). Peripheral left upper lobe collapse. **A:** PA radiograph. There is considerable radiographic density along the lateral aspect of the left upper lobe, a finding suggesting possible loculated pleural fluid. Note slight shift of the trachea to the left. **B–E:** Sequential sections through the left upper lobe, imaged with wide windows. There is dense consolidation of the lateral portion of the left upper lobe, in a configuration suggestive of an axillary subsegment. Airway patency is easily confirmed. The consolidated lung is bordered both anteriorly and posteriorly by hyperaerated lung in the anterior segment of the left upper lobe and the posterior segment of the left lower lobe, respectively. Note that the consolidated segment has a triangular configuration with the apex pointing medially. These findings account for the increased density seen along the lateral margin of the left upper lobe in A, due to the wider band of consolidated lung present laterally as compared with medially. **F,G:** Section through the left upper lobe, both before and after the administration of i.v. contrast. Note that there is uniform enhancement of the consolidated portion of the left upper lobe. No pleural fluid is present.

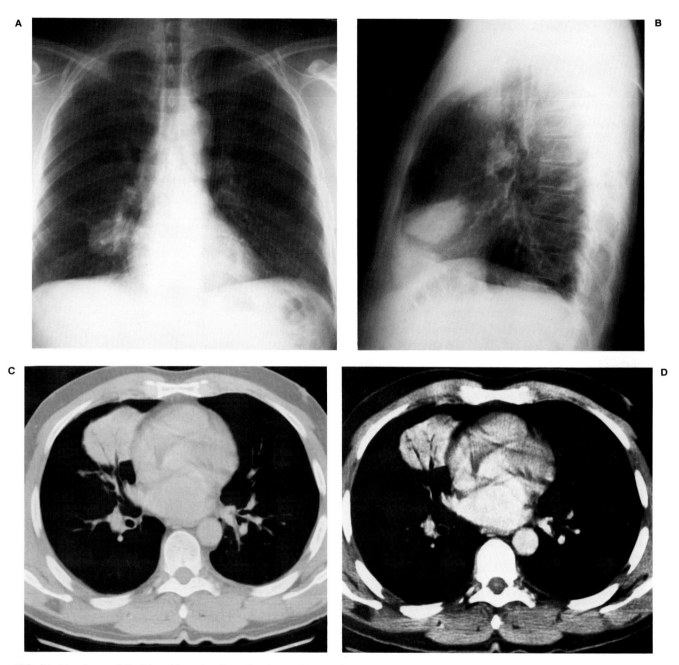

FIG. 31. Lymphoma. **A,B:** PA and lateral radiographs show evidence of a mass in the region of the middle lobe. On the lateral film there is a suggestion of volume loss in the middle lobe. **C,D:** Section through the middle lobe bronchus, imaged with wide and narrow windows respectively, following a bolus of i.v. contrast media. A poorly marginated mass is present within the middle lobe, within which distinct air-bronchograms can be identified. Note that the middle lobe bronchus and its segmental subdivisions are patent. While nonspecific, this appearance, when chronic, should suggest a diagnosis of either lymphoma or alveolar cell carcinoma. Subsequently biopsy proved pulmonary lymphoma.

CT is equally efficacious in differentiating these various forms of collapse.

Invariably, any discussion of lobar collapse will lead to the diagnostic dilemma posed by alveolar cell carcinoma and pulmonary parenchymal lymphoma. In these cases, there may be radiographic evidence of collapse associated with patent bronchi. In the evaluation of these patients, CT has proven to be valuable, especially in clarifying the patterns of parenchymal involvement in patients with pulmonary lymphoma (Fig. 31). In these cases, parenchymal masses frequently appear to have a lobar configuration, and, further, are frequently associated with air-bronchograms. CT clarifies the pattern of lymphomatous infiltration that is only partially lobar in distribution.

The role of MR in assessing pulmonary atelectasis is more controversial. Clearly, in cases in which knowledge of the extent of tumor is important and intravenous contrast material cannot be administered, MR represents an excellent alternative imaging modality (Fig. 8). MR may also play a complementary role to CT in cases in which dynamic CT is unsuccessful in differentiating tumor from collapsed lung. The potential use of MR contrast agents in the evaluation of bronchial neoplasia and pulmonary atelectasis should also be noted (Fig. 28). The role of MR in assessing parenchymal changes following radiation, although intriguing, must await further evaluation.

REFERENCES

1. Robbins LL, Hale EH, Merril OE. The roentgen appearance of lobar and segmental collapse of the lung. I. Technique of examination. *Radiology* 1945;44:471–476.
2. Robbins LL, Hale CH. The roentgen appearance of lobar and segmental collapse of the lung. II. The normal chest as it pertains to collapse. *Radiology* 1945;44:543–547.
3. Robbins LL, Hale CH. The roentgen appearance of lobar and segmental collapse of the lung. III. Collapse of an entire lung or the major part thereof. *Radiology* 1945;45:23–26.
4. Robbins LL, Hale CH. The roentgen appearance of lobar and segmental collapse of the lung. IV. Collapse of the lower lobes. *Radiology* 1945;45:120–127.
5. Robbins LL, Hale CH. The roentgen appearance of lobar and segmental collapse of the lung. V. Collapse of the right middle lobe. *Radiology* 1945;45:260–266.
6. Robbins LL, Hale CH. The roentgen appearance of lobar and segmental collapse of the lung. VI. Collapse of the upper lobes. *Radiology* 1945;45:347–355.
7. Lubert M, Krause FR. Patterns of lobar collapse as observed radiologically. *Radiology* 1951;56:165–182.
8. Krause GR, Lubert M. Gross anatomic spatial changes occurring in lobar collapse: a demonstration by means of three-dimensional plastic models. *AJR* 1958;79:258–268.
9. Proto AV, Tocino I. Radiographic manifestations of lobar collapse. *Semin Roentgenol* 1980;15:117–173.
10. Naidich DP, Khouri NF, McCauley DI, Leitman BS, Hulnick D, Siegelman SS. Computed tomography of lobar collapse: Part I. Endobronchial obstruction *J Comput Assist Tomogr* 1983;7:745–757.
11. Naidich DP, Khouri NF, McCauley DI, Leitman BS, Hulnick D, Siegelman SS. Computed tomography of lobar collapse: Part II. Collapse in the absence of endobronchial obstruction. *J Comput Assist Tomogr* 1983;7:758–767.
12. Naidich DP, Ettenger N, Leitman BS, McCauley DI. CT of lobar collapse. *Semin Roentgenol* 1984;19:222–235.
13. Raasch BN, Heitzman ER, Carsky EW, Lane EJ, Berlow ME, Witwer G. A computed tomographic study of bronchopulmonary collapse. *Radiographics* 1984;4:195–232.
14. Glazer HS, Aronberg DJ, Van Dyke JA, Siegel SS. Computed tomographic manifestation of pulmonary collapse. In: Siegelman SS, ed. *Computed tomography of the chest.* New York: Churchill Livingstone, 1984;81–121.
15. Khoury MB, Godwin JD, Halvorsen RA, Putman CE. CT of lobar collapse. *Invest Radiol* 1985;20:708–716.
16. Mintzer RA, Sakowicz BA, Blonder JA. Lobar collapse. Usual and unusual forms. *Chest* 1988;94:615–620.
17. Webb WR, Gamsu G, Speckman JM. Computed tomography of the pulmonary hilum in patients with bronchogenic carcinoma. *J Comput Assist Tomogr* 1983;7:219–225.
18. Naidich DP, Lee JJ, Garay SM, McCauley DI, Aranda CP, Boyd AD. Comparison of CT and fiberoptic bronchoscopy in the evaluation of bronchial disease. *AJR* 1987;148:1–7.
19. Henschke CI, David SD, Auh Y, et al. Detection of bronchial abnormalities: comparison of CT and bronchoscopy. *J Comput Assist Tomogr* 1987;11:432–435.
20. Mayr B, Heywang SH, Ingrisch H, Huber RM, Haussinger K, Lissner J. Comparison of CT with MR imaging of endobronchial tumors. *J Comput Assist Tomogr* 1987;11:43–48.
21. Woodring JH. Determining the cause of pulmonary atelectasis: a comparison of plain radiography and CT. *AJR* 1988;150:757–763.
22. Shepard JO, Dedrick CG, Spizarny DL, McLoud TC. Technical note. Dynamic incremental computed tomography of the pulmonary hila using a flow-rate injector. *J Comput Assist Tomogr* 1986;10:369–371.
23. Tobler J, Levitt RG, Glazer HS, Moran J, Crouch E, Evens RG. Differentiation of proximal bronchogenic carcinoma from post-obstructive lobar collapse by magnetic resonance imaging. Comparison with computed tomography. *Invest Radiol* 1987;22:538–543.
24. Glazer GM, Francis IR, Gebarski K, Samuels BI, Sorenson KW. Dynamic incremental tomography in the evaluation of the pulmonary hila. *J Comput Assist Tomogr* 1983;7:59–64.
25. Fraser RG, Pare JA. *Diagnosis of diseases of the chest.* 2nd ed. Philadelphia: W.B. Saunders, 1979.
26. Fishman EK, Freeland HS, Wang KP, Siegelman SS. Case report. Intrabronchial lesion on computed tomography secondary to blood clot. *J Comput Assist Tomogr* 1984;8:547–549.
27. Golden R. The effect of bronchostenosis upon the roentgen ray shadows in carcinoma of the bronchus. *AJR* 1925;13:21–30.
28. Burke M, Fraser R. Obstructive pneumonitis: a pathologic and pathogenetic reappraisal. *Radiology* 1988;166:699–704.
29. Cohen AM, Solomon EH, Alfidi RJ. Computed tomography in bronchial atresia. *AJR* 1980;135:1097–1099.
30. Kowal LE, Goodman LR, Zarro VJ, Haskin ME. Case report. CT diagnosis of broncholithiasis. *J Comput Assist Tomogr* 1983;7:321–323.
31. Shin MS, Ho KJ. Broncholithiasis: its detection by computed tomography in patients with recurrent hemoptysis of unknown etiology. *J Comput Assist Tomogr* 1983;7:189–193.
32. Berger PE, Kuhn KP, Kuhns LR. Computed tomography and the occult tracheobronchial foreign body. *Radiology* 1980;134:133–135.
33. Felson B. Lung torsion: radiographic findings in nine cases. *Radiology* 1987;162:631–638.
34. Moser ES, Proto AV. Lung torsion: case report and literature review. *Radiology* 1987;162:639–643.
35. Berkman YM. Uncomplicated torsion of the right upper lobe secondary to spontaneous pneumothorax. *Chest* 1985;87:695–697.
36. Pinstein ML, Winer-Muram H, Eastridge C, Scott R. Middle lobe torsion following right upper lobectomy. *Radiology* 1985;155:580.
37. Rosenbloom SA, Ravin CE, Putman CE, Sealy WC, Vock P, Clark TJ, Godwin JD, Chen JT, Baber C. Peripheral middle lobe syndrome. *Radiology* 1983;149:17–21.
38. Clinicopathologic Conference. Right middle lobe syndrome progressing to death in a 77 year old woman. *Am J Med* 1987;82:471–480.

39. Tannenberg J, Pinner M. Atelectasis and bronchiectasis. *J Thorac Cardiovasc Surg* 1942;11:571–616.
40. Croxatto OC, Lanarie A. Pathogenesis of bronchiectasis. Experimental study and anatomic findings. *J Thorac Cardiovasc Surg* 1954;27:514–528.
41. Spencer H. *Pathology of the lung.* Oxford: Pergamon Press, 1968.
42. Nabawi P, Mantrauaot R, Breyer D, Capek V. Case report: computed tomography of radiation-induced lung injuries. *J Comput Assist Tomogr* 1981;5:568–570.
43. Pagani JJ, Libshitz HI. CT manifestations of radiation-induced change in chest tissue. *J Comput Assist Tomogr* 1982;6:243–248.
44. Mah K, Poon PY, Dyk JV, Keane T, Majesky IF, Rideout DF. Assessment of acute radiation-induced pulmonary changes using computed tomography. *J Comput Assist Tomogr* 1986;10:736–743.
45. Holbert JM, Chasen MH, Libshitz HI, Mountain CF. The postlobectomy chest: anatomic considerations. *Radiographics* 1987;7:889–911.
46. Mahoney MC, Shipley RT. Neofissure after right upper lobectomy: radiographic evaluation. *Radiology* 1988;166:721–723.
47. Cohen AM, Creviston S, LiPuma JP, et al. Nuclear magnetic resonance imaging of the mediastinum and hili: early impressions of its efficacy. *AJR* 1983;141:1163–1169.
48. Axel L, Kressel HY, Thickman D, et al. NMR imaging of the chest at 0.12 T: initial clinical experience with a resistive magnet. *AJR* 1983;141:1157–1162.
49. Levitt RG, Glazer HS, Roper CL, Lee JKT, Murphy WA. Magnetic resonance imaging of mediastinal and hilar masses: comparison with CT. *AJR* 1985;145:9–14.
50. Webb WR, Jensen BG, Sollitto R, de Geer G, McCowin M, Gamsu G, Moore E. Bronchogenic carcinoma: staging with MR compared with staging with CT and surgery. *Radiology* 1985;156:117–124.
51. Glazer GM, Gross BH, Aisen AM, Quint LE, Francis IR, Orringer MB. Imaging of the pulmonary hilum: a prospective comparative study in patients with lung cancer. *AJR* 1985;145:245–248.
52. Huber DJ, Kobzik L, Melanson G, Adams DF. The detection of inflammation in collapsed lung by alterations in proton nuclear magnetic relaxation times. *Invest Radiol* 1985;20:460–464.
53. Tobler J, Levitt RG, Glazer HS, Moran J, Crouch E, Evens RG. Differentiation of proximal bronchogenic carcinoma from postobstructive lobar collapse by magnetic resonance imaging. Comparison with computed tomography. *Invest Radiol* 1987;22:538–543.
54. Shioya S, Haida M, Ono Y, Fukuzaki M, Yamabayashi H. Lung cancer: differentiation of tumor, necrosis, and atelectasis by means of T1 and T2 values measured *in vitro. Radiology* 1988;167:105–109.
55. Glazer HS, Levitt RG, Lee JKT, Emami B, Gronemeyer S, Murphy WA. Differentiation of radiation fibrosis from recurrent pulmonary neoplasms by magnetic resonance imaging. *AJR* 1984;143:729–730.
56. Zeitler E, Kaiser W, Feyrer E, Feyrer R. Magnetic resonance imaging with and without Gd-DTPA, of bronchial carcinoma. In: Runge VM, Claus C, Roland F, Everette JA, eds. *Contrast agents in magnetic resonance imaging. Proceedings of an international workshop.* Amsterdam: Excerpta Medica, 1986.
57. Wang KP. Flexible transbronchial needle aspiration biopsy for histological specimens. *Chest* 1985;88:860–864.
58. Shure D, Fedillo PF. Transbronchial needle aspiration in the diagnosis of submucosal and peribronchial bronchogenic carcinoma. *Chest* 1985;88:49–51.
59. Shure D, Astarita RW. Bronchogenic carcinoma presenting as an endobronchial mass. Optimal number of biopsy specimens for diagnosis. *Chest* 1983;83:865–867.
60. Emami B, Melo A, Carter BL, Munzenrider JE, Piro AJ. Value of computed tomography in radiotherapy of lung cancer. *AJR* 1978;131:63–67.
61. Goitein M, Wittenberg J, Mondiondo M, Doucette J, Friedberg C, Ferrucci J, Gunderson L, Linggood R, Shipley W, Fineberg HJ. The value of CT scanning in radiation therapy treatment planning: a prospective study. *Int J Radiat Oncol Biol Phys* 1979;5:1787–1798.
62. Smith V, Parker DL, Stanley JH, Phillips TL, Boyd DP, Kan PT. Development of a computed tomographic scanner for radiation therapy treatment planning. *Radiology* 1980;136:489–493.
63. Barrett A, Dodds HJ, Husband JE. The value of computed tomography in radiation therapy. *Computed Tomography* 1981;5:217–218.
64. Zinreich ES, Baker RR, Ettenger DS, Order SE. New frontiers in the treatment of lung cancer. *CRC Crit Rev Oncol Hematol* 1985;3:279–308.
65. Babcock PC. The role of computed tomography in the planning of radiotherapy fields. *Radiology* 1983;147:214–244.
66. Kvale PA, Eichenhorn MS, Radke JR, Miks V. YAG laser photoresection of lesions obstructing the central airways. *Chest* 1985;3:283–288.
67. Brutinel WM, Cortese DA, McDougall JC, Gillio RG, Bergstradlh EJ. A two-year experience with the neodymium-YAG laser in endobronchial obstruction. *Chest* 1987;2:159–165.
68. Desai SJ, Mehta AC, Medendorp SV, Golish JA, Ahmad M. Survival experience following Nd:YAG laser photoresection for primary bronchogenic carcinoma. *Chest* 1988;5:939–944.
69. Pearlberg JL, Sandler MA, Kvale P, Beute GH, Madrazo BL. Computed-tomographic and conventional linear-tomographic evaluation of tracheobronchial lesions for laser photoresection. *Radiology* 1985;154:759–762.
70. Lam S, Muller NL, Miller RR, Kostashuk EC, Szasz IJ, LeRiche JC, Lee-Chuy E. Predicting the response of obstructive endobronchial tumors to photodynamic therapy. *Cancer* 1986;58:2298–2306.
71. Saterfiel JL, Virapongse C, Clore FC. Computed tomography of combined right upper and middle lobe collapse. *J Comput Assist Tomogr* 1988;12:383–387.
72. Adler J, Cameron DC. Case report. CT correlation in peripheral right upper lobe collapse. *J Comput Assist Tomogr* 1988;12:510–511.
73. Don C, Desmarais R. Peripheral upper lobe collapse in adults. *Radiology* 1989;170:657–659.
74. Naidich DP. CT/MR correlation in the evaluation of trachea bronchial neoplasms. *Radiol Clin North Am* 1990;28:555–571.

Pulmonary Hila

The critical factors in accurate interpretation of computed tomographic (CT) and magnetic resonance (MR) scans of the pulmonary hila are detailed knowledge of normal cross-sectional anatomy, coupled with careful attention to the techniques of scanning (1–11). The purpose of this chapter is to review pertinent normal CT and MR anatomy, as well as explore how this knowledge can be applied to interpreting hilar abnormalities.

GENERAL PRINCIPLES AND METHODOLOGY

CT of Pulmonary Hila

The pulmonary hila are comprised of airways, including segmental and in some cases subsegmental bronchi, and pulmonary arteries and veins. As will be discussed, there is a fairly constant relationship between these structures that allow for immediate identification at given levels. In most cases, pulmonary lymphatic vessels are not visualized, and hence they present no problems in evaluation. On rare occasion, bronchial arteries may be visualized (12).

Technically, the hila can be evaluated either with or without the use of intravenous (i.v.) contrast media (Figs. 1–4). Without contrast, analysis centers around the bronchial tree and the interface between the pulmonary parenchyma and the soft-tissue structures of the hila (Figs. 3 and 4). These parameters are best evaluated with wide windows (generally window ranges of 1,500–2,000 HU[1]). Without the use of i.v. contrast, accurate interpretation of the hila requires thorough familiarity with normal cross-sectional anatomy (1,2).

Alternatively, the hila can be studied following the administration of i.v. contrast. Although opacification of hilar vessels simplifies interpretation, it should be emphasized that there is no one best strategy for contrast utilization. It is our contention that each case should be individualized methodologically. Consideration must be given to the nature of the problem to be investigated, the status of the patient, and especially the capabilities and limitations of the particular equipment available.

Optimal evaluation requires dense opacification of hilar vessels (Figs. 1, 2, and 4). Whenever possible, dynamic scanning should be utilized, either with multiple images at a single preselected level to evaluate focal abnormalities (dynamic static scanning) or through multiple levels to evaluate diffuse disease (dynamic incremental scanning). The use of power injectors should be encouraged when available, provided adequate venous access has been assured, and there is careful monitoring by a physician (10,11). In our experience, mechanical delivery optimally of approximately 60% iodinated contrast material (generally 1.5–2.0 cc/sec) ensures uniform opacification of all hilar vessels, simplifying interpretation. As previously noted, iodine content should be suf-

---

[1] HU, Hounsfield Unit(s).

A

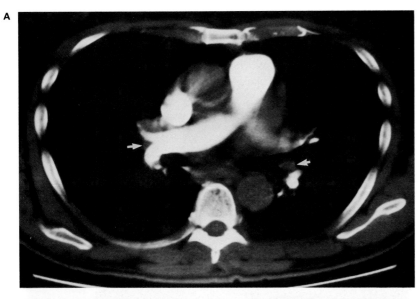

B

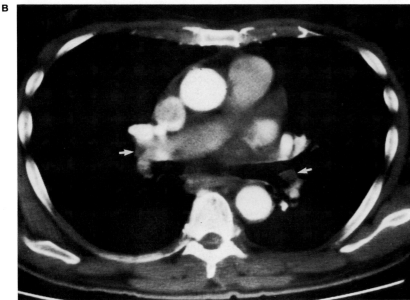

FIG. 1. Hilar CT dynamic-static scanning. **A:** Dynamic CT section through the right main pulmonary artery obtained following the bolus administration of 60 cc of i.v. contrast media. This image was obtained during the phase of maximal opacification of the pulmonary arteries, which are easily identifiable. **B:** Section at the same level as A, obtained ~10 sec later, during the phase of maximal aortic opacification. Contrast in the pulmonary arteries is still present, although diminished. Pulmonary veins are now brightly enhanced, as is the aorta. Note that hilar nodes as small as a few millimeters in size are easily identified with this technique due to their lack of significant enhancement (*arrows* in A and B).

                                                                                                         →

FIG. 2. Hilar CT dynamic-static scanning. **A–I:** Dynamic CT sections through the right main pulmonary artery obtained sequentially during the administration of 50 cc of i.v. contrast media delivered at 2.0 cc/sec using a power injector. In this case, contrast appears simultaneously in the superior vena cava and pulmonary arteries due to a 10 sec delay in image acquisition following initiation of the bolus. Note that the passage of contrast is easily followed from the superior vena cava and pulmonary arteries, to the pulmonary veins, left atrial appendage (*arrow* in B), and the aorta. If properly timed, circulation time can be measured. **J:** Graphic representation of time differentials in the absolute degree of contrast opacification within the aorta (1), pulmonary artery (2), and left atrial appendage (3), respectively. Note that peak opacification of the left atrium clearly precedes peak opacification within the aorta. Unfortunately, with routinely available scanners, insufficient data are usually accumulated within allowable time to generate truly accurate flow measurements, particularly in the pulmonary arteries. These limitations, however, do not apply to subsecond scanners presently available commercially.

A 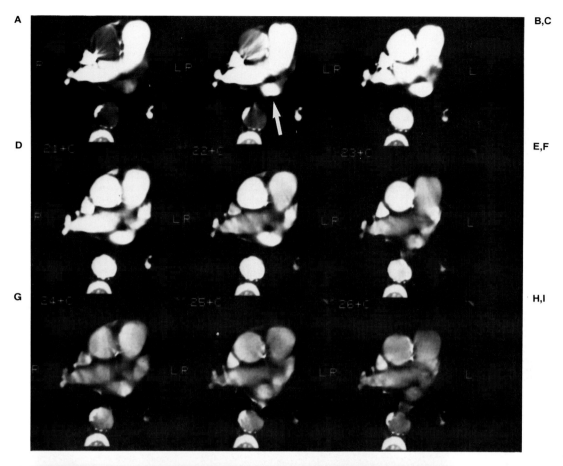 B,C

D E,F

G H,I

J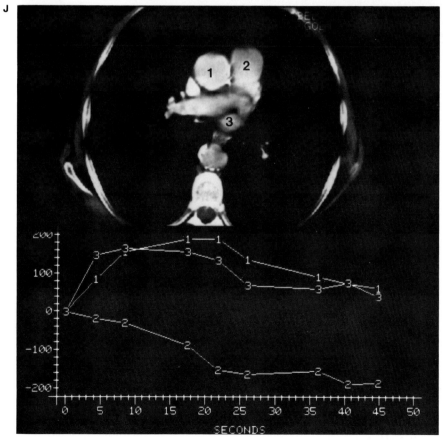

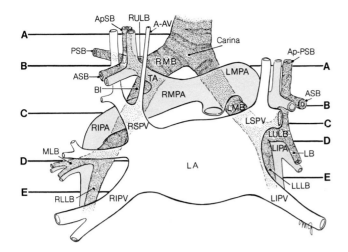

FIG. 3. Schematic representation of the pulmonary hila derived from AP hilar tomograms, as described by Yamashita (7) (see text). Characteristic sections are labeled **A–E.**

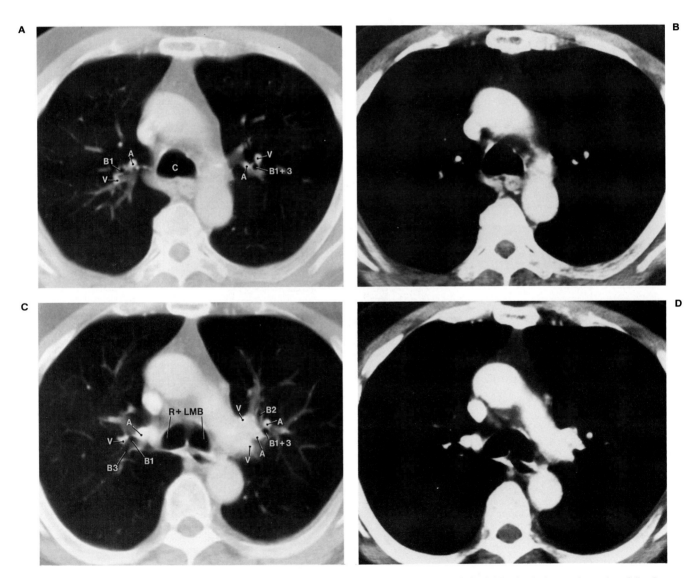

FIG. 4(A–N). Hilar CT: dynamic-incremental scanning. Sequential 10-mm thick sections through both hila, beginning at the carina, following a bolus of i.v. contrast material. Each section is imaged both with wide and narrow windows, respectively, to allow side by side comparison. These images should be analyzed in conjunction with Fig. 3. **A,B:** Section through the distal trachea/proximal carina (C). B1, apical segmental bronchus of the right upper lobe; B1 + 3, apical-posterior segmental bronchus of the left upper lobe; A and V, apical branches of the upper lobe pulmonary arteries and veins, respectively. Note that, at this level, only the largest vascular structures, surrounding the apical segmental bronchi, can be identified in B. **C,D:** Section obtained 1 cm caudad to A, through the proximal right and left main-stem bronchi (R + LMB). B1, apical segmental bronchus; B3, posterior segmental bronchus of the right upper lobe; B1 + 3, apical-posterior segmental bronchus; B2, anterior segmental bronchus of the left upper lobe; A and V, branches of upper lobe arteries and veins, respectively. Again, note that in D only the largest and most central veins are identifiable when narrow windows are used.

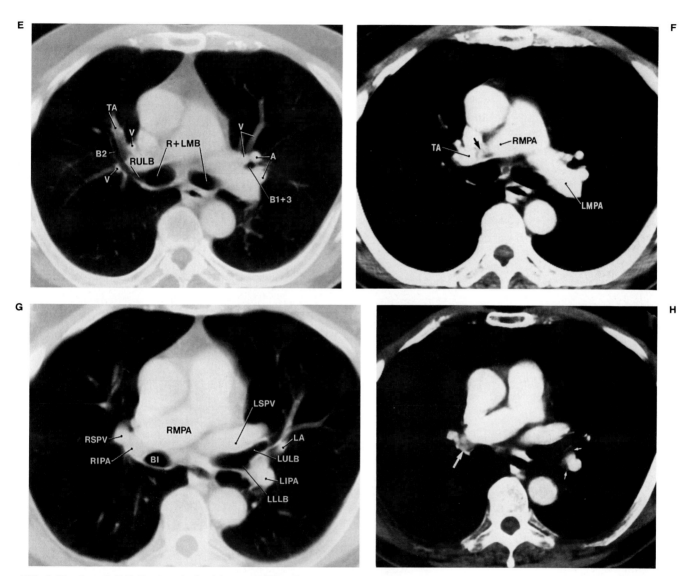

FIG. 4. (*Continued*) **E,F:** Section obtained 1 cm caudad to C, through the right and left main-stem bronchi (R + LMB). RULB, right upper lobe bronchus; B2, anterior segmental bronchus of the right upper lobe; TA, truncus anterior; B1 + 3, apical-posterior segmental bronchus of the left upper lobe; A and V, branches of the upper lobe pulmonary arteries and veins, respectively. Apparent filling defect in the right main pulmonary artery (*arrow* in F) is due to partial volume averaging (compare with the appearance of the right main pulmonary artery in Fig. 4H). **G,H:** Section obtained 1 cm caudad to E, through the upper portion of the bronchus intermedius (BI). RMPA, right main pulmonary artery; RSPV, right superior pulmonary vein; RIPA, superior aspect of the right interlobar pulmonary artery; LSPV, left superior pulmonary vein; LULB, left upper lobe bronchus; LIPA, left interlobar pulmonary artery; LLLB, left lower lobe bronchus; LA, lingular artery. *Arrow* on right points to a region of low density characteristically identified in the right hilum at this level, caused in part by partial voluming of the adjacent right main pulmonary artery as it curves inferiorly to become the interlobar pulmonary artery and, in part, due to hilar fat. *Small arrows* on left point to small left hilar lymph nodes.

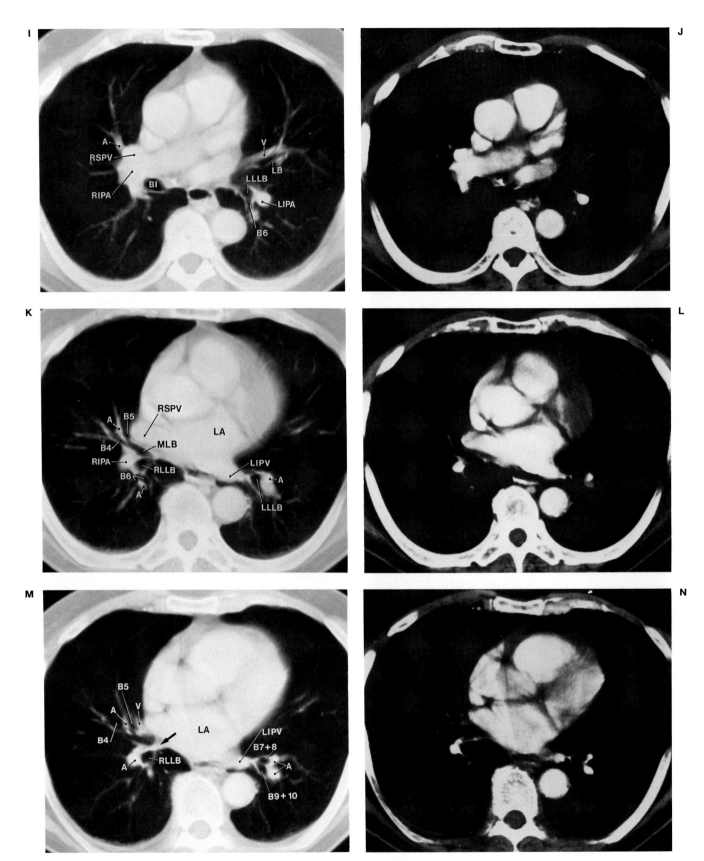

FIG. 4. (*Continued*) **I,J:** Section obtained 1 cm caudad to G, through the lower portion of the bronchus intermedius (BI). RIPA, right interlobar pulmonary artery; RSPV, right superior pulmonary vein; LLLB, left lower lobe bronchus; LB, lingular bronchus; B6, superior segmental bronchus of the left lower lobe. A and V, central pulmonary arteries and veins, respectively. **K,L:** Section obtained 1 cm caudad to I, through the middle lobe bronchus (MLB) and right lower lobe bronchus (RLLB). LA, left atrium; B4 and B5, the lateral and medial segmental bronchi of the right middle lobe, respectively; RIPA, right interlobar pulmonary artery; LIPV, left inferior pulmonary vein; A, segmental pulmonary arteries. **M,N:** Section obtained 1 cm caudad to L. LA, left atrium; B7 + 8, anteromedial basilar segmental bronchus; B9 + 10, common trunk of the lateral and posterior basilar segmental bronchi; A and V, segmental arteries and veins. *Arrow* points to the superior aspect of the right inferior pulmonary vein, which characteristically runs in a horizontal plane.

ficient to cause dense vascular opacification (see Chapter 1).

In general, the degree of opacification that is obtained following only rapid drip infusion of i.v. contrast material rarely results in adequate visualization of hilar vessels, and, consequently, routine utilization of this technique should be discouraged.

In our experience, when dynamic scan capability is unavailable, at best only one or two images can be obtained with intense opacification of vessels following the routine injection of i.v. contrast media. In this setting, consequently, we advocate an alternative approach. This involves obtaining an initial series of nonenhanced images acquired first through a region of interest predetermined by correlation with either a routine or digital chest radiograph (scanogram). Following this, a bolus of i.v. contrast media is administered at a precise level or at most a few levels previously selected from the nonenhanced sections.

Although it may seem that the hila should always be studied following i.v. contrast, evaluation of the hila based on the interpretation of nonenhanced images has some distinct advantages. In a significant percentage of cases, the study actually may be completed noninvasively. Additionally, the ability to interpret nonenhanced images is of obvious value in patients who have known allergy to i.v. contrast media or renal insufficiency. Uncooperative patients may also cause problems in interpretation. When there is significant respiratory motion, contrast enhancement is of less value; in these cases, information is generally best obtained by imaging the hila with wide windows.

MR of Pulmonary Hila

Compared with CT, MR offers several potentially important advantages for evaluating the hilum (see

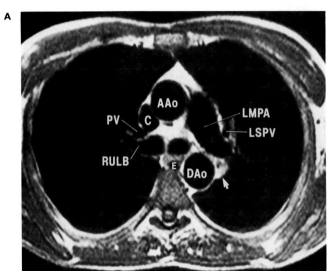

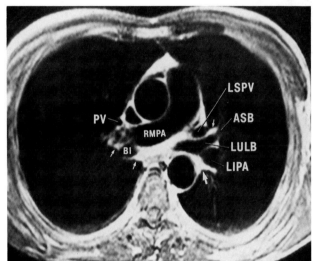

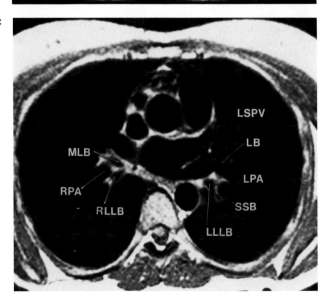

FIG. 5. Normal hilar anatomy: MR. Every-beat gated, axial SE images. **A:** Section through the carina (compare with Fig. 4C–F). RULB, right upper lobe bronchus; PV, right superior pulmonary vein; C, superior vena cava; AAo, ascending aorta; DAo, descending aorta; E, esophagus; LMPA, left main pulmonary artery. LSPV, left superior pulmonary vein. Note the relative lack of signal from the hila on either side, due to the presence of air within the airways and adjacent lung, and flow-void from the hilar vessels. **B:** Section through the bronchus intermedius (BI) (compare with Fig. 4G and H). RMPA, right main pulmonary artery; LULB, left upper lobe bronchus; ASB, anterior segmental bronchus. LIPA, left interlobar pulmonary artery. **C:** Section through the middle lobe bronchus (MLB) (compare with Fig. 4K and L). RLLB, right lower lobe bronchus; RPA, right pulmonary artery; LB, lingular bronchus; LPA, left interlobar pulmonary artery; SSB, superior segmental bronchus. Note that at all levels (*arrows* in A–B), focal areas of intermediate signal can be identified within the hila, bilaterally. Although ostensibly due to focal deposits of fat, differentiation from small hilar nodes is clearly difficult.

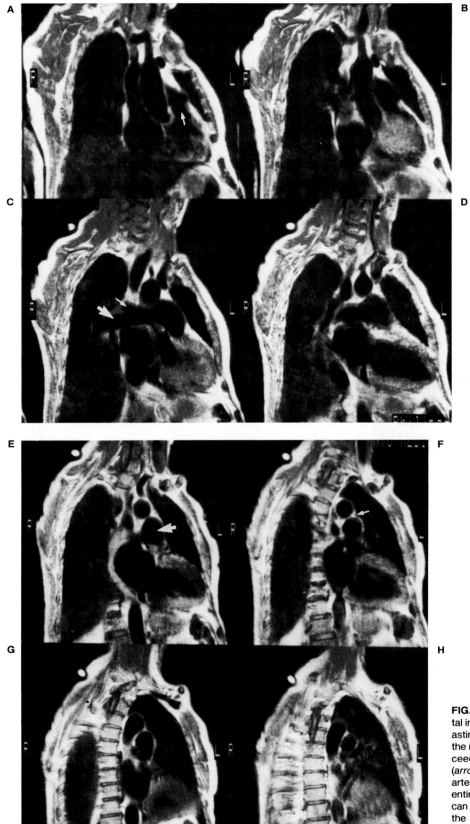

FIG. 6. Hilar anatomy: MR. **A–H:** Oblique sagittal images, from front to back, through the mediastinum and hila, beginning at a plane through the main pulmonary artery (*arrows* in A) and proceeding sequentially, first through the right (*arrow* in C) and then the left main pulmonary artery (*arrow* in E). Note that in this plane, the entire length of the right main pulmonary artery can be visualized, including the point of origin of the truncus anterior (*small arrow* in C). The left main pulmonary artery, cut in cross-section, appears circular; the aorticopulmonary window is also seen to good advantage (*small arrow* in F).

Chapter 1) (13–20). In addition to a lack of ionizing radiation, these include multiplanar scan capability and, in particular, a lack of reliance on i.v. contrast to identify hilar vessels. Routine evaluation is best accomplished with multislice, axial spin-echo (SE) images (Fig. 5). Typically, we use 10-mm thick sections, two to four data acquisitions, and a 256 × 256 display matrix, although a reduced (128 × 256) matrix may provide adequate anatomic delineation of the hila when attempting to minimize the time of the study. Cardiac gating should be considered mandatory in order to minimize transmitted cardiac pulsations (21,22). Respiratory gating may improve image quality as well (23); however, in most cases it unnecessarily prolongs the time of examination.

As a general rule, there is no need to obtain routine sagittal or coronal images; these may be obtained as indicated to further clarify otherwise confusing anatomic relationships. Oblique parasagittal images, in particular, may prove of value when attempting to visualize the central pulmonary arteries (Fig. 6). With cardiac gating, the effective repetition-time (TR) is equal to the R-R interval, (which generally ranges between 500 and 700 msec). Depending on the clinical indication, either single or multi-echo sequences can be obtained. Multislice, multi-echo SE sequences are particularly valuable for differentiating intravascular pathology from flow-related artifacts, especially when even-echoes [for example, echo-time (TE) 30, 60] are obtained.

Alternate strategies have been proposed, including the use of a rotating-gated, multi-phasic technique (24). With this approach, routine multi-level SE images are repeated four or five times, each time rotating the temporal order in which images from each level are obtained. This results in the acquisition of images at four or five phases of the cardiac cycle at each of four or five levels through the hilum. Unfortunately, this approach is time consuming and, although potentially of value, especially in analyzing pulmonary artery hypertension, in our judgment, rarely indicated.

Gated T2-weighted images are easily obtained by acquiring data every-other or even every-third beat; their use, however, should be selective. When indicated to further characterize select hilar pathology, for example, such as identification of a suspected bronchogenic cyst, single level, multi-echo T2-weighted pulse sequences (TR 1,500–2,200/TE 30, 60, 90, 120) at levels preselected from initial T1-weighted scans, in our experience, have proven especially useful (25).

Dynamic "fast field" echo imaging, using gradient refocused echoes and small flip angles, allow cine display of cardiac and vascular anatomy (see Chapter 1); although, as yet, this technique has not proven of routine clinical value, cine-gradient-refocused MR has significant potential in the evaluation of pulmonary vascular disease (26).

ANATOMY

Evaluation of the hila, both without and with i.v. contrast media, is facilitated by detailed knowledge of cross-sectional anatomy. The key to the CT anatomy of the pulmonary hila is cross-sectional bronchial anatomy. Because air within the lumen serves as a natural contrast agent, the bronchi serve as convenient, easily identifiable reference points that allow immediate anatomic orientation. They also form a lattice on which the pulmonary arteries and veins are draped in a characteristic fashion.

Evaluation of the hila is simplified by the use of characteristic sections (Fig. 3). These are easily definable by reference to the bronchial tree. On the right side, these include sections through the carina and apical segmental bronchus of the right upper lobe; the right upper lobe bronchus; the bronchus intermedius; the middle lobe bronchus; and the right lower lobe basilar segmental bronchi, respectively. On the left side, these include sections through the apical-posterior segmental bronchus of the left upper lobe; the upper portion of the left upper lobe bronchus; the lower portion of the left upper lobe bronchus, at the level of the left upper lobe spur; and through the left lower lobe basilar segmental bronchi, respectively.

In a routine sequence of eight 10-mm thick sections obtained through the hila following a bolus of i.v. contrast media, using dynamic incremental scanning, it can be anticipated that most if not all of these characteristic sections will be identifiable (Fig. 4). As will be illustrated, because of characteristic relationships between bronchi and hilar vessels at each of these levels, recognition of airways may allow routine identification of specific hilar vessels, even without i.v. contrast administration. Due to their importance, these anatomic relationships are reviewed in detail in the following section.

Right Hilum

At the level of the carina, the right upper lobe pulmonary arteries (segmental branches to the apical segment of the right upper lobe) and the right superior pulmonary veins (segmental branches draining the apical segment of the right upper lobe) course vertically, adjacent to the apical segmental bronchus; typically, arteries lie just medial to and the veins just lateral to the apical segmental bronchus (Fig. 4A and B).

At the level of the right upper lobe bronchus, the truncus anterior is usually identifiable. This large vessel is the first major branch of the right main pulmonary artery, arising within the pericardium (Fig. 7) and characteristically lies just anterior to the right upper lobe bronchus (Fig. 4E and F). Typically, a large branch of

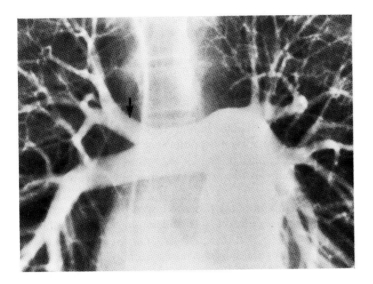

FIG. 7. PA view; normal pulmonary angiogram. The first branch of the main right pulmonary artery arises from within the pericardium, the truncus anterior (*arrow*). (Compare with CT appearance in Fig. 4E and F.)

the right superior pulmonary vein lies within the angle formed by the bifurcation of the right upper lobe bronchus into anterior and posterior segmental bronchi. Additionally, anterior and medial to the truncus anterior, there frequently is a small convexity that represents another right upper lobe vein (the apical-anterior vein), which also may characteristically be found in this location without the need for i.v. contrast media.

At the level of the bronchus intermedius, inferiorly, the right superior pulmonary vein lies alongside the lateral border of the right interlobar pulmonary artery, causing the right hilum at this level to have a slightly nodular contour. Frequently, multiple veins can be identified in this location; these should not be mistaken for adenopathy (Fig. 4G–J).

Once the right main pulmonary artery reaches the lateral border of the bronchus intermedius, it is not unusual for this artery to have a triangular and somewhat irregular configuration. This normal variation is caused by a change in the course of the right pulmonary artery as it turns inferiorly and becomes the right interlobar pulmonary artery (Fig. 8). The sudden change in the course of the right pulmonary artery as it assumes an interlobar position is evident; when viewed in cross-section, at the point at which it turns inferiorly, this artery will have a triangular configuration (Fig. 4I and J).

At the level of the middle lobe bronchus, the interlobar pulmonary artery lies immediately lateral to the lateral borders of both the middle and lower lobe bronchi. The interlobar artery at this point is vertically oriented and is thus seen in cross-section as an oval structure. The right superior pulmonary vein lies medial to the middle lobe bronchus and can be seen entering the upper portion of the left atrium (Fig. 4K and L).

At the level of the basilar segmental bronchi, below the anatomic limits of the right hilum, the right interlo-

bar pulmonary artery bifurcates into the various basilar segmental pulmonary arteries. These have a characteristic, rounded configuration, lying posterolateral to the proximal portions of the basilar segmental bronchi (Fig. 4M and N). Unlike the basilar pulmonary arteries, inferior pulmonary veins are oriented horizontally and routinely can be traced into, first, the right inferior pulmo-

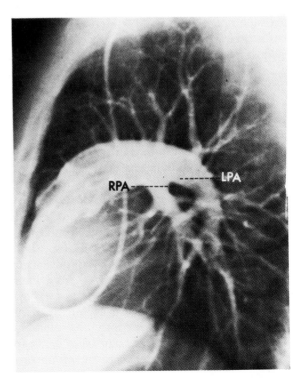

FIG. 8. Lateral radiograph from pulmonary angiogram shown in Fig. 7. The proximal right and left interlobar pulmonary arteries (RPA, LPA) are labeled. (Compare with Fig. 4E and F on the left, and Fig. 4I and J on the right.)

nary vein and, subsequently, into the lower portion of the left atrium.

Left Hilum

On the left side, although characteristic relationships between vessels and airways are also present, there is far more anatomic variation.

Corresponding to the anatomy on the right side, the superior pulmonary veins tend to be located anteriorly. At the level of the carina, the apical-posterior segmental bronchus is separated from the left main bronchus by the main left pulmonary artery, which courses over the left upper lobe bronchus at this level. The left superior pulmonary vein (the branch draining the apical-posterior segment of the left upper lobe) and the left upper lobe pulmonary artery (the main branch to the left upper lobe) can be recognized as two distinct vessels. In general, at this level the left upper lobe pulmonary artery can be traced to its origin from the main left pulmonary artery and lies posterolateral to the left superior pulmonary vein (Fig. 4A–D).

At the level of the upper portion of the left upper bronchus, above the spur, the posterior wall of the left upper lobe bronchus is slightly convex because it is indented superiorly and posteriorly by the left main pulmonary artery as it courses over the left upper lobe bronchus (Fig. 4E and F, and Fig. 6). Posterior to the left upper lobe bronchus, the left pulmonary artery continues as the left interlobar pulmonary artery, which typically appears triangular and even slightly irregular at this level. This normal variation is caused by a change in the course of the left pulmonary artery as it turns to descend toward the lower lung segments (Fig. 8). The left superior pulmonary vein invariably lies in front of the left upper lobe bronchus as it courses toward the left atrium and, frequently, has a horizontal course; distinct branching usually can be identified peripherally within the pulmonary parenchyma.

At the level of the lower portion of the left upper lobe bronchus, through the left upper lobe spur, the left interlobar pulmonary artery has a nearly vertical course and always lies just lateral to the spur. The interface between the artery and the adjacent pulmonary parenchyma is generally smooth and rounded (Fig. 4I and J). Adjacent and just lateral to the origin of the lingular bronchus, the pulmonary artery to the lingula frequently can be identified. Anteriorly, the inferior portion of the left superior pulmonary vein also can be recognized lying directly anterior to the left upper lobe bronchus.

Characteristically, pulmonary parenchyma can be seen between the pulmonary artery and the descending aorta at the level of the left upper lobe bronchus (Fig. 4G

and H). Webb and Gamsu (27) have shown that this portion of lung frequently comes in close proximity to the posteromedial wall of the left upper and lower lobe bronchi at this level. Thickening and/or nodularity of this left "retrobronchial stripe" is a sensitive sign for tumor infiltration and/or adenopathy in the left hilum, and should be searched for routinely.

At the level of the basilar segmental bronchi, the anatomy of the inferior portion of the left hilum is essentially a mirror image of that on the right side. Branches of the pulmonary artery to the left lower lobe lie lateral and posterior to the left lower lobe basilar bronchi. The left inferior pulmonary vein is oriented horizontally and can routinely be traced into the lower portion of the left atrium. The left inferior pulmonary vein courses alongside the lateral border of the descending aorta.

Despite significant variation in their appearance, identification of most small hilar vessels is generally possible by following their course on sequential images into larger vessels. These anatomic relationships may be appreciated on almost every scan illustrated in this section and is an important principle in evaluating hilar and parenchymal disease.

Normal Hilar Anatomy: MR

Anatomically, the appearance of the hila with MR is identical to CT when visualized in cross-section. Unlike CT, however, identification of hilar vessels with MR is not dependent on the use of i.v. contrast media. Typically, flowing blood within hilar vessels generates no signal; since no signal is generated by air within the bronchi and little if any signal is generated by the adjacent pulmonary parenchyma, only the walls of these structures can be distinguished. As a consequence, due to the relatively poor spatial resolution of MR as compared with CT, normal structures within the hila usually are identifiable only on the basis of prior knowledge of normal cross-sectional hilar anatomy (Fig. 5).

Using routine, electrocardiogram (ECG) gated, SE pulse sequences, most abnormalities within the hila are easily identifiable as foci of intermediate signal intensity. Unfortunately, on relatively T1-weighted, SE images through normal hila, signal generated by soft tissues prominent enough to be confused with enlarged nodes or masses may be identified in a significant percentage of cases (Fig. 5). These probably represent focal hilar fat and small, normal-sized lymph nodes, and occur most frequently in the right hilum at the point at which the right main pulmonary artery crosses in front of the bronchus intermedius to become the right interlobar pulmonary artery (Fig. 5B); at the level of the middle lobe bronchus, anterolaterally (Fig. 5C); and on the left side, through the left upper lobe bronchus, especially at the level of the left upper lobe spur (Fig. 5B and C). Similar problems in the interpretation of CT scans also have been encountered (28).

It should be emphasized that signal from within the hila also may be vascular in origin; although this may be of potential diagnostic value—as in the diagnosis of pulmonary hypertension, or intrapulmonary thrombi and tumor—this finding may also be seen in normal vessels, depending on a number of variables, including the phase of the cardiac cycle at which the image was acquired (see Chapter 1). As will be discussed, in individual cases, differentiating normal flow-related intravascular signal from abnormal intravascular signal is generally not problematic.

Similar constraints, as described above, apply to the interpretation of both coronal and sagittal hilar images. Relatively poor spatial resolution, coupled with a lack of familiarity with normal anatomic relationships in the coronal and sagittal planes, may make interpretation difficult (Fig. 9). As these images are of little routine clinical value and their acquisition is time consuming, they are not routinely indicated. Exceptionally, in the evaluation of subcarinal masses, both coronal and sagittal images may prove invaluable by more clearly delineating anatomic relationships, especially between subcarinal masses and the roof of the left atrium (16–20).

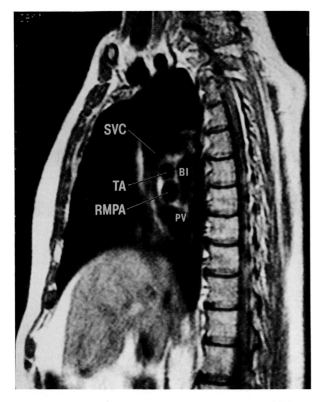

FIG. 9. Hilar anatomy: sagittal MR. Every-beat gated, SE image through the right hilum. SVC, superior vena cava; TA, truncus anterior; BI, bronchus intermedius; RMPA, right main pulmonary artery; PV, confluence of pulmonary veins. Despite clear delineation of hilar structures, sagittal images are rarely necessary.

PULMONARY VASCULAR DISEASE

Differentiation between enlarged vessels and hilar adenopathy and/or hilar masses is frequently difficult with plain radiography. By virtue of the clarity of detail obtained with cross-sectional imaging, both CT and MR play important roles in differentiating pulmonary vascular disease from other significant hilar pathology.

Pulmonary Artery Hypertension

The use of radiographic measurements in predicting pulmonary artery hypertension (PAH) has proven of limited value only, in part due to technical difficulties in obtaining accurate radiographic measurements (29).

Normal ranges in the size of both the main and interlobar pulmonary arteries have been measured in cross-section (30,31). Using computer-generated CT density profiles to accurately measure pulmonary artery diameters, in evaluating 26 normal controls, Kuriyama et al. (31) found that the upper limit of normal diameters, plus or minus two standard deviations, was as follows: the main pulmonary artery, 28.6 mm; the left pulmonary artery, 28 mm; and the proximal right pulmonary artery, 24.3 mm.

Utilizing size criteria, CT is of value in predicting pulmonary artery hypertension (Fig. 10). As documented by Kuriyama et al. (31), in an evaluation of 32 adults with known cardiopulmonary disease, 20 of whom had documented mean pulmonary artery pressures > 18 mm Hg, CT proved 82% accurate in predicting PAH based on a measurement of the diameter of the main pulmonary artery. Unfortunately, although enlargement of the main pulmonary artery has been shown to be highly specific, significant hypertension may be associated with normal-sized pulmonary arteries. In the series of Kuriyama et al. (31), CT proved only moderately sensitive in predicting PAH, failing to identify five of 16 cases. When the main pulmonary artery is enlarged, correlation between the diameter of the main pulmonary artery and mean pulmonary artery pressure has been established, especially when normalized for body surface area.

Occasionally, the configuration of the pulmonary outflow tract and the left pulmonary artery may appear to be abnormal in a normal patient. Mencini and Proto (32) have called attention to a variation in the configuration of the pulmonary outflow tract and the main left pulmonary artery in which these structures are higher than usual, lying adjacent and to the left of the aortic arch. This appearance may simulate a mediastinal mass. In cases in which the configuration of the pulmonary artery is unusual (particularly when associated with a paucity of mediastinal fat), the injection of a bolus of i.v. contrast medium may be indispensable.

A
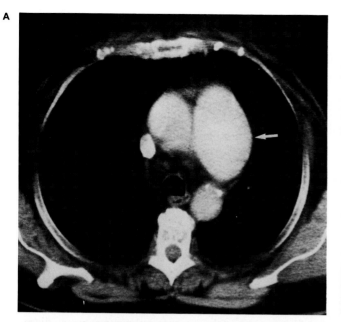

B
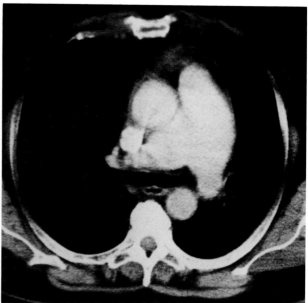

C
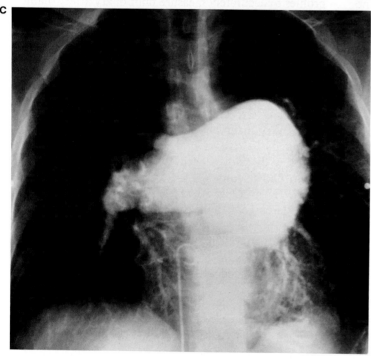

FIG. 10. Pulmonary hypertension. CT evaluation. **A,B:** CT sections through the main and right and left main pulmonary arteries, respectively, following a bolus of i.v. contrast media. There is aneurysmal dilatation of the main pulmonary artery (*arrow* in A) as well as both the proximal right and left pulmonary arteries in this patient with documented pulmonary hypertension. **C:** Corresponding pulmonary arteriogram.

ECG-gated MR imaging has also been utilized to evaluate patients with pulmonary artery hypertension (33–35). As compared with CT, MR has several inherent advantages. These include the potential for noninvasive evaluation of pulmonary blood flow, as well as simultaneous assessment of right ventricular function and morphology. As shown by Bouchard et al. (34), in a retrospective study of 25 patients with documented pulmonary artery hypertension, with and without superimposed pulmonary emboli, the presence of intraluminal signal during systole correlated well with moderate to severe grades of pulmonary hypertension, identifiable in all 19 patients (100%) with systolic pressures ≥80 mm

Hg (Fig. 11). Unfortunately, in patients with moderately severe degrees of pulmonary hypertension, i.e., with pressures between 65 and 80 mm Hg, MR proved positive in only three of five (60%) cases. MR proved equally insensitive when mean pulmonary artery pressures were evaluated.

Significantly, MR can be used to measure right ventricular wall thickness, and paradoxical septal motion by assessing interventricular septal curvature; it is unlikely, however, that these measurements will prove of routine value in the detection of patients with early or mild pulmonary hypertension. MR may be of considerable additional value in the identification of patients whose

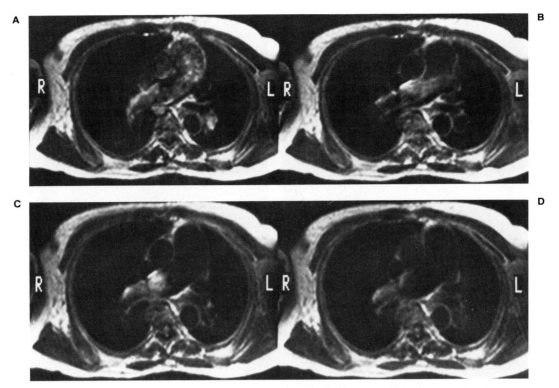

FIG. 11. Pulmonary hypertension. MR evaluation. **A–D:** MR images obtained at a single level through the right main pulmonary artery acquired at evenly spaced intervals throughout the R-R interval, from a rotating-gated, multiphasic study. Persistent signal can be identified in the distal portion of the right main pulmonary artery throughout both the late diastolic and systolic portions of the cardiac cycle. Note absence of flow-related signal in all other vascular structures, especially obvious in systole (B and C). At cardiac catheterization, main pulmonary artery pressure measured 65/27 mm Hg, with a mean pressure of 40 mm Hg.

pulmonary hypertension is secondary to intracardiac pathology, such as shunts.

Pulmonary Artery Aneurysms

The role of CT in the evaluation of pulmonary artery aneurysms has been well documented (Fig. 12). Al- though rare, pulmonary artery aneurysms are seen in a wide variety of conditions and have been associated with infection; congenital heart disease, especially, patent ductus arteriosus, atrial and ventricular septal defects, and congenital abnormalities of the pulmonary valve; primary vascular diseases, congenital and acquired, in- cluding both cystic medial necrosis and atherosclerosis;

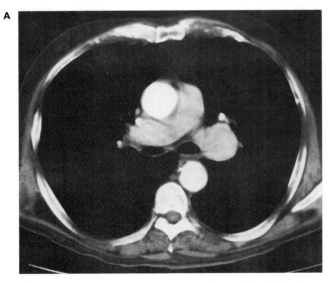
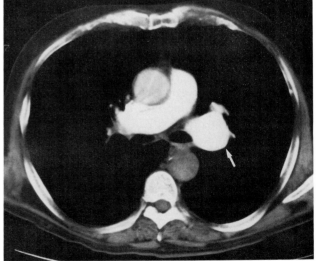

FIG. 12. Pulmonary artery aneurysm. **A,B:** Sequential sections from a dynamic-static contrast-enhanced sequence obtained at the level of the right main pulmonary artery in a patient with a left hilar mass identified on a routine chest radiograph (not shown). The interlobar pulmonary artery is aneurysmally dilated (*arrow* in B).

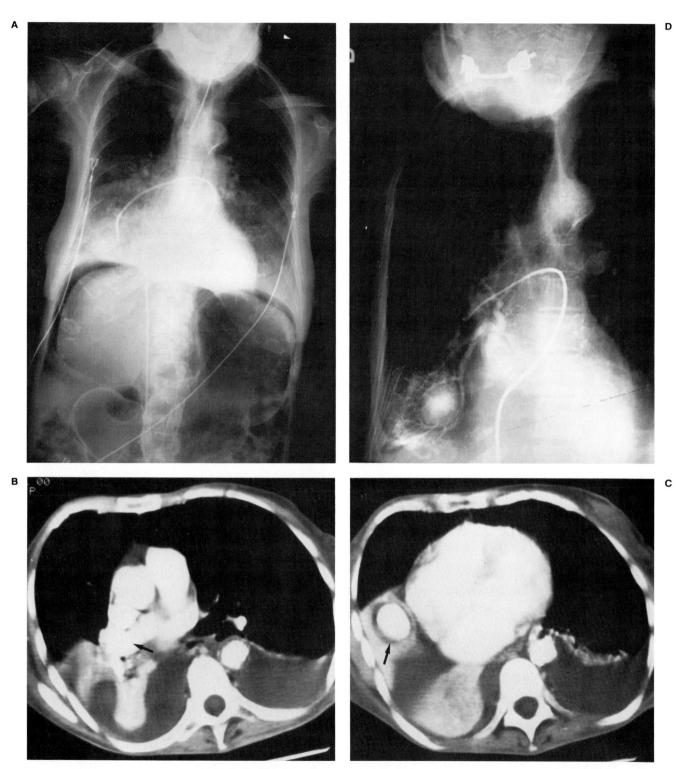

FIG. 13. Posttraumatic pulmonary artery aneurysm. **A:** PA radiograph shows the presence of a malpositioned Swan-Ganz catheter with its tip directed towards the base of the right lower lobe. Pneumoperitoneum is due to abdominal surgery. **B,C:** Sequential CT sections through the right main pulmonary artery (*arrow* in B) and the right lower lobe, respectively. A large pleural effusion is present, causing compression atelectasis of both the middle and right lower lobes. Within the collapsed middle lobe, marked contrast enhancement can be identified within an apparent vascular structure (*arrow*). **D:** Coned-down view from a selective right pulmonary artery arteriogram shows a peripheral pulmonary artery aneurysm corresponding in location to the tip of the Swan-Ganz catheter shown in A, and the large peripheral vascular structure identified within the middle lobe in C. (Case courtesy of Deborrah Reede, M.D., Long Island College Hospital, New York.)

congenital abnormalities, both isolated, and associated with hereditary hemorrhagic telangiectasia; and as a result of both penetrating and nonpenetrating trauma (Fig. 13) (36–38). Pulmonary artery aneurysms also are associated with generalized vasculitis, as occurs in Behçet's disease, Hughes Stovin syndrome, and even giant cell arteritis. Interestingly, the leading cause of pulmonary artery aneurysms is probably cystic medial necrosis, in association with both congenital and acquired cardiovascular disease, accompanied by pulmonary hypertension.

Radiologic diagnosis is frequently problematic (36). Although pulmonary artery aneurysms are generally visible, their appearance is rarely specific. Peripheral aneurysms may be mistaken for parenchymal nodules or metastases, unless accompanying vessels are identified; central lesions are easily confused with hilar adenopathy, masses, or even aortic aneurysms. As a consequence, definitive diagnosis traditionally has required pulmonary angiography. Presently, contrast-enhanced CT and MR have been shown to be reliable methods for diagnosing both central and peripheral aneurysms, obviating the need for more invasive studies in all cases, save those for which therapeutic intervention is planned (9,39–41).

Pulmonary Thromboembolism

Numerous reports have documented both the potential uses and limitations of CT in the evaluation of patients with suspected pulmonary thromboembolism (42–48). Overfors et al. (44) have shown experimentally that peripheral pulmonary emboli could be diagnosed in the descending pulmonary arteries in four of five living dogs. However, in a retrospective study of 18 patients with pulmonary thromboembolism evaluated with contrast-enhanced dynamic incremental CT, Chintapalli et al. (47) were able to identify central pulmonary arterial thrombi in only seven of 18 cases. Rarely, thrombi may be detectable in segmental arteries < 1 cm in size (46). When visualized, pulmonary emboli appear as filling defects within the pulmonary arteries on bolus contrast-enhanced scans (Fig. 14).

The potential of MR in the evaluation of pulmonary thromboembolism has also been evaluated (Fig. 14) (49–54). Pope et al. (49), in an experimental study of 30 dogs, using routine SE sequences, showed that MR had a sensitivity of 82% and a specificity of 88% in diagnosing pulmonary emboli. Gamsu et al. (50) showed that pulmonary emboli labeled with nonmagnetic barium threads could be identified with MR in 12 of 19 sites (63%) documented to have emboli by corresponding CT scans. Recently, MR has also been shown to be of value in diagnosing pulmonary artery sarcomas, especially following i.v. injection of gadolinium-DTPA (122).

On SE images, central pulmonary emboli appear as areas of bright signal within corresponding pulmonary arteries; peripherally, emboli are identifiable as discrete foci of relatively high-signal intensity, usually present on contiguous scans, without evidence of branching (Figs. 14 and 16) (50). From a practical standpoint, intravascular signal resulting from thrombi within central arteries is usually easily differentiable from flow-related signal enhancement by the use of either multi-phase cardiac gating, or double-echo pulse sequences; charac-

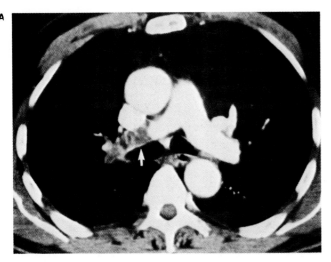

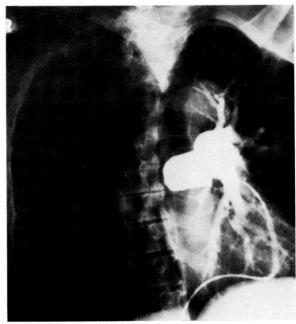

FIG. 14. Pulmonary embolus. Right main pulmonary artery. **A:** A large, filling defect is apparent in this contrast-enhanced section through the right main pulmonary artery (*arrow*). There is no evidence of tumor surrounding the artery. **B:** Oblique projection; main pulmonary arteriogram. Obstruction of the right main pulmonary artery is confirmed. The angiographic appearance suggested tumor occlusion: none was found at surgery.

A

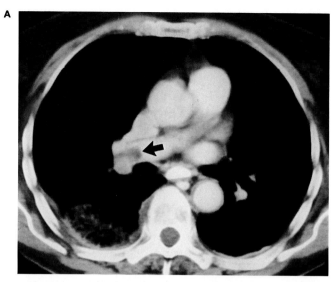

B

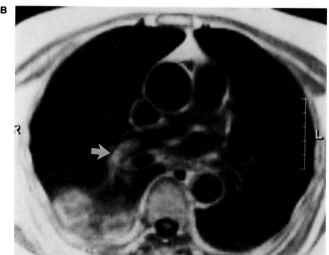

C

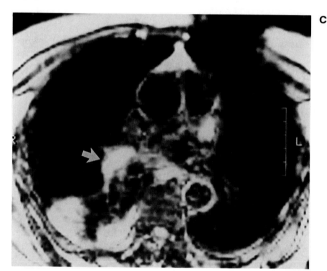

FIG. 15. Pulmonary artery thrombus. **A:** Contrast enhanced CT image shows filling defect in the right main pulmonary artery (*arrow*). Note the presence of fluffy, peripheral infiltrates in the superior segment of the right lower lobe, due to pulmonary infarction. **B,C:** Routine gated SE image and gradient refocused image, respectively, through the right hilum. Note that in both images thrombus within the right main pulmonary artery is easily identified (*arrows, B,C*) as an area of increased signal intensity, especially marked in the gradient refocused scan. Two separate peripheral infarcts are also easily identified in the right lower lobe. (Case courtesy of Deborah Reede, MD, Long Island College Hospital, NY.)

teristically, on second echo images, emboli show little if any change in signal intensity, whereas flow-related signal will be markedly enhanced (Fig. 17). Even in patients with pulmonary artery hypertension in whom increased signal within pulmonary arteries is routinely visualized, utilizing the technique of even-echo rephasing, central thrombus can still be differentiated from flow-related artifacts (35,54).

Unlike central thrombi, peripheral emboli are more difficult to identify; in part, this is due to limited spatial resolution and respiratory motion artifacts. Additionally, signal from peripheral emboli may be difficult to differentiate from that caused by focal areas of parenchymal consolidation or mucous plugging (55).

As an alternative to routine SE sequences, the pulmonary arteries may be evaluated with cine-gradient-refocused images (Fig. 15). Comparing this technique with SE images, Posteraro et al. (26), in a retrospective study of 11 patients with documented pulmonary emboli, found cine-gradient-refocused images to be more sensi-

tive, identifying thrombi in all cases. As discussed in Chapter 1, on images obtained with gradient-refocused echoes, flowing blood has a much higher signal intensity than soft tissues, simulating the appearance of routine angiography. Using the criteria of low-intensity intraluminal filling defects or abrupt vascular cutoff with high-intensity peripheral flow versus vascular cutoff without high-intensity capping or intravascular webs, Posteraro et al. (26) have postulated that acute and chronic emboli, respectively, may be differentiable using gradient-refocused echoes. Although intriguing, the real value of this technique remains to be established.

Despite initial enthusiasm, the roles of both CT and MR in the evaluation of pulmonary thromboembolism are limited; pulmonary arteriography remains the gold standard. This is due not only to the greater sensitivity of pulmonary angiography, but to the simultaneous ability to derive physiologic data. The diagnosis of peripheral emboli in particular remains elusive. In patients for whom angiography is contraindicated, however, or as a

A

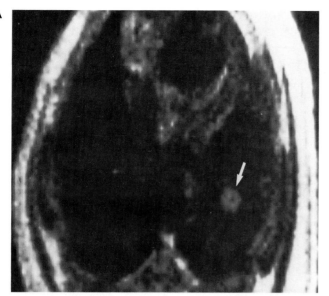

B

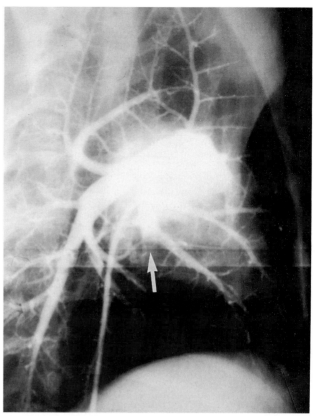

FIG. 16. Experimental pulmonary artery thrombus: MR. **A:** Every-beat gated, axial section through the lower lobes in a dog whose pulmonary arteries were injected with autologous clot. Signal can be identified in the left lower lobe (*arrow*), within otherwise featureless lung fields. **B:** Pulmonary artery arteriogram in the same animal shows thrombus obstructing a left lower lobe pulmonary artery (*arrow*), corresponding in location to the area of signal seen in A. (Images courtesy of Jeffrey Weinreb, M.D., New York University Medical Center, New York, NY.)

A

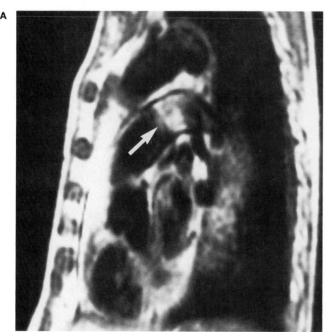

B

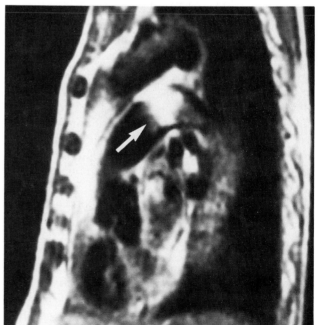

FIG. 17. Flow-related signal: MR. **A,B:** Every-beat gated, sagittal sections through the main pulmonary artery obtained with symmetrical TE's of 30 and 60 msec, respectively. Note that although intraluminal signal can be identified in the apex of the main pulmonary artery in the image obtained with a 30-msec TE (*arrow* in A), this significantly increases in the image obtained with a 60-msec TE (*arrow* in B). This increase in signal intensity is due to even-echo rephasing, a finding extremely helpful in differentiating flow-related signal from true intravascular pathology.

means for follow-up in patients with known chronic emboli, especially when these are central, both CT and especially MR may play a valuable role.

Vascular Neoplasia

In addition to pulmonary embolism and thrombus, intravascular filling defects may also result from both primary or secondary (metastatic) tumors (Figs. 18,19). Although primary vascular tumors arising in the pulmonary arteries are rare, they are not unknown (56,57). Typically sarcomatous, these may originate either within the right ventricle and extend through the valve into the main pulmonary arteries, or, alternatively, they may arise directly within the pulmonary arteries themselves. Histologically, pulmonary artery sarcomas are most frequently undifferentiated: specific subtypes in-

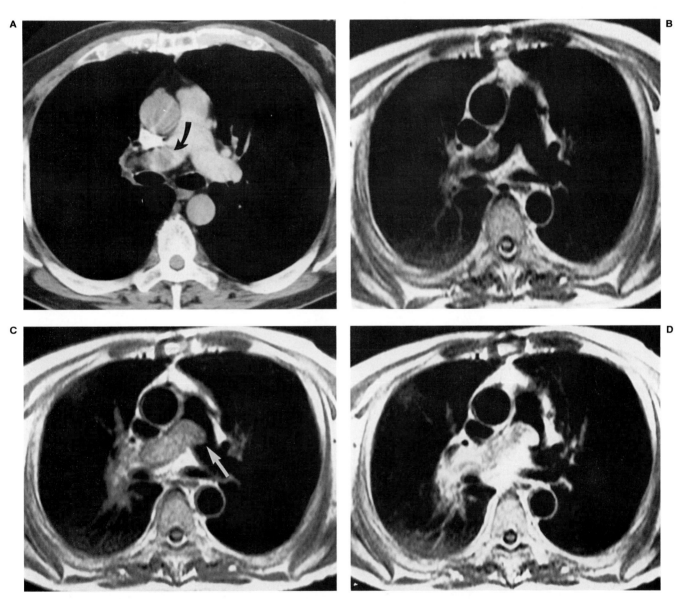

FIG. 18. A: CT scan at the level of the carina following a bolus injection of i.v. contrast medium shows a focal filling defect within the right main pulmonary artery (*arrow*). This appearance is nonspecific and may result from either tumor or thrombus. **B:** Every-beat gated, noncontrast-enhanced SE MR section at the level of the carina shows an eccentric, slightly nodular intravascular filling defect within the right main pulmonary artery (compare with A). Additionally, note that there is a subtle increase in signal intensity within the right lung as compared with the left lung, presumably reflecting vascular stasis and congestion. **C:** Every-beat gated, noncontrast-enhanced SE MR image at the same level as shown in A and B, 3 months later. A lobular mass of intermediate signal intensity is now clearly identifiable filling most of the lumen of the right main pulmonary artery, extending medially to partially obstruct the lumen of the left main pulmonary artery (*arrow*). A significant increase in the size of this lesion is apparent. **D:** Every-beat gated SE MR image at the same level as shown in C obtained 1 minute after i.v. injection of Gd-DTPA. Note that there is a marked increase in the signal intensity of the intraluminal filling defect within the right main pulmonary artery as compared with the precontrast-enhanced image (compare with C). This is consistent with the presence of vascularized tissue as occurs within tumor as distinct from a nonvascularized intraluminal thrombus. Again, note the presence of increased signal within the right lung, which also shows considerable signal enhancement following the i.v. injection of Gd-DTPA (compare with C). Surgically verified pulmonary artery sarcoma. (From Weinreb et al., ref. 122.)

clude, most commonly, leiomyosarcomas and myxo-sarcomas, with rhabdomyosarcomas, fibrosarcomas, chondrosarcomas, and malignant mesenchymomas accounting for the remainder. Significantly, there is considerable overlap both in the CT and MR appearance of tumor within a pulmonary artery and other potential filling defects, specifically, chronic intrapulmonary arterial thrombi. The diagnosis of a pulmonary artery sarcoma is usually made at autopsy.

In addition to primary vascular tumors, tumor within pulmonary arteries may be caused by tumor arising either within the lung, hilum, or mediastinum. Although most cases are secondary to bronchogenic carcinoma, both extrathoracic metastases as well as primary intra-

cardiac tumors may invade or cause obstruction of both pulmonary arteries and veins. Although rare, this type of tumor extension is easily identifiable with both contrast-enhanced CT and MR (Fig. 19) (58,59).

With CT, tumor encasement of hilar vessels and mediastinal invasion due to bronchogenic carcinoma optimally requires the administration of a bolus of i.v. contrast media (Fig. 20). As discussed in Chapter 6, encasement of the main pulmonary arteries is an absolute contraindication to resection in patients with bronchogenic carcinoma (Fig. 21). Although identification of pulmonary artery encasement is usually not problematic, overinterpretation should be avoided. Specifically, the finding of tumor adjacent to the main pulmonary

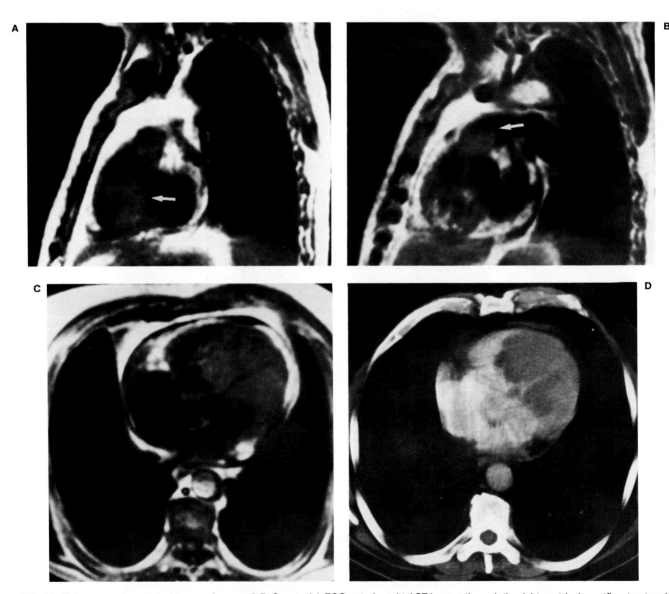

FIG. 19. Pulmonary artery metastases: melanoma. **A,B:** Sequential, ECG-gated, sagittal SE images through the right ventricular outflow tract and main pulmonary artery, respectively, show intermediate signal throughout the right ventricle (*arrow* in A) and within the proximal main pulmonary artery (*arrow* in B). **C,D:** ECG-gated axial SE image and corresponding contrast-enhanced axial CT section through the right and left ventricles confirms extensive intracardiac tumor. Biopsy confirmed metastatic melanoma.

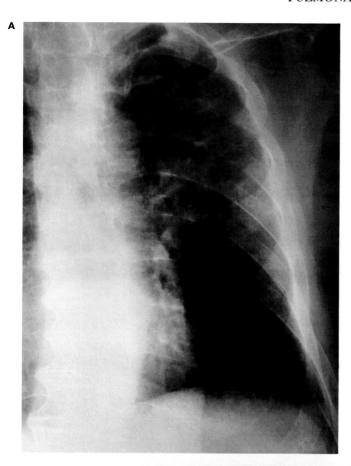

A

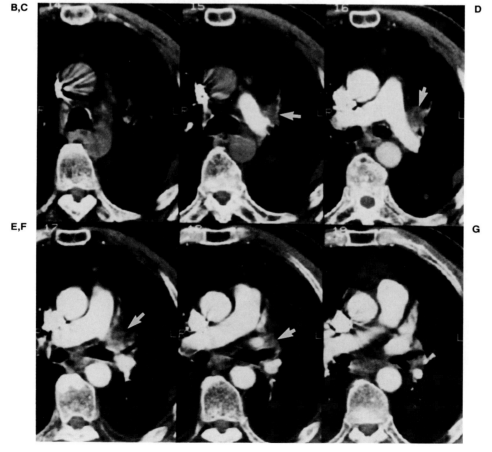

FIG. 20. Bronchogenic carcinoma: left hilum. **A:** Coned-down view from a PA radiograph shows fullness of the left hilum and a peripheral, left upper lobe infiltrate. **B–G:** Sequential CT sections obtained through the left hilum from above down during administration of 150 cc of i.v. contrast medium injected at a rate of 2 cc/sec using a power injector. Extensive tumor and adenopathy are diffusely present throughout the left hilum, easily differentiated from hilar vessels due to a lack of contrast enhancement (*arrows* in C–F). Enlarged, nonenhancing subcarinal nodes are present as well. Note precise delineation between normal bronchi, and adjacent tumor and blood vessels, providing a detailed road map for either bronchoscopy or transthoracic needle biopsy.

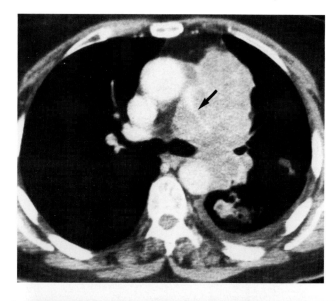

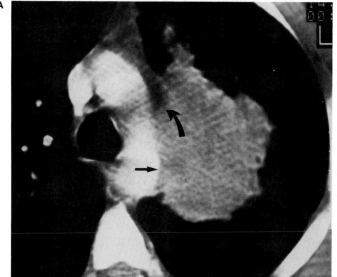

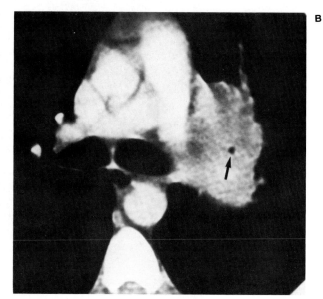

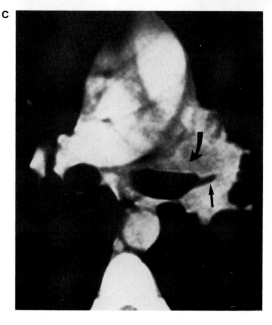

FIG. 21. Bronchogenic carcinoma: left hilum. CT section through the left hilum following a bolus of i.v. contrast medium. Extensive tumor has infiltrated the hilum and mediastinum, encasing the left main pulmonary artery (*arrow*). A small pleural effusion is present as well. In this case, CT allows precise staging, excluding attempted resection.

FIG. 22. Bronchogenic carcinoma: left hilum. **A–C:** Enlargements of sequential CT scans through the left hilum, beginning at the level of the aorticopulmonary window and preceding caudally. A large tumor is present in the left hilum, surrounding and narrowing the apical-posterior segmental bronchus (*arrow* in B), and narrowing and nearly obstructing the origin of the left upper lobe bronchus (*arrow* in C). Tumor abuts the descending aorta (*arrow* in A), seemingly infiltrating posterior mediastinal fat (*curved arrow* in A). More inferiorly, tumor has obliterated the left superior pulmonary vein, which is usually identifiable immediately anterior to the left upper lobe bronchus (*curved arrow* in C). Despite these findings, a pneumonectomy was successfully performed.

arteries, regardless of how extensive, should not be interpreted as definitive evidence of unresectability (Fig. 22).

Although tumor obstruction of hilar vessels is most often secondary to bronchogenic carcinoma, other lesions, both benign and malignant, have been reported to cause pulmonary arterial obstruction (60–63). The CT appearance of pulmonary artery obstruction secondary to fibrosing mediastinitis, in particular, has been noted (Fig. 23) (64–67). This disorder causes a wide spectrum of clinical and radiographic changes, from incidental, asymptomatic disease to life-threatening pulmonary hy-

pertension. The result of granulomatous disease, especially histoplasmosis, a characteristic appearance of widespread mediastinal and hilar calcifications causing narrowing or obliteration of both pulmonary arteries and veins should suggest the diagnosis (Fig. 23). Although alterations in the configuration of mediastinal and hilar vessels secondary to fibrosing mediastinitis have been documented with MR, the inability of MR to detect calcifications is a clear disadvantage (67).

Pulmonary artery compression secondary to aneurysms of both the ascending and descending aorta correctly identified by CT also has been reported (Fig. 24)

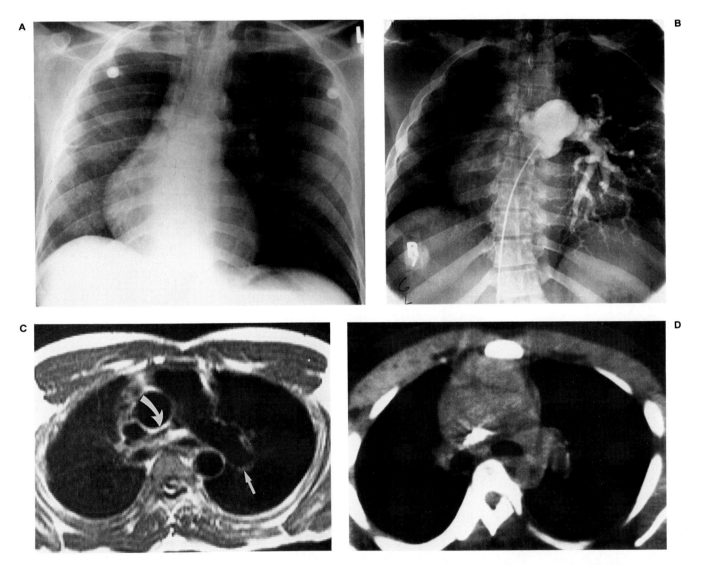

FIG. 23. Fibrosing mediastinitis. **A:** PA radiograph shows markedly diminished ventilation in the right lung, associated with a shift of the heart and mediastinum to the right. Right hilar structures are difficult to identify. **B:** Pulmonary angiogram shows abrupt cutoff of the right main pulmonary artery, raising the possibility of obstruction secondary to tumor. **C:** Every-beat gated, axial SE MR scan obtained just below the carina. The left pulmonary artery is slightly enlarged (*arrow*). The right main pulmonary artery is markedly attenuated (*curved arrow*). Although there is a slight increase in the signal within the mediastinum adjacent to the right main pulmonary artery, this is nonspecific in appearance. There is no obvious mediastinal mass seen. **D:** Nonenhanced CT scan at the same level as C, showing extensive mediastinal calcification in the region surrounding the right main pulmonary artery. Extensive mediastinal and hilar calcifications were present as well at numerous other levels (not shown). (Case courtesy of Jerry Patt, M.D., Union Memorial Hospital, Baltimore, MD.)

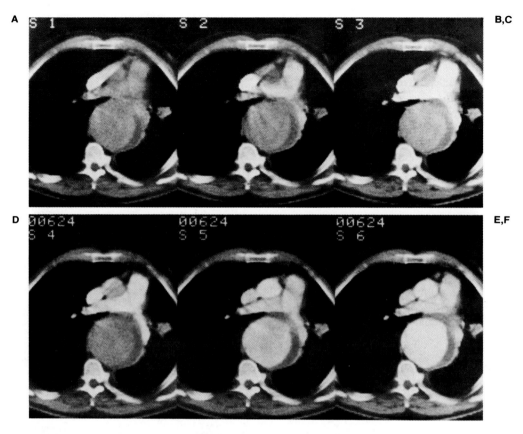

FIG. 24. Pulmonary artery compression: aortic aneurysm. **A–F:** Dynamic-static CT sections at the level of the right upper lobe bronchus show marked compression of the proximal left main pulmonary artery by a large aneurysm of the descending aorta.

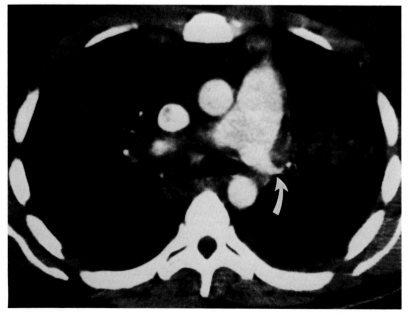

FIG. 25. Sarcoidosis. CT section through the carina, following a bolus of i.v. contrast, in a patient with histologically documented pulmonary sarcoidosis. There is marked narrowing of the left main pulmonary artery (*arrow*) due to extrinsic compression from enlarged hilar nodes. Infiltrate is present within the left upper lobe, associated with a moderate left pleural effusion, partly loculated in the lateral portion of the oblique fissure. Enlarged subcarinal nodes can be identified as well. These findings mimic the appearance of carcinomatous involvement of the hilum and pleura. (From Hamper et al., ref. 123.)

(68). Unfortunately, in cases in which the etiology is other than vascular, accurate diagnosis usually necessitates histologic evaluation (Fig. 25).

Pulmonary Venous Disease

CT has proven to be a sensitive, noninvasive method for establishing the diagnosis of a pulmonary varix, obviating the need for angiography (69,70). Varices are easily identifiable as enlarged but otherwise normal pulmonary vein(s) that directly drain into the left atrium, typically involving the right lower lobe, less commonly the left upper lobe and lingula (Fig. 26). Although commonly found in association with acquired heart disease, left atrial enlargement, and pulmonary venous hyper-

tension, pulmonary varices also rarely occur as congenital local dilatations of a segment of a pulmonary vein in otherwise normal patients. In those cases in which a pulmonary varix masquerades either as a discrete pulmonary nodule or even an arteriovenous malformation (AVM), bolus contrast administration is essential in order to show continuity between the varix and associated pulmonary veins. Characteristically, unlike typical AVMs, isolated pulmonary varices enhance only during the phase of maximal venous opacification.

CT findings in patients with pulmonary veno-occlusive disease have also been reported (71,72). In this entity, diffuse endothelial proliferation results in the occlusion of small pulmonary veins, especially in otherwise healthy young patients, resulting in severe

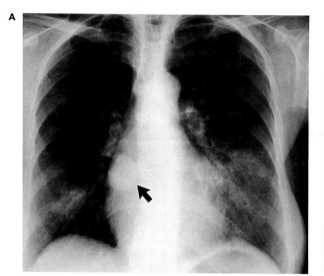
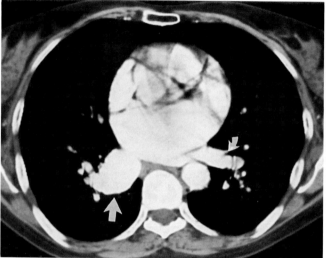

FIG. 26. Pulmonary varix. **A:** PA radiograph shows sharply defined right hilar mass (*arrow*). **B:** Contrast-enhanced CT section through the inferior right hilum shows aneurysmal dilatation of the right inferior pulmonary vein (*curved arrow*) contiguous with the left atrium. (Compare with appearance of normal left inferior pulmonary vein (*arrow*).) This appearance is diagnostic of a pulmonary varix.

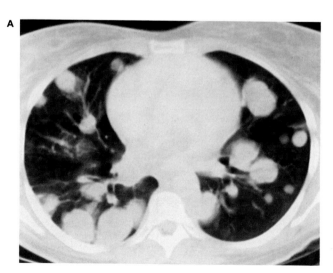
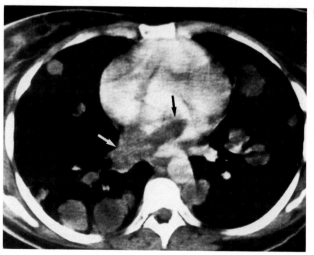

FIG. 27. Invasive (metastatic) uterine leiomyomatosis. **A,B:** CT section through the right inferior pulmonary vein, imaged with wide and narrow windows, respectively, following a bolus of i.v. contrast medium. Multiple nodules are present in both lungs of varying sizes, many clearly related to adjacent blood vessels (A). A large filling defect is also present within the left atrium and left inferior pulmonary vein, representing extension of tumor from the lungs into the left heart (*arrows* in B). (Case courtesy of Ira Tyler, MD, Albert Einstein Medical Center, Bronx, NY.)

pulmonary hypertension. With CT, prominent hila can be shown to be due to enlarged pulmonary arteries; in conjunction with the findings of small-calibered central pulmonary veins, a normal- or small-sized left atrium, and an absence of mediastinal fibrosis, a correct diagnosis of veno-occlusive disease should be suggested.

Involvement of the pulmonary veins with tumor also has been documented both with CT and MR. Although typically the result of direct invasion by bronchogenic carcinoma, occasionally metastatic tumor may extend into the left atrium via the pulmonary veins (Fig. 27).

Congenital Anomalies

A wide range of congenital abnormalities may affect both the main and right and left pulmonary arteries, with and without associated cardiac abnormalities (Fig. 28) (73–75).

The radiologic features of "absence," or agenesis, of a pulmonary artery are frequently characteristic and include a small hemithorax, ipsilateral displacement of the mediastinum, absence of the corresponding pulmonary artery, and reticular densities in the lung, usually attrib-

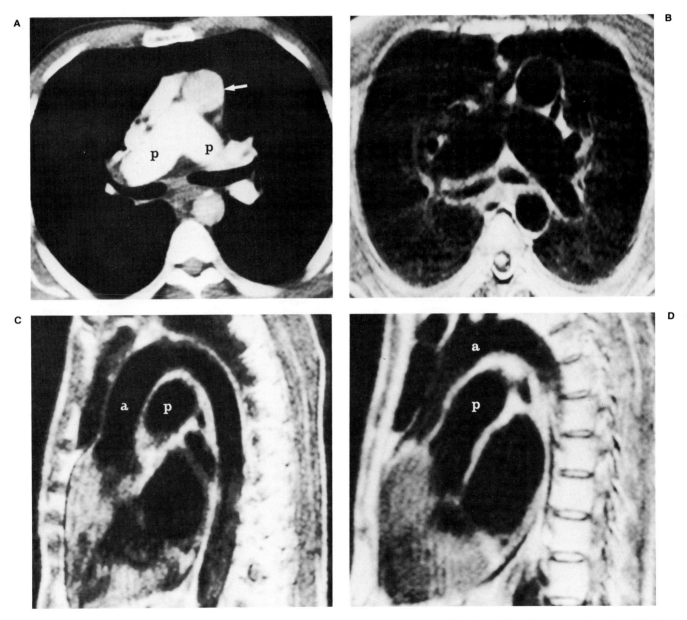

FIG. 28. Corrected L-transposition. **A:** CT section at the level of the right upper lobe bronchus following a bolus of i.v. contrast medium. Both the right and left main pulmonary arteries are dilated and occupy the same axial plane (p's). They are clearly anomalous in position, lying posterior, and slightly to the right of the ascending aorta (*arrow*). **B:** Every-beat gated, axial MR section at the same level as B, showing identical anatomic relationships (compare with B). **C,D:** Every-beat gated, sagittal MR sections through the root of the aorta and origin of the main pulmonary artery, respectively. Note that in both sections the aorta (a's in C and D) lies anterior to the main pulmonary artery (p's) and is related to the anterior ventricle.

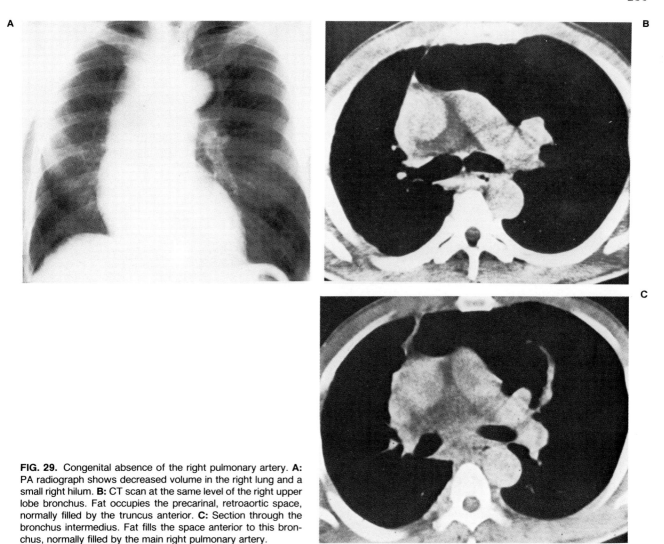

FIG. 29. Congenital absence of the right pulmonary artery. **A:** PA radiograph shows decreased volume in the right lung and a small right hilum. **B:** CT scan at the same level of the right upper lobe bronchus. Fat occupies the precarinal, retroaortic space, normally filled by the truncus anterior. **C:** Section through the bronchus intermedius. Fat fills the space anterior to this bronchus, normally filled by the main right pulmonary artery.

uted to bronchial collateral circulation (Fig. 29). Resulting from embryologic disappearance of the proximal portions of either the right or the left sixth arch, respectively, agenesis of a pulmonary artery may occur either as an isolated event or in association with congenital heart disease, typically tetralogy of Fallot.

Both absent and hypoplastic pulmonary arteries are easily identified with CT (Figs. 29 and 30) (76). In select cases, not only can the diagnosis be established, but additional information concerning the presence and extent of collateral circulation may also be evaluated (Fig. 30).

Anomalies of the right pulmonary artery may be seen in association with the scimitar syndrome, so named for the association of hypoplasia of the right lung with partial anomalous pulmonary venous return, usually to the inferior vena cava (Fig. 31) (25).

Another rare pulmonary arterial anomaly is the pulmonary artery sling, or anomalous left pulmonary artery (77–79). In this condition, an anomalous, retrotracheal left pulmonary artery arises from the extraperi-

cardial segment of the right pulmonary artery and wraps around the junction of the trachea and right main-stem bronchus to pass in front of the esophagus on its way to the left lung (Fig. 32). En route the anomalous artery may cause compression of the right main-stem bronchus and result in chronic stridor. In these cases, respiratory symptoms may be dramatically relieved by surgical repair of the anomalous artery. Berden et al. (79) have coined the term "ring-sling complex" to describe the association of an aberrant left pulmonary artery with diffuse long segment tracheal stenosis. In these cases, tracheal stenosis is due to complete cartilage rings with absence of any significant pars membranacea. Unlike cases of isolated aberrant left pulmonary arteries, in cases with the ring-sling complex, repair of the anomalous pulmonary artery does not lead to symptomatic relief of stridor.

Identification of anomalies of the pulmonary arteries is especially important in the evaluation of patients with cyanotic congenital heart disease (80,81). In these cases,

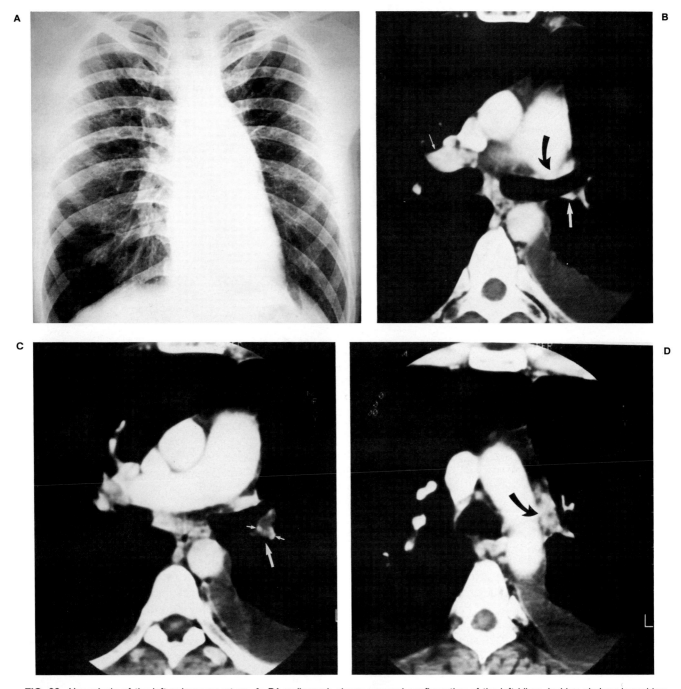

FIG. 30. Hypoplasia of the left pulmonary artery. **A:** PA radiograph shows unusual configuration of the left hilum, lacking obvious branching vessels. **B,C:** Enlargements of sections through the main and right pulmonary arteries, respectively. Note marked narrowing of the origin of the left main pulmonary artery (*curved arrow* in B) and absence of a definable left interlobar pulmonary artery in its normal location behind the left upper lobe bronchus (*straight arrows* in B and C). The right main pulmonary artery and truncus anterior (*small straight arrow* in B) are enlarged. **D:** Section at the level of the aortic arch. There are numerous small opacifying vessels (*curved arrow* in D) in the anterior mediastinum to the left of the aortic arch. These presumably represent enlarged bronchial collaterals, probably present in the left hilum as well (see *small arrows* in C). (Case courtesy of Sam Berenbaum, M.D., New York, NY.)

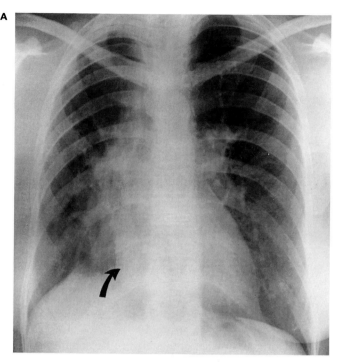

FIG. 31. Scimitar (hypogenetic lung) syndrome. **A:** Postero-anterior chest radiograph shows volume loss on the right side, with shift of the heart and mediastinum. An ill-defined linear density is apparent in the right lower lobe, medially, suggesting aberrant venous drainage (*arrow*). **B–D:** Every-beat gated axial images through the carina, and the mid and lower thorax, respectively. Marked volume loss is apparent on the right. The right main pulmonary artery is well defined and normal in caliber (*arrow* in B). The right inferior pulmonary vein cannot be identified in its normal location (compare with the normal left inferior pulmonary vein, *arrow* in C). Instead, there is anomalous drainage of the right inferior pulmonary vein into the inferior vena cava (*arrow* in D). **E:** CT scan through the right lower lobe, imaged with lung windows, shows enlarged inferior pulmonary veins coalescing within the right lower lobe (*arrow* in E). Note that these are easily defined with CT, unlike MR (compare with C). (From Naidich et al., ref. 25.)

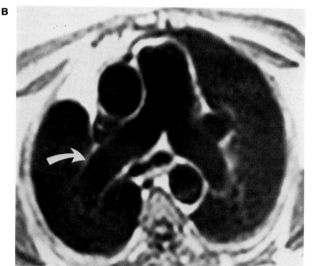

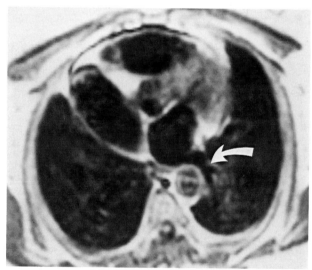

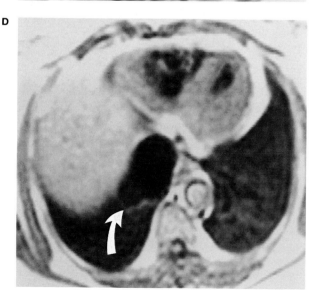

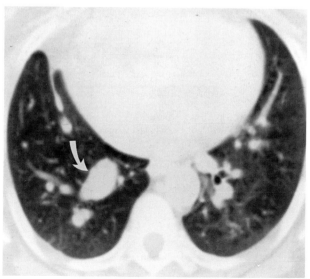

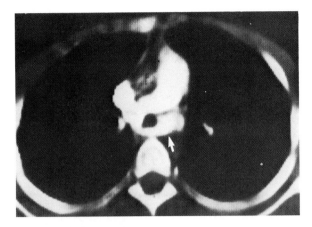

FIG. 32. Anomalous left pulmonary artery. Contrast-enhanced scan outlining the anomalous course of the left pulmonary artery swinging behind the trachea to reach the left hilum (*arrow*). (From Moncado et al., ref. 78, with permission.)

information concerning the presence and size of the pulmonary arteries is frequently of vital importance in determining operative strategy. As discussed in greater de-

tail in Chapter 11, both CT and MR in particular play a particularly valuable role in both the initial and follow-up assessments of patients receiving palliative systemic-pulmonary artery shunts (81).

HILAR MASSES

CT Evaluation

CT is extremely accurate in the detection of hilar masses and adenopathy (82–84). As a practical matter, hilar pathology is most easily evaluated using dynamic incremental scanning following a bolus of i.v. contrast media (Figs. 1, 2, and 4). By densely opacifying vessels, enlarged lymph nodes and masses stand out in stark contrast, greatly simplifying interpretation (Figs. 20 and 21).

Despite the advantages of i.v. contrast administration, however, detailed knowledge of cross-sectional hilar anatomy is still requisite. In cases in which i.v. contrast cannot be utilized or in which contrast administration is

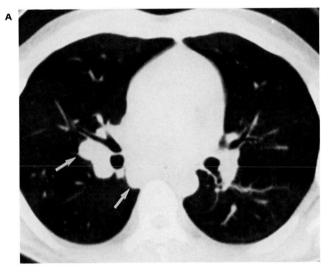

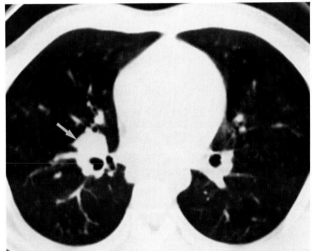

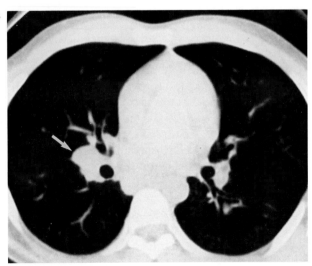

FIG. 33. Hilar adenopathy: sarcoidosis. **A–C:** Sequential images through hila, from above down. At each level, bilaterally enlarged lymph nodes can be identified, without the use of i.v. contrast medium. The key to identification of adenopathy is the change in the normal contour of the lung/hilum interface (*arrows*). Such alterations are easiest to identify when sections are obtained through characteristic levels, as shown in Fig. 3.

A

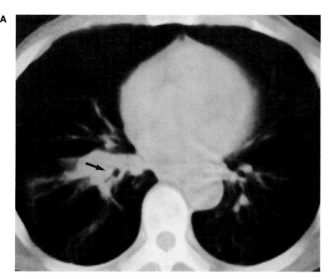
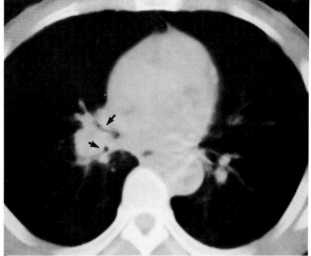

B

FIG. 34. Metastatic renal cell carcinoma. **A,B:** Sequential sections through the hila obtained in a patient with known renal cell carcinoma. Intravenous contrast could not be administered due to renal failure. In this case, alterations in the normal appearance of the airways (*arrows*) allowed confident diagnosis of tumor, subsequently confirmed bronchoscopically.

suboptimal, interpretation based on anatomic alterations is still of enormous value. The same criteria applicable in the interpretation of routine tomography [both anteroposterior (AP) and 55° oblique hilar tomography] apply as well in CT (85–88). The criteria are as follows: generalized hilar enlargement; focal hilar enlargement (focal hilar mass); compression, displacement, and/or infiltration of the bronchial tree; and nodularity in the contour of the hilum, usually indicating hilar lymph node enlargement.

In our experience, most abnormalities may be detected either as a consequence of distortion of the general configuration of the hilum (i.e., a change in the nature of the lung/hilum interface) (Fig. 33) or of alterations in the bronchial tree (Fig. 34). In both cases, as previously emphasized, the emphasis is on visualization of structures and/or interfaces that are best seen with wide windows. Bronchial alterations, in particular, may be exceedingly subtle and may represent the only clear abnormality in an otherwise normal-appearing hilum. Especially significant are abrupt changes in the overall caliber of the bronchial tree, which may be indicative of diffuse, circumferential, submucosal tumor infiltration.

Identification of bronchial pathology may be of value in determining the best diagnostic approach to hilar masses. In patients in whom no significant alteration in the airways can be identified, CT-guided transthoracic needle aspiration may be preferred. As reported by Sider and David (89), in their evaluation of CT-guided transthoracic needle biopsies in 20 patients with hilar masses following nondiagnostic bronchoscopies, a cytological diagnosis of cancer was obtained using a 22-gauge needle in 19 of 20 (95%) cases. Similar results detailing transthoracic needle biopsy of the hila have been re-

ported (90–92). Visualization of bronchial pathology is also an important component in the assessment of patients with hilar masses causing segmental or lobar collapse. In these cases, identification of abnormal airways may be of diagnostic value in determining the etiology of collapse, especially in patients in whom clear differentiation of a mass or tumor cannot be visualized following i.v. contrast (93–95).

Hilar Adenopathy

CT is efficacious in defining the presence and extent of tumor involvement in the pulmonary hila and mediastinum. Although differentiation between mass per se and massively enlarged, tumor-filled hilar lymph nodes may be problematic, in most cases the significance of this differentiation is of little consequence (Fig. 20).

Of greater clinical concern is the value of CT in identifying the presence of diffuse, or generalized, hilar adenopathy. Differentiation between pulmonary vascular "prominence" and adenopathy probably accounts, more than any other indication, for the necessity of further study of the hila beyond routine radiographs.

The hallmark of hilar adenopathy on CT is the finding of nodularity in the contour of the hilum (Fig. 33). Confirmation of the presence of adenopathy is easily obtained following i.v. contrast administration (Figs. 1 and 4).

Adenopathy need not be apparent on plain radiographs to be easily visualized with CT, especially unsuspected posterior hilar adenopathy. This is because the posterior hilar/lung interface seen in cross-section is especially characteristic (Fig. 4). Alterations in this portion of the hila, such as, for example, effacement of the posterior wall of the right upper lobe bronchus, the bronchus intermedius, or obliteration of the azygoesophageal recess or the left retrobronchial stripe, may be exceedingly subtle yet still distinctive when seen in cross-section. Additionally, posterior hilar adenopathy does not distort the lateral margin of the hila and, hence, is usually not definable on either PA or lateral radiographs. Significantly, adenopathy restricted to the anterior portions of the hila is more difficult to define than are posterior nodes, especially without i.v. contrast, because the pulmonary/hilar interface anteriorly is somewhat less characteristic than these same interfaces posteriorly (Fig. 4) (1,2).

A standard nomenclature for regional lymph nodes, including hilar nodes, has been proposed by the American Thoracic Society for the purpose of staging lung cancer (96). As discussed in greater detail in Chapter 6, right hilar nodes are now included in the right tracheobronchial lymph node grouping (10R), whereas left hilar nodes are included in the left peribronchial grouping (10L). The use of a standard nomenclature for lung cancer staging clearly should be encouraged.

In select cases, the appearance of hilar nodes is sufficiently characteristic to suggest the appropriate diagnosis. Tuberculous lymphadenopathy, in particular, has been noted to have a suggestive appearance (97,98). Following i.v. contrast administration, acutely enlarged, tuberculous lymph nodes frequently show evidence of low central density (Fig. 35). This appearance has been reported in patients with metastatic nodes—in particular, in patients with testicular carcinoma—but it is a less common cause than tuberculous adenitis (99). In our experience, low-density nodes have been an especially common finding in tuberculous patients with acquired immune deficiency syndromes (AIDS). Although other fungal infections, such as cryptococcus, may also have a similar appearance, especially in this population, only rarely are low-density lymph nodes encountered in AIDS patients either with Kaposi's sarcoma or with lymphoma.

The diagnosis of tuberculous hilar lymphadenopathy is further suggested when hilar nodes are seen to cavitate. As shown in Fig. 36, the finding of cavitated hilar nodes associated with acinar lung disease is particularly characteristic.

Calcification within hilar and mediastinal nodes is easily identified with CT and, as has been discussed, represents a significant advantage of CT compared with MR in evaluating the hila. Occasionally, the pattern of calcification within nodes is characteristic. In particular, the finding of peripheral calcification, so-called eggshell calcification, commonly occurs in patients with silicosis, coal-worker's pneumoconiosis, sarcoidosis, postirradiation Hodgkin's disease, and granulomatous infections such as histoplasmosis and blastomycosis (100). Less

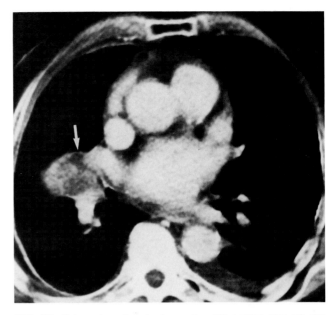

FIG. 35. Tuberculous lymphadenopathy. CT section through the right hilum at the level of the origin of the middle lobe bronchus following a bolus of contrast medium. Massively enlarged, low-density lymph nodes are present in the right hilum (*arrow*). A small left-sided pleural effusion is present as well. Although nonspecific, in the proper clinical setting, enlarged, low-density nodes, either hilar or mediastinal, should suggest the diagnosis of possible tuberculous adenopathy.

frequent causes include scleroderma and amyloid. As shown in Fig. 37, identification of this distinctive pattern is greatly facilitated by CT.

In addition to the value of CT in detecting adenopathy, CT occasionally can be used to differentiate "ordinary" from "vascular" lymph nodes (101). In select cases, this may suggest a specific diagnosis (Fig. 38) (102). It should be emphasized that the distribution of i.v. contrast medium within tumors, in particular, is a reflection of several parameters, including blood flow, total quantity and concentration of contrast medium, distribution between the vascular and extravascular spaces, and renal function. These matters are considered in detail in Chapter 1. Marked enhancement of lymph nodes following i.v. contrast medium administration has been noted in a variety of tumors, including hypervascular lymph nodes in cases of small cell carcinoma of the lung, vascular metastases from renal cell and papillary thyroid carcinoma, as well as in patients with angio-immunoblastic lymphadenopathy viral infections, vaccinations, and even drug reactions (102). A similar appearance of enhancing lymph nodes has been described in Castleman's disease as well (103).

Although the appearance of nodes in select cases may be diagnostic, it must be emphasized that in most cases, hilar nodes are nonspecific in appearance. CT is essentially an anatomic imaging modality; it is usually impossible to differentiate inflammatory, reactive adenopathy from other causes of enlarged nodes, specifically tumor.

A

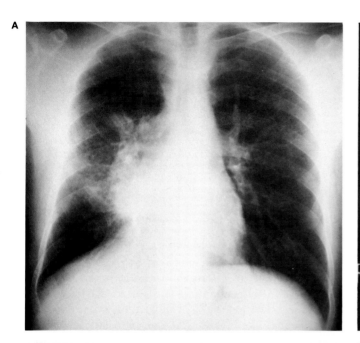

C

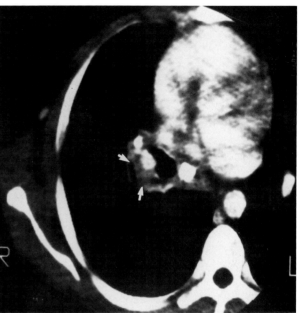

B

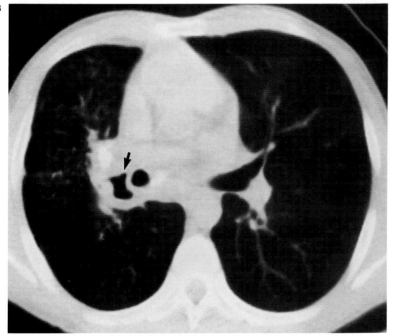

FIG. 36. Tuberculous lymphadenopathy. **A:** PA radiograph shows markedly enlarged right hilum, associated with an infiltrate in the right mid lung field. **B:** Enlargement of a section through the right hilum, following a bolus of i.v. contrast medium. A calcified lymph node is present adjacent to the origin of the right lower lobe bronchus, medially. Laterally, confluent, low-density lymph nodes can be defined, easily separable from the hilar vessels (*arrow*). **C:** CT section at the level of the bronchus intermedius shows both calcification and cavitation of lymph nodes in the right hilum (*arrows*) not apparent on the PA chest radiograph (compare with A). Note that within the right lung anteriorly, numerous poorly defined, airspace nodules can be defined, characteristic of acinar TB. In this case, cavitation of tuberculous hilar nodes led to endobronchial spread of TB preferentially into the anterior segment of the right upper lobe.

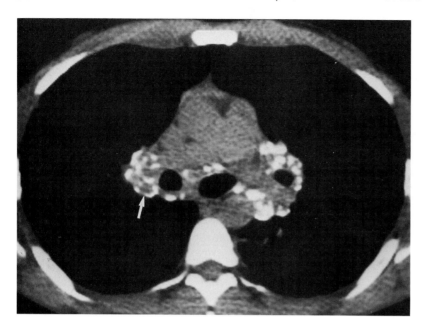

FIG. 37. Eggshell calcification: sarcoidosis. CT section at the level of the bronchus intermedius in a patient with documented sarcoidosis, imaged with narrow windows. Note the extensively calcified hilar and subcarinal lymph nodes, many of which have a distinctly peripheral or circular pattern (*arrow*).

As nodes as small as 3 mm may be defined routinely with bolus technique, interpretation, especially in an older population of patients, can be problematic (Fig. 1). Clearly, detection of hilar lymphadenopathy per se is of limited value without careful clinical correlation.

As a practical matter, how do we define "significant" adenopathy? In our experience, nodes should be considered significant in a routine setting if adenopathy is sufficiently large to deform or distort the contour of the lung/hilar interface. In general, this corresponds to lymph nodes that are at least 1–1.5 cm in size. Designating nodes of this size as abnormal is in keeping with

most reports of established criteria for significant mediastinal adenopathy (see Chapter 6), considering that the range in size of normal hilar nodes is usually considered slightly greater than that for mediastinal nodes. This size criterion is also of value in the interpretation of MR scans. Although the presence of foci of intermediate signal intensity may be anticipated even within normal hila, as already discussed, these are rarely greater than 1 cm in size.

Despite the clinical utility of the criteria outlined above for differentiating normal from abnormal hilar nodes, it cannot be overemphasized that any definition that depends on the size of lymph nodes is intentionally "practicable" and subject to limitations. The significance of hilar nodes can only be interpreted with reference to the clinical history; absolute verification of the significance of any size lymph node ultimately requires histologic correlation.

CT/MR Correlations

Numerous studies have compared the efficacy of CT with MR in evaluating the pulmonary hila, especially in patients with bronchogenic carcinoma. As a general rule, the two modalities are similar in their abilities to detect significant pathology (Fig. 39) (104–112).

In their analysis of 44 patients with bronchogenic carcinoma prospectively evaluated with both CT and MR, Musset et al. (112) found no statistical difference between the two imaging modalities in the evaluation of either tumor extent or node involvement. Levitt et al. (107), in a comparison of CT and MR of both the mediastinum and hila in the staging of 37 patients with lung cancer, found that CT staged 35 of 37 cases appropri-

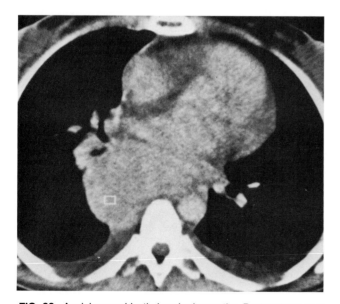

FIG. 38. Angioimmunoblastic lymphadenopathy. Postcontrast scan at level of the middle lobe bronchus. Massive adenopathy is present, showing significant contrast enhancement (compare, visually, the density of these nodes with the superior vena cava).

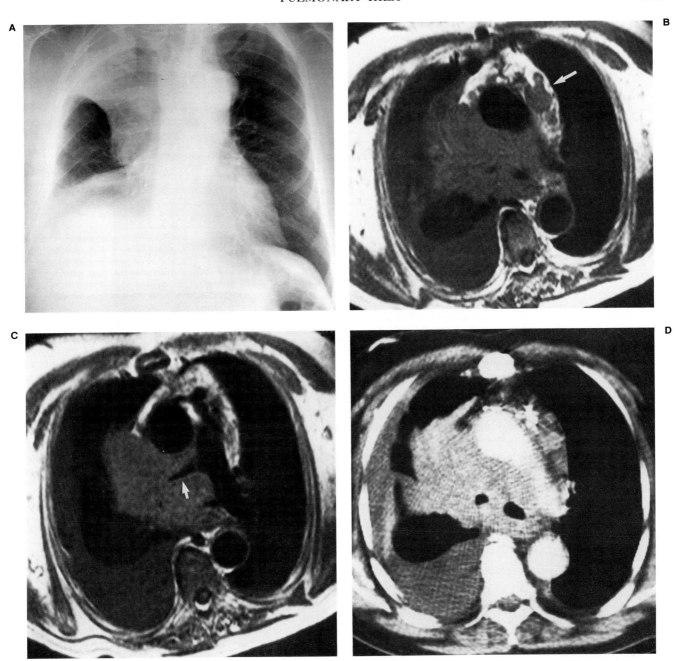

FIG. 39(A–D). Bronchogenic carcinoma: right upper lobe collapse. **A:** PA radiograph shows collapse of the right upper lobe. **B,C:** Every-beat gated, axial SE MR scans at the level of the aorticopulmonary window and the right main pulmonary artery, respectively. Extensive tumor can be identified in the right hilum, directly invading the mediastinum. The right main pulmonary artery is encased (*arrow* in C), and the right and left main-stem bronchi are narrowed. Extensive prevascular lymphadenopathy can be identified (*arrow* in B), as well as a large right-sided pleural effusion. **D:** Contrast-enhanced CT scan at the same level as B, showing identical findings.

ately, whereas MR correctly staged 36 of 37 cases. Glazer et al. (108), in a prospective study comparing 55° oblique tomography, dynamic CT, and MR in evaluating the pulmonary hila in 19 patients with lung cancer in whom surgical confirmation was available, found no significant differences between these modalities in overall accuracy. Although CT and MR were found to be significantly more sensitive than 55° oblique tomography in detecting involved nodes, both CT and MR

proved to have relatively low specificity, due to detection of minimally enlarged, subsequently surgically confirmed benign hilar nodes. On the basis of this data, it was concluded by these investigators that MR, CT, and routine tomography all are incapable of accurately staging the hila in patients with lung cancer, primarily due to low specificity.

As compared with dynamic CT, MR suffers two distinct disadvantages in evaluating the pulmonary hila.

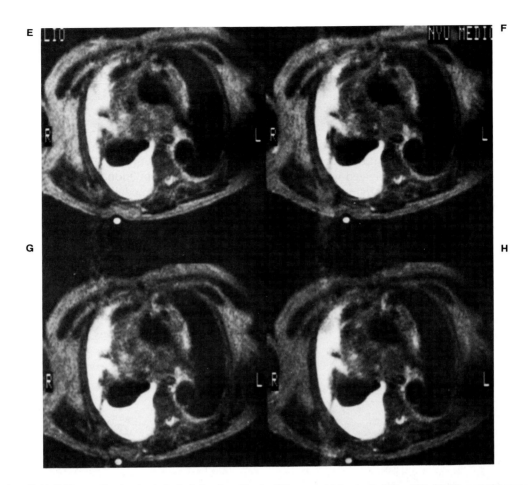

FIG. 39. (*Continued*) **E–H:** Every-other beat gated, single-level, multi-echo SE scans obtained with TE's of 30, 60, 90, and 120 msec, respectively. This sequence was utilized to ensure heavy T2-weighting. Note the marked increase in signal associated with fluid in the pleural space (compare with B and C). In this case, despite heavily T2-weighted imaging, no clear distinction can be made between central obstructing tumor and peripheral collapsed lung.

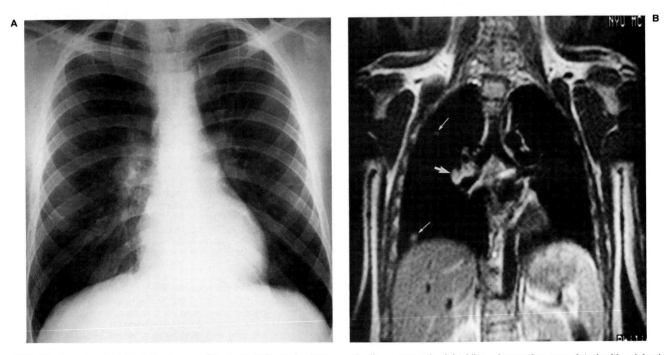

FIG. 40. Sarcoidosis: MR evaluation. **A:** PA chest radiograph shows markedly asymmetric right hilar adenopathy, associated with minimal widening of the mediastinum, and normal-appearing parenchyma. **B:** Every-beat gated, coronal MR scan through the carina shows characteristic appearance of enlarged hilar lymph nodes, identifiable as foci of intermediate signal within the region of the hilum (*arrow*). The left hilum is normal, without identifiable signal. Two discrete pulmonary nodules can be seen in the right lung (*small arrows*), which even retrospectively cannot be identified on the PA radiograph obtained the same day. These findings are nonspecific. In this case, a transbronchial biopsy proved negative, necessitating a diagnostic thoracotomy.

First, as previously noted, calcification within nodes usually cannot be detected with MR. This is of obvious significance in attempting to differentiate benign from malignant nodes or when evaluating such diseases as fibrosing mediastinitis (Fig. 23).

Second, because of decreased spatial resolution, small, adjacent lymph nodes, easily identified separately by CT, may appear conglomerately enlarged with MR. MR also is clearly inferior to CT in identifying bronchial abnormalities. As has been repeatedly stressed, this is an especially important component of hilar evaluation. Mayr et al. (113), in an evaluation of 29 patients suspected of having an endobronchial mass, evaluated with both CT and MR, found that only ∼70% of pathologically confirmed abnormal airways and in 45% of normal airways could be accurately identified with MR, as compared with the nearly 100% accuracy of CT (113). Similar limitations also have been reported by Webb et al. (111).

Which modality should be utilized—CT or MR? In our judgment, this decision ideally should be individualized. As previously discussed, unfortunately, in most cases neither CT nor MR provides tissue-specific diagnoses (Fig. 40). Consequently, given differences in cost and availability, as well as limitations in the detection of calcification and bronchial abnormalities, for routine evaluation of the pulmonary hila, at present, CT remains the imaging modality of choice.

What indications are there for the use of MR? MR is clearly superior to non–contrast-enhanced CT scans for evaluating the pulmonary hila. Additionally, due to its superior delineation of both hilar and mediastinal vessels, as well as cardiac structures, MR should be considered superior to CT in the evaluation of patients suspected of both congenital and acquired pulmonary vascular disease. MR may also be superior in evaluating suspected cystic abnormalities such as bronchogenic cysts and central mucoid impaction (Fig. 41) (25,114).

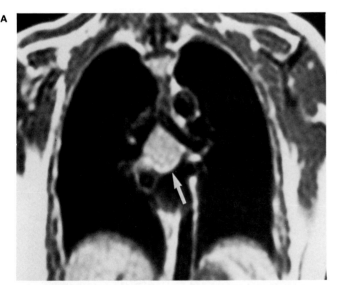

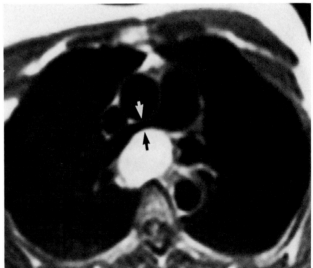

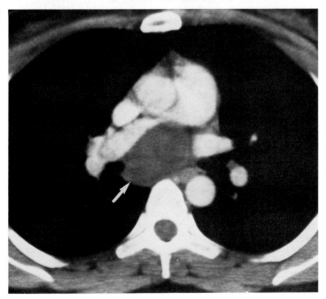

FIG. 41. Bronchogenic cyst. **A:** Every-beat gated, coronal MR scan through the carina. There is a well-defined, rounded mass in the subcarinal space, within which intermediate signal can be identified (*arrow*). In this case, MR was obtained to evaluate a patient complaining of increasingly severe dyspnea with a normal chest radiograph (not shown). A marked decrease in both ventilation and perfusion were subsequently noted on nuclear medicine scans. **B:** Every-other beat ECG-gated axial SE scan obtained at the level of the right main pulmonary artery. A subcarinal mass is present, within which considerable signal can be identified uniformly, characteristic of a fluid-containing mass. Note that the mass is causing considerable extrinsic compression of the right main pulmonary artery (*arrows* in B). These findings taken together are diagnostic of a subcarinal bronchogenic cyst. The intermediate signal observed within the cyst on the T1-weighted coronal scan reflects elevated protein content within the cyst fluid, which proved to be hemorrhagic at surgery. **C:** CT scan obtained at the same level as B, following a bolus of i.v. contrast. A large, fluid-filled mass is present in the subcarinal space, causing marked compression of the adjacent right main pulmonary artery. Although bronchogenic cysts frequently have densities higher than water on nonenhanced CT scans, a definite diagnosis usually can be established with a carefully performed study utilizing i.v. contrast if it can be demonstrated that there is virtually no evidence of enhancement.

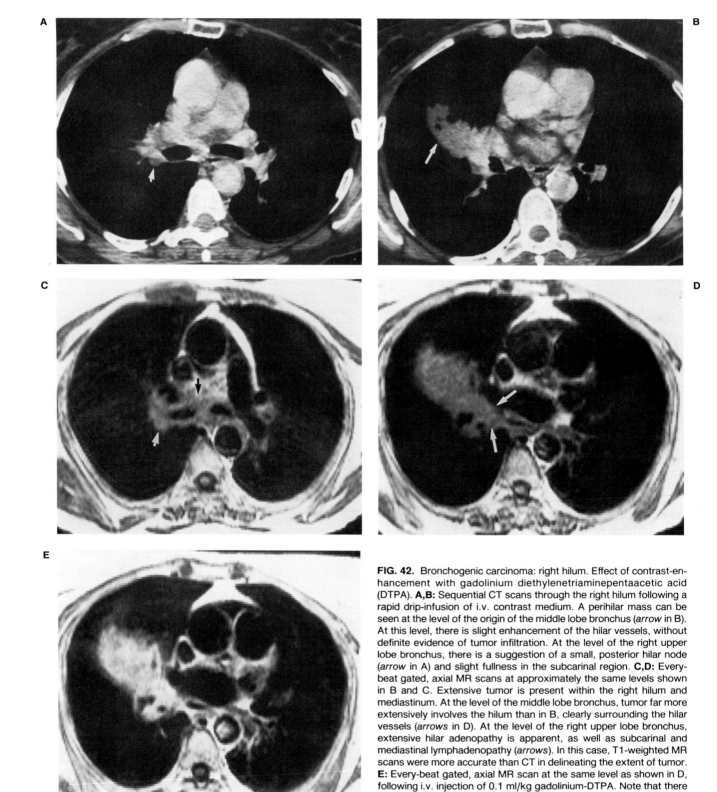

FIG. 42. Bronchogenic carcinoma: right hilum. Effect of contrast-en-hancement with gadolinium diethylenetriaminepentaacetic acid (DTPA). **A,B:** Sequential CT scans through the right hilum following a rapid drip-infusion of i.v. contrast medium. A perihilar mass can be seen at the level of the origin of the middle lobe bronchus (*arrow* in B). At this level, there is slight enhancement of the hilar vessels, without definite evidence of tumor infiltration. At the level of the right upper lobe bronchus, there is a suggestion of a small, posterior hilar node (*arrow* in A) and slight fullness in the subcarinal region. **C,D:** Every-beat gated, axial MR scans at approximately the same levels shown in B and C. Extensive tumor is present within the right hilum and mediastinum. At the level of the middle lobe bronchus, tumor far more extensively involves the hilum than in B, clearly surrounding the hilar vessels (*arrows* in D). At the level of the right upper lobe bronchus, extensive hilar adenopathy is apparent, as well as subcarinal and mediastinal lymphadenopathy (*arrows*). In this case, T1-weighted MR scans were more accurate than CT in delineating the extent of tumor. **E:** Every-beat gated, axial MR scan at the same level as shown in D, following i.v. injection of 0.1 ml/kg gadolinium-DTPA. Note that there is considerable increase in the amount of signal present within the tumor as compared to D, consequent to the T1 shortening effect of gadolinium.

Although contrast-enhanced CT scans remain the standard, it should be emphasized, that unlike CT, technological improvements in MR continue to evolve at a rapid pace. This includes significant evolution in the development of MR-specific contrast agents (Fig. 42) (115). It may be anticipated that in the foreseeable future, indications for the use of MR will continue to expand.

Invariably, any discussion of CT of the pulmonary hila raises questions about the efficacy of both CT and MR as compared to routine tomography (both AP and 55° oblique). Although initial comparisons were critical of CT, these studies are generally invalid, since many of them were performed with older units (frequently with 18-sec scan times) and, more important, were conducted prior to detailed anatomic evaluation of normal cross-sectional hilar anatomy (116–121).

In our opinion, whatever the limitations of CT and MR as compared with routine tomography, these are more than compensated for by the exquisite depiction of normal hilar anatomy and the correspondingly high sensitivity of both these modalities for detecting hilar pathology. The ability to visualize the hilum without intervening or superimposed structures allows precise visualization and evaluation of structures that previously were difficult to assess. There is little comparison between routine tomography and either CT or MR in the degree of certainty with which subtle alterations within the hila can be analyzed.

As importantly, compared with routine tomography, both CT and MR have the inherent advantage that every image provides detailed information about the entire thorax, with equivalent clarity. This frequently provides critical information that otherwise might have been overlooked, allowing a more refined and definitive evaluation of hilar pathology, as well as providing an important advantage in determining the best diagnostic approach for patients requiring a tissue diagnosis.

Finally, although routine tissue characterization is not possible, at least in select cases both CT and MR can provide histologically specific diagnoses, generally not obtainable with routine tomography, by means either of differential density measurements or characteristic changes in relative signal intensities identified (Fig. 41).

REFERENCES

1. Naidich DP, Khouri NF, Scott WW, Wang KP, Siegelman SS. Computed tomography of the pulmonary hila: 1. Normal anatomy. *J Comput Assist Tomogr* 1981;5:459–467.
2. Naidich DP, Khouri NF, Stitik FP, McCauley DI, Siegelman SS. Computed tomography of the pulmanary hila: 2. Abnormal anatomy. *J Comput Assist Tomogr* 1981;5:468–475.
3. Webb WR, Glazer F, Gamsu G. Computed tomography of the normal pulmonary hilum. *J Comput Assist Tomogr* 1981;5:476–484.
4. Webb WR, Gamsu G, Glazer G. Computed tomography of the abnormal pulmonary hilum. *J Comput Assist Tomogr* 1981;5:485–490.
5. Jardin M, Remy J. Segmental bronchovascular anatomy of the lower lobes: CT analysis. *Radiology* 1986;147:457–468.
6. Naidich DP, Terry PB, Stitik FP, Siegelman SS. Computed tomography of the bronchi: 1. Normal anatomy. *J Comput Assist Tomogr* 1980;4:746–753.
7. Yamashita H. *Roentgenologic anatomy of the lung.* Tokyo: Igaku-Shoin, 1978.
8. Glazer G, Francis IR, Gebarski K, Samuels BI, Sorensen KW. Dynamic incremental computed tomography in evaluation of the pulmonary hila. *J Comput Assist Tomogr* 1983;7:59–64.
9. Godwin JD, Webb RW. Dynamic computed tomography in the evaluation of vascular lung lesions. *Radiology* 1981;138:629–635.
10. Shepard JO, Dedrick CG, Spizarny DL, McLoud TC. Technical note. Dynamic incremental computed tomography of the pulmonary hila using a flow-rate injector. *J Comput Assist Tomogr* 1986;10:369–371.
11. Price DB, Nardi P, Teitcher J. Venous air embolization as a complication of pressure injection of contrast media: CT findings. *J Comput Assist Tomogr* 1987;11:294–295.
12. Furuse M, Saito K, Kunieda E, Aihara T, Touei H, Ohara T, Fukushima K. Bronchial arteries: CT demonstration with arteriographic correlation. *Radiology* 1987;162:393–398.
13. Axel L, Kressel HY, Thickman D, Epstein DM, Edelstein W, Bottomley P, Redington R, Baum S. NMR imaging of the chest at 0.12 T: initial clinical experience with a resistive magnet. *AJR* 1983;141:1157–1162.
14. Cohen AM, Creviston S, LiPuma JP, Bryan PJ, Lieberman J, Haaga JR, Alfidi RJ. Nuclear magnetic resonance imaging of the mediastinum and hili: early impressions of its efficacy. *AJR* 1983;141:1163–1169.
15. Webb WR, Gamsu G, Stark DD, Moore EH. Magnetic resonance imaging of the normal and abnormal pulmonary hila. *Radiology* 1984;152:89–94.
16. Webb WR, Jensen BG, Gamsu G, Sollitto R, Moore EH. Coronal magnetic resonance imaging of the chest: normal and abnormal. *Radiology* 1984;153:729–735.
17. O'Donovan PB, Ross JS, Sivak ED, O'Donnell JK, Meaney TF. Pictorial essay. Magnetic resonance imaging of the thorax: the advantages of coronal and sagittal planes. *AJR* 1984;143:1183–1188.
18. Webb WR, Gamsu G, Crooks LE. Multisection sagittal and coronal magnetic resonance imaging of the mediastinum and hila. Work in progress. *Radiology* 1984;150:475–478.
19. Webb WR, Jensen BG, Gamsu G, Sollitto R, Moore EH. Sagittal MR imaging of the chest: normal and abnormal. *J Comput Assist Tomogr* 1985;9:471–479.
20. Batra P, Brown K, Steckel RJ, Collins JD, Ovenfors CO, Aberle D. MR imaging of the thorax: a comparison of axial, coronal, and sagittal imaging planes. *J Comput Assist Tomogr* 1988;12:75–81.
21. Westcott JL, Henschke CI, Berkmen Y. MR imaging of the hilum and mediastinum: effects of cardiac gating. *J Comput Assist Tomogr* 1985;9:1073–1078.
22. Mazer MJ, Carroll FE, Falke THM. Practical aspects of gated magnetic resonance imaging of the pulmonary artery. *J Thorac Imaging* 1988;3:73–84.
23. Ehman RL, McNamara MT, Pallack M, Hricak H, Higgins CB. Magnetic resonance imaging with respiratory gating: techniques and advantages. *AJR* 1984;143:1175–1182.
24. Crooks LE, Barker B, Chang H, et al. Magnetic resonance imaging strategies for heart studies. *Radiology* 1984;154:459–465.
25. Naidich DP, Rumancik WM, Ettenger NA, Feiner HD, Schulman MH, Spatz EM, Toder ST, Genieser NB. Congenital anomalies of the lungs in adults: MR diagnosis. *AJR* 1988;151:13–19.
26. Posteraro RH, Sostman HD, Spritzer CE, Herfkens RJ. Cine-gradient-refocused MR imaging of central pulmonary emboli. *AJR* 1989;152:465–468.
27. Webb WR, Gamsu G. Computed tomography of the left retrobronchial stripe. *J Comput Assist Tomogr* 1983;7:65–69.
28. Ashida C, Zerhouni EA, Fishman EK. CT demonstration of prominent right hilar soft tissue collections. *J Comput Assist Tomogr* 1987;11:57–59.
29. Bush A, Gray H, Denison DM. Diagnosis of pulmonary artery hypertension from radiographic estimates of pulmonary arterial size. *Thorax* 1988;43:127–131.

30. O'Callaghan JP, Heitzman ER, Somogyi JW, Spirty BA. CT evaluation of pulmonary artery size. *J Comput Assist Tomogr* 1982;6:101–104.

31. Kuriyama K, Gamsu G, Stern RG, Cann CE, Herfkens RJ, Brundage BH. CT-determined pulmonary artery diameters in predicting pulmonary hypertension. *Invest Radiol* 1984;19:16–22.

32. Mencini RA, Proto AV. The high left and main pulmonary arteries: a CT pitfall. *J Comput Assist Tomogr* 1982;6:452–459.

33. von Schulthess GD, Fisher MR, Higgins CB. Pathologic blood flow in pulmonary vascular disease as shown by gated magnetic resonance imaging. *Ann Intern Med* 1985;103:317–323.

34. Bouchard A, Higgins CB, Byrd B, Amparo EG, Osaki L, Axelrod R. Magnetic resonance imaging in pulmonary artery hypertension. *Am J Cardiol* 1985;56:938–942.

35. White RD, Winkler ML, Higgins CB. MR imaging of pulmonary arterial hypertension and pulmonary emboli. *AJR* 1987;149:15–21.

36. Bartter T, Irwin RS, Nash G. Review. Aneurysms of the pulmonary arteries. *Chest* 1988;94:1065–1079.

37. Butto F, Lucas RV, Edwards JE. Pulmonary arterial aneurysm. A pathologic study of five cases. *Chest* 1987;91:237–241.

38. SanDretto MA, Scanlon GT. Multiple mycotic pulmonary artery aneurysms secondary to intravenous drug use. *AJR* 1984;143:89–90.

39. Shin MS, Ceballos R, Bini RM, Ho KJ. Case report. CT diagnosis of false aneurysm of the pulmonary artery not demonstrated by angiography. *J Comput Assist Tomogr* 1983;7:524–526.

40. Daykin EL, Irwin GAL, Harrison DA. Case report. CT demonstration of a traumatic aneurysm of the pulmonary artery. *J Comput Assist Tomogr* 1986;10:323–324.

41. Jeang MK, Adyanthaya A, Kuo L, Schweppe I, Hallman G, Adams P. Multiple pulmonary artery aneurysms. New use for magnetic resonance imaging. *Am J Med* 1986;81:1001–1004.

42. Dunnick NR, Doppman JL, Pevsner PH. Failure of computer assisted tomography to detect experimental acute obstruction of major pulmonary arteries. *J Comput Assist Tomogr* 1977;1:330–332.

43. Sinner WN. Computed tomographic patterns of pulmonary thromboembolism and infarction. *J Comput Assist Tomogr* 1978;2:395–399.

44. Overfors C-O, Godwin JD, Brito BS. Diagnosis of peripheral pulmonary emboli by computed tomography in the living dog. Work in progress. *Radiology* 1981;141:519–523.

45. Lourie GL, Pizzo SV, Ravin C, Putnam C, Thompson WM. Experimental pulmonary infarction in dogs. A comparison of chest radiography and computed tomography. *Invest Radiol* 1982;17:224–232.

46. Godwin JD, Webb WR, Gamsu G, Overfors C-O. Computed tomography of pulmonary embolism. *AJR* 1980;135:691–695.

47. Chintapalli K, Thorsen MK, Olson DL, Goodman LR, Gurney J. Computed tomography of pulmonary thromboembolism and infarction. *J Comput Assist Tomogr* 1988;12:553–559.

48. Breatnach E, Stanley R. Case report. CT diagnosis of segmental pulmonary artery embolus. *J Comput Assist Tomogr* 1984;8:762–764.

49. Pope CF, Sostman D, Carbo P, Gore JC, Holcomb W. The detection of pulmonary emboli by magnetic resonance imaging. Evaluation of imaging parameters. *Invest Radiol* 1987;22:937–946.

50. Gamsu G, Hirji M, Moore EH, Webb WR, Brito A. Experimental pulmonary emboli detected using magnetic resonance. *Radiology* 1984;153:467–470.

51. Moore EH, Gamsu G, Webb WR, Stulbarg MS. Pulmonary embolus: detection and follow-up using magnetic resonance. *Radiology* 1984;153:471–472.

52. Thickman D, Kressel HY, Axel L. Demonstration of pulmonary embolism by magnetic resonance imaging. *AJR* 1984;142:921–922.

53. Stein MG, Crues JV, Bradley WG, et al. MR imaging of pulmonary emboli; an experimental study in dogs. *AJR* 1986;147:1133–1137.

54. Fisher MR, Higgins CB. Central thrombi in pulmonary arterial hypertension detected by MR imaging. *Radiology* 1986;158:223–226.

55. Brasch RC, Gooding CA, Lallemand DP, Wesbey GE. Magnetic resonance imaging of the thorax in childhood. *Radiology* 1984;150:463–467.

56. Bleisch VR, Kraus FT. Polypoid sarcoma of the pulmonary trunk: analysis of the literature and report of a case with leptomeric organelles and ultrastructural features of rhabdomyosarcoma. *Cancer* 1980;46:314–324.

57. Olsson HE, Spitzer RM, Erston WF. Primary and secondary pulmonary artery neoplasia mimicking acute pulmonary embolism. *Radiology* 1976;118:49–53.

58. Chul B, Woldenber LS, Kim KT. Pulmonary vein tumor thrombosis and left atrial extension in lung cancer. *Computed Tomography* 1984;8:331–336.

59. Dore R, Alerci M, D'Andrea F, Giulio GD, Agostini AD, Volpato G. Intracardiac extension of lung cancer via pulmonary veins: CT diagnosis. *J Comput Assist Tomogr* 1988;12:565–568.

60. Shields JJ, Cho KJ, Geisinger KR. Pulmonary artery constriction by mediastinal lymphoma simulating pulmonary embolus. *AJR* 1980;135:147–150.

61. Marshall ME, Trump DL. Acquired extrinsic pulmonic stenosis caused by mediastinal tumors. *Cancer* 1982;49:1496–1499.

62. Hamper UM, Fishman EK, Khouri NF, Johns CJ, Wang KP, Siegelman SS. Typical and atypical CT manifestations of pulmonary sarcoidosis. *J Comput Assist Tomogr* 1986;10:928–936.

63. Berkowitz KA, Fleischman JK, Smith RL. Bronchogenic cyst causing a unilateral ventilation-perfusion defect on lung scan. *Chest* 1988;93:1292–1293.

64. Weinstein JB, Aronberg DJ, Sagel SS. CT of fibrosing mediastinitis: findings and their utility. *AJR* 1983;141:247–251.

65. Berry DF, Buccigrossi D, Peabody J, Peterson KL, Moser KM. Review. Pulmonary vascular occlusion and fibrosing mediastinitis. *Chest* 1986;89:296–301.

66. Wieder S, White TJ, Salazar J, Gold RE, Moinddin M, Tonkin I. Pulmonary artery occlusion due to histoplasmosis. *AJR* 1982;138:243–251.

67. Farmer DW, Moore E, Amparo E, Webb WR, Gamsu G, Higgins CB. Calcific fibrosing mediastinitis: demonstration of pulmonary vascular obstruction by magnetic resonance imaging. *AJR* 1984;143:1189–1191.

68. Cramer M, Foley WD, Palmer TE. Compression of the right pulmonary artery by aortic aneurysms: CT demonstration. *J Comput Assist Tomogr* 1985;9:310–314.

69. Borokowski GP, O'Donovan PB, Troup BR. Pulmonary varix: CT findings. *J Comput Assist Tomogr* 1981;5:827–829.

70. Chaise LS, Soulen RL, Teplick S, Patrick H. Computed tomographic diagnosis of pulmonary varix. *J Comput Assist Tomogr* 1983;7:281–284.

71. Matsumoto AH, Parker LA, Delany D. CT demonstration of central pulmonary venous and arterial occlusive diseases. *J Comput Assist Tomogr* 1987;11:640–644.

72. Lombard CM, Churg A, Winokur S. Pulmonary veno-occlusive disease following therapy for malignant neoplasms. *Chest* 1987;92:871–876.

73. Sherrick DW, DuShane JW. Agenesis of a main branch of the pulmonary artery. *AJR* 1962;87:917–928.

74. Kieffer SA, Amplatz K, Anderson RC, Lillehei CW. Proximal interruption of a pulmonary artery. *AJR* 1965;95:592–597.

75. Sotomora RF, Edwards JE. Anatomic identification of so-called absent pulmonary artery. *Circulation* 1978;57:624–633.

76. Sondheimer HM, Oliphant M, Schneider B, Kavey RW, Blackman MS, Parker F. Computerized axial tomography of the chest for visualization of "absent" pulmonary arteries. *Circulation* 1982;65:1020–1025.

77. Stone DN, Bein ME, Garris JB. Anomalous left pulmonary artery: two new adult cases. *AJR* 1980;135:1259–1263.

78. Moncado R, Demos TC, Churchill R, Reynes C. Case report. Chronic stridor in a child: CT diagnosis of pulmonary vascular sling. *J Comput Assist Tomogr* 1983;7:713–715.

79. Berden WE, Baker DH, Wung JT, et al. Complete cartilage-ring tracheal stenosis associated with anomalous left pulmonary artery: the ring-sling complex. *Radiology* 1984;152:57–64.

80. Hernandez RJ, Bank ER, Shaffer EM, Snider AR, Rosenthal A. Comparative evaluation of the pulmonary arteries in patients with right ventricular outflow tract obstructive lesions. *AJR* 1987;148:1189–1194.

81. Jacobstein MD, Fletcher BD, Nelson AD, Clampitt M, Alfidi RJ, Riemenschneider TA. Magnetic resonance imaging: evaluation of palliative systemic-pulmonary artery shunts. *Circulation* 1984;70:650–656.

82. Webb WR, Gamsu G, Speckman JM. Computed tomography of the pulmonary hilum in patients with bronchogenic carcinoma. *J Comput Assist Tomogr* 1983;7:219–225.

83. Glazer GM, Francis IR, Shirazi KK, et al. Evaluation of the pulmonary hilum: comparison of conventional radiography, 55 degree posterior oblique tomography, and dynamic computed tomography. *J Comput Assist Tomogr* 1983;7:983–989.

84. Sone S, Higashira T, Marimoto S, et al. CT anatomy of hilar lymphadenopathy. *AJR* 1983;140:887–892.

85. Favez G, Willa C, Heinzer F. Posterior oblique tomography at an angle of 55 degrees in chest roentgenology. *AJR* 1974;120:907–915.

86. McLeod RA, Brown LR, Miller WE, DeRenee RA. Evaluation of the pulmonary hila by tomography. *Radiol Clin North Am* 1976;14:51–84.

87. Genereux GP. Review. Conventional tomographic hilar anatomy emphasizing the pulmonary veins. *AJR* 1983;141:1241–1257.

88. Chasen MH, Yrizarry JM. Tomography of the pulmonary hili. Anatomical reassessment of the conventional 55 degree posterior oblique view. *Radiology* 1983;149:365–369.

89. Sider L, David TM. Hilar masses: evaluation with CT-guided biopsy after negative bronchoscopic examination. *Radiology* 1987;164:107–109.

90. Westcott JL. Percutaneous needle aspiration of hilar and mediastinal masses. *Radiology* 1981;141:323–329.

91. Westcott JL. Percutaneous transthoracic needle biopsy. *Radiology* 1988;169:593–601.

92. Perlmutt LM, Johnston WW, Dunnick NR. Percutaneous transthoracic needle aspiration: a review. *AJR* 1989;152:451–455.

93. Naidich DP, Ettenger N, Leitman BS, McCauley DI. CT of lobar collapse. *Semin Roentgenol* 1984;19:222–235.

94. Woodring JH. Determining the cause of pulmonary atelectasis: a comparison of plain radiography and CT. *AJR* 1988;150:757–763.

95. Tobler J, Levitt RG, Glazer HS, Moran J, Crouch E, Evens RG. Differentiation of proximal bronchogenic carcinoma from post-obstructive lobar collapse by magnetic resonance imaging. Comparison with computed tomography. *Invest Radiol* 1987;22:538–543.

96. Tisi GM, Friedman PJ, Peters RM, et al. Clinical staging of primary lung cancer. Official statement of the American Thoracic Society. *Am Rev Respir Dis* 1983;127:659–664.

97. Im JG, Song KS, Kang HS, Park JH, Yeon KM, Han MC, Kim CW. Mediastinal tuberculous lymphadenitis: CT manifestations. *Radiology* 1987;164:115–119.

98. Reede DL, Bergeron RT. Cervical tuberculous adenitis: CT manifestations. *Radiology* 1985;154:701–704.

99. Scatarige JC, Fishman EK, Kuhajda FP, Taylor GA, Siegelman SS. Low attenuation nodal metastases in testicular carcinoma. *J Comput Assist Tomogr* 1983;7:682–687.

100. Gross BH, Schneider HJ, Proto AV. Eggshell calcification of lymph nodes: an update. *AJR* 1980;135:1265–1268.

101. Shapeero LG, Blank N, Young SW. Contrast enhancement in mediastinal and cervical lymph nodes. *J Comput Assist Tomogr* 1983;7:242–244.

102. Khouri NF, Eggelston JE, Siegelman SS. Angioimmunoblastic lymphadenopathy: a cause for mediastinal nodal enlargement. *Am J Roentgenol* 1978;130:1186–1188.

103. Fiore D, Biondetti PR, Calabro F, Rea F. Case report. CT demonstration of bilateral Castleman tumors in the mediastinum. *J Comput Assist Tomogr* 1983;7:719–720.

104. Cohen AM, Creiston S, LiPuma JP, Bryan PJ, Haaga JR, Alfidi RJ. NMR evaluation of hilar and mediastinal lymphadenopathy. *Radiology* 1983;148:739–742.

105. Dooms GC, Hricak H, Crooks LE, Higgins CB. Magnetic resonance imaging of the lymph nodes: comparison with CT. *Radiology* 1984;153:719–728.

106. Berquist TH, Brown LR, May GR, Jett JR, Bernatz PE. Magnetic resonance imaging of the chest: a diagnostic comparison with computed tomography and hilar tomography. *Magn Reson Imaging* 1984;2:315–327.

107. Levitt RG, Glazer HS, Roper CL, Lee JKT, Murphy WA. Magnetic resonance imaging of mediastinal and hilar masses: comparison with CT. *AJR* 1985;145:9–14.

108. Glazer GM, Gross BH, Aisen AM, Quint LE, Francis IR, Orringer MB. Imaging of the pulmonary hilum: a prospective comparative study in patients with lung cancer. *AJR* 1985;145:245–248.

109. Muller NL, Webb WR. Radiographic imaging of the pulmonary hila. *Invest Radiol* 1985;20:661–671.

110. Heelan RT, Martini N, Westcott JW, Bains MS, Watson RC, Caravelli JF, et al. Carcinomatous involvement of the hilum and mediastinum: computed tomographic and magnetic resonance evaluation. *Radiology* 1985;156:111–115.

111. Webb WR, Jensen BG, Sollitto R, de Geer G, McCowin M, Gamsu G, Moore E. Bronchogenic carcinoma: staging with MR compared with staging with CT and surgery. *Radiology* 1985;156:117–124.

112. Musset D, Grenier P, Carette MF, Frija G, Hauuy MP, Desbleds MT, Girard P, Bigot JM, Lallemand D. Primary lung cancer staging: prospective comparative study of MR imaging with CT. *Radiology* 1986;160:607–611.

113. Mayr B, Heywang SH, Ingrisch H, Huber RM, Haussinger K, Lissner J. Comparison of CT with MR imaging of endobronchial tumors. *J Comput Assist Tomogr* 1987;11:43–48.

114. Mendelson DS, Rose JS, Efremidis SC, Kirschner PA, Cohen BA. Bronchogenic cysts with high CT numbers. *AJR* 1983;140:463–465.

115. Zeitler E, Kaiser W, Feyrer E, Feyrer R, Holik B. Magnetic resonance imaging with and without Gd-DTPA, of bronchial carcinoma. In: Runge VM, Claussen C, Roland F, James AE, eds. *Contrast agents in magnetic resonance imaging. Proceedings of an international workshop, January 1986, San Diego, California.* Amsterdam: Excerpta Medica, 1986.

116. Hughes RL, Mintzer RA, Shields TW, Jensik RJ, Cugell DW. Management of the hilar mass. Clinical conference in pulmonary disease. *Chest* 1981;79:85–91.

117. Mintzer RA, Malave SR, Neuman HL, et al. Computed vs. conventional tomography in evaluation of primary and secondary pulmonary neoplasms. *Radiology* 1979;132:653–659.

118. McCloud TC, Wittenberg J, Ferrucci JT. Computed tomography of the thorax and standard radiographic evaluation of the chest: a comparative study. *J Comput Assist Tomogr* 1979;3:170–180.

119. Hirleman J, Yiu-Chiv V, Chiv L, Shapiro R. The resectability of primary lung carcinoma: a diagnostic staging review. *Computed Tomography* 1980;4:146–163.

120. Osborne DR, Korobkin M, Ravin CE, Putman CE, Wolfe WG, Sealy WC, Young WG, Breiman R, Heaston D, Ram P, Halber M. Comparison of plain radiography, conventional tomography, and computed tomography in detecting intrathoracic lymph node metastases from lung carcinoma. *Radiology* 1982;143:157–161.

121. Inouye SK, Sox HC. Standard and computed tomography in the evaluation of neoplasms of the chest: a comparative efficacy assessment. *Ann Intern Med* 1986;105:906–924.

122. Weinreb JC, Davis SD, Berkmen YM, Isom W, Naidich DP. Pulmonary artery sarcoma: evaluation using Gd-DTPA. *J Comput Assist Tomogr* 1990;14(4):647–649.

123. Hamper UM, Fishman EK, Khour, Johns CJ, Wang KP, Siegelman SS. Typical and atypical CT manifestations of pulmonary sarcoidosis. *J Comput Assist Tomogr* 1986;10:928–936.

Chapter 6

Lung Cancer

Lung cancer is the leading cause of cancer death in the world. In the United States, 93,000 men and 46,000 women died of this disease in 1988. Although the death rate from lung cancer in men is decreasing, a rapid increase in mortality rates for women has been observed. Recently lung cancer surpassed breast cancer as the most common cause of cancer death in females. Unfortunately, results of lung cancer treatment have remained disappointing, leading to more aggressive therapeutic approaches and more vigorous staging procedures.

Accurate staging is critical in the selection of treatment and in the evaluation of prognosis of patients with bronchogenic carcinoma. Computed tomographic (CT) examination of the thorax is only one of the many tests used for staging. The surgeon, pulmonologist, radiologist, and pathologist share the responsibility for accurate staging. A uniform staging system enables every participant in the management of the patient to communicate results unambiguously. Familiarity with the staging system now used for lung cancer is essential to an understanding of CT's role in lung cancer. The staging system devised for lung cancer has evolved over the past 30 years, following the establishment of the American Joint Committee on Cancer and End Results Reporting (AJCC) in 1959. In 1970, the task force on lung cancer of the AJCC adopted the T, N, M system originally proposed by Pierre Denoix (1). The initial classification scheme was published in 1973 and a modified version appeared in 1979 (2,3). In 1985, the staging system was updated to reflect modern treatment strategies and to resolve differences with other systems used in Europe and in Japan. At the World Conference on Lung Cancer

in 1985, a new uniform international staging system was adopted (4). The current system has two major components: anatomic extent of disease (TNM) and cell typing. The new system is based largely on the prior AJCC formulation but has been modified to reflect recent changes in the surgical approach to lung cancer (5).

STAGING OF THE PRIMARY TUMOR EXTENT (T)

T is the descriptor given to the primary tumor and its local complications. The precise definitions are given in Table 1. T staging is subdivided in four groups: T1 to T4. T1 and T2 subgroups have remained unchanged from the previous AJCC system.

The former T3 subgroup has been subdivided into two categories. The previous T3 descriptor encompassed lesions deemed unresectable. However, surgical experience has documented that some of these tumors are potentially resectable. Specifically, patients with cancer involving the chest wall (in the absence of distant or nodal metastases) have a relatively good survival rate ranging from 30–40% with and without adjuvant radiotherapy (6–11). With the development of modern reconstructive techniques, large portions of the chest wall can now be resected with no untoward functional effects. For example, Pancoast tumors, which were considered unresectable in the past, are now considered resectable provided vertebral bodies and major structures such as the brachial plexus are not involved. With the advent of bronchial reconstruction procedures, select

TABLE 1. *Definition of primary tumor (T) characteristics in lung cancer according to TNM system*

Descriptor	Definition
TX	Tumor proved by the presence of malignant cells in bronchopulmonary secretions but not visualized roentgenographically or bronchoscopically, or any tumor that cannot be assessed as in a retreatment staging.
T0	No evidence of primary tumor.
TIS	Carcinoma in situ.
T1	A tumor that is 3.0 cm or less in greatest dimension, surrounded by lung or visceral pleura, and without evidence of invasion proximal to a lobar bronchus at bronchoscopy.[a]
T2	A tumor more than 3.0 cm in greatest dimension, or a tumor of any size that either invades the visceral pleura or has associated atelectasis or obstructive pneumonitis extending to the hilar region. At bronchoscopy, the proximal extent of demonstrable tumor must be within a lobar bronchus or at least 2.0 cm distal to the carina. Any associated atelectasis or obstructive pneumonitis must involve less than an entire lung.
T3	A tumor of any size with direct extension into the chest wall (including superior sulcus tumors), diaphragm, or the mediastinal pleura or pericardium without involving the heart, great vessels, trachea, esophagus, or vertebral body, or a tumor in the main bronchus within 2 cm of the carina without involving the carina.
T4	A tumor of any size with invasion of the mediastinum or involving heart, great vessels, trachea, esophagus, vertebral body, or carina, or presence of malignant pleural effusion.[b]

[a] The uncommon superficial tumor of any size with its invasive component limited to the bronchial wall that may extend proximal to the main bronchus is classified as T1.

[b] Most pleural effusions associated with lung cancer are due to tumor. There are, however, a few patients in whom cytopathologic examination of pleural fluid (on more than one specimen) is negative for tumor; the fluid is nonbloody and is not an exudate. In such cases where these elements and clinical judgment dictate that the effusion is not related to the tumor, the cancer should be staged T1, T2, or T3, excluding effusion as a staging element.

patients whose tumors are within 2 cm of the carina also can now undergo curative resection (12,13). In addition, minimal invasion of the pericardium or mediastinal pleura without invasion of the underlying major structures has been found to be surgically manageable with potentially improved survival, especially in patients with squamous cell carcinoma. As a consequence, a major modification of the previous AJCC system includes the separation of advanced lesions considered potentially resectable by today's standards (now defined as T3) from those extensive lesions that are generally not resectable (now defined as T4).

An important footnote to the new international staging system relates to the presence of pleural effusions. A pleural effusion generally predicts a poor prognosis for patients with lung cancer, justifying a T4 classification. However, the possibility that a pleural effusion is only reactive (as may occur in patients with obstructive atelectasis, underlying pneumonia, or possible obstruction of the lymphatics) requires that the malignant nature of any effusion be proven before considering a patient unresectable. In particular, otherwise unsuspected small pleural effusions may be seen on thoracic CT; these should not be considered prima facie evidence of unresectability until malignant cells have been documented within the effusion.

The trend toward more aggressive surgical therapy and the inclusion of previously unresectable groups has changed the way thoracic CT scans are interpreted when assessing the primary tumor. The most important role of the radiologist in T staging is to assess whether a T4 classification is warranted on the basis of unequivocal CT findings. Indeed, CT staging should support curative surgery in potentially resectable tumors. CT can reliably determine the presence of mediastinal soft-tissue invasion or involvement of major mediastinal structures, such as the heart, great vessels, trachea, esophagus, and vertebral bodies. However, definite involvement should only be considered if clear-cut destruction and interdigitation of the tumor with the given structure is demonstrated. A CT diagnosis of T4 status applies to the following situations:

1. Tumors involving the trachea or narrowing of the carina, usually involving both sides of the carina (Figs. 1 and 2; see also Figs. 35, Chapter 3 and Fig. 2, Chapter 4). Lesions implicating the proximal portion of the major bronchi only are classified as T3 only if the carina is spared (see Fig. 22, Chapter 5).
2. Tumors surrounding, narrowing, or compressing the superior vena cava, the aorta, main pulmonary artery, right or left pulmonary artery beyond the mediastinal pleural reflection, or a major branch of any vessel within the mediastinal fat (Figs. 1 and 2; see also Figs. 21 and 39, Chapter 5).
3. Tumors extending into the soft tissues of the mediastinum. These tumors are characterized by irregular interdigitations of tumor tissue with mediastinal fat or protrusions of tumor displacing or encasing mediastinal structures (Figs. 1–3).

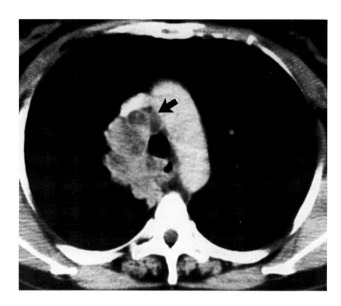

FIG. 1. Stage 3B disease: mediastinal invasion. Contrast-enhanced CT scan through the aortic arch shows tumor (T4) infiltrating into the mediastinum just behind the vena cava (*arrow*) which is compressed posteriorly.

4. Pleural masses, pleural effusion, or extensive invasion of the chest wall (Figs. 3 and 4). Because the prognosis for patients with lung cancer and pleural effusion is poor, pleural effusion can only be dismissed on CT if it is small. In addition, there should be no associated pleural thickening, pleural cytology should be negative, and there should be a plausible clinical explanation for the presence of pleural fluid

(for example, congestive heart failure or pneumonia), and no other criteria for T4 status should be met.
5. Erosion of a vertebral body (Fig. 5).

The interpretation of a CT examination in patients with T4 lesions is generally not difficult. Often, multiple findings which would indicate a T4 status co-exist. Tumors surrounding blood vessels also implicate the

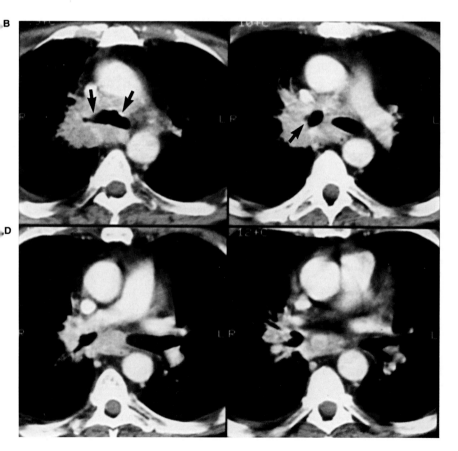

FIG. 2. Stage 3B disease: mediastinal invasion. **A–D:** Enlargements of sequential contrast-enhanced CT sections through the mediastinum show the presence of extensive tumor (T4) encasing the carina and mainstem bronchi, associated with enlarged subcarinal lymph nodes. Note that the contours of both main-stem bronchi are nodular, indicating invasion and fixation of the central airways (*arrows* in A and B).

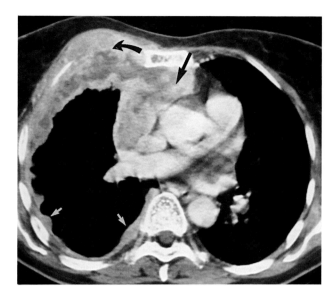

FIG. 3. Stage 3B disease: mediastinal and chest wall invasion. Contrast-enhanced CT section at the level of the right main pulmonary artery shows extensive tumor (T4) infiltrating the mediastinum (*black arrow*) as well as the chest wall (*curved arrow*). Note that the pleura circumferentially on the right side is thickened, nodular, and irregular due to extensive infiltration by tumor (*white arrows*).

soft tissues of the mediastinum. Patients with T4 lesions are also more apt to demonstrate advanced nodal disease, as well as distant metastases. It cannot be overemphasized, however, that when interpreting CT scans for staging, difficulties may be encountered if findings prove less than unequivocal. This is especially true in anatomic areas where partial volume effects may blur boundaries, such as superior sulcus tumors or central masses, including medially located lower lobe masses (see Fig. 22, Chapter 5). CT is not accurate in defining invasion when only thickening of the boundaries between the tumor and the pleura or pericardium or chest wall is seen. A lesion that abuts or makes only limited contact with such structures cannot confidently be diagnosed as being invasive because associated desmoplastic

reactions and inflammation can simulate tumor extension into an adjacent structure (Fig. 6). Likewise, microscopic invasion may be completely missed. The low reliability of CT in this context has been documented by several authors (14–16). Baron et al., for example, describe several patients with tumors adjacent to zones of pleural or pericardial thickening where subsequent surgery showed no spread of tumor (16).

In an attempt to increase specificity, Glazer et al. have described three criteria that help identify patients with indeterminate mediastinal or pleural invasion whose lesions are likely to be technically resectable (17). These criteria include: (a) less than 3 cm of tumor contact between the tumor and the adjacent mediastinum; (b) less than 90° circumferential contact between the tumor

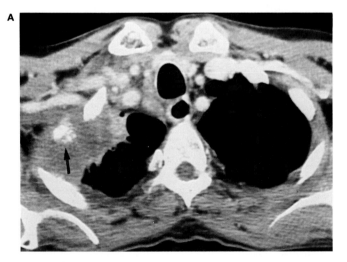
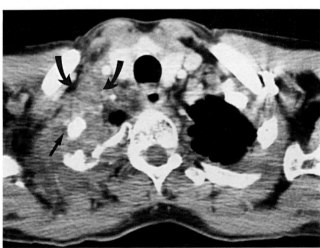

FIG. 4. Stage 3B disease: invasion of the chest wall and brachial plexus. **A, B:** Sequential contrast-enhanced CT scans through the thoracic inlet. An irregular, heterogeneous low-density mass is present in the right upper lobe, clearly invading the chest wall associated with lytic destruction of the first three ribs (*arrows* in A and B). Note that superiorly the tumor (T4) has extended into the base of the neck where it has obliterated all normal landmarks (*curved arrows* in B). Clinically this patient had evidence of brachial plexus involvement.

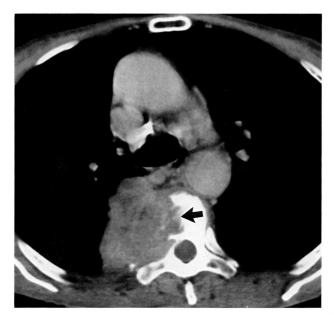

FIG. 5. Stage 3B disease: invasion of the thoracic spine. Contrast-enhanced CT section shows a large tumor (T4) in the right lower lobe directly invading the adjacent vertebral body (*arrow*).

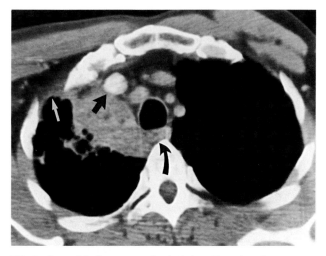

FIG. 6. Stage 3A disease: mediastinal pleural invasion. Contrast-enhanced CT scan shows a tumor (T3) in the right upper lobe that abuts the entire length of the mediastinum. Note that mediastinal fat planes are well preserved except anteriorly adjacent to the lateral aspect of the superior vena cava (*black arrow*), and posteriorly in the region of the posterior wall of the trachea and adjacent esophagus (*curved arrow*). This appearance is nonspecific, as is evidence of subtle pleural thickening along the anterolateral pleural surface (*white arrow*). At surgery there was no evidence of mediastinal invasion.

and the aorta; and (c) the presence of mediastinal fat between the mass and adjacent mediastinal structures. In their study, 36 out of 37 masses with one or more of these CT findings were technically resectable (17). Fortunately, with advances in surgical management, this issue is not as critical as it was in the past—even patients with limited tumor involvement of pleura or pericardium are classified as T3 and are not disqualified from surgical resection (Fig. 6).

In select cases, many of these difficulties may be obviated by the use of thin-section CT scans to define better the relationship of the tumor to the surrounding structures. Contrast enhancement is also critical in all cases where the relationship of major vessels to tumor is questioned (Fig. 7). Although difficulties may be encountered when tumors are associated with pneumonitis or obstructive atelectasis, due to blurring of the boundaries between the tumor and surrounding in-

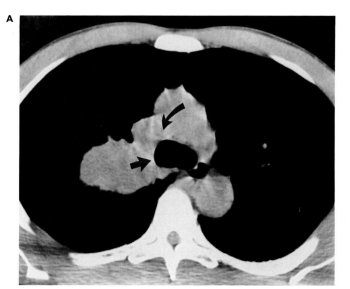

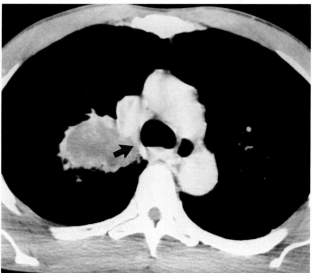

FIG. 7. The role of contrast enhancement in accurate CT staging. **A, B:** CT sections through the carina, obtained pre and postadministration of i.v. contrast media, respectively. Note that without contrast enhancement, the tumor appears to abut the lateral wall of the right main-stem bronchus (*arrow* in A); furthermore, delineation of mediastinal fascial planes is limited and adenopathy cannot be excluded (*curved arrow* in A). Following contrast enhancement, the tumor clearly lies lateral to the azygos vein (*arrow* in B). No mediastinal adenopathy is identified. Surgery documented T2N1 disease.

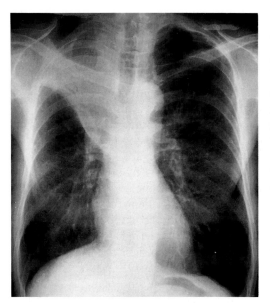
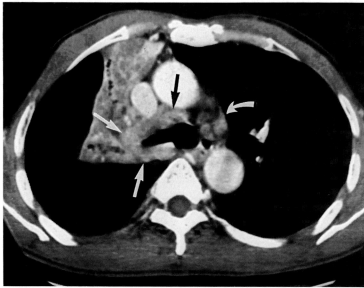

FIG. 8. Stage 3B disease: encasement of the carina; contralateral mediastinal adenopathy. **A:** Posteroanterior radiograph shows classic appearance of right upper lobe collapse, limiting evaluation of the hilum and mediastinum. There is no radiographic evidence to suggest this lesion is unresectable. **B:** Contrast-enhanced CT section through the carina shows classic CT appearance of right upper lobe collapse. In addition to evidence of tumor (T4) encasing the right main-stem bronchus (*straight arrows*), there are enlarged contralateral mediastinal lymph nodes easily identified within the aorticopulmonary window (*curved arrow*). Involvement of the carina and right main-stem bronchus was confirmed bronchoscopically.

flamed parenchyma, contrast-enhanced studies often can resolve the uncertainty (Fig. 8).

The diagnosis of T4 status is perhaps the most valuable contribution of CT to the management of patients with advanced lung cancers. This contribution has not been stressed in the literature because such patients rarely undergo surgery. However, it is one of the main reasons stated by surgeons to justify the use of CT in lung cancer staging (18). In a recent prospective cooperative trial involving 250 patients, only two patients underwent a thoracotomy and were found to harbor T4 disease undetected by both CT and magnetic resonance (MR) (19). CT therefore appears to be an effective method for preventing unnecessary thoracotomies in unequivocal T4 disease.

NODAL STAGING (N)

The descriptor N refers to the presence or absence of regional lymph node metastasis. The definitions used in the new international system are listed in Table 2. N0 indicates no demonstrable metastases to regional lymph nodes. This group demonstrates a better prognosis with every T status. N1 status is characterized by metastatic disease to peribronchial or hilar nodes. These nodes are all within the lung and are completely covered by pleura. N1 status may necessitate a pneumonectomy (rather than a lobectomy) for total removal of disease (Fig. 9).

In the previous staging system, N2 status referred to any metastasis to mediastinal lymph nodes. It indicated a very poor prognosis regardless of the chosen therapeutic option. However, several reports suggest that complete resection of the primary tumor and ipsilateral mediastinal lymph nodes, with or without adjuvant radiotherapy, may improve prognosis. Mountain and Naruke et al. have advocated thoracotomy and resection for patients with N2 disease (7,20,21). Five-year survival rates ranging from 14–42% have been reported. The best prognosis appears to be in the group of patients in whom

TABLE 2. *Definition of nodal involvement (N) in lung cancer by TNM classification*

Descriptor	Definition
N0	No demonstrable metastases to regional lymph nodes.
N1	Metastases to lymph nodes in the peribronchial or the ipsilateral hilar region, or both, including direct extension.
N2	Metastases to ipsilateral mediastinal lymph nodes and subcarinal lymph nodes.
N3	Metastases to contralateral mediastinal lymph nodes, contralateral hilar lymph nodes, ipsilateral or contralateral scalene, or supraclavicular lymph nodes.

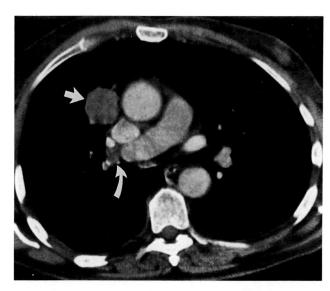

FIG. 9. Stage 2 disease: ipsilateral hilar adenopathy. Contrast-enhanced CT scan shows a well-defined right upper lobe mass abutting the mediastinum without evidence of invasion (*arrow*), associated with an enlarged right hilar (11R) node (N1) (*curved arrow*).

only low ipsilateral lymph nodes are involved and in patients with squamous cell carcinoma. Other authors do not find a significant dependence on cell type (22,23). The extent of nodal involvement by tumor has an impact on prognosis. It seems that when metastatic disease is discovered only at thoracotomy (especially after a negative mediastinoscopy), the prognosis and chance of complete surgical removal are better than when metastases to mediastinal lymph nodes are identified at mediastinoscopy (24).

It is logical to think that prognosis is a function of the degree of dissemination of disease prior to diagnosis. When cancer enters a mediastinal node, there is obviously an early microscopic phase in which the tumor is confined by the node. Such nodes are likely to be normal in size and undetectable by mediastinoscopy or surgical palpation. With tumor growth, permeation of the node and eventual extension through the capsule along with enlargement and induration may be observed. It would appear that capsular penetration is a likely indication that tumor has spread to other nodes or entered the systemic circulation. Bergh and Schersten reported 43% survival in 35 patients when resected cancer was entirely intranodal as opposed to 4.3% survival in 47 patients with malignancy extending through the capsule (25). Other investigators have cited similar statistics (26). Given the evidence that some subgroup of N2 disease may exhibit a better prognosis, a subdivision of the N2 group into N2 and N3 was deemed necessary and was included in the new international staging system.

The new N2 category includes all patients with ipsilateral mediastinal lymph nodes and subcarinal lymph

nodes. However, controversy remains about the significance of subcarinal lymph nodes (Fig. 10). In a few series, when careful nodal analysis was undertaken, metastases to the subcarinal lymph nodes carried a poor prognosis (20,23,27). In fact, subcarinal lymph nodes could easily be considered contralateral because they are located in the midline. There is also disagreement about the meaning of uppermost ipsilateral mediastinal lymph node involvement (see Fig. 49, Chapter 2), which is listed as a contraindication for surgical resection by some authors (24,28) but not by others (23).

If controversy surrounds the interpretation of N2 disease, there is general agreement that N3 status implies nonresectability. It should be emphasized that in select cases, N3 status may be conferred as the result of clinical sequelae, as in patients with signs of recurrent laryngeal nerve involvement (see Fig. 49, Chapter 2). It should also be noted that in the current staging system, supraclavicular and scalene nodes have been included as "regional" nodes because radiotherapists can include them in a radiation therapy portal. Consequently, metastases to the scalene and supraclavicular nodes which were previously considered evidence of distant metastatic disease are now classified as N3.

Clearly, the significance of mediastinal nodal disease is being actively reassessed. With the changing surgical attitude toward the management of mediastinal nodes, interpretation of nodal staging by CT requires adaptability to the predominant philosophy at a given institution. To ensure uniformity of studies as well as better understanding of nodal spread of disease patterns, the American Thoracic Society (ATS) proposed a standard lymph

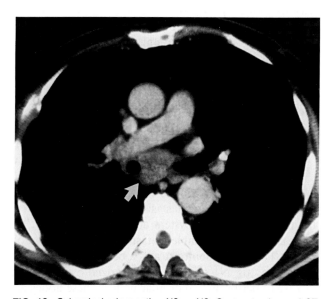

FIG. 10. Subcarinal adenopathy: N2 vs N3. Contrast-enhanced CT scan shows extensive subcarinal adenopathy (*arrow*). Although technically not considered evidence of contralateral disease (see Table 2), the significance of subcarinal adenopathy in staging lung cancer is controversial.

node map in 1983 (Table 3 and Fig. 11) (29). The ATS system is based on the concept that thoracic nodes are better defined if their relationship to fixed anatomic structures (such as the azygous vein, bronchi, or aortic arch) can be described. Such anatomic structures are easily recognizable at surgery, mediastinoscopy, and on CT scans. A major goal of the ATS system was to improve the separation of so-called hilar (N1) from mediastinal (N2) nodes. The AJCC definition for N1 nodes includes all nodes within the pleural reflection at surgery. This definition is somewhat arbitrary since the visceral pleura cannot always be visualized and some nodes may be partially covered by visceral pleura even though they are anatomically within the hilum. The ATS classification describes nodal stations based on the identification of the major anatomic structures of the mediastinum (Table 3 and Fig. 11). Thirteen nodal stations have thus been defined.

After polling thoracic surgeons at major university hospitals, it was determined that the mediastinoscopist should be able to characterize nodes in the following stations: 2R, 2L, 4R, 4L, 10R, 10L and 7. Nodal stations 5 and 6 are not accessible to the mediastinoscope (see Fig. 49, Chapter 2) (29). Note that the words hilar and mediastinal are not used in the ATS system. In 1988, Friedman and the ATS committee on lung cancer suggested that station 10R should be considered hilar, but 10L should be considered mediastinal (30). Friedman also recommended combining nodal stations 8 (the para-esophageal group) and 9 (the pulmonary ligament group), as a single nodal station. He also recommended adding nodal station 14 for supradiaphragmatic nodes, which should be included in the N2 category if ipsilateral. Nodal station 1 was redefined to include scalene and supraclavicular nodes which are now considered N3 in the new AJCC system. Because the emphasis in the future will be to assess differences in prognosis for patients undergoing extensive lymph node resections, it is

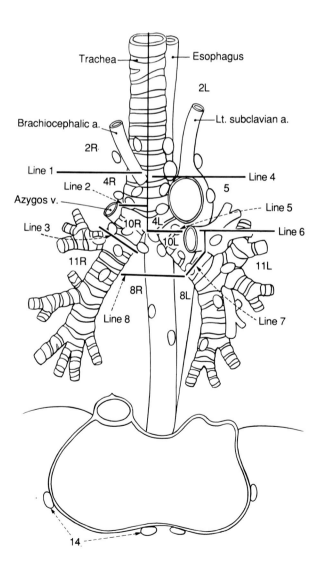

FIG. 11. Standard lymph node map proposed by the American Thoracic Society, 1983 (ref. 29). **Right side:** Line 1 represents the top of the aortic arch. Right paratracheal nodes above this line are classified as 2R (right upper paratracheal). Line 2 is at the level of the arch of the azygos vein. Nodes to the right of the midline between lines 1 and 2 are classified as 4R (right lower paratracheal). Line 3 extends across the right main bronchus at the level of the origin of the right upper lobe bronchus. Right-sided nodes positioned along the right main-stem bronchus below line 2 and above line 3 are classified as 10R (right tracheobronchial). Nodes along lobar bronchi distal to line 3 are classified as 11R (intrapulmonary). Nodes in the mediastinum more than 3 cm caudal to the carina and located adjacent to the esophagus or within the right pulmonary ligament are classified as 8R (right para-esophageal). **Left side:** Line 4 represents the top of the distal aortic arch. Left paratracheal nodes above this line are classified as 2L (left upper paratracheal). Line 5 represents the level of the carina. Line 6 represents the top of the left pulmonary artery. Left paratracheal nodes located between lines 4 and 5 are classified as 4L (left lower paratracheal). Nodes in the mediastinum located in the aorticopulmonary window, lateral to the ligamentum arteriosum and between lines 4 and 6, are classified as 5 (aorticopulmonary window nodes). Line 7, analogous to line 3 on the right side, represents the point of division of the left main bronchus. Nodes along and around the left bronchus from the carina to the origin of the left upper lobe bronchus are classified as 10L (left peribronchial). Directly analogous to the right side, left-sided mediastinal nodes more than 3 cm caudal to the carina and located adjacent to the esophagus or within the left pulmonary ligament are classified as 8L (left para-esophageal). **Midline:** Nodes in the subcarinal region in the triangle formed by the medial aspects of the right and left main bronchi and line 8 are classified as 7 (subcarinal). Line 8 is placed 2 cm below the carina. Not shown on the diagram are nodes in the anterior mediastinum, anterior to the ascending aorta and its proximal branches. Such nodes are classified as 6 (anterior mediastinal).

TABLE 3. *Definitions of regional nodal stations for prethoracotomy staging*

Station	Definition
X	Supraclavicular nodes.
2R	Right upper paratracheal (suprainnominate) nodes: nodes to the right of the midline of the trachea between the intersection of the caudal margin of the innominate artery with the trachea and the apex of the lung. (Includes highest R mediastinal node.) (Radiologists may use the same caudal margin as in 2L.)
2L	Left upper paratracheal (supra-aortic) nodes: nodes to the left of the midline of the trachea between the top of the aortic arch and the apex of the lung. (Includes highest L mediastinal node.)
4R	Right lower paratracheal nodes: nodes to the right of the midline of the trachea between the cephalic border of the azygos vein and the intersection of the caudal margin of the brachiocephalic artery with the right side of the trachea. (Includes some pretracheal and paracaval nodes.) (Radiologists may use the same cephalic margin as in 4L.)
4L	Left lower paratracheal nodes: nodes to the left of the midline of the trachea between the top of the aortic arch and the level of the carina, medial to the ligamentum arteriosum. (Includes some pretracheal nodes.)
5	Aorticopulmonary nodes: subaortic and para-aortic nodes, lateral to the ligamentum arteriosum or the aorta or left pulmonary artery, proximal to the first branch of the left pulmonary artery.
6	Anterior mediastinal nodes: nodes anterior to the ascending aorta or the innominate artery. (Includes some pretracheal and preaortic nodes.)
7	Subcarinal nodes: nodes arising caudal to the carina of the trachea but not associated with the lower lobe bronchi or arteries within the lung.
8	Para-esophageal nodes: nodes dorsal to the posterior wall of the trachea and to the right or left of the midline of the esophagus. (Includes retrotracheal, but not subcarinal nodes.)
9	Right or left pulmonary ligament nodes: nodes within the right or left pulmonary ligament.
10R	Right tracheobronchial nodes: nodes to the right of the midline of the trachea from the level of the cephalic border of the azygos vein to the origin of the right upper lobe bronchus.
10L	Left peribronchial nodes: nodes to the left of the midline of the trachea between the carina and the left upper lobe bronchus, medial to the ligamentum arteriosum.
11	Intrapulmonary nodes: nodes removed in the right or left lung specimen plus those distal to the main-stem bronchi or secondary carina. (Includes interlobar, lobar, and segmental nodes.)

From American Thoracic Society Clinical staging of primary lung cancer. *Am Rev Respir Dis* 1983; 127:659, with permission.

important for the radiologist interpreting CT scans to become very familiar with this new classification. This system is rapidly becoming the worldwide standard.

Role of CT

CT Technique

The detectability of hilar nodes correlates directly with the amount of mediastinal fat that provides a natural contrasting background (Fig. 9). With reduced amounts of mediastinal fat, interpretation may be difficult. Another problem is related to the partial volume effect in anatomic areas oriented obliquely relative to the plane of scanning (see Chapter 1). Quint et al. compared lymph node size and number in five cadavers imaged by CT and followed by lymph node dissection (31). An excellent correlation between CT and pathology was found for right-sided mediastinal lymph nodes. However, CT was less accurate on the left side, most particularly in region 10L, where it detected only four of fourteen lymph nodes found on dissection. Genereux also found that CT was less accurate for assessing normal nodes in the aorticopulmonary window and the subcarinal region, including regions 7 and 10L (32). Clearly, there is a risk of understaging lymph nodes on

the left side of the mediastinum. In addition, it is often difficult to distinguish lymph nodes from hilar vessels without the use of contrast media. These considerations have led to a change in the imaging strategy for the mediastinum. For regions where the orientation of anatomic structures is essentially perpendicular to the plane of scanning, 8–10 mm sections are adequate. However, thinner 5-mm sections may need to be obtained from the top of the aortic arch through the subcarinal regions. In addition, contrast enhancement, preferably using dynamic incremental scanning, is recommended for better definition of low mediastinal and aorticopulmonary window nodes. Critical areas where contrast enhancement is most often useful are:

1. The region of the aorticopulmonary window where the inferior margin of a prominent distal aortic arch or the superior aspect of the main pulmonary artery may be misinterpreted as a nodal mass (Fig. 8);

2. The right pulmonary artery as it passes around the bronchus intermedius, and the left pulmonary artery as it arches over the left upper lobe bronchus, where nodes adjacent to the vessels may be misinterpreted as nodular portions of the pulmonary artery (Fig. 9);

3. The truncus anterior, the first branch of the right pulmonary artery, as it courses through the mediastinum en route to the right upper lobe. It may be confused

with a node when it is seen in cross-section. Small collections of connective tissue near the truncus anterior may mimic nodes; however, the fatty density of these collections should be a clue to the true nature of this normal variant (33).

Blood vessels, such as a tortuous innominate artery or a persistent left superior vena cava, are most apt to be mistaken for mediastinal nodes. The recesses of the pericardium also present an additional potential source of confusion. The superior sinus, the most prominent of the pericardial recesses, may be visualized as a soft-tissue structure in the mediastinum anterior to the tracheal bifurcation and directly posterior to the ascending aorta (34). The key feature that distinguishes the superior sinus from a lymph node is the near-water density of this structure.

Accuracy of Lymph Node Staging by CT

A large number of studies has assessed CT accuracy in staging nodal disease in lung cancer patients. The majority of studies have used nodal size alone as the diagnostic criterion. To date, there is no definite evidence that characteristics other than size (such as shape, appearance of borders, or node density) are of value in staging lung cancer. Although correlating lymph node size with presence or absence of metastatic disease would seem to constitute a straightforward study design, the reported accuracies of CT in assessing metastatic nodal disease cover a bewildering range of values, ranging from the low 40% to the high 90% (19,46–58).

Normal Mediastinal Nodes

Because the primary goal of nodal staging is to determine the presence or absence of metastatic lymphadenopathy, knowledge of normal nodal anatomy is important. Only a few studies have been performed on normal patients to characterize size and number of normal nodes. Beck and Beattie found an average of 64 mediastinal lymph nodes in human cadavers (35). Schnyder and Gamsu examined 127 normal subjects from Switzerland. They found that the diameter of nodes in the pretracheal retrocaval space (which corresponds to region 10R of the ATS map) was 5.5 mm ± 2.8 (36). Nodes were detected in 80% of the scans. In addition, while lymph node size appeared to increase slightly with the patient's age, almost all nodes were smaller than 11 mm. Glazer et al. performed a thorough investigation of lymph node size by CT in 56 normal subjects (37). They measured the longest and shortest axes in the transverse plane. Short axis was the most reliable parameter of nodal size because it is less dependent on the spatial orientation of the node relative to the

transaxial scan. They found that the largest nodes in normal individuals were subcarinal (region 7), where the mean short axis was 6.2 mm ± 2.2 and right tracheobronchial (region 10R), and where the mean short axis was 5.9 ± 2.1. Based on their data, they concluded that 10 mm is the short axis measurement above which a node should be considered enlarged (37).

A more recent study on 40 adult cadavers from Japan by Kiyono et al. substantially coincides with the results of Glazer et al. in the United States, and Schnyder and Gamsu in Swiss subjects (38). Kyono et al. clearly showed much greater variation in the range of normal long axis diameters than with maximum short axis measurements. They also observed that nodes occur most frequently in regions 4, 7, and 10, where they can be demonstrated in 90–100% of subjects. The mean short diameter of nodes in their transverse plane range from 2.4 to 5.6 mm. The largest nodes were subcarinal (region 7), with 25% of cadavers demonstrating nodes larger than 10 mm in short axis in that region. For the subcarinal region, using mean +2 standard deviations, these authors found a value of 12.3 mm as the upper limit of normal. In region 10R the upper limit of normal was 10.8 mm. For all other regions, the mean plus two standard deviations did not exceed 10 mm. They also found that upper paratracheal nodes are smaller than lower paratracheal nodes and left paratracheal nodes are smaller and less numerous than right paratracheal nodes. The major findings of these studies have been summarized in Table 4.

Existing data indicate that the short axis measurement of lymph nodes is the least variable measure of enlargement. The normal size of lymph nodes varies depending on its location in the mediastinum. A threshold value of 10 mm appears to represent two standard deviations for the population studied, except in the subcarinal region where a 12 mm value can be used. However, these findings should not be interpreted too rigidly.

TABLE 4. *Lymph node size by ATS nodal station*

Nodal station	Shot axis diameter		Proposed threshold (mm)
	CT (mm)	PATH (mm)	
2R	3.5 ± 1.3	3.7	8
2L	3.3 ± 1.6	2.9	7
4R	5.0 ± 2.0	4.0	10
4L	4.7 ± 1.9	4.1	10
5	4.7 ± 2.1	3.6	10
6	4.1 ± 1.7	3.3	8
7	6.2 ± 2.2	5.6	11
8R	4.4 ± 2.6	3.7	10
8L	3.8 ± 1.7	2.9	8
10R	5.9 ± 2.1	4.5	10
10L	4.0 ± 1.1	3.5	7

Modified from refs. 37 and 38.

First, the sample size is small. Also, age-related and environmentally related variations may exist. Thus, threshold values should be considered only as guidelines. Further, it has been suggested that defining node size in a given region relative to other regions may be a more reliable parameter for detecting nodal disease. This method was suggested by Buy et al. who demonstrated increased accuracy in detecting nodal pathology when nodes were defined as abnormal only when larger than 10 mm in the short axis, and if a difference could be documented between these same nodes and the largest node identifiable in other territories (39). Their working hypothesis was that size comparison between regions may decrease false positive diagnoses due to underlying inflammatory disease. Further studies correlating not only the absolute size of nodes but the distribution patterns and relative sizes between nodal stations should prove valuable.

Patterns of Nodal Spread

A knowledge of the patterns of metastatic spread to locoregional lymph nodes is valuable when interpreting CT findings. Rouviere was the first to systematically study the lymphatic drainage of the lung (40). Typically, lymph flows into intrapulmonary nodes around segmental bronchi, then to lobar or interlobar nodes, and then to lymph nodes at the hilar areas. The spread of lung cancer generally follows the same pathway. The lymphatic pathways from the individual lobes to the mediastinum are constant.

In 1952, Borrie described more precisely the mechanisms of lymph drainage (41). In the right lung, a collection of intrapulmonary lymph nodes that lie between the upper lobe bronchus and the superior segmental or middle lobe bronchi appeared to be the common drainage pathway for all three lobes. In addition, the right upper lobe drains to nodes in the region of the azygos vein, also called the superior tracheobronchial nodes, contiguous with nodes in the lower paratracheal area. The middle and lower lobes also drain to the subcarinal nodes and to nodes in the pulmonary ligament and adjacent to the esophagus (42). A group of lymph nodes located between the left upper lobe bronchus and the left superior segmental bronchus drains both the left upper and left lower lobes. In addition, the left upper lobe drains to nodes in the aorticopulmonary window, the anterior mediastinum, the left paratracheal area, and the subcarinal nodes. As on the right side, the left lower lobe exhibits preferential drainage to the subcarinal nodes, para-esophageal nodes, and nodes of the pulmonary ligament.

An important consideration is the pattern of lymphatic spread. Does it occur in an orderly manner or can some proximal nodes be spared while more distal nodes

are involved by disease? Studies by Libshitz et al. and Martini et al. suggest that the latter is true. Nearly 30% of patients with lung cancer had "skipped" metastases to mediastinal lymph nodes with no involvement of lobar or hilar nodes (43,44). Thus, one should not assume that absence of hilar nodes indicates the absence of disease in the mediastinal nodes. Likewise, it is important to understand differences in the patterns of tumor spread throughout the various pulmonary lobes. Although as a rule bronchogenic carcinoma tends to spread to ipsilateral mediastinal lymph nodes, significant exceptions occur.

In a study by Nohl-Oser, contralateral spread was observed in 3.6% of patients with right upper lobe tumors, 3.7% in those with right lower lobe tumors, 11% in patients with left upper lobe tumors, and 25% in patients with left lower lobe tumors (45). Left lung tumors appear to have a higher propensity for contralateral spread than right lung tumors. Right lung cancers spread mainly to the ipsilateral mediastinal nodes. Nodal stations 10R and 4R are most commonly involved and extend to the higher paratracheal node stations 2R and finally to the scalene or inferior deep cervical nodes. Tumors in the right lower and middle lobe frequently spread to subcarinal nodal station 7 and tracheobronchial and paratracheal nodal stations 10R and 4R. It should be noted that subcarinal nodes are midline nodes connected to both right and left lymphatic systems and from which contralateral spread can occur. Although the new staging system classifies subcarinal nodes as ipsilateral and resectable, the ATS believes that "carinal involvement should be considered bilateral." This unresolved controversy will require further study. Contralateral lymphatic spread is more common with left lung tumors, especially those in the left lower lobe. Regional lymph node stations 4L and 10L are commonly involved. Left upper lobe tumors often metastasize to subcarinal station 7, the aorticopulmonary window station 5, and intramediastinal node station 6. The left lower lobe lesions are the ones most likely to spread contralaterally via the subcarinal node station 7 to the right paratracheal regions and to the pulmonary ligament and para-esophageal stations.

After 10 years of investigation, a more coherent picture of the exact role and limitations of CT in the staging of mediastinal lymph nodes is emerging. A review of the literature indicates that variations in accuracy can be attributed to the methodologies used by investigators. First, numerous size criteria have been used to define enlarged nodes. Most authors agree that lymph nodes less than 1 cm in diameter are probably normal even though they may still harbor microscopic metastases; however, there is considerable variation in the size criteria used to identify abnormal nodes. While lymph nodes greater than 15 mm are generally considered abnormal by most authors, lymph nodes between 11–15 mm have been variably categorized. Second, the problem of defining abnormal size criteria has been further compounded by the use of different criteria for measuring lymph node size. Although Glazer et al. (37) and Kiyono et al. (38) advocate the use of the short axis measurement, a recent study by Staples et al. found that a long axis measurement greater than 10 mm was the best criterion on CT (59). These differences in size criteria mean that the sensitivity and specificity of the test will vary.

The absence of a uniform size criterion among studies only partially explains the wide disparity in results. Most studies have involved small series of patients—usually 50 or less—leading to considerable statistical variation. Also, populations within reported series have not been homogeneous in terms of disease severity. Indeed, the prevalence of nodal metastasis is known to vary depending on the T stage of the tumor, with the likelihood of negative nodes much higher in patients with stage T1 disease. Thus a negative test is more likely to be correct in that group of patients than in patients with more advanced disease. Because of the increased likelihood of finding enlarged reactive inflammatory nodes in advanced cases (more often associated with atelectasis and postobstructive pneumonitis) (46,60), in can be anticipated that specificity will be lower in patients with T3 lesions than in patients with T1 lesions.

Another confounding variable has been the lack of uniformity in the measure of truth used by investigators. Some studies have relied on surgical as well as pathologic correlation to establish the accuracy of CT interpretations. Many early studies, however, did not include a thorough exploration of the mediastinum at the time of thoracotomy. As a result, small lymph nodes that appeared normal macroscopically and at palpation could easily have been overlooked at the time of surgery, and consequently, be called negative even though they harbored microscopic disease. Obviously, this would tend to reduce the number of false negative studies and improve the apparent sensitivity of the test. Moreover, surgeons cannot sample contralateral nodes at the time of surgery. In some studies, mediastinoscopy was used to verify the status of contralateral nodes. In others, however, a negative CT scan was considered sufficient to avoid preoperative mediastinoscopy.

These problems were appreciated early on by a few investigators. In 1984, Libshitz and McKenna studied 86 patients with bronchogenic carcinoma who had mediastinal CT and full nodal sampling (46). In 33% of cases, metastases involved nodes less than 1 cm in diameter. These nodes were either missed or classified as normal using CT. In an extension of this study (61), the same authors found a 10% incidence of metastatic disease in lymph nodes smaller than 1 cm. In the group of patients with metastatic disease (25 of 102 patients), CT detected only 60% of lesions using 1 cm as a threshold

value. Similarly, in 1988, Staples et al. reported results from a series of patients who underwent preoperative mediastinoscopy and thorough mediastinal exploration (59). In this study, the authors tried to match nodal stations examined by CT with nodal stations examined by mediastinoscopy or surgery. They documented a sensitivity of only 79% and a specificity of 65%. Additionally, these authors found that in 7 of 44 patients, tumor was absent in the enlarged nodes seen on CT but was present in normal-sized lymph nodes located in a different nodal station. Thus the overall sensitivity of CT in predicting the number of patients with mediastinal metastasis was 79%, whereas the sensitivity for individual lymph nodes was only 66%.

More recent prospective studies have confirmed the limited accuracy of CT when compared with thorough pathologic correlation. McCloud et al. reported a CT sensitivity of 41% and a specificity of 84% (62). Likewise, Grenier et al. found a sensitivity of 46% and a specificity of 79% (63). In a multi-center cooperative study of the Radiology Diagnostic Oncology Group that included prospective blinded readings and systematic surgical sampling, the sensitivity of CT was 52% and specificity was 69% (19). Clearly, all recent studies document a lower accuracy than was previously reported for CT. It is probable that this is primarily the result of improved measures of truth, that is, careful, systematic pathologic examination of all accessible lymph nodes. Lower sensitivity can be explained by the increasing number of normal-sized lymph nodes with microscopic disease found in those studies. Lower specificity is directly related to the number of enlarged nodes that do not harbor disease. As mentioned previously, Libshitz and McKenna examined this problem in patients with lung cancer and concomitant atelectasis, pneumonitis, or evidence of granulomatous disease (46). Of their 86 patients, 39 had associated pneumonia or atelectasis; of these 39, 54% had lymph nodes larger than 1 cm. Ten of these patients harbored metastatic disease, but 11 had reactive enlarged lymph nodes. Likewise, Hirleman et al. found that five of seven patients with a false positive reading from CT images had evidence of postobstructive atelectasis or pneumonia (60).

What conclusions can be drawn about the role of CT in mediastinal nodal staging? Clearly, there are serious limitations in the use of CT for assessing mediastinal nodal involvement by tumor. Indeed, Libshitz and McKenna have questioned whether CT has any utility in evaluating mediastinal lymph nodes. Other investigators value CT as a noninvasive mapping procedure to guide mediastinoscopy or surgical sampling (59). In our opinion, CT remains the primary noninvasive modality for staging local invasion and nodal status. One should be keenly aware that staging issues constantly evolve as results of different therapeutic approaches become known. For example, the evidence that patients with N2 disease have a better prognosis following extensive lymph node dissection is still being evaluated. Clinical data now support the hypothesis that survival of such patients depends on the underlying character of the nodal involvement. Bergh and Schersten reported a 43% survival rate when resected cancer was entirely intranodal, as opposed to a 4.3% survival rate when malignancy extended through the capsule (25). Similarly, it has been shown that patients in whom nodal disease is not detected during mediastinoscopy but only at thoracotomy have a better prospect of survival (64,65). Such findings suggest that normal-sized lymph nodes harboring metastatic disease may not have the same prognostic significance as larger positive nodes with penetration of tumor through the capsule (Fig. 12). In this context, false negative CT examinations in normal-sized lymph nodes may not be a limiting factor since these patients are now considered candidates for surgery. As removal of all nodes becomes important, CT is valuable for its ability to visualize all nodes, whether normal or abnormal. In addition, if patients with varied prognoses can be segregated according to the degree of abnormal node involvement, detailed CT analysis of the morphologic features of lymph nodes may become important (Fig. 13). If CT scans show no enlarged lymph nodes and no

evidence of capsular penetration, it would seem reasonable to bypass surgical staging procedures (such as mediastinoscopy) and proceed directly to thoracotomy.

Unfortunately, CT will never provide histologic specificity. As previously stressed, enlarged nodes may simply be the result of benign reactive changes. In the context of advanced disease with associated pneumonitis, atelectasis, or inflammation, preoperative sampling of these nodes becomes essential for two reasons: (a) to prove the presence of disease; and (b) to evaluate the presence of nodal disease in the contralateral mediastinum rather than in the ipsilateral nodes which are all accessible during thoracotomy. This last point is especially important in the context of the new staging system. A valid question would be to determine the accuracy of CT in assessing the contralateral mediastinum. This could prove especially important in the management of left-sided lung tumors, particularly left lower lobe lesions, which have a higher propensity for contralateral spread. It is possible that contralateral disease distant from the primary site may be less affected by the problem of false positive diagnoses related to associated inflammation.

In brief, the interpretation of mediastinal or nodal sampling by CT should be flexible and adaptable to the specific management philosophy of one's institution. In

A
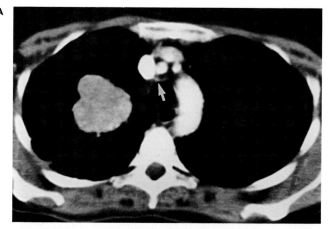

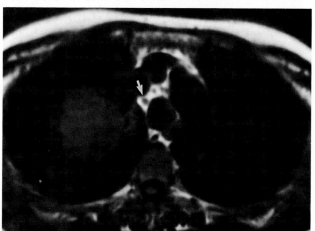
B

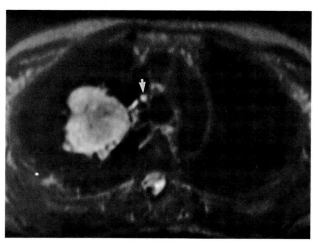
C

FIG. 12. Stage 3A disease: ipsilateral mediastinal metastases. **A:** Contrast-enhanced CT scan shows a lobulated mass in the right upper lobe. A very small pretracheal lymph node (*arrow*) corresponding to region 2R can just be identified. Similar-sized mediastinal nodes were seen throughout the mediastinum and right hilum (not shown). **B, C:** T1- and T2-weighted MR images at approximately the same level as A, respectively. Pretracheal lymph nodes are shown to good advantage, embedded in mediastinal fat (*arrow* in B). Note that the T2-weighted image shows bright signal within nodes identified on the T1-weighted scan (*arrow* in C). At surgery, these nodes proved positive. Unfortunately, signal intensity within nodes is nonspecific; a similar appearance may be seen as well in hyperplastic lymph nodes.

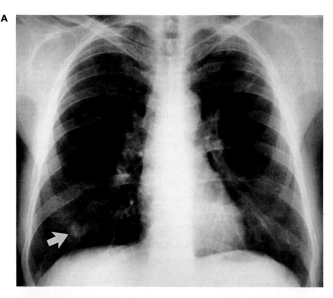

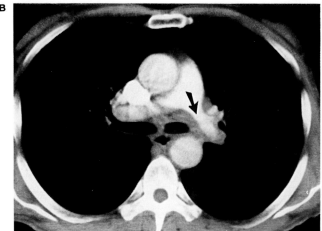

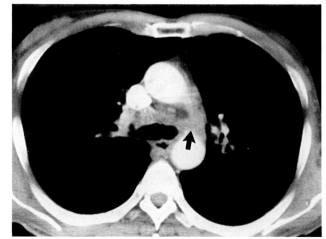

FIG. 13. Radiographic T1N0M0 disease: the role of CT. **A:** Posteroanterior radiograph shows a nodule in the right lower lobe (*arrow*). The hilar and mediastinal contours are normal. **B, C:** Sequential contrast-enhanced CT scans show extensive tumor throughout the mediastinum. This appearance is consistent with extranodal spread of disease (*arrow* in C). Note that the left main pulmonary artery is encased (*arrow* in B). This case shows the value of CT in more precisely defining the extent of disease prior to attempting surgical resection.

addition, as management philosophies evolve the role of CT will undoubtedly change. Further research and refinement in the methods of analyzing lymph node disease may provide new applications for CT, such as the potential use of high resolution CT to assess such features as node clustering, border sharpness and, as suggested by Buy et al. (39), assessment of relative sizes between nodal stations.

STAGING OF DISTANT METASTASIS (M)

The descriptor M relates to the presence of distant metastases (M1) or their absence (M0) (Table 5). Patients with distant metastases carry a very poor prognosis and are generally treated with chemotherapy, radiotherapy, or both. For didactic purposes, the TM system is described in an orderly pathophysiologic progression from local extension T to distant metastasis M. In fact, the clinical work-up of a patient with lung cancer generally proceeds in the opposite direction, that is, from M to T. Initial clinical evaluation and laboratory

tests strive to detect M1 disease, which will preclude more aggressive and expensive work-up and therapy. Biopsies are performed for suspicious skin lesions or palpable lymph nodes. Abnormal biochemical tests may indicate the necessity for imaging of the liver or bones to detect distant metastasis. Neurologic findings may indicate central nervous system disease, to be confirmed by CT. Thoracic CT becomes important in the staging process only when these initial steps are negative. Often, clinically silent sites of distant metastatic disease can be discovered. Mathews et al. studied 200 patients who died within 30 days of presumed curative surgery. At autopsy, 48 of these patients (23.4%) had metastasis, 18 of them to the adrenal gland and 16 to the liver (66). In a

TABLE 5. *Definition of distant metastases (M) in lung cancer by TNM classification*

Descriptor	Definition
M0	No (known) distant metastases.
M1	Distant metastases present—specify site(s).

comparable population, a 26% incidence of extrathoracic metastasis was found at autopsy (67). It is therefore common practice to obtain scans of the upper abdomen after examination of the thorax to evaluate the liver and adrenal glands for clinically silent metastatic disease. CT examination of the upper abdominal examination is most important in the following settings:

1. In patients with undifferentiated carcinomas, because the risk of distant metastases in this population is generally higher.
2. In patients with T3 lesions, because justification for thoracotomy may be borderline, and in these cases, again, there is a higher likelihood of distant metastases. This is true even with patients who demonstrate no evidence of mediastinal adenopathy since only 70% of patients with distant metastatic disease demonstrate lymph node involvement in the mediastinum.
3. In patients with N2 disease, particularly when the histology is other than squamous cell carcinoma.
4. In patients with questionable physiologic status who may not withstand surgical resection.

It cannot be overemphasized that the accuracy of CT in detecting upper abdominal pathology directly correlates with scan technique, especially when evaluating the liver. Proper examination of the liver by CT is in itself an exacting task. In the thorax, parenchymal lesions and lymph nodes are accentuated either by surrounding aerated lung or mediastinal fat. Liver metastases can be detected only by virtue of a difference in attenuation between tumor and adjacent normal liver. A bolus of intravenous contrast media increases the ability to identify metastases, which typically exhibit less enhancement than normal liver and consequently are seen as "filling defects." The accuracy of CT in detecting liver metastases is a function of the quality of the CT examination. In patients in whom there is a strong suspicion of hepatic disease (based on clinical evidence either of hepatomegaly or abnormal liver function), the abdomen should be examined prior to the thorax. In this setting, hepatic scanning is best performed with 12 to 20 contiguous sections utilizing dynamic incrementation, following administration of 150 to 180 ml of 60% iodinated contrast media, preferrably using a power injector. In our experience, a biphasic injection first delivering a bolus of 50 cc at 5 cc per sec, followed by the remainder at approximately 1 cc per sec provides optimal differential enhancement between normal liver and metastases, especially when scans are obtained following an initial delay of about 25 sec.

As with thoracic lesions, the nature of hepatic and adrenal masses must be histologically confirmed before a patient is declared unresectable. This is especially true

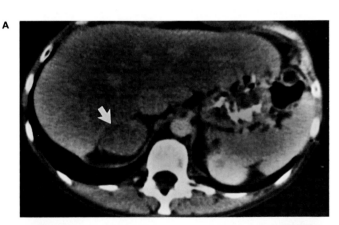

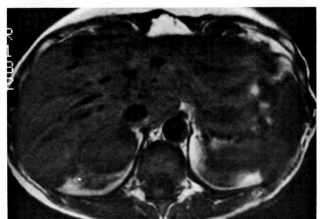

FIG. 14. Stage 4 disease: adrenal metastases. **A:** Contrast-enhanced CT scan through the adrenals shows an approximately 3 × 3 cm mass in the right adrenal gland (*arrow*) in a patient with known adenocarcinoma of the lung metastatic to mediastinal lymph nodes. **B, C:** T1- and T2-weighted MR images at the same level as in A, respectively. The right adrenal mass appears moderately hyperintense on the T2-weighted image relative to liver with slight heterogeneity, features suggestive of metastatic disease (histologically confirmed adrenal metastasis).

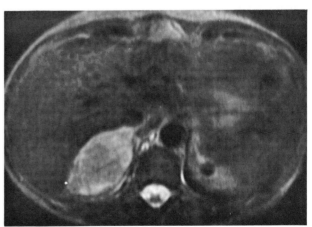

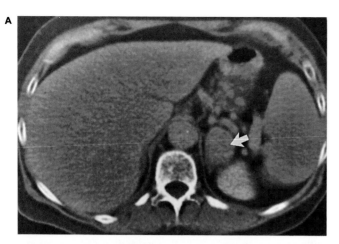

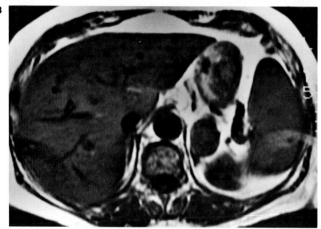

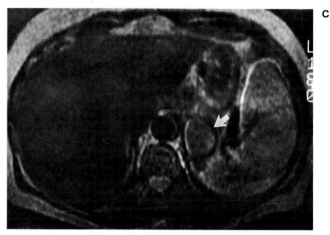

FIG. 15. Adrenal adenoma: CT/MR correlation. **A:** Contrast-enhanced CT scan through the upper abdomen shows an approximately 2 × 3 cm homogeneous left adrenal mass (*arrow*) incidentally discovered in a patient with known bronchogenic carcinoma. **B, C:** T1- and T2-weighted MR images at the same level as A, respectively. With T1 weighting, the mass is well defined and homogeneous; with T2 weighting, the mass has relatively low signal intensity (*arrow* in C) (compare with Fig. 14). Note the chemical shift artifact causing the adrenal mass to be seemingly etched in white, medially, and outlined in black, laterally. Given the size of the lesion and slight heterogeneity, this appearance was interpreted as nonspecific; at surgery this proved to be a benign adrenal adenoma. This case illustrates some of the difficulties that may be experienced in characterizing adrenal masses by MRI.

for small adrenal masses (Figs. 14 and 15). The adrenal gland may be biopsied using CT monitoring (68). A fair proportion of cases of nodular adrenal enlargement will be found to represent benign adrenal adenomas or adrenal hyperplasia (69).

STAGE GROUPINGS

Based on comparable extent of disease, anticipated treatment, and prognosis, TNM subsets have been defined corresponding to 4 stages of disease (Table 6). These groupings into stages are largely the result of careful studies by Mountain (4) of the prognostic factors and treatment outcomes in 3,753 patients. The best prognosis is found in patients with Stage 0, i.e. carcinoma in situ, or Stage 1 (T1N0M0 or T2N0M0) disease. In the old staging system, T1N1M0 lesions were considered Stage 1 as well. However, with the increased recognition that the presence of any positive pulmonary nodes worsens prognosis, this group of patients has been reclassified as Stage 2, along with the T2N1M0 lesions. Consequently, Stage 1 is reserved for all patients without evidence of nodal metastasis, while Stage 2 denotes metastases to the intrapulmonary lymph node stations (11R, 10R, and 11L).

Stage 3 has been subdivided into two subgroups. Stage 3A (T3N0M0, T3N1M0, or T1-T3N2M0) represents patients with advanced disease in whom extensive surgery (including resection of all ipsilateral and subcarinal lymph nodes) may be of value, especially if adjuvant radiotherapy or chemotherapy is used. Stage 3B includes all cases of more advanced disease without distant metastasis. Stage 4 represents any patient with evidence of distant metastasis.

TABLE 6. *TNM stage grouping for lung cancer*

Stage		TNM subsets	
Occult cancer	TX	N0	M0
0	TIS	Carcinoma in situ	
1	T1	N0	M0
	T2	N0	M0
2	T1	N1	M0
	T2	N1	M0
3A	T3	N0	M0
	T3	N1	M0
	T1–3	N2	M0
3B	Any T	N3	M0
	T4	Any N	M0
4	Any T	Any N	M1

Patients with Stage 3B disease may benefit from radiation therapy, often in conjunction with chemotherapy. This group is often referred to as the extensive radiotherapy group. Patients with Stage 4 disease are generally treated with chemotherapy with limited use of palliative radiotherapy. This group is referred to as the chemotherapy group. The radiologist interpreting CT scans needs to be familiar with the staging groups and their implications to enhance both the technical quality of studies and the quality of interpretation.

It is worth noting that there is no optimal CT technique to stage lung cancer. Instead, each study should reflect an initial estimate of the probable stage of disease based on routine chest radiographs, as well as an estimate of the patient's clinical status. For example, in patients suspected of Stage 1 disease, especially T1N0M0 lesions, in whom a diagnosis of malignancy has not yet been established, initial scans should be obtained prior to the administration of intravenous contrast, utilizing thin (1.5 to 2 mm) sections in order to accurately measure tissue density (see Chapter 8). As already discussed, this approach differs fundamentally from patients in whom a diagnosis of lung cancer has already been established and in whom distant metastases are suspected, especially within the liver. In cases in which tumor appears primarily central, especially when associated with peripheral atelectasis, initial attention should be paid to the region of the pulmonary hilum. As discussed in detail in Chapters 2, 4, and 5, evaluation of the hilum is best achieved using dynamic incremental scans following a bolus of approximately 100 to 150 cc's of 60% iodinated contrast media. This allows optimal differentiation between central obstructing lesions and peripherally collapsed lung (see Fig. 8). In patients in whom evaluation centers on differentiating Stage 3A from 3B disease, a similar technique as described for the hilum also can be used, with scans initially obtained either through the center of lesions suspected of invading either the chest wall or mediastinum, or from the level of the thoracic inlet to the carina in patients for whom the critical question is evaluation of mediastinal nodal disease. As already noted, in each case scan technique optimization is based on an initial assessment of the probable disease stage based largely on radiographic appearances. It should be emphasized that regardless of technique, all patients in whom lung cancer is suspected should have additional images obtained through the upper abdomen to include the adrenal glands as part of a routine chest CT study. This requires very little extra time and is of sufficient benefit to warrant routine acquisition of these few extra images.

INFLUENCE OF CELL TYPE

There are four major lung cancer cell types: squamous cell carcinoma, adenocarcinoma, large cell undifferentiated carcinoma, and small cell undifferentiated carcinoma (SCLC). Patients with SCLC are generally considered Stage 4 at the time of presentation. As a consequence, for patients with SCLC, a simplified classification of "limited" or "extensive" disease is employed. Limited disease refers to tumor confined to a single hemithorax without associated pleural effusion. Extensive disease indicates spread to the contralateral hemithorax or extrathoracic metastases. CT is of value in this group of patients mainly as a monitoring tool to assess the response of the disease to either chemotherapy or radiotherapy (Fig. 16). As newer chemotherapeutic and adjuvant surgical protocols are introduced, more accurate staging of these patients may be helpful in the future (70).

The other cell types demonstrate a generally better prognostic trend with the best chances of survival being observed in patients with squamous cell carcinoma (although this is only statistically significant in the lower stage groups). Adenocarcinoma and large cell undifferentiated carcinoma tend to metastasize earlier than squamous cell carcinoma. Consequently, a histologic diagnosis of adenocarcinoma or large cell undifferentiated carcinoma should prompt extreme caution, with more careful evaluation of the mediastinum both noninvasively as well as either preoperative mediastinoscopy or mediastinotomy, as indicated. Likewise, a search for occult metastatic disease prior to surgery and needle biopsy sampling of all suspicious extrathoracic sites is justified in these cell types.

ROLE OF MR IN STAGING LUNG CANCER

Since the advent of MR, numerous studies have been performed to assess its value relative to CT in the management of patients with lung cancer (48,63,71–73). MR offers inherent advantages that may be of use in lung cancer staging. First, the delineation of mediastinal and hilar vessels does not require the administration of intravenous contrast medium. Second, direct coronal, sagittal, and oblique imaging provides superb anatomic detail in regions difficult to study with CT, such as the lung apex, the aorticopulmonary window, and the supradiaphragmatic regions. Third, the increased soft-tissue differentiation achievable with MR may also be helpful in differentiating tumor from other processes.

It should be emphasized that MR also exhibits significant disadvantages relative to CT. It is costly and time-consuming, and the spatial resolution is less than that achievable with CT. Artifacts and blurring of structures related to respiratory and cardiac motion are a potential problem, although this has been greatly reduced by the advent of motion compensation techniques and the systematic use of cardiac gating. The general consensus at present is that MR and CT have similar accuracies, therefore in our opinion, CT remains the imaging mo-

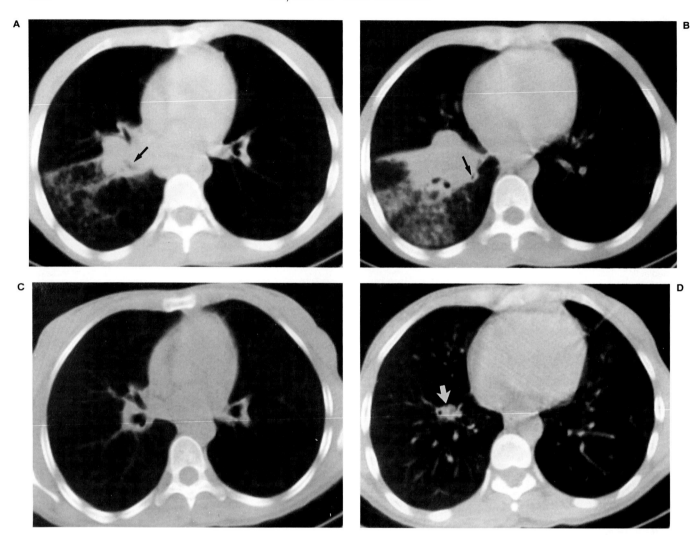

FIG. 16. Small-cell lung cancer: CT evaluation. **A, B:** Sequential CT sections through the right hilum show extensive tumor deforming both the middle lobe and right lower lobe bronchi (*arrows* in A and B), causing distal consolidation and atelectasis. Diagnosis established by transbronchial biopsy. **C, D:** CT scans through the same levels as shown in A and B, following 6 months of chemotherapy. Note that there has been near complete regression of tumor, although there is a small, residual, soft-tissue density adjacent to the basilar bronchi (*arrow* in D). CT allows precise evaluation of response to therapy in these cases, allowing for close monitoring and potentially early detection of tumor recurrence.

dality of choice both for assessing patients with abnormal chest radiographs suspected of having lung cancer, and staging patients with documented bronchogenic carcinoma. Nonetheless, as will be discussed in detail, in select cases MR can play a significant complementary role in the evaluation and staging of lung cancer.

Role of MR in Assessment of Mediastinal and Chest Wall Invasion

Chest wall invasion adjacent to a lung tumor may be better demonstrated by MR than by CT. This is because MR provides better tissue contrast, particularly on T2-weighted images, between tumor, chest wall, fat, and muscles (48,74). A thin layer of extrapleural fat separating the tumor mass from the chest wall can almost always be seen on high quality MR images. This thin

layer of extrapleural fat, located beneath the parietal pleura, may be effaced in the presence of early invasion (Fig. 17). Using conventional CT, this fat layer is more difficult to see. Although plain radiographs generally demonstrate rib destruction better than MR, MR most clearly demonstrates the mass within the chest wall. In addition, MR images in the sagittal or coronal planes are advantageous in imaging superior sulcus tumors (Figs. 18 and 19) (75). Sagittal or coronal plane images often show the extent of chest wall invasion and involvement of the subclavian artery or brachial plexus better than either transaxial CT or MR images (77,78).

A significant advantage of MR is its ability to demonstrate the relationship between tumor and major mediastinal vascular structures without the need for administration of intravenous contrast media. Indeed, with MR, good contrast is generally observed between the flow void within blood vessels and the high signal inten-

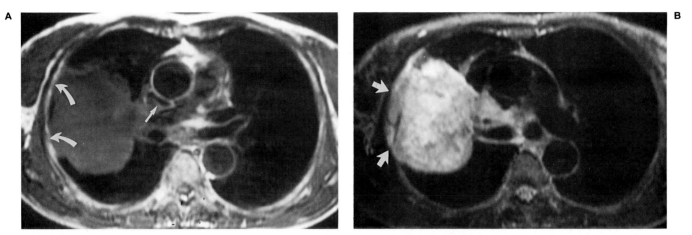

FIG. 17. Stage 3A disease: ipsilateral mediastinal adenopathy/chest wall invasion. **A:** T1-weighted MR scan shows a right hilar mass with apparent extension into the mediastinum, causing compression of the superior vena cava (*straight arrow*). Laterally, there is a suggestion that tumor has infiltrated extrapleural fat, identifiable as focal areas of decreased signal intensity (*curved arrows*). **B:** T2-weighted MR scan, at a level slightly higher than A. Tumor clearly extends into the chest wall (*arrows*). At surgery, the vena cava was found not to be invaded. Hilar and mediastinal nodes proved positive, without evidence of mediastinal invasion. The tumor was successfully resected despite chest wall invasion.

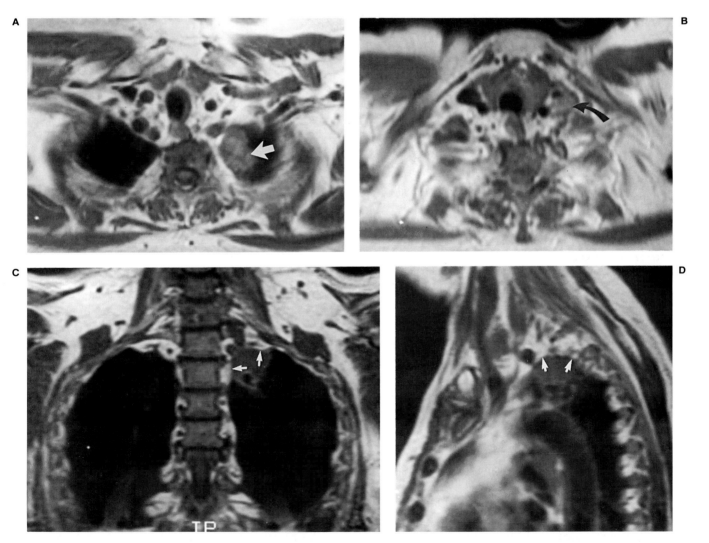

FIG. 18. Stage 3A disease: Pancoast tumor. **A, B:** Sequential MR images through the thoracic inlet from below-upward show a lobular mass in the left lung apex (*arrow* in A). Note that the medial border of the tumor is well delineated by fat. A large supraclavicular lymph node is present on the left, as well, just posterior to the left jugular vein and lateral to the left carotid artery (*arrow* in B). **C, D:** Coronal and sagittal images through the lung apex, respectively, show sharp demarcation between the tumor and adjacent mediastinal and extrapleural fat along most of the course of the tumor-pleural interface (*arrows* in C and D). No contact is seen with the spine. Although these findings suggested a lack of gross chest wall invasion, at surgery microscopic invasion was documented with minimal tumor extension into the subpleural fat. The supraclavicular node shown in A proved to be positive.

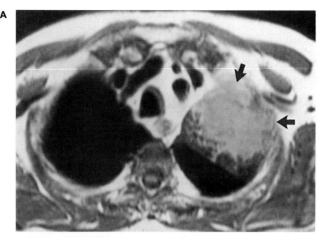

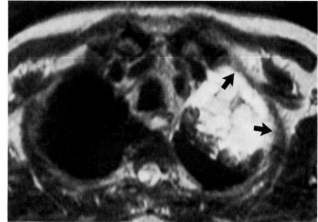

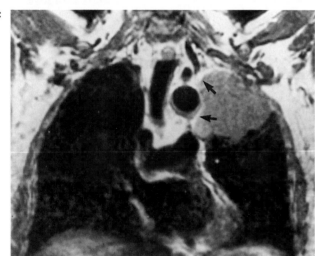

FIG. 19. Stage 3A disease: chest wall invasion. **A, B:** T1- and T2-weighted axial MR images through the left lung apex show a poorly marginated tumor mass extending laterally into the chest wall (*arrows*). Note that medially the mediastinal fat is well preserved. **C:** Coronal MR image again shows that the mass is invading the chest wall laterally. Although the mass clearly parallels a considerable portion of the mediastinum, the mediastinal fat remains intact (*arrows*). At surgery, chest wall invasion was confirmed; the mediastinum proved to be normal.

sity mediastinal fat and the mediastinal pleural margins. In addition, the pericardium is routinely demonstrated, identifiable as a line of hypointensity surrounding the heart and the base of the major vessels. Although neither MR nor CT are capable of demonstrating minimal invasion of either the mediastinal pleura or mediastinal fat, significant obliteration of mediastinal fat planes or compression or encasement of mediastinal vessels appear better demonstrated by MR than CT. In a prospective study by the Radiologic Diagnostic Oncology Group (15), no statistically significant differences were observed in the relative accuracies of CT and MR in staging lung cancer, except for significantly better delineation of mediastinal and chest wall invasion by MR (19). The specific instances in which we believe MR to be useful are as follows:

1. Superior sulcus tumors (chest wall invasion). MR shows extent of chest wall invasion and proximity to spine, spinal canal, nerves (including the recurrent laryngeal nerves as well as the brachial plexus), and the spinal cord in an exquisite fashion (Figs. 18 and 19).

2. Tumor in contact with the heart, in particular the left atrium. MR is helpful in determining pericardial involvement (T3 disease) versus pericardial and cardiac muscle involvement (T4 disease).

3. Central tumor with direct extension in the subcarinal region. In this setting, coronal images in particular are extremely valuable in determining the precise extent of tumor, especially in relation to the carina (Figs. 20 and 21).

4. Tumor extension into the aorticopulmonary window. Again, coronal images may be extremely helpful in determining encasement of the pulmonary artery and aorta (Fig. 22).

5. Invasion of the superior vena cava and adjacent me-

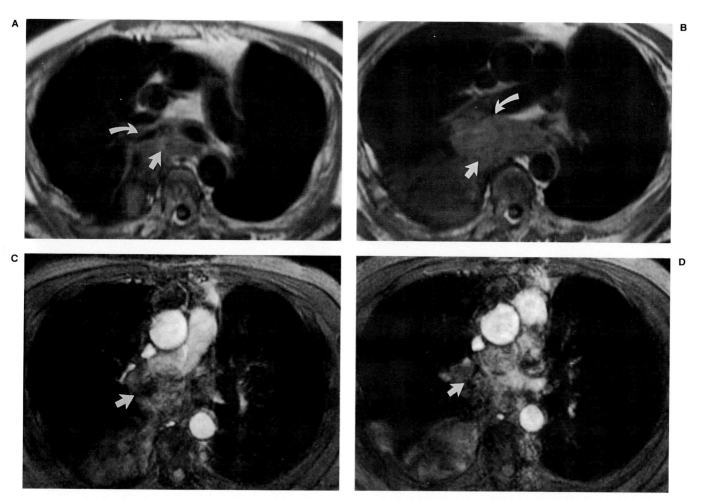

FIG. 20. Stage 3B disease: mediastinal invasion. **A, B:** T1-weighted axial MR images at the level of the carina and right main pulmonary artery, respectively, show mass extending from the right lower lobe into the subcarinal space (*arrows* in A and B), resulting in encasement of the right main-stem bronchus (*curved arrow* in A). There is considerable contact between the mass and the posterior wall of the right main pulmonary artery (*curved arrow* in B). **C, D:** Gradient-refocused images at and just above the level shown in B. These flow-sensitive images show that the right pulmonary artery and right hilar structures are encased by tumor (*arrows* in C and D). Despite these findings, surgery was attempted; the lesion, however, proved unresectable.

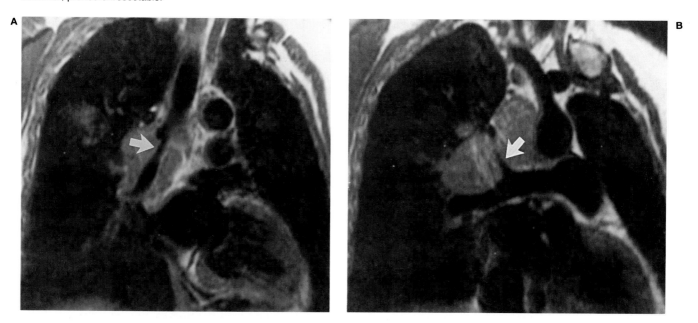

FIG. 21. Stage 3B disease: mediastinal adenopathy coronal images. **A, B:** Sequential coronal MR images through the mediastinum show extensive adenopathy surrounding and narrowing the bronchus intermedius (*arrow* in A), as well as encasing the truncus anterior (*arrow* in B). Note the extensive paratracheal adenopathy, especially well seen in B. In select cases, coronal images may be of particular value in determining the true extent of disease.

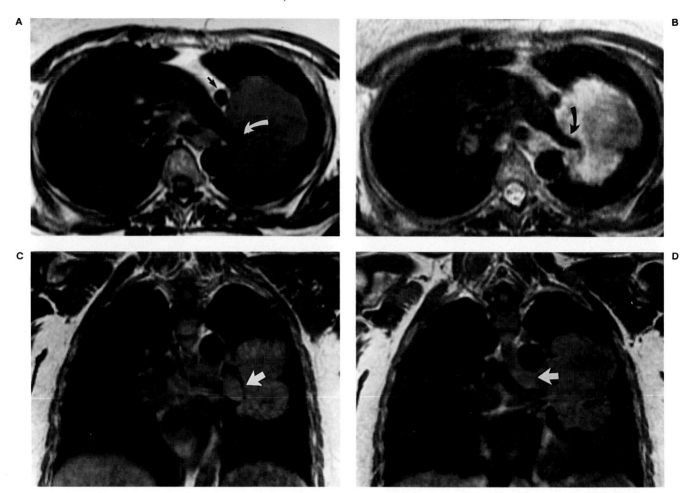

FIG. 22. Stage 3B disease: mediastinal invasion. **A, B:** Axial T1- and T2-weighted MR images at the same level through the carina in a patient with squamous cell carcinoma. Tumor clearly encases the left main pulmonary artery (*curved arrows* in A and B). Note the presence of a persistent left superior vena cava, a normal variant (*straight arrow* in A). **C, D:** Coronal T1-weighted images show encasement of the left main pulmonary artery to better advantage (*arrow* in C). Note the presence of enlarged aorticopulmonary and left paratracheal lymph nodes (*arrow* in D).

diastinal soft tissues in patients with otherwise radiographically resectable right hilar disease (Fig. 23).

6. Tumor located in the cardiophrenic angles and in the medial aspect of the lower lobes. MR is helpful in determining invasion of the aorta and para-esophageal tissues as well as determining pericardial versus cardiac involvement.

MR in the Evaluation of the Hila

Contrast-enhanced CT and MR are both accurate in detecting hilar masses and adenopathy (see Chapter 5). However, in patients in whom there is a contraindication to the intravenous administration of contrast media or with poor vascular opacification, MR may allow a more confident diagnosis, especially of hilar invasion. On occasion, MR can demonstrate node enlargement invisible with CT, especially when partial volume effects between adjacent vessels and nodes prevent identification (see Fig. 42, Chapter 5). Because blood vessels usually have a low signal and nodes have a relatively higher signal, such a confusion is less likely with MR (Fig. 24). It should be noted, however, that slow flow in hilar vessels may be associated with significant signal, even in normal individuals. Additionally, MR is unable to detect nodal calcifications. These drawbacks render MR unsuitable as a routine imaging modality for evaluating the pulmonary hila. In select cases, MR may aid surgical planning by determining the extent of invasion of both central pulmonary arteries or veins. This may be of particular value in deciding whether a patient requires a pneumonectomy or, instead, special reconstructive techniques.

Because of its better spatial resolution, CT is superior to MR in determining the presence or extent of endobronchial tumors (79). As discussed in Chapter 4, in select cases in which proximal bronchial obstruction is associated with postobstructive pneumonitis, MR can help by differentiating the obstructing carcinoma from surrounding atelectatic lung, especially on T2-weighted

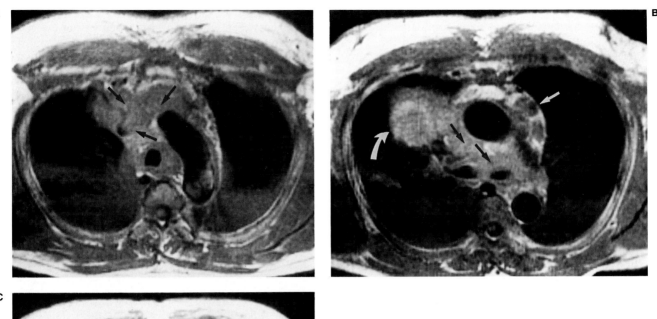

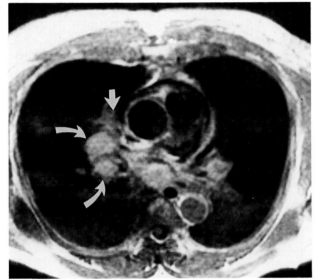

FIG. 23. Stage 3B disease: superior vena caval obstruction; contralateral, extranodal adenopathy. **A–C:** Sequential MR images show extensive metastatic lymphadenopathy in a patient with a primary right upper lobe lung cancer (*curved arrow* in B). Note transcapular extension of disease from the nodes into surrounding fat, as well as encasement of the superior vena cava (*black arrows* in A and B). In addition, contralateral mediastinal lymph nodes are identifiable in B, just anterior to the left main pulmonary artery (*straight white arrow*), as well as enlarged subcarinal node and right hilar nodes surrounding the bronchus intermedius (*curved arrows* in C). Note that there are bilateral pleural effusions as well as a small pericardial effusion, the latter probably secondary to direct extension of tumor (*straight arrow* in C).

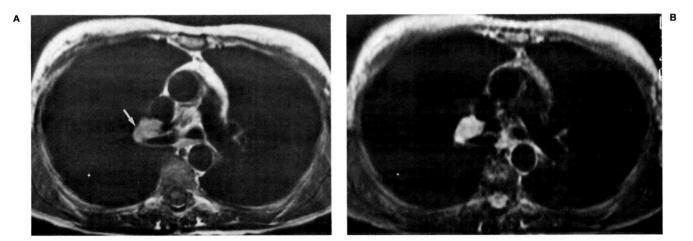

FIG. 24. Hilar adenopathy: MR evaluation. **A:** T1-weighted MR image through the right hilum shows evidence of moderately enlarged right hilar nodes just anterior to the right upper lobe bronchus (*arrow*), identifiable as a focal area of intermediate signal intensity (compare with the normal appearing left hilum). **B:** T2-weighted MR scan at approximately the same level as in A shows considerably enhanced signal within the right hilum, again confirming the presence of enlarged nodes. Unfortunately, there is nothing in the appearance of these nodes that allows differentiation between benign and malignant adenopathy. Surgically proven metastatic lymph nodes in a patient with a right upper lobe tumor (not shown).

or gadolinium-enhanced images (see Figs. 26 and 28, Chapter 4). In such patients, the consolidated lung typically exhibits a higher signal intensity than the central hilar mass (80,81).

Role of MR in Nodal Staging

Differentiation between mediastinal lymph nodes and mediastinal fat is easily accomplished on T1-weighted MR sequences. In general, MR is similar to CT in its ability to detect and define mediastinal lymph nodes (see Fig. 12) (19). However, with the limited spatial resolution of MR and its inability to obtain scans at suspended respiration, blurring of structures may occur. On occasion, several small lymph nodes have been mistaken by MR for a single, large, abnormal node mass (79). As already noted, MR is significantly disadvantaged due to its inability to detect calcification within mediastinal or hilar nodes. Although coronal or sagittal MR may be helpful in studying aorticopulmonary window or subcarinal nodes, this is only occasionally indicated and clearly does not justify the routine use of MR.

With the advent of MR, it was hoped that malignant and benign nodes could be differentiated based on differences in relaxation times. In a study by De Geer et al., a difference was found in the T1 values of nodes enlarged due to sarcoidosis (mean, 544 ms) compared with nodes enlarged because of metastatic tumor (mean, 769 ms); unfortunately, however, considerable overlap between these groups existed (82). Glazer et al. performed an *in vitro* study of freshly resected nodes in patients with lung cancer (83). They found that although groups of involved and uninvolved nodes differed in average T1 values, with metastatic nodes exhibiting a longer T1 (mean, 640 ms versus 566 ms), there was too much overlap between the groups to allow differentiation. Recent studies in Europe using gadolinium-DTPA contrast enhancement also do not appear to allow confident differentiation between benign and malignant lymph nodes.

The Role of MR in the Assessment of Distant Metastasis

Because of the examination length and the cost, MR is not recommended for routine staging of distant metastases in the upper abdomen. However, it may be used to characterize potential adrenal masses found on CT (Figs. 14 and 15). The radiologic appearance of adrenal metastasis generally is nonspecific. Although these lesions tend to be large, a significant number may appear as either small unilateral or bilateral lesions. Generally, metastases present as solid masses. When less than 3 cm in diameter, they typically appear homogeneous on CT. Larger lesions may show central necrosis or areas of hemorrhage. In most cases, adrenal metastases cannot be clearly distinguished from benign lesions (such as an adenoma, hematoma, pheochromocytoma, or inflammatory masses) on the basis of morphology alone. Features that suggest a malignant lesion include large size (greater than 3 cm); irregular margins, with or without invasion of adjacent structures; inhomogeneous CT density; and a thick, irregular, enhancing rim (84). Small ovoid lesions with a thin rim and homogeneous density are more likely to be benign.

MR, owing to its high tissue signal differentiation, can be useful in select cases in differentiating metastatic disease from benign adenomas. Typically, metastases have a higher signal intensity than most adenomas on T2-weighted sequences. Ratios of the intensity of the adrenal tumor to adjacent liver, muscle, or fat have been used (85–87). Metastatic lesions tend to have a higher signal intensity than that of liver or muscle and near or higher than that of fat, while benign adenomas have signal intensities similar to or less than that of liver. Pheochromocytomas characteristically exhibit very high T2-weighted signal intensity. Unfortunately, some overlap can be observed in the relaxation times of benign and malignant masses (88). In our experience, one-third of cases with positive adrenal findings present with small (<1.5 cm) adrenal masses with low signal intensity on T2-weighted scans, a typical presentation of nonfunctioning cortical adenomas. In another one-third of cases, lesions demonstrate a combination of features including large size, irregular margins, and heterogeneity, although predominantly high intensity, on T2-weighted scans; these findings all suggest metastatic disease. In the majority of these cases, intrathoracic disease is almost always advanced, generally involving T2 or T3 lesions associated with evidence of enlarged mediastinal nodes. Finally, in one-third of cases, lesions measure between 1.5 and 2.5 cm in size, morphologic or signal features are not characteristic, and needle biopsies are required for further diagnosis.

ROLE OF MR AND CT IN THE FOLLOW-UP OF TREATED LUNG CANCER

In select cases, MR seems to be able to differentiate tumor from fibrosis (see Chapter 1). In patients who have undergone radiation therapy for treatment of carcinoma, radiation-induced fibrosis in a recurrent tumor can be difficult to differentiate with CT. It has been reported that recurrent tumor can be distinguished from posttreatment radiation fibrosis by using T2-weighted MR pulse sequences (89). In 12 patients studied by Glazer et al., posttreatment fibrosis had a low signal intensity on both T1- and T2-weighted images, while tumor showed relatively increased intensity on T2-weighted sequences. Unfortunately, such differentiation

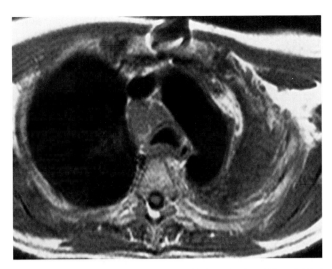

FIG. 25. Postpneumonectomy space: MR evaluation. T1-weighted MR image through the mediastinum shows enlarged pretracheal nodes following a left-sided pneumonectomy. MR should replace CT in patients with extensive surgical clips, or in whom i.v. contrast is contraindicated.

is difficult in patients who have recently completed treatment because inflammatory reaction secondary to radiation therapy may also lead to high signal intensity on T2-weighted sequences. In addition, associated inflammatory disease from other causes cannot be differentiated from recurrent tumor. Another problem encountered in attempting to differentiate postradiation fibrosis from tumor recurrence within the lung is that retained secretions within airways can simulate recurrent tumor. It is presumed that destruction of the ciliated epithelium in the paramediastinal regions of the lung following radiation therapy prevents effective clearance of secretions. These secretions generate high T2-weighted signal because of their high free-water content (see chapter 4, Fig. 27).

A far more prosaic use of MR is in the evaluation of patients following lobectomy or pneumonectomy. Although CT is generally used to detect recurrent disease, MR may be especially valuable (a) in patients in whom extensive surgical clips limit CT interpretation, and (b) in patients unable to receive intravenous contrast (Fig. 25). In the setting of patients who require multiple follow-up examinations, MR can replace CT as the imaging method of choice.

SUMMARY

It is apparent that the use of CT in staging patients with lung cancer has gained wide acceptance. In 1986, Pearson reported on the lung cancer incidences in Toronto over the past 25 years (90). In his experience, the number of thoracotomies for unresectable disease had decreased from 25% to 5%, with operative mortality decreasing from 10% to 3%, and 5-year survival increasing

from 23% to 40%. Pearson cited better selection of surgical candidates due to both invasive and noninvasive techniques as the major factor for these improved statistics. That CT has had a significant impact on lung cancer staging has also been documented by Epstein et al. (14). In a survey of over 500 thoracic surgeons, 98% of the responding surgeons advocated the use of CT, and more than one-third said they used it routinely. Surgeons cited the determination of resectability in patients with a central mass, with or without associated atelectasis, a prominent hilum, or an abnormal mediastinum on plain chest radiography as the most important indications. These results appear to indicate that for most surgeons, the major contribution of CT staging lies in its use as a diagnostic tool preventing unnecessary thoracotomies, excluding advanced cases of lung cancer from surgical consideration. Significantly, only 57% of surgeons agreed that a negative CT examination of the mediastinum obviated the need for mediastinoscopy.

It is our belief, too, that the first and foremost contribution of CT staging is to exclude patients with clear-cut invasion of major structures or evidence of otherwise unsuspected metastatic disease from surgical consideration. New prospective studies with carefully controlled patient populations and pathologic correlation indicate a lower accuracy for CT in the staging of nodal metastases. This lower accuracy, foreseen by earlier investigators, has been confirmed by several independent groups. As the role of CT has been assessed, the staging system itself has been revised. This revision was prompted by new evidence indicating that aggressive surgery, with or without adjuvant forms of therapy, may offer improved prospects for patients with lung cancer. Resection of ipsilateral lymph node metastases, when confined to normal-sized nodes in particular, appears to enhance survival. As a consequence, in our opinion, a negative CT examination (with normal-sized nodes less than 10 mm in diameter) can be construed as justification to bypass preoperative staging procedures including mediastinoscopy. However, this statement should be tempered by the fact that left-sided lung lesions have a higher propensity for contralateral nodal metastases. Because of partial volume effects in the region of the aorticopulmonary window and subcarinal space, these lesions may be more difficult to stage with conventional CT. Thus, careful examination of the contralateral mediastinum, especially in left-sided lesions, is mandatory. Significantly, the accuracy of CT in staging distant sites, such as contralateral nodal stations, has not been addressed by prospective studies. For now, a reasonable solution to this problem would be to initiate preoperative mediastinal exploration whenever enlarged nodes are found in the mediastinum contralateral to a known tumor.

Although small-sized positive nodes should not influence management, enlarged lymph nodes should always be aggressively pursued. Patients should never be denied a potentially curative resection based solely on the radiographic appearance of lymph nodes. Because they may represent benign disease, enlarged nodes should always be assessed histologically. This policy will provide a firm rationale for decisions about curative resection. Although evidence suggests that grossly enlarged nodes are more likely to exhibit capsular penetration, a poor prognostic indicator, until more data is accumulated concerning the accuracy of CT in predicting capsular invasion, in most cases histologic proof is still strongly recommended for any enlarged mediastinal nodes, especially those in regions 4R, 2R, 10L, 4L, and 2L.

It should be emphasized that in the report by Epstein et al., only 10% of surgeons indicated that CT was useful in patients with small peripheral nodules (14). Indeed, there is some controversy about the utility of CT in patients with small peripheral nodules and an apparently normal mediastinum on plain chest radiographs. Pearlberg et al. found that CT contributed useful information in only 1 of 23 patients with T1N0M0 lesions (91). On the other hand, Heavey et al. found significant findings in 5 of 31 patients with peripheral nodules (92,93).

It should be emphasized that the role of CT in evaluating patients with solitary pulmonary nodules depends on whether or not a diagnosis of cancer has or has not been established. In patients in whom a diagnosis of cancer has not been established, CT may be of considerable value by detecting the presence of either significant calcification or fat, findings indicative of benign disease. CT may also help in determining the best approach to obtaining histology by predicting the likely results of transbronchial biopsy versus transthoracic needle aspiration or biopsy. In our judgment, in patients with undiagnosed disease, CT should always be obtained prior to surgical resection (see Chapter 8). In patients in whom a diagnosis of cancer has already been established, as already indicated, the role of CT is more controversial. Although no dogmatic advice can be offered, in our experience, patients with peripheral adenocarcinomas and small cell undifferentiated carcinomas exhibit a higher incidence of mediastinal nodal disease than patients with squamous cell cancers. Consequently, we recommend that CT scans be obtained when tumors of these cell types are identified (see Fig. 13). In addition, given the propensity for contralateral metastasis in left-sided lesions, it may be prudent to scan all left-sided T1N0M0 lesions regardless of cell type.

The main role of MR at this time is as a problem-solving tool. Limited and focused MR examinations should be used to evaluate or to resolve specific questions related to invasion of the chest wall or mediastinum, especially in the evaluation of vascular or neural invasion. MR may also be valuable, albeit to a lesser

extent, in adrenal mass characterization. Finally, MR should be considered an alternative for all patients who cannot tolerate the administration of intravenous contrast media.

REFERENCES

1. Denoix PF. Enquete permanent dans les centres anticancereux. *Bull Inst Nat Hyg* 1946;1:70.
2. American Joint Committee for Cancer Staging and End Results Reporting. *Clinical staging system for carcinoma of the lung.* Philadelphia: JB Lippincott, 1973.
3. Staging of Lung Cancer 1979. American Joint Committee for Cancer Staging and End-results Reporting: Task Force on Lung Cancer, Chicago, IL, 1979.
4. Mountain CF. A new international staging system for lung cancer. *Chest* 1986;89:225S–233S.
5. Mountain CF. Prognostic implications of the International Staging System for Lung Cancer. *Semin Oncol* 1988;15:236–245.
6. McCaughan BC, Martini N, Bains MS, McCormack PM. Chest wall invasion in carcinoma of the lung: Therapeutic and prognostic implications. *J Thorac Cardiovasc Surg* 1985;89:836–841.
7. Mountain CF. The biological operability of stage III non-small cell lung cancer. *Ann Thorac Surg* 1985;40:60–64.
8. Paone JF, Spees EK, Newton CG, et al. An appraisal of en bloc resection of peripheral bronchogenic carcinoma involving the thoracic wall. *Chest* 1981;81:203.
9. Paulson DL. Carcinomas in the superior pulmonary sulcus. *J Thorac Cardiovasc Surg* 1975;70:1095.
10. Piehler JM, Pairolero PC, Weiland LH, et al. Bronchogenic carcinoma with chest wall invasion: factors affecting survival following en bloc resection. *Ann Thorac Surg* 1982;34:684–691.
11. Trastek VF, Pairolero PC, Piehler JM, et al. En bloc (non-chest wall) resection for bronchogenic carcinoma with parietal fixation: factors affecting survival. *J Thorac Cardiovasc Surg* 1984;87:352–358.
12. Gilbert A, Deslauriers JJ, McLish A, Piraux M. Tracheal sleeve pneumonectomy for carcinoma of the proximal left main bronchus. *Can J Surg* 1984;27:583–585.
13. Jensik RJ, Faber LP, Kittle CF, et al. Survival in patients undergoing tracheal sleeve pneumonectomy for bronchogenic carcinoma. *J Thorac Cardiovasc Surg* 1982;84:489–496.
14. Epstein DM, Stephenson LW, Gefter WB, et al. Value of CT in the preoperative assessment of lung cancer: a survey of thoracic surgeons. *Radiology* 1986;161:423–427.
15. Webb RW, Gatsonis C, Zerhouni EA, Heelan RT, Glazer GM, Francis IR, McNeil BJ. CT and MR in staging non-small cell bronchogenic carcinoma: report of the radiological diagnostic oncology group. *Radiology* 1990; in press.
16. Baron RL, Levitt RG, Sagel SS, et al. Computed tomography in the preoperative evaluation of bronchogenic carcinoma. *Radiology* 1982;145:727–732.
17. Glazer HS, Duncan-Meyer J, Aronberg DJ, et al. Pleural and chest wall invasion in bronchogenic carcinoma: CT evaluation. *Radiology* 1985;157:191–194.
18. Pennes DR, Glazer GM, Wimbish KJ, et al. Chest wall invasion by lung cancer: limitations of CT evaluation. *AJR* 1985;144:507–511.
19. Glazer HS, Kaiser LR, Anderson DJ, Molina PL, Emami B, Roper CL, Sagel SS. Indeterminate mediastinal invasion in bronchogenic carcinoma: CT evaluation. *Radiology* 1989;173:37–42.
20. Naruke T, Goya T, Tsuchiya R, Suemasu K. The importance of surgery to non-small cell carcinoma of lung with mediastinal lymph node metastasis. *Ann Thorac Surg* 1988;46:603–610.
21. Naruke T, Goya T, Tsuchiya R, Suemasu K. Prognosis and survival in resected lung carcinoma based on the new international staging system. *J Thorac Cardiovasc Surg* 1988;96:440–447.
22. Kirschner PA. Lung cancer: Preoperative radiation therapy and surgery. *NY State J Med* 1981;81:339.
23. Martini N, Flehinger BJ, Zaman MB, Beattie EJ. Results of resection in non-oat cell carcinoma of the lung with mediastinal lymph node metastases. *Ann Surg* 1983;198:386–397.

24. Pearson FG, DeLarue NC, Ilves R, et al. Significance of positive superior mediastinal nodes identified at mediastinoscopy in patients with resectable cancer of the lung. *J Thorac Cardiovasc Surg* 1982;83:1.

25. Bergh NP, Schersten T. Bronchogenic carcinoma: a follow-up study of a surgically treated series with special reference to the prognostic significance of lymph node metastasis. *Acta Chir Scand (Suppl)* 1965;341:1.

26. Little AG, DeMeester TR, MacMahon H. The staging of lung cancer. *Semin Oncol* 1983;10:56–70.

27. Kirsh MM, Sloan H. Mediastinal metastases in bronchogenic carcinoma: influence of postoperative irradiation, cell type, and location. *Ann Thorac Surg* 1982;33:459.

28. Smith RA. The importance of mediastinal lymph node invasion by pulmonary carcinoma in selection of patients for resection. *Ann Thorac Surg* 1978;25:5.

29. Tisi GM, Friedman PJ, Peters RM, et al. Clinical staging of primary lung cancer. *Am Rev Respir Dis* 1983;127:659.

30. Friedman PJ. Lung cancer: update on staging classifications. *AJR* 1988;150:261–264.

31. Quint LE, Glazer GM, Orringer MB, et al. Mediastinal lymph node detection and sizing at CT and autopsy. *AJR* 1986;147:469–472.

32. Genereux GP, Howie JL. Normal mediastinal lymph node size and number: CT and anatomic study. *AJR* 1984;142:1095–1100.

33. Ashida C, Zerhouni EA, Fishman EK. CT demonstration of prominent right hilar soft tissue collections. *J Comput Assist Tomogr* 1987;11:57–59.

34. Aronberg DJ, Peterson RR, Glazer HS, Sagel SS. The superior sinus of the pericardium: CT appearance. *Radiology* 1985;153:489.

35. Beck E, Beattie EJ Jr. The lymph nodes in the mediastinum. *J Int Coll Surg* 1958;29:247.

36. Schnyder PA, Gamsu G. CT of the pretracheal retrocaval space. *AJR* 1981;136:303.

37. Glazer GM, Gross BH, Quint LE, Francis IR, Bookstein FL, Orringer MB. Normal mediastinal lymph nodes: number and size according to American Thoracic Society mapping. *AJR* 1985;144:261–265.

38. Kiyono K, Sone S, Sakai F, et al. The number and size of normal mediastinal lymph nodes: a postmortem study. *AJR* 1988;150:771–776.

39. Buy JN, Ghossain MA, Poirson F, et al. Computed tomography of mediastinal lymph nodes in nonsmall cell lung cancer, a new approach based on the lymphatic pathway of tumor spread. *J Comput Assist Tomogr* 1988;12:545–552.

40. Rouviere H. *Anatomy of the human lymphatic system.* Ann Arbor, MI: Edwards, 1938.

41. Borrie J. Primary carcinoma of the bronchus: prognoses following surgical resection. *Ann R Coll Surg Engl* 1952;10:165.

42. Nohl-Oser HC. Lymphatics of the lung. In: Shields TW, ed. *General thoracic surgery.* Philadelphia: Lea & Febiger, 1989.

43. Libshitz HI, McKenna RJ Jr, Mountain CF. Patterns of mediastinal metastases in bronchogenic carcinoma. *Chest* 1986;90:229–232.

44. Martini N, Flehinger BJ, Zaman MB, et al. Results in resection in non-oat cell carcinoma of the lung with mediastinal lymph node metastases. *Ann Surg* 1983;198:386–397.

45. Nohl-Oser HC. An investigation of the anatomy of the lymphatic drainage of the lungs. *Ann R Coll Surg Engl* 1972;51:157.

46. Libshitz HI, McKenna RJ Jr. Mediastinal lymph node size in lung cancer. *AJR* 1984;143:715–718.

47. Faling LJ, Pugatch RD, Jung-Legg Y, et al. Computed tomographic scanning of the mediastinum in the staging of bronchogenic carcinoma. *Am Rev Resp Dis* 1981;124:690.

48. Musset D, Grenier P, Carette MF, et al. Primary lung cancer staging: prospective comparative study of MR imaging with CT. *Radiology* 1986;160:607–611.

49. Breyer RH, Karstaedt N, Mills SA, et al. Computed tomography for evaluation of mediastinal lymph nodes in lung cancer: correlation with surgical staging. *Ann Thorac Surg* 1984;38:215–220.

50. Brion JP, Depauw L, Kuhn G, et al. Role of computed tomography and mediastinoscopy in preoperative staging of lung carcinoma. *J Comput Assist Tomogr* 1985;9:480–484.

51. Daly BD, Faling LJ, Bite G, et al. Mediastinal lymph node evaluation by computed tomography in lung cancer. *J Thorac Cardiovasc Surg* 1987;94:664–672.

52. Daly BD, Pugatch RD, Gale ME, et al. Computed tomography, an effective technique for mediastinal staging in lung cancer. *J Thorac Cardiovasc Surg* 1984;88:486–494.

53. Libshitz HI, McKenna RJ, Haynie TP, et al. Mediastinal evaluation in lung cancer. *Radiology* 1984;151:295–299.

54. Rhoads AC, Thomas JH, Hermreck AS, et al. Comparative studies of computerized tomography and mediastinoscopy for the staging of bronchogenic carcinoma. *Am J Surg* 1986;152:587–591.

55. Moak GD, Cockerill EM, Farber MO, et al. Computed tomography vs standard radiology in the evaluation of mediastinal adenopathy. *Chest* 1982;82:69.

56. Glazer GM, Orringer MB, Gross BH, Quint LE. The mediastinum in non-small cell lung cancer: CT-surgical correlation. *AJR* 1984;142:1101–1105.

57. Osborne DR, Korobkin M, Ravin CE, et al. Comparison of plain radiography, conventional tomography, and computed tomography in detecting intrathoracic lymph node metastases from lung carcinoma. *Radiology* 1982;142:157.

58. Lewis JW Jr, Madrazo BL, Gross SC, et al. The value of radiographic and computed tomography in the staging of lung carcinoma. *Ann Thorac Surg* 1982;34:553–558.

59. Staples CA, Miller NL, Miller RR, Evans KG, Nelems B. Mediastinal nodes in bronchogenic carcinoma: comparison between CT and mediastinoscopy. *Radiology* 1988;167:367–372.

60. Hirleman MR, Yin-Chin VS, Chin LC, Schapero RL. The resectability of primary lung carcinoma: a diagnostic staging review. *CT* 1980;4:146.

61. McKenna RJ, Libshitz HI, Mountain CF. Roentgenographic evaluation of mediastinal nodes for preoperative assessment in lung cancer. *Chest* 1985;88:206–210.

62. McCloud TC, Kosiuk JP, Templeton PA, Shepard JO, Moore EH, Mathisen DJ, Wain JC, Grillo HC. CT in the staging of bronchogenic carcinoma: update of analysis by correlative lymph node mapping and sampling. *Radiology* 1989;173(P):69.

63. Grenier P, Dubray B, Carette MF, Frija G, Musset D, Chastan GC. Preoperative thoracic staging of lung cancer: CT and MR evaluation. *Diagn Inter Radiol* 1989;173(P):69.

64. Pearson FG. Use of mediastinoscopy in selection of patients for lung cancer operations. *Ann Thorac Surg* 1980;30:295.

65. Ashraf MH, Milsom PL, Walesby RK. Selection by mediastinoscopy and long-term survival in bronchial carcinoma. *Ann Thorac Surg* 1980;30:208.

66. Mathews MJ, Kanhouwa S, Peckren J, Robinette D. Frequency of residual and metastatic tumor in patients undergoing curative surgical resection in lung cancer. *Chem Rep* 1973;4:63.

67. Winstanley DP. Fruitless resections. *Thorax* 1968;23:327.

68. Bernardino ME, McClennan MW, Phillips VM, et al. CT guided adrenal biopsy: accuracy, safety, and indications. *AJR* 1985;144:67–69.

69. Oliver TW, Bernardino ME, Miller JL, et al. Isolated adrenal masses in nonsmall cell bronchogenic carcinoma. *Radiology* 1984;153:217–218.

70. Meyer JA. Effect of histologically verified TNM stage on disease control in treated small cell carcinoma of the lung. *Cancer* 1985;55:1747–1752.

71. Martini N, Heelan R, Westcott J, et al. Comparative merits of conventional, computed tomographic, and magnetic resonance imaging in assessing mediastinal involvement in surgically confirmed lung cancer. *J Thorac Cardiovasc Surg* 1985;90:639–648.

72. Patterson GA, Ginsberg RJ, Poon PY, et al. A prospective evaluation of magnetic resonance imaging, computed tomography, and mediastinoscopy in the preoperative assessment of mediastinal node status in bronchogenic carcinoma. *J Thorac Cardiovasc Surg* 1987;94:679–84.

73. Poon PY, Bronskill MJ, Henkelman RM, et al. Mediastinal lymph node metastases from bronchogenic carcinoma: detection with MR imaging and CT. *Radiology* 1987;162:651–656.

74. Haggar AM, Pearlberg JL, Froelich JW, et al. Chest wall invasion by carcinoma of the lung: detection by MR imaging. *AJR* 1987;148:1075–1078.

75. Heelan RT, Demas BE, Caravelli JF, et al. Superior sulcus tumors: CT and MR imaging. *Radiology* 1989;170:637–641.

76. Webb WR, Jensen BJ, Gamsu G, Sollitto R, Moore EH. Sagittal MR imaging of the chest: normal and abnormal. *J Comput Assist Tomogr* 1985;9:471–479.

77. Blair DN, Rapoport S, Sostman HD, Blair OC. Normal brachial plexus: MR imaging. *Radiology* 1987;165:763–767.

78. Castagno AA, Shuman WP. MR imaging in clinically suspected brachioplexus tumor. *AJR* 1987;149:1219–1222.

79. Webb WR, Jensen BJ, Sollitto R, et al. Bronchogenic carcinoma: staging with MR compared with staging with CT and surgery. *Radiology* 1985;156:117–124.

80. Webb WR, Kameda K, Adachi S, Kono M. Detection of T factor in lung cancer using MRI and CT. *J Thorac Imag* 1988;3:73–80.

81. Tobler JA, Levitt RG, Glazer HS, Moran J, Crouch E, Evans RG. Differentiation of proximal bronchogenic carcinoma from post-obstructive lobar collapse by magnetic resonance imaging: comparison with computed tomography. *Invest Radiol* 1987;22:538–543.

82. De Geer G, Webb WR, Sollitto R, Golden J. MR characteristics of benign lymph node enlargement in sarcoidosis and Castleman's disease. *Eur J Radiol* 1986;6:145–148.

83. Glazer G, Orringer MB, Chenevert TL, et al. Mediastinal lymph nodes: relaxation time/pathologic correlation and implications in staging of lung cancer with MR imaging. *Radiology* 1988;168:429–431.

84. Berland LL, Koslin DB, Kenney PJ, et al. Differentiation between small benign and malignant adrenal masses with dynamic incremented CT. *AJR* 1988;151:95–101.

85. Reinig JW, Doppman JL, Dwyer AJ, Frank J. MRI of indeterminate adrenal masses. *AJR* 1986;147:493–496.

86. Glazer GM, Woolsey EJ, Borrello J, et al. Adrenal tissue characterization using MR imaging. *Radiology* 1986;158:73–79.

87. Chang A, Glazer HS, Lee JKT, et al. Adrenal gland: MR imaging. *Radiology* 1987;163:123–128.

88. Chezmar JL, Robbins SM, Nelson JRC, et al. Adrenal masses: characterization with T1-weighted MR imaging. *Radiology* 1988;166:357–359.

89. Glazer HS, Lee JKT, Levitt RL, et al. Radiation fibrosis: differentiation from recurrent tumor by MR imaging. *Radiology* 1985;156:721–726.

90. Pearson FG. Lung cancer: the past 25 years. *Chest* 1986;89:200S–205S.

91. Pearlberg JL, Sandler MA, Beute GH, Madrazo BL. T1 N0 M0 bronchogenic carcinoma: assessment by CT. *Radiology* 1985;157:187–190.

92. Heavey LR, Glazer GM, Gross BH, Francis IR, Orringer MB. The role of CT in staging radiographic T1 N0 M0 lung cancer. *AJR* 1986;146:285–290.

93. Conces DJ, Klink JF, Tarver RD, Moak GD. T1 N0 M0 lung cancer: evaluation with CT. *Radiology* (in press).

Chapter 7

Focal Lung Disease

Assessment of a localized parenchymal abnormality detected on plain radiographs presents one of the most challenging problems in pulmonology. Given the many causes of focal lung disease, accurate noninvasive diagnosis is essential to reduce the need for invasive approaches. The development of scanners which permit thin-section studies at suspended respiration has led to increased use of computed tomography (CT) for such an assessment. Initially, efforts were concentrated on *densitometric* analyses that could provide specific information by detecting calcification or fat within nodules. More recently, CT has been found to provide unique *morphologic* clues that help characterize many focal pulmonary processes.

The application of magnetic resonance (MR) to focal lung disease is still in its infancy. Respiratory motion remains a major impediment to the evaluation of the pulmonary parenchyma. There are, however, several indications for using MR as an adjunct modality, primarily in patients with suspected vascular pathology.

GENERAL CONSIDERATIONS

Focal lung disease is manifested in most cases by nodular lesions or localized areas of pulmonary infiltration and consolidation. Several attributes unique to CT make it especially useful in assessing focal lung disease.

CT offers the advantage of imaging the lung unimpeded by superimposed structures. In addition, the high contrast achieved between normal parenchyma and focal processes facilitates both visualization and analysis. With proper electronic window settings, the conspicuity of nodules is much higher than with plain radiographic techniques and detectability of lesions is greatly enhanced. For example, the limit of visibility for noncalcified nodules is approximately 6 mm on plain radiographs, whereas CT can demonstrate nodules as small as 1 mm.

CT is by far the most sensitive technique in the detection of focal parenchymal disease. Thus, whenever the clinical situation suggests a high likelihood of an undetected pulmonary abnormality—even when the chest radiograph is negative—CT should be given strong consideration. For example, the search for metastatic nodules too small to be seen by plain radiography or potentially obscured by overlying structures is now a routine indication for chest CT. More recently, the rising incidence of immune system deficiency in the patient population secondary to the expanding use of organ transplantation, chemotherapy, and AIDS has fostered the use of CT as a sensitive method for the early detection of infectious complications.

CT can more precisely define the morphology and the relationship of a given pulmonary lesion to airways and vessels. In many cases, such a determination is of great value in reaching a specific diagnosis. For example, the demonstration of a connection between a pulmonary artery branch and a nodular lesion may be a strong clue to a vascular or hematogenous etiology. The relationship to airways is helpful not only in determining the best bronchoscopic approach, but also in suggesting a specific etiology, as in a bronchial carcinoid.

CT permits density discrimination in an order of magnitude greater than that achieved by conventional radiographic methods. In addition, density measurements by CT can be quantified whereas subjective assessment is the rule with conventional methods. Consequently, densitometric analyses have come to play a major diagnostic role in the assessment of pulmonary nodules.

Throughout this chapter we will demonstrate how these characteristic advantages of CT can be utilized to achieve optimal diagnostic performance for the clinical entities commonly encountered in daily practice.

THE SOLITARY PULMONARY NODULE

The term solitary pulmonary nodule refers to a focal, rounded, or ovoid lesion of the lung parenchyma less than 6 cm in diameter. The pulmonary nodule is one of the most common radiologic findings, occurring in about 1 to 2 per 1,000 chest radiographs. Clinically, this finding is most often made in an asymptomatic patient during routine screening radiography. Other common situations include the patient with a known extrathoracic malignancy in whom a surveillance film demonstrates a nodule, the immunocompromised patient who presents with a lesion (with or without fever), and the patient with apparent extrathoracic metastases and a pulmonary mass. The lung is an organ in open contact with the atmosphere and is therefore constantly subjected to potentially noxious agents. Not surprisingly, then, most nodules represent reactive benign processes such as granulomas. Unfortunately, a solitary nodule is also the most common presentation for asymptomatic bronchogenic carcinoma. In a review of 1,267 lung cancers by Theros (1), 507 or 40% of cases initially presented as peripheral lung masses. A bronchogenic carcinoma is even more likely to present as a peripheral lung nodule in asymptomatic individuals. This was true in

72% of the patients with asymptomatic lung cancer detected with radiographic screening by Stitik and Tockman (2).

Despite advances in the assessment of pulmonary nodules with conventional radiography, bronchoscopy, and percutaneous biopsy, surgical resection is still required in many patients with benign lesions in order to exclude the possibility of malignancy. For instance, Keagy et al. (3) reviewed 303 thoracotomies for suspected but preoperatively unconfirmed malignancies. They found that 79 of 122 patients who underwent a minor resection (biopsy, wedge resection, or segmentectomy) and 33 of 102 who underwent a major resection (lobectomy or pneumonectomy) "were shown to have benign disease despite the preoperative suspicion of cancer." The distinction between a benign and a malignant nodule is, therefore, the primary goal of diagnostic evaluation.

Benign granulomas and primary bronchogenic carcinomas constitute the majority of all resected pulmonary nodules, accounting for over 80% of cases. The exact percentage of granulomas versus malignancies in resected nodules varies depending on the reported series, with malignancies representing 40–60% of all resected lesions (4,5). Other etiologies include hamartoma (5–7%), solitary metastases (4–5%), bronchial carcinoid (2%), organizing pneumonia, pulmonary infarct, and arteriovenous malformation, in order of decreasing frequency.

The diagnostic approach to a pulmonary nodule should be an orderly process proceeding from conventional radiographs to more sophisticated invasive techniques. Careful use of all available diagnostic options should lead to optimal segregation of patients requiring no intervention from those requiring thoracotomy. First and foremost, the intraparenchymal nature of any nodular abnormality needs to be confirmed. Second, an assessment of the likely nature of a nodule should be undertaken. This assessment is based on clinical information and prior studies to define the characteristics of the nodule and its growth rate. Finally, densitometric CT analysis can help detect calcification or fat and specific morphologic features, if present.

Confirmation of the Intraparenchymal Nature of the Nodule

When an abnormality is detected on a chest radiograph, the first duty of the radiologist is to determine the exact location of the lesion. Indeed, superimposition of structures on the plain radiograph may lead to uncer-

→

FIG. 2. Limitations of conventional radiography: extrapleural lesions. **A:** Radiographs showing a semicircular density on the lateral aspect of left chest (*arrow*). **B:** CT demonstrates a pleural mass with smooth margins and obtuse angles. The CT numbers were low and a lipoma was diagnosed. No confirmation was obtained. By clearly showing the extrapulmonary locations of radiographic abnormalities, CT obviates the need for more invasive testing.

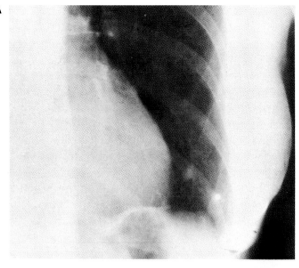

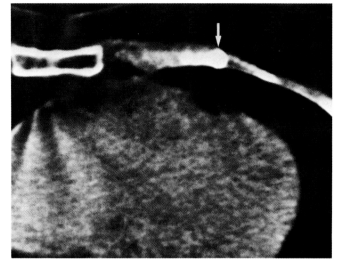

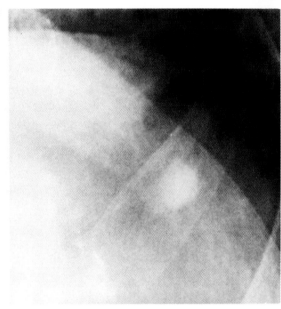

FIG. 1. Limitations of conventional radiography: chest wall lesions (58-year-old female with history of right mastectomy for carcinoma and an apparently new left lower lobe nodule). **A:** Chest radiography with nipple marker. A definite nodule density is present in the lower left lung field. **B:** CT scan. No lung nodule is seen, but in the projected area of the radiographic abnormality, a focal density in the overlying rib is noted (*arrow*). A diagnosis of bone island was suggested. **C:** Fluorographic spot view. The diagnosis of bone island is confirmed.

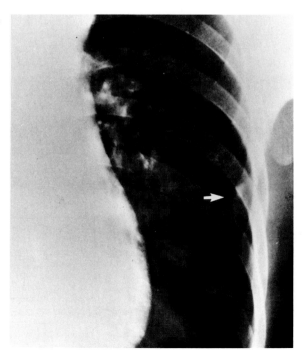

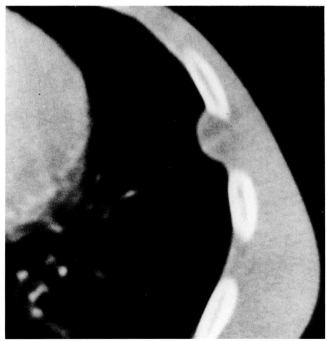

tainty about the exact location of a perceived abnormality. The most common causes of pseudo-nodules on plain films are:

1. a bone island in a rib (Fig. 1);
2. a protruding structure such as a pleural-based mass or plaque (Figs. 2 and 3);
3. a tortuous branch vessel of the aorta (Fig. 4);
4. a prominent pulmonary vein; or
5. a surface structure such as a mole on the skin.

Ten to twenty percent of small or subtle lesions interpreted as possible nodules on the initial radiograph are not actual intraparenchymal nodules. This problem can be resolved by a variety of approaches. Repeat radiographs with nipple markers and/or oblique views, as well as fluoroscopy with or without spot views, are helpful. If uncertainty remains, CT can be used to determine the exact location of the abnormality. CT is particularly helpful for lesions located in complex anatomic regions (the apices and the paraspinal, perihilar, and paracardiac areas).

At the time of the CT examination, the plain radiographic findings must be correlated to ensure that the proper area has been examined. This is particularly im-

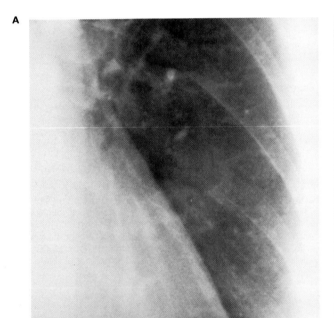

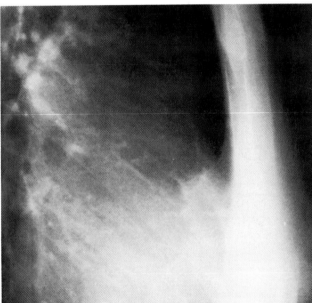

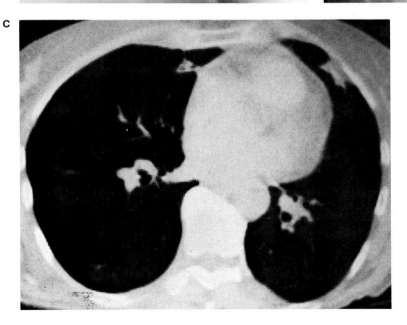

FIG. 3. Limitations of conventional radiography: pleural plaque and fibrosis. **A,B:** PA and lateral radiographs, coned down views. An irregular, spiculated, round density is seen on both views which gives the impression of a mass. **C:** CT definitely demonstrates that the mass is, in fact, an irregular, flat, pleural plaque, which does not warrant suspicion of carcinoma and should be followed conservatively. It is because the plaque is obliquely oriented relative to the PA as well as the lateral axis that it appears mass-like on PA and lateral plain films.

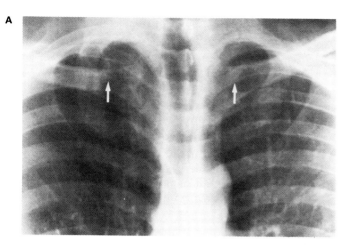
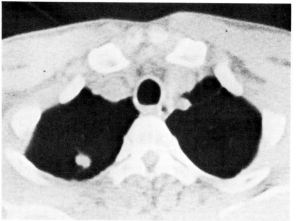

FIG. 4. CT in questionable abnormalities (42-year-old asymptomatic male smoker). **A:** Close-up view of apices reveals a small density on the right side and a similar one on the left (*arrows*). **B:** CT reveals that the right density represents a true intrapulmonary lesion, which subsequently was proved to be an adenocarcinoma, and that the left lesion represents a tortuous subclavian artery.

portant for nodules located in the perihilar regions. With CT, centrally located vessels running perpendicularly to the scanning plane can hamper the recognition of adjacent nodules. However, careful and orderly analysis of adjacent contiguous scans resolves this problem. The possibility of misdiagnosing a nodule also exists when the junction of the first rib with the sternum is made prominent by osteophytes that protrude in the anterior aspect of the upper lobes, simulating a nodule (Fig. 5). The most significant diagnostic pitfall of CT, however, is the possibility of missing a pulmonary nodule because of unequal respiratory cycles or undetected patient dis-

placement during the examination (6). Extreme care should be exercised to ensure that breathing instructions are understood by the patient. To identify discrepancies in anatomic levels, careful analysis of the CT images in a sequential manner is necessary. Control of respiratory excursion by feedback monitoring devices has been proposed but has not gained practical acceptance (7). A new method includes the rapid acquisition of a series of scans during a single breath-hold to avoid all possibility of spurious displacement between scans. This is easily done using a dynamic incremental scanning technique (8,9).

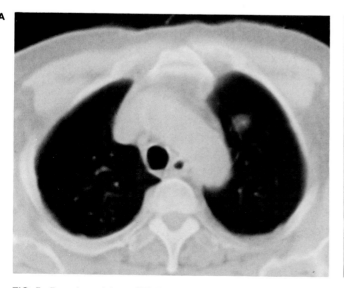
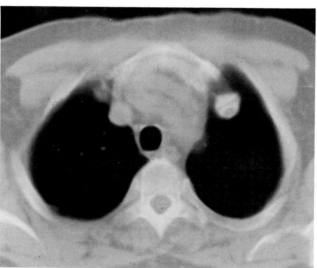

FIG. 5. Pseudo-nodule on CT. **A:** An apparent nodule is seen in the left upper lobe. **B:** Adjacent scan located more cranially reveals that nodule seen in A represents a prominent osteophytic junction of the first rib with the sternum. This is a common cause of pseudo-nodule on CT.

Determining the Nature of an Intraparenchymal Nodule

Once the intraparenchymal location of a suspected pulmonary nodule has been shown, the next objective is to define its exact etiology. The morphologic features of a nodule, although often suggestive, are not reliable enough because of significant overlap in the appearance of benign and malignant lesions. But, as demonstrated by Cummings et al. (10) who used bayesian analysis, the combination of several morphologic and clinical characteristics can be helpful. By combining the estimated likelihoods of malignancy as a function of size, shape, contour, smoking history, and patient age, it is possible to define subsets of patients for whom the possibility of malignancy is so high or so low that management is decisively affected. For example, patients over 35 years of age with a significant smoking history of over 5 to 10 years and a lesion over 2.5 cm in diameter that appears spiculated and is located in the upper lobes, have a very high likelihood of malignancy. In such patients, aggressive diagnosis with needle biopsy, bronchoscopy, or surgery, if necessary, is indicated. Conversely, asymptomatic nonsmokers less than 35 years old presenting with a round, smooth, less than 2-cm diameter lesion of the lower lobes represent a patient group with a low likelihood of malignancy. Noninvasive approaches, including CT if necessary, are warranted in such cases.

Although large size indicates a high likelihood of malignancy, small size is not a reliable indicator for benign disease. With the emphasis on early detection and the increasing use of chest radiography, more malignancies are now diagnosed at an earlier stage. In one study, 6.4% of the primary malignancies were 1 cm or less in diameter (11). Another multi-center cooperative study found 15% of the primary cancers in that size range (12). The

appearance of edges is also not characteristic of a specific etiology. Although spiculation is most common in malignancies, up to 35% of malignancies may have smooth, slightly lobulated edges (12,13).

There are few absolute noninvasive criteria for certifying a pulmonary nodule as benign. The most convincing evidence of benign disease is the unequivocal demonstration of absence of growth for at least two years. Thus, comparison with old studies, if available, should be the first step in the evaluation of any nodule. The second best criterion of benignancy is the finding of intranodular calcification distributed in a diffuse, central, or laminated pattern. Multiple series have demonstrated that the radiographic detection of calcification in pulmonary nodules indicates a high probability of benign disease. In the 1950s, when aggressive surgical management of pulmonary nodules was the rule, large numbers of resected calcified solitary masses proved to be benign (14,15). A careful analysis of specimen radiographs of lung nodules by O'Keefe et al. (16) revealed four different calcification patterns: a) laminated and concentric; b) dense central nidus; c) "popcorn" type; and d) punctate (Fig. 6).

The first three types were found to be characteristic of benign lesions. The fourth type could be seen in unusual cases of malignancy. Calcification is much less common in malignancies. Theros found only seven radiographically calcified cancers in a series of 1,267 cases of pulmonary nodules (1). These findings prompted the widespread use of conventional tomography techniques in the 1960s and 1970s to characterize pulmonary nodules. Despite the introduction of conventional tomography in the assessment of nodules, a large number of benign lesions remained undetected, leading to a high percentage of unnecessary thoracotomies. In a ten-year study

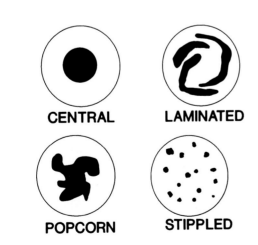

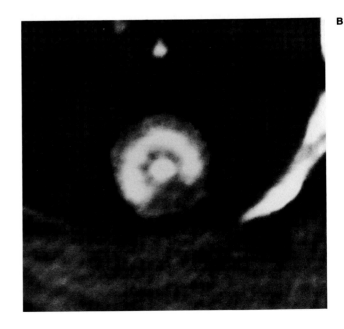

FIG. 6. Patterns of calcification. **A:** Central, laminated, and popcorn-like calcification patterns are characteristic of benign nodules. The stippled pattern can be seen in both benign and malignant lesions. **B:** Example of laminated calcification in a granuloma.

Higgins et al. (11) found that 36% of resected nodules were malignant. In individuals over 50 years of age, the percentage rose to 55%. In a series by Stitik and Tockman, linear tomography showed unsuspected benign calcification in less than 4% of cases (2). In a study by Good (14), less than 2% of 294 masses considered noncalcified by standard chest roentgenography revealed unsuspected calcium deposits with linear tomography. Clearly, a more sensitive technique to assess calcification of nodules was needed. CT, with its greater density resolution, serves this purpose.

Detecting Calcification by CT Densitometry

Three basic assumptions support the use of CT to distinguish benign from malignant nodules. First, granulomas contain more calcium more often than do malignant tumors. Second, a large number of calcified granulomas cannot be identified as such by conventional techniques. And third, CT densitometric measurements are more sensitive and reliable than those obtained by conventional methods.

Dystrophic calcification, the most common type found in granulomas, is a common end result of many types of tissue injuries. Suppurative liquefaction, coagulation, and enzymatic necrosis can all lead to deposition of calcium salts, mostly calcium carbonates, and calcium phosphates (17). Calcium and phosphorus, elements with high atomic numbers, increase attenuation coefficients and lead to higher CT numbers for calcified nodules. Sagel et al. (18) first reported this phenomenon in an asymptomatic patient with two nodules that appeared uncalcified on conventional tomography. One of the nodules, a granuloma, had CT numbers indicating a much higher density than that of the other nodule, a carcinoma. Similar observations were made in subsequent series by Jost et al. (19), Muhm et al. (20), and McLoud et al. (21). Raptopoulos et al. (22), in the first systematic analysis of CT density in 31 solitary lung nodules, found five high-density nodules in which no calcification was apparent on conventional tomography. All of the high-density nodules were benign. These early studies confirmed the potential of CT in evaluating pulmonary nodules, but accurate determination of CT density in the smaller nodules was hampered by the lack of thin sections.

Partial volume averaging of surrounding air using thick sections prevents "true" density assessment. Consequently, reliable measurements of nodule density require thin sections and selection of pixels with the highest CT numbers, ensuring that only nodule material is represented. This concept led to the first proposal by Siegelman et al. (23) for systematically using CT to replace conventional tomography. After locating the nodule with thick sections, a series of thin-section scans at suspended respiration are obtained throughout the nodule. By averaging the 32 highest-valued contiguous pixels, a representative CT number of the nodule can be generated (Fig. 7). *A very important caveat is that injection of iodinated contrast is contraindicated when performing such studies.* Iodine is a high atomic number element which, like calcium, is highly attenuating and can artificially increase the CT number of a pulmonary nodule. This can lead to a false diagnosis of calcification (24).

In the first study of 91 nodules by Siegelman et al. (23), 33 benign nodules were identified by virtue of a representative CT number greater than 164 Hounsfield units (HU). All 58 malignant nodules had representative CT numbers lower than 147 HU, and 20 of the 33 benign lesions had representative CT numbers greater than 164 HU. These investigators concluded that CT was more objective and sensitive than conventional techniques in assessing the density of solitary pulmonary nodules. The representative number method was subsequently tried by other investigators but results were mixed. Godwin et al. (25) examined 36 nodules using 165 HU as the threshold. All 14 malignant lesions had low CT numbers. Five nodules that appeared calcified on conventional tomography also appeared calcified on CT. However, only one of the 17 benign nodules that did not contain apparent calcification on conventional studies was deemed calcified by CT. The finding of unsuspected calcification in only one of 36 cases led Godwin and co-workers to conclude that the incremental gain offered by CT was not large enough to justify replacing conventional tomography.

The apparent discrepancy between these well-conducted studies led to the hypothesis that patient selection factors related to geographic and institutional variations may have been at play. For example, conventional tomography techniques were not standardized and the criteria for interpreting such studies were subjective. Thus, solitary pulmonary nodules that would have been considered calcified by one group of investigators may have been deemed noncalcified by another group. Likewise, the prevalence of granulomatous disease may have been different. These biases could have falsely increased the sensitivity level of CT compared to conventional tomography at one institution but not at others.

Other researchers hypothesized that equipment-related differences could explain the observed discrepancies. This prompted more research into the fundamentals of CT densitometry for pulmonary nodules and, in turn, revealed that in the chain of events needed to generate CT numbers for pulmonary nodules, several sources of variance can be introduced. CT numbers cannot therefore be considered to represent absolute measures of x-ray attenuation. McCullough showed that even though CT numbers are defined relative to physically constant substances such as water or air, many

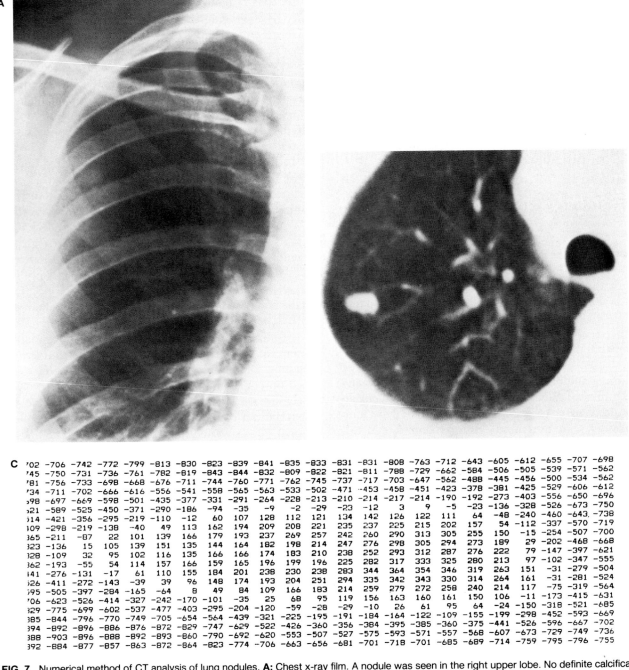

FIG. 7. Numerical method of CT analysis of lung nodules. **A:** Chest x-ray film. A nodule was seen in the right upper lobe. No definite calcification was appreciated on plain films or tomography. **B:** CT scan of a 4-mm–thick section. Several sections of the nodule are obtained at suspended respiration. The section in which the highest CT numbers are observed is selected for analysis. **C:** A printout of the CT numbers representing the nodules is obtained. The highest numbers are identified within the section and the average of the 32 highest contiguous numbers is calculated; when above 164 HU, the nodule can be considered benign, as in this case.

variables can influence the measured CT density of a given structure within the body (26). Zerhouni et al. were the first to systematically analyze all factors potentially influencing quantitative CT measurements of solitary pulmonary nodules (27). By performing a series of experiments on different scanners, large variations in the CT numbers of simulated pulmonary nodules were observed. These variations prevented direct comparison of results from scanner to scanner. Several factors were found to be critical to the performance of CT densitometry.

The algorithm of reconstruction used to compute CT numbers can have a profound influence on the apparent CT numbers of nodules of different size (Fig. 8). Recon-

A 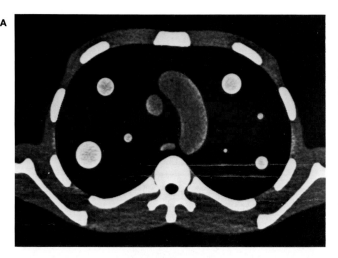 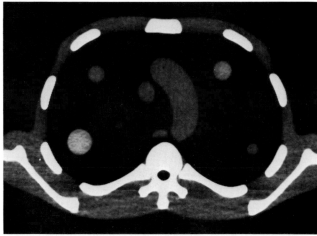 B

FIG. 8. Influence of algorithm of reconstruction on CT numbers of pulmonary nodules. **A** and **B** represent the same scan of an anthropomorphic phantom containing simulated nodules of different sizes but identical composition. Image A was processed using high *spatial* resolution reconstruction software. Note the high density of the nodules relative to the simulated aortic arch. Image B was processed using a high *contrast* resolution reconstruction software. Note the much lower apparent density of the nodules. The decrease in density affects the smaller nodule to a greater extent. The smaller nodules now appear of lower density than the aorta. This experiment demonstrates the relativity of CT numbers and their dependence on software which may result in widely divergent CT density measurements depending on nodule size. Note also that comparing density of a nodule to a known structure such as the aorta is potentially misleading.

struction algorithms that are designed to enhance *spatial* resolution tend to increase the CT numbers of smaller nodules. On the other hand, algorithms designed to enhance *contrast* resolution rely on "smoothing" techniques which are based on averaging the density of neighboring pixels. In the lung such algorithms have the effect of artificially decreasing the CT number of nodules, thereby preventing sensitive detection of calcification. The effect of differences in reconstruction software is most pronounced with smaller nodules, which also are most likely to be benign. The CT number to use as a calcification threshold may thus vary for different scanners and for nodules of different sizes. Therefore, no *universal* threshold CT number can be used to differentiate calcified from noncalcified nodules.

Another important source of variation is the effect of surrounding structures on the ultimate measurement of a given nodule's density. For example, in patients with thick chest walls, more attenuation of the x-ray beam as it traverses the patient leads to a change in the effective energy spectrum of the beam. This effect, known as beam hardening, can lead to decreased density measurements for nodules (28) (Fig. 9). Manufacturers may apply corrections for the beam hardening effect based on the expected attenuation properties of the body part scanned. These corrections are effective for the head or abdomen, which are of homogeneous density. However, in the chest where there are wide differences in density of the chest walls and lungs, corrections are less effective.

The influence of the nodule position within the field of scanning is another important variable. Ideally, the same object should exhibit identical CT numbers regardless of the position of the object within the field of view of the scanner. However, this is not observed in each scanner. Often, differences of 40–50 HU can be seen between the density of a nodule measured at the center of the field of view compared to a measure obtained at the edge of the field of view (27,29).

Other investigations by Levi et al. showed the unreliability of CT numbers as absolute values (30). Subsequent investigations by McCullough and Morin (31) suggested that CT densitometry of lung nodules could not be reproducibly performed unless the effects of thoracic geometry were taken into account. Zerhouni et al. (27) reached similar conclusions and established that no single, generally valid threshold CT number can be defined for densitometry of solitary pulmonary nodules. The critical number of 164 HU originally described by Siegelman et al. (23) applied only to the particular scanner used.

It became rapidly apparent in the early 1980s that the use of CT for evaluating pulmonary nodules would depend on finding ways of correcting for the many sources of variance affecting CT densitometry. Three methods can be used to achieve such a goal. First, one can study a number of patients to establish a threshold value (or values) for the particular scanner used, ensuring stability of measurements by careful calibration and monitoring. The main drawback of this method is the requirement of an initial experimental group of patients and the need to redefine a new threshold CT number every time a modification is implemented on the scanner. Proto and Thomas (32) followed this method and examined 149

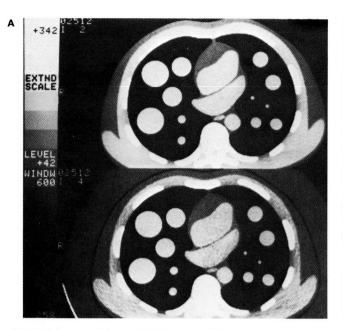
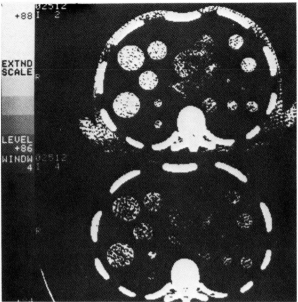

FIG. 9. Influence of chest wall thickness on CT numbers. **A:** Phantom containing simulated nodules of identical composition was scanned without (*top*) and with (*bottom*) additional ring of fatty equivalent material to simulate a thin versus an obese patient. **B:** Narrow window settings image of A shows greater apparent density of simulated nodules in "thin" phantom. This experiment shows that CT numbers may be affected by surrounding material, thus complicating accurate densitometry.

solitary pulmonary nodules for which they found a CT threshold value of 200 HU. Seventy-seven of the 149 nodules were malignant; all measured less than 151 HU. Twenty-six of the 72 benign lesions had a representative CT number over 200 HU. Of these twenty-six, 21 had no detectable calcification on conventional tomography. Sagel (33), using a threshold CT number of 140 HU, was able to diagnose benign disease in 15% of all cases in which conventional tomography did not suggest calcification.

Dual energy scanning is another technique that can overcome the problem of densitometry. Theoretically, this method offers the potential of generating absolute and reliable assessments of calcium content. Cann et al. (34) performed experiments with phantoms specifically designed to simulate lung nodules. They found dual energy CT more sensitive than single energy CT in detecting as well as quantifying calcification. However, this method has been applied to only a few patients and no documented clinical trial has been reported to date. Technical problems in the implementation of the method and the need for substantial hardware and software modifications are major impediments to progress.

The Reference Phantom Method

Other investigators sought a standardization method to permit widespread use of CT densitometry for nodules. A standard reference device to determine nodule density independently of scanner performance was proposed (35). Fullerton and White were the first to demonstrate the need for anthropomorphic test objects for CT densitometry (36). White et al. (37) suggested the use of specially formulated resins to duplicate the shape and x-ray properties of body parts for all densitometric analyses. Based on these concepts, Zerhouni et al. developed a reference phantom that can simulate the shape, dimensions, and radiographic density of the thoracic cage in most patients (35).

Cylinders that can be located anywhere within the lung cavity of the phantom are used to simulate the size and position of the patient's nodule (Fig. 10). The aim is to simulate as closely as possible the conditions of measurement within the patient to provide a meaningful comparison of density, independent of equipment-related or patient-related variations. The density of the reference cylinders is adjusted to correspond to a density

FIG. 11. Example of calcified benign nodule. **A:** Eight-mm right upper lobe nodule with patient scan (*top*) and phantom simulation (*bottom*). **B:** Comparison of images in A with minimum window width shows a group of several pixels of higher density than that of the reference nodule which is no longer visible at a level of 54 HU.

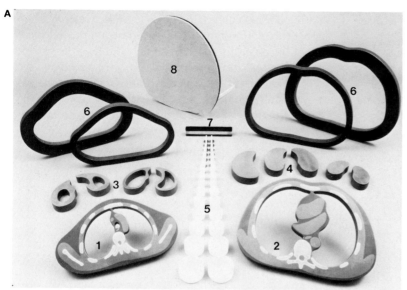

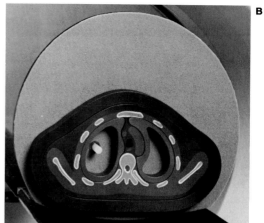

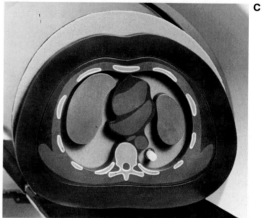

FIG. 10. Reference phantom for pulmonary nodule densitometry. **A:** Components of the phantom are basic anatomic sections with 1 and 2, representing upper and lower thorax, made of special tissue-equivalent material. Inserts to simulate apices (3), spleen and liver (4), nodules (5), and chest wall thickness (6) are provided along with a slice thickness gauge (7) to check for accuracy of slice thickness and a support board (8). These components can be used to simulate most patients and to provide a reference comparison. **B:** Example of simulation of a 1-cm nodule in the right upper lobe. **C:** Example of simulation of a 1-cm nodule in left costophrenic angle.

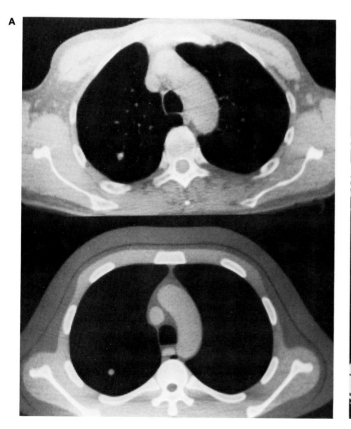

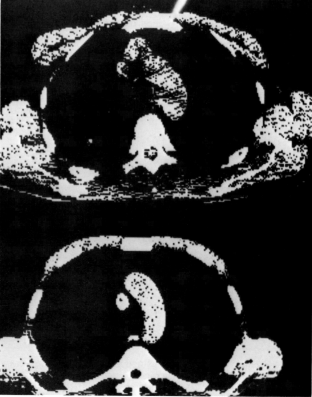

slightly higher than the 164 HU threshold value originally found by Siegelman et al. (23). The use of a reference phantom greatly simplifies the task of measuring pulmonary nodule density. The method consists of scanning the patient with thin sections and then selecting the part of the phantom that best represents the patient anatomy. Adjustments for chest wall thickness correct for beam hardening artifacts and a reference cylinder (of appropriate size) is placed within the lung cavity of the phantom to simulate the nodule of the patient in size and position within the gantry (Fig. 10 B and C). The phantom is then scanned immediately after the patient, using identical technical factors. The density of the patient nodule and that of the reference phantom nod-

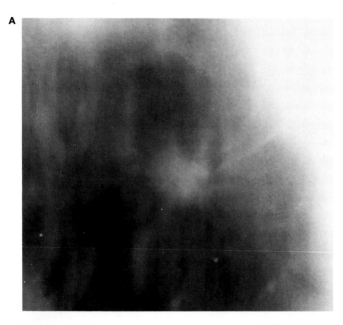

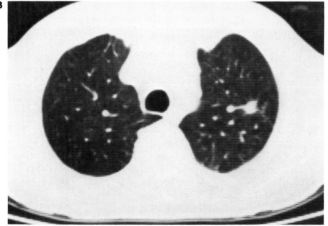

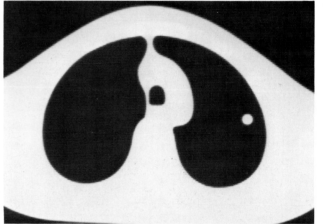

FIG. 12. A: Tomogram of 1.4-cm left upper lobe nodule shows no calcification. **B,C:** Thin section CT scans of patient (B) and phantom simulation (C). **D,E:** Same as B with narrow window width of 2 HU and level of 94 HU. The reference nodule (D) is no longer visible whereas a large group of centrally located pixels is still seen in the patient nodule (E) indicating a central nucleus of calcification and a high likelihood of benignancy. Follow up over two years showed no change in this presumed granuloma.

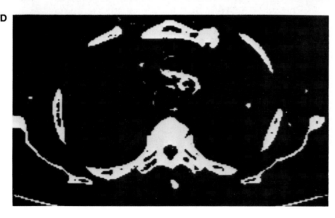

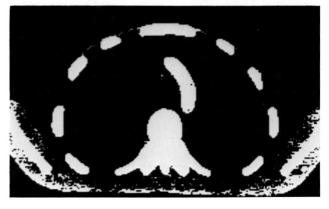

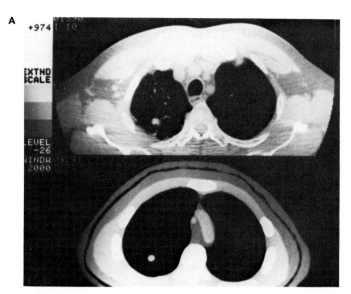
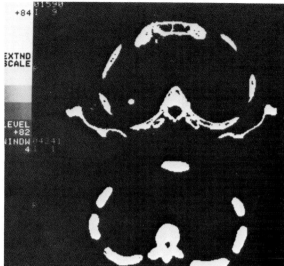

FIG. 13. Benign nodule: Sixty-three-year-old patient with right upper lobe nodule found on routine examination. **A:** Patient scan (*top*) and phantom simulation (*bottom*). No gross calcification is noted. **B:** Comparison at narrow window width shows that almost entire patient nodule contains pixels of greater density than reference nodule and is thus calcified. In about half of benign nodule cases, thin section CT alone does not reveal visually obvious calcification; comparison with reference phantom is needed for sensitive detection.

ule can then be compared. Calcification in nodules is detected when a group of adjacent pixels is found to be of greater density than the densest pixel of the reference nodule (Figs. 11–13).

Such a phantom was tested in an initial series of 41 nodules, enabling detection of 11 of 17 benign lesions.

None of the 24 malignant lesions had attenuation values above those of the reference nodule (35) (Figs. 14–16). Subsequently, a larger multi-center cooperative trial involving 10 institutions throughout the United States was undertaken (12). Using six different types of scanners, 384 nodules considered noncalcified by conventional

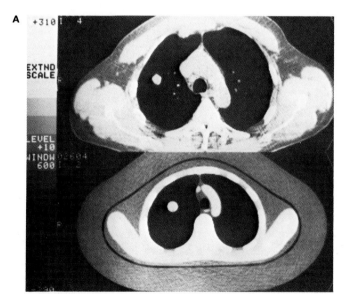
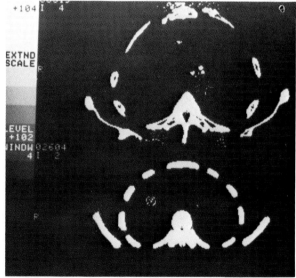

FIG. 14. Phantom method for CT analysis of lung nodules (53-year-old male with right upper lobe adenocarcinoma). **A:** The patient's scan is displayed in the upper image. The scan of the reference phantom with "reference nodule" in position is shown in the lower image. A fat-equivalent ring of appropriate thickness was added to the upper thorax section of the phantom to simulate the chest wall thickness of the patient. The same technical factors were used to scan patient and phantom. The phantom was scanned immediately after completion of the patient's study to avoid time-related drifts. To interpret the images no computer printouts are needed. **B:** Method of interpretation. The same image as in (A) is displayed, but the window width is reduced to a minimum, 4 HU in this case. The window level is then progressively moved up until either the patient's nodule or the phantom's nodule disappears from view. In the case illustrated, the patient's nodule is no longer visible at 102 HU, whereas the phantom's nodule is still visible. This indicates that the patient's nodule is not sufficiently dense to be considered benign and should be investigated further. If simultaneous double display is not available on the scanner, the phantom can be viewed first, and the window level moved up until the reference nodule disappears; then the patient's images are displayed using that particular window level and the narrowest window width.

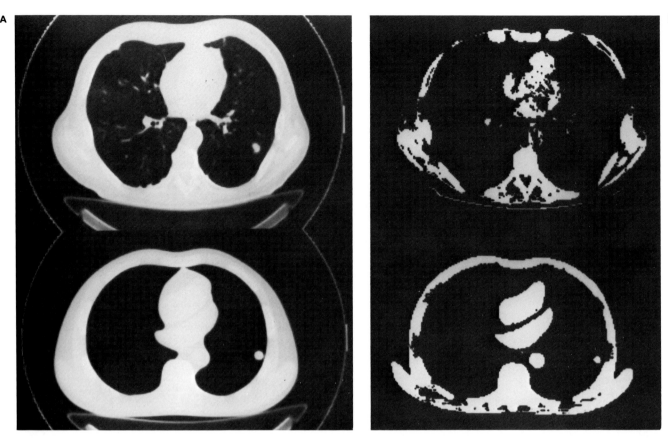

FIG. 15. 1.3-cm adenocarcinoma, left lower lobe. **A:** Scan of patient and reference phantom. **B:** Comparison at narrow window width. Patient nodule contains no pixel of greater density than reference nodule.

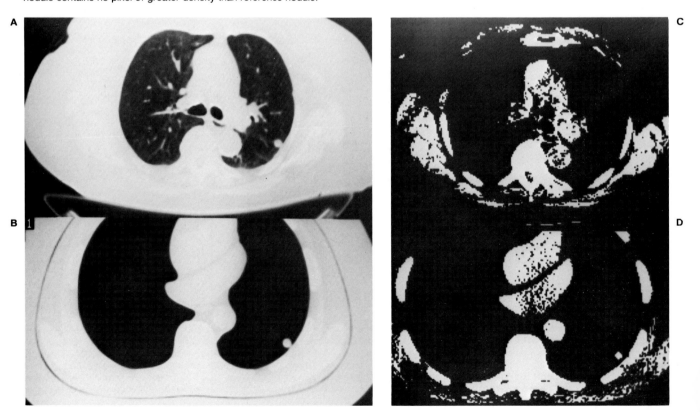

FIG. 16. 1.1-cm metastatic adenocarcinoma to left lower lobe. **A:** Patient scan. **B:** Reference phantom scan. **C,D:** Comparison shows no evidence of calcification in this patient nodule.

methods were examined. One hundred eighteen of these nodules proved to be benign. In 65 of these (55%), unsuspected calcification was demonstrated with thin-section CT aided by the reference phantom. Detailed analysis of these 65 cases demonstrated that in 28, obvious calcification could be identified by simple inspection of the scans at narrow window settings. In the remaining 37 cases, calcification could not be clearly demonstrated without careful comparison with the reference phantom. This study effectively ended the controversy surrounding the use of CT densitometry in pulmonary nodules. The authors concluded that thin-section CT was indicated in the evaluation of pulmonary nodules. In slightly less than half of the calcified benign nodules, obvious calcification could be made evident by thin-section scanning without the need for comparison with a reference standard. In the other half, sensitive and reliable detection of calcification required the use of a reference phantom.

The reference phantom offers a simple way of performing CT densitometry for pulmonary nodules on any scanner and does not require advanced expertise. Several groups of independent investigators subsequently reported their experience and have confirmed the usefulness of this method. Khan et al. (38) pointed out the robustness and reliability of the method in a series of patients in whom benign nodules were uniquely demonstrated by phantom-aided densitometry. Huston and Muhm (39) at the Mayo Clinic studied 112 solitary pulmonary nodules that were indeterminate on plain film tomography. Of the 112 nodules, 33 were more attenuating than the reference phantom. In 32 of these 33, the nodule was determined to be benign by follow-up studies of up to 4.5 years or by surgical sampling. One of the 33 nodules represented a calcified metastatic lesion from endometrial carcinoma. Jones et al. (40) from the Cleveland Clinic successfully categorized 10 nodules as benign in a series of 31 nodules. One lesion, an adenocarcinoma, was falsely called benign using the technique. The authors concluded that the excellent density discrimination achieved with CT makes it a superior tool for nodule analysis and that the reference phantom greatly simplified the technique. They also stressed the fact that calcification was not a feature unique to benign lesions, and successful clinical application required cautious interpretation of results. Ward et al. (41) reviewed their first three years of experience using phantom-aided CT. They studied 50 consecutive patients in whom a nodule was discovered on screening chest radiography and who were considered candidates for surgery. Twenty patients (40%) clearly met the phantom CT criteria for benign nodules. They stressed the fact that only one of the 20 patients would have met standard x-ray criteria for benign disease. Thirty patients who had lesions with densities less than the phantom nodule underwent thoracotomy and in 17 (57%)

the lesions were malignant. No patient in their series who had a "benign" reading on the phantom-aided CT study had a malignancy at surgery or during follow-up. The authors concluded that CT densitometry may prevent unnecessary thoracotomy in a significant percentage of patients.

It appears, then, that CT densitometry can be generalized and is effective, regardless of population type and geographic differences. Even in Japan, as reported by Shimizu et al. (42), phantom-aided CT densitometry has resulted in improved characterization of benign nodules. Other investigators have suggested that improvements in scanner technology have made CT densitometric measurements more reliable on modern scanners, reducing the need for external reference standards and further simplifying the technique. DeGeer et al. (43) found limited variability on their GE 9800 scanner using a reference phantom for testing.

Although progress has been made in improving the reliability of CT scanners, one should remain careful. A study by Cann (29) compared advanced scanners and still found significant variability in densitometric measurements. Although CT densitometry can be performed without a phantom, the use of an external reference standard remains the surest and simplest way of sensitively detecting calcification. In practice, CT densitometry of lung nodules, with or without the aid of a phantom, has replaced conventional tomography at most institutions.

The Problem of the Calcified Carcinoma

Calcification in a solitary pulmonary nodule is not a histospecific sign of benignancy. A cancer may develop near a pre-existing calcified scar or granuloma (Fig. 17).

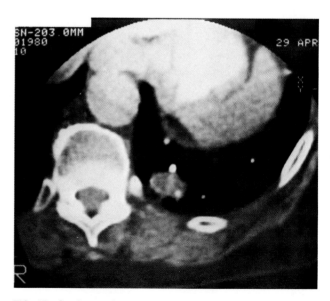

FIG. 17. Carcinoma developing in patient with pre-existing calcified granulomata from prior chicken pox pneumonia. The tumor has engulfed a nearby granuloma.

A

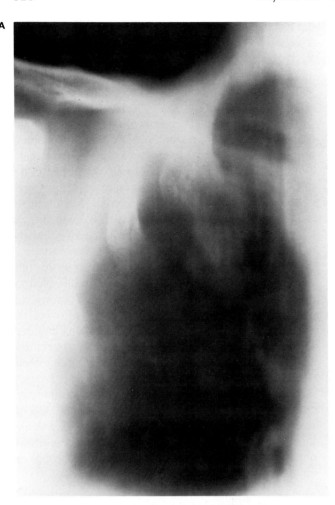

B

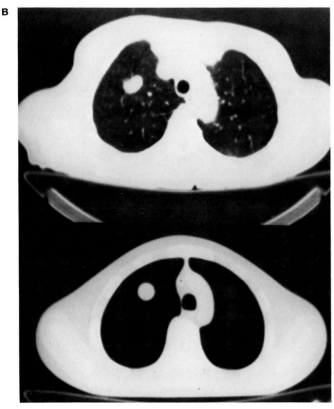

FIG. 18. Calcified cancer. Example of intrinsically calcified adenocarcinoma. **A:** Tomogram reveals a 3.5-cm nodule of right upper lobe without obvious calcification. **B:** CT scan of patient (*top*) and phantom simulation (*bottom*). **C:** Comparison at narrow window width reveals a cluster of calcified pixels within the lesion. **D:** Xerogram of specimen confirms presence of intrinsic calcification within lesion. CT densitometry of nodules larger than 3 cm should be interpreted with extreme caution as the majority of such lesions are not benign. (From Zerhouni et al., ref. 12, with permission. Case courtesy of Robert Woolfitt, M.D., Norfolk General Hospital, Norfolk, VA.)

D

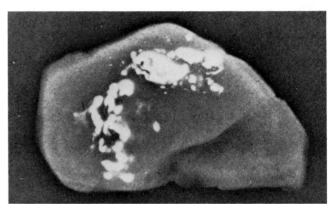

C

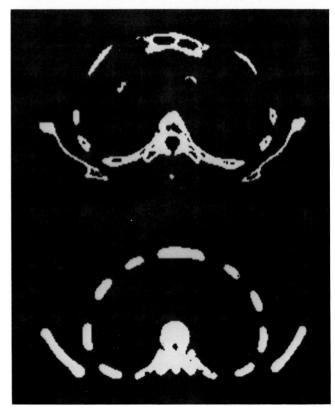

Intrinsic calcifications can also be found. Histologic studies indicate that up to 14% of cancers may contain some calcification. Although these calcifications are rarely seen by radiography, as demonstrated by Theros who found calcification in only seven of 1,267 cases (1), CT demonstrates some evidence of calcification in a greater percentage of cases. In the cooperative study by Zerhouni et al. (12), 7% of malignancies demonstrated evidence of calcification on CT. Siegelman et al. (13), in an extended study of 634 solitary pulmonary nodules, found that 13.4% of primary lung cancers contained some evidence of localized calcification with CT. In each of the studies of Huston and Muhm (39), Jones et al. (40), and Zerhouni et al. (12), one case of a calcified nodule was misdiagnosed as a benign granuloma and represented a calcified malignant lesion (Fig. 18). This points out the need for developing criteria other than presence or absence of calcification in order to establish the benign nature of a nodule.

Major differences in the calcification pattern of benign and malignant lesions allow a confident diagnosis in most cases. The lesion tends to be very large in most instances of calcified malignancies (Fig. 19). In a review by Mahoney et al. (44) of CT records of 353 malignancies, 20 (6%) exhibited calcification. Fourteen of the lesions were 5 cm or greater and three were between 3 and 5 cm. Only three lesions were 2 cm or smaller. In the cooperative study of Zerhouni et al. (12), 12 malignant nodules contained some calcification and all but one were larger than 3 cm. In the study of Siegelman et al. (13), 38 of 283 malignancies showed calcification, but only six were less than 2 cm in diameter.

The pattern of calcification is also a helpful diagnostic indicator. Most cancers exhibit punctate or peripheral scattered calcifications with no large concentration of calcified areas. Calcification occupies a very small proportion of malignant tumor volume. In benign lesions, at least 10% of the nodule is calcified, with most cases exhibiting 50% or more calcification by volume. Thus, a benign pattern of calcification is distinctly unusual in small cancers. However, anecdotal cases of central as well as diffuse calcification have been reported in malignancy (45).

To further increase specificity, morphologic characteristics have also been studied. An analysis of the lesion margins is helpful when considered in combination with the calcification patterns.

Siegelman et al. (13) defined four categories of nodular edges:

1. Sharp and smooth.
2. Moderately smooth with some lobulation.
3. Irregular undulation or slight spiculation.
4. Grossly irregular with spiculation.

Most benign nodules fell into category 1 or 2, whereas malignant nodules typically showed a type 3 or 4 edge

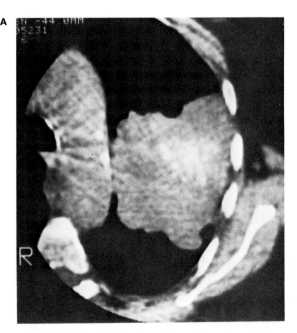 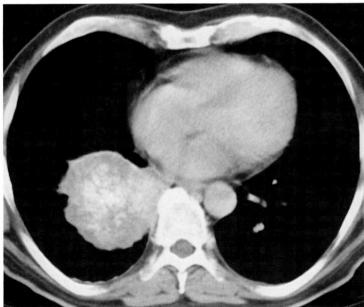

FIG. 19. Examples of calcified carcinoma. The majority of carcinomas harboring calcification by CT are large lesions as illustrated. **A:** Squamous cell carcinoma, left upper lobe. **B:** Adenocarcinoma, right lower lobe, probably metastatic from mucin-producing adenocarcinoma of colon.

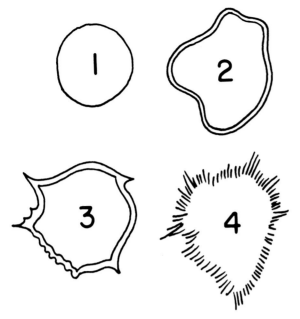

FIG. 20. Edge analysis. The appearance of edges is a helpful adjunctive sign to be considered in calcified nodules. Smooth (1) or slightly lobulated (2) edges are typical of benign lesions. Malignant lesions tend to demonstrate irregular (3) or spiculated (4) edges. Thus, a calcified nodule with a type 3 or 4 edge should be cautiously interpreted. (From Siegelman et al., ref. 13, with permission.)

(Fig. 20). Similar results were reported in the national cooperative study on pulmonary nodules, where 91 lesions had a spiculated appearance (type 3 or 4 edge). Eleven of these 91 were benign and only two of these 11 exhibited a benign pattern of calcification (12). These two lesions were smaller than 1.5 cm in diameter. Thus, spiculated lesions larger than 1.5 cm should be viewed with extreme caution, even if gross calcification is present. Interpretation guidelines are summarized in Fig. 21. In all cases, the possibility of misdiagnosis mandates close follow-up with repeat chest radiographs at 3, 6, 12, and 24 months to ensure that the calcified lesion does not grow.

Recommendations for Using CT Densitometry

With the experience accumulated over the past 10 years, it is now possible to better define the role of CT densitometry in the evaluation of the pulmonary nodule. Clearly, CT is of most value in smaller nodules less than 2 cm in diameter. Lesions larger than 3 cm in diameter are very likely to represent malignancy. CT densitometry adds little to the management of these patients. More definitive and invasive tests should be em-

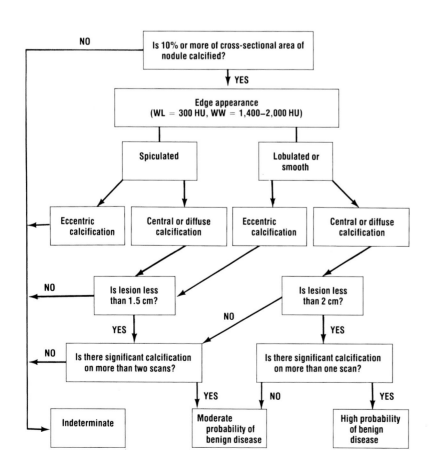

FIG. 21. Interpretation guidelines for CT of lung nodules. (From Zerhouni et al., ref. 12, with permission.)

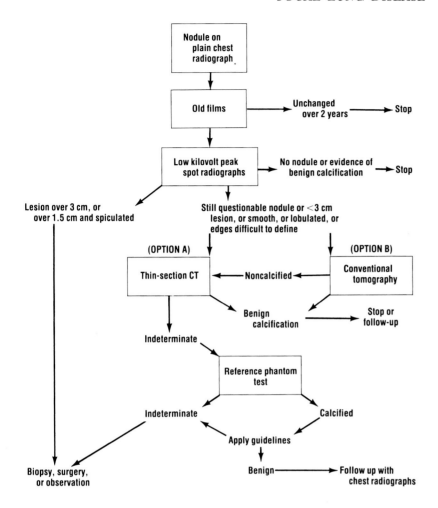

FIG. 22. Suggested diagnostic algorithm for pulmonary nodules. (From Zerhouni et al., ref. 12, with permission.)

ployed in these cases. CT is most valuable in assessing lesions with smooth or slightly lobulated borders. The finding of calcium deposits, representing a significant volume of the nodule (at least 10–20% in volume) and located in the center of the nodule, are reliable indicators of benignancy.

The following management protocol is suggested for a newly discovered solitary pulmonary nodule in an otherwise normal patient (Fig. 22). If the mass is less than 3 cm in diameter and has not been present for more than two years, low kilovolts peak (kVp) spot radiographs under fluoroscopic guidance may be performed. If no definite calcification is identified, proceed to thin-section CT. If no gross calcification is readily apparent on the thin-section scans, proceed with a reference phantom comparison of the density of the patient's nodule with that of the reference standard. If calcification is detected by CT, the interpretation guidelines outlined in Fig. 21 should be followed. For lesions with spiculated edges, we suggest a CT study only if the lesion is 1.5–2.0 cm in maximum diameter and if the clinical presentation suggests a reasonable possibility of benign disease. A young patient with no smoking history or a patient from an endemic zone of granulomatous disease is one

example of this instance. For any lesion larger than 3 cm, we do not recommend CT scanning unless there is a strong clinical suggestion of benign disease. In larger lesions, directly proceeding to bronchoscopy or percutaneous needle aspiration biopsy is an appropriate initial step.

PULMONARY CARCINOID TUMORS

As a subset of malignant lesions, these tumors exhibit features that are easily recognized in most cases. The pulmonary carcinoid tumor is slow-growing but is considered a low grade malignancy. Metastases are rare. The resectability and curability of these tumors exceeds that of other primary pulmonary malignancies. The 10-year survival is 88% for the typical lesion (46,47). Unlike bronchial carcinomas, carcinoid tumors have a high incidence of calcification. In a series of 12 such lesions, Magid et al. found focal calcifications in four (48). Three of these lesions were centrally located near lobar or segmental bronchial bifurcations. Calcification was most often distributed at the periphery of the nodule. The CT appearance of these nodules was characterized by a smooth, round contour in most cases. Many of these tumors demonstrate a close proximity to a bronchial bifurcation (Fig. 23). Typically, the tumor may compress and splay the adjacent bronchi but does not destroy them. In some cases, the lesion partially or completely obstructs the bronchi and may appear as a focal mass within the bronchial lumen. Dense calcification of such lesions has been reported. Confusion with calcified hilar lymph nodes is the main diagnostic pitfall. Pulmonary carcinoid tumors were originally called bronchial adenomas. However, the term adenoma is no longer accepted because these tumors are not always glandular

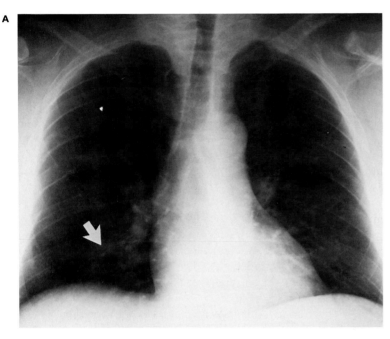

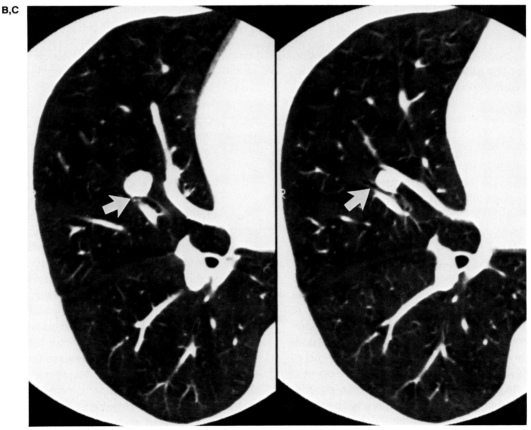

FIG. 23. Carcinoid tumor. **A:** 1.5-cm nodule in right middle lobe (*arrow*). **B,C:** Thin-section CT shows typical location at bronchial bifurcation, smooth contours, and deformation without destruction of the adjacent bronchus (*arrows*). (Compare with Figs. 44 and 45, Chapter 3.)

in origin and they are no longer considered benign (49,50). Most carcinoid tumors are centrally located near bronchial bifurcations. Presumably, the preferential distribution of Kulchitsky's cells near such locations accounts for the predominant location of these lesions near bronchial bifurcations. The Kulchitsky's cell is most probably the cell of origin for carcinoid tumors.

About 20% of pulmonary carcinoids present as peripheral pulmonary lesions. Even when peripheral, the nodule can be seen to abut subsegmental bronchi on thin-section scans. Peripheral carcinoids tend to exhibit more malignant behavior than do centrally located lesions. It has been suggested that carcinoid tumors probably should be subdivided into two distinct subgroups. The classic carcinoid tumors are usually found proximal to subsegmental bronchi and are smaller at presentation. The atypical carcinoids are usually larger, more peripheral, and are seen in an older population. Some investigators consider atypical peripheral carcinoids a variant of small cell lung cancer, mandating aggressive management (46,47) (see Chapter 3, Fig. 46).

Carcinoid tumors are considered part of the amine precursor uptake and decarboxylation (APUD) spectrum of neuroendocrine tumors, but *pulmonary* carcinoids are relatively inactive biologically. These tumors demonstrate little neurosecretory activity or associated desmoplastic reaction, unlike their intestinal counterparts. Histologic studies of these lesions have shown islands of calcification or ossification in up to 30% of cases. One hypothesis is that this tumor produces some osteogenic factor or hormone-inducing local ossification (51). Thus, pulmonary carcinoid can be recognized by CT if the lesion appears smooth, round, is located in close proximity to a bronchial bifurcation, and exhibits peripherally distributed calcification or ossification.

THE PULMONARY HAMARTOMA

As work continued in the 1980s on CT evaluation of the solitary pulmonary nodule, it became apparent that several subsets of lesions could be identified, even in the absence of calcification. The best example of such a subset is represented by pulmonary hamartomas, which can be specifically recognized when focal deposits of fat are identified by a CT number in the −80 to −120 HU range (Fig. 24). Hamartomas are lesions composed of normal tissues arranged in a disorderly pattern. They are the most common benign tumors of the lung and are believed to arise from embryologic rests. Hamartomas represent a very small proportion of all pulmonary nodules, but because they are frequently not recognized preoperatively, they account for 6–8% of all resected pulmonary nodules. They occur most often in the fifth to sixth decade of life. Cartilage is generally the dominant mesenchymal component of the lesion, often leading to calcification. De Rooij et al. (52) reviewed their experience in 20 resected solitary hamartomas of the lung. Analyzing the lesions histologically, they found fatty tissue in 7 cases and chondroid tissue in 13 of 20.

In a study of 47 patients by Siegelman et al. (53), 30 hamartomas were diagnosed as benign with detection of calcification in 2, fat without calcification in 18, or calcification and fat in 10 (Figs. 25 and 26). The authors concluded that nodules measuring 2.5 cm or less with smooth edges and demonstrating focal collections of fat (or fat alternating with areas of calcification) warranted a firm diagnosis of hamartoma and should be conservatively managed. In rare instances, hamartomas can be multiple (Fig. 27). Other fatty-like tissues can also be characterized by CT densitometry. For example, the detection of oily substances with a CT number in the range of fatty tissues in a pulmonary infiltrate is a pathognomic sign of lipoid pneumonia (Fig. 28).

METASTATIC DISEASE

Evaluation of patients with known extrathoracic malignancies is the prime example of the superior ability of CT to confidently detect focal lung disease. It has become one of the most common indications for thoracic CT.

The superior sensitivity of CT in the detection of metastatic pulmonary nodules was documented soon after its introduction. Generally, CT should be used when the discovery of an occult pulmonary metastasis may have an impact on clinical management. The propensity of certain tumors to metastasize to the lung varies and should be taken into account. Gilbert and Kagan (54) have studied the estimated incidences of lung metastases for various primary neoplasms at presentation and autopsy. Choriocarcinoma, renal cell carcinoma, and bone and soft tissue sarcomas are the primary cancers most likely to metastasize to the lung. CT is of greater benefit in patients with such tumors (Table 1). In addition to its advantageous cross-sectional display of anatomy and high contrast, the high sensitivity of CT is underscored by pathologic data on the preferential distribution and size of metastases. Metastatic lesions tend to be subpleural in location, a region difficult to examine by plain radiography. In a study of serial sections of resected lungs containing metastatic nodules, Scholten and Kreel (55) found that 60% of the lesions were in an immediate pleural or subpleural location and an additional 25% were located in the outer third of the lung. Two-thirds of metastatic lesions occur in the lower lobes.

In another pathologic study by Crow et al. (56), 59% of metastatic lesions measured 5 mm or less, a size rarely detected with standard radiography. Muhm et al. (57), in a clinical series of 91 patients, found more nodules with CT (35%) than with whole lung tomography. In

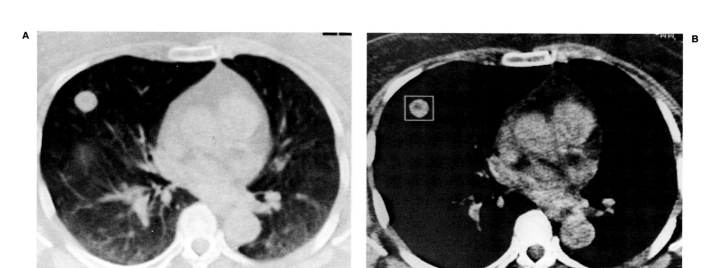

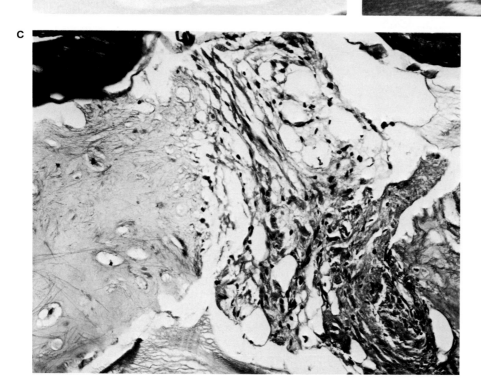

FIG. 24. Hamartoma containing fat in 32-year-old woman with incidentally discovered nodule. **A:** CT scan shows smooth, round nodule, right middle lobe. **B:** Same scan at narrower window shows zone of low attenuation in the range of fat in center of nodule. **C:** Specimen from needle biopsy shows typical features of hamartoma with noncalcified cartilage and abundant fat. (From Siegelman et al., ref. 53, with permission.)

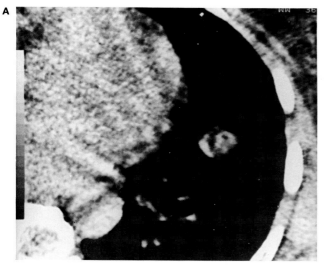

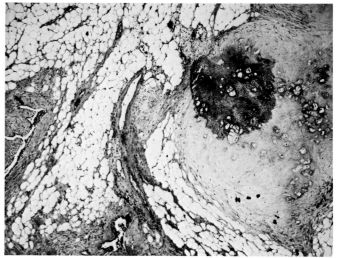

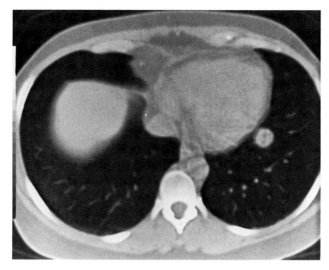

FIG. 26. Example of hamartoma with central deposits of fat and peripheral calcification. Note again smooth contours.

TABLE 1. *Incidence of pulmonary metastases from extrathoracic primaries (at presentation and autopsy)*[a]

Primary lesion	Presentation %	Autopsy %
Choriocarcinoma (female)	60	70–100
Kidney	5–30	50–75
Rhabdomyosarcoma	21	25
Wilm's tumor	20	60
Ewing's sarcoma	18	77
Osteosarcoma	15	75
Testicular (germinal)	12	70–80
Melanoma	5	66–80
Thyroid	5–10	65
Breast	5	60
Hodgkin's lymphoma	5	50–70
Colon/rectum	5	25–40
Head and neck	5	13–40
Bladder	5–10	25–30
Prostate	5	13–53
Non-Hodgkin's lymphoma	1–10	30–40

[a] Modified from Gilbert and Kagen, ref. 54.

A
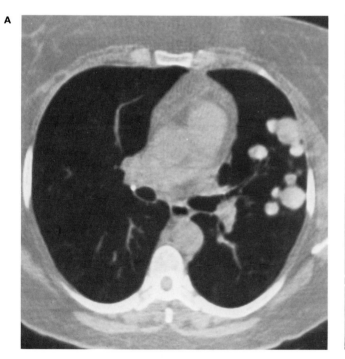

B
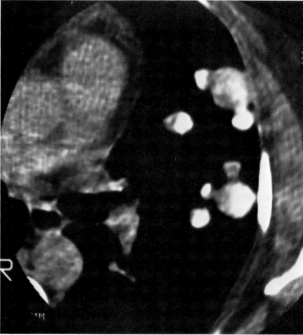

FIG. 27. Multiple hamartomas. **A:** Note multiple, smooth, round nodules in lingula. **B:** Scan at narrow window settings reveals intrinsic areas of calcification but no clearly definable fat deposits. Confirmed by needle biopsy of largest lesion.

←

FIG. 25. Hamartoma containing calcification and fat in 60-year-old woman. **A:** CT scan shows 2.5-cm nodule in lingula. High and low attenuation areas corresponding to areas of calcification and fat, respectively, can be seen. **B:** Specimen from needle biopsy shows characteristic combination of fat, cartilage, and ossified cartilage (*dark area*). (From Siegelman et al., ref. 53, with permission.)

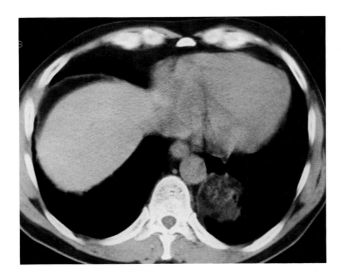

FIG. 28. Lipoid pneumonia. Left lower lobe mass in elderly patient using oily drops for nasal dryness. Note focal infiltrate with large areas of low attenuation in the range of fatty tissues typical of this entity. (Case courtesy of Dr. Norman Ettenger, Manhattan V.A. Hospital, NY.)

14% of cases, bilateral nodules were detected when conventional tomography showed only unilateral disease. Nodules were detected in 6% of cases where none were seen with conventional techniques. Eighty-three percent of the additional nodules detected with CT were found at surgery to represent metastatic disease. Schaner et al. (58), in a prospective radiologic pathologic study, confirmed that CT defined more nodules than did conventional tomography. CT was much more effective for nodules in the 3–6 mm range. But a disturbing finding of these authors was that 60% of the additional nodules detected by CT proved to be granulomas and pleural-based lymph nodes at resection. In addition, nearly one-third of the nodules discovered by CT could not be found by the surgeon. Indeed, small lesions pose a real dilemma. They are difficult to biopsy percutaneously and may not be palpable at surgery. Furthermore, in the population of patients with extrathoracic malignancies, the prevalence of granulomas and superimposed infections is higher than in the normal population. Consequently, the increased sensitivity of CT leads to the discovery of many incidental focal pulmonary densities. Detection of such abnormalities in the oncologic patient raises the issue of determining whether these lesions represent metastatic disease or incidental findings.

Metastatic lesions are morphologically similar to benign nodules. Most metastatic lesions are smaller than 2 cm and have a smooth, round contour. However, unless the primary carcinoma exhibits a tendency to calcification, as in bone sarcomas or mucin-producing carcinomas, metastatic lesions are rarely calcified (Fig. 29B). CT densitometry can be helpful in these instances. A constellation of morphologic findings can also enhance diagnostic specificity. In a study of patients with cancer and multiple pulmonary nodules detected by CT, Gross

et al. (59) found that metastatic lesions are more likely to be spherical or ovoid in shape. Linear, triangular, irregularly shaped, or multiple ill-defined lesions, especially when centrally located, are less likely to represent metastases. They also found that if noncalcified round lesions larger than 2.5 cm were present or if more than 10 lesions were visualized in any one patient, the likelihood of metastatic disease was very high.

More recently, new and potentially valuable morphologic clues have come to light. For example, a frequently observed sign is the demonstration of a connection between the metastatic nodule and an adjacent branch of the pulmonary artery. This sign is most often seen when vessels are oriented in a plane parallel to the plane of scanning. Pathologic correlations in inflated lung specimens have shown the frequent presence of a pulmonary vessel leading to the center of metastatic lesions (60). In a study by Milne and Zerhouni (61), the connection between pulmonary arteries and nodules seen by CT was confirmed by microangiographic studies. A vascular connection cannot always be demonstrated with CT because of the different orientations of the scanned plane and the vessel leading to the metastatic lesion, but the presence of such a sign is helpful for distinguishing hematogenous metastases from either primary carcinomas or granulomatous lesions (Fig. 29). A major potential pitfall in using this *mass-vessel sign* is the possibility of partial volume effects making a lesion appear connected to an adjacent but unrelated vessel. Thin sections are thus preferred to assess this sign.

Another sign we have found helpful is the presence of a zone of hypodensity distal to the metastatic nodule, presumably representing a zone of hypoperfusion distal to the pulmonary vessel occluded by the metastasis (Fig. 30). Even after successful chemotherapy of metastatic

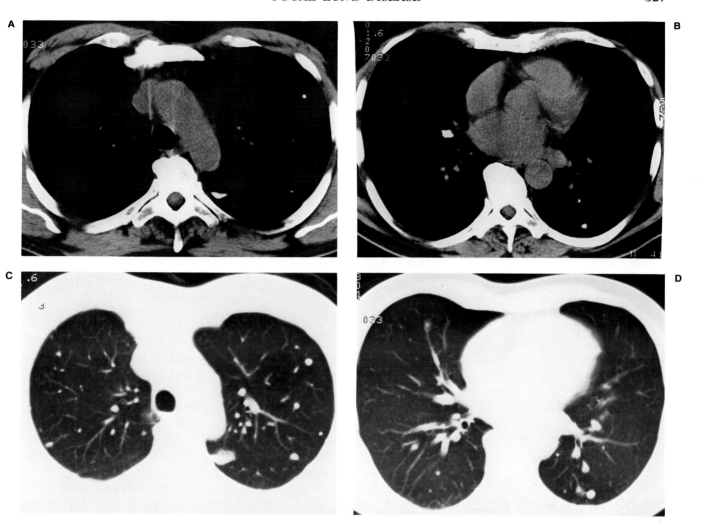

FIG. 29. Metastatic osteosarcoma. **A,B:** Scans at narrow window settings reveal multiple calcified lung nodules which would be consistent with calcified granulomata. **C,D:** Scans at wide window settings show that several of these nodules are connected to vessels. This vessel-mass sign is helpful in suggesting the diagnosis of hematogenous metastases.

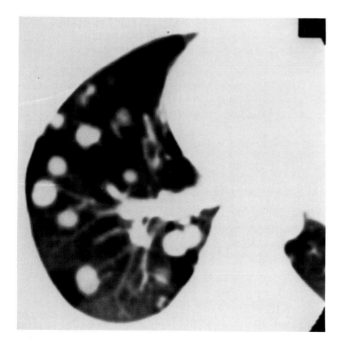

FIG. 30. Distal hypoperfusion sign. Metastatic nodules. Several nodules appear connected to vessels. A zone of hypodensity can be seen distal to the nodules in the lower lobe posteriorly. This sign is presumably due to hypoperfusion of parenchyma due to occlusion of the feeding artery by the metastasis. This finding is helpful in confirming that a nodule and an adjacent vessel are truly connected but it can only be seen at narrow window settings.

lung disease, a mass-vessel connection can still be seen (Fig. 31). The frequent presence of reticular changes surrounding metastatic lesions is also a helpful diagnostic sign. The pathologic basis for this appearance is growth of neoplastic cells in capillaries and lymphatic vessels with secondary perivascular and interstitial

edema and fibrosis. In a study of inflated lung specimens by Ren et al. (62), interstitial changes were observed in 69% of cases of metastatic lung disease. These changes were characterized by beaded septa due to direct tumor growth in pulmonary capillaries and lymphatics within the septal interstitium. This beaded septal change was

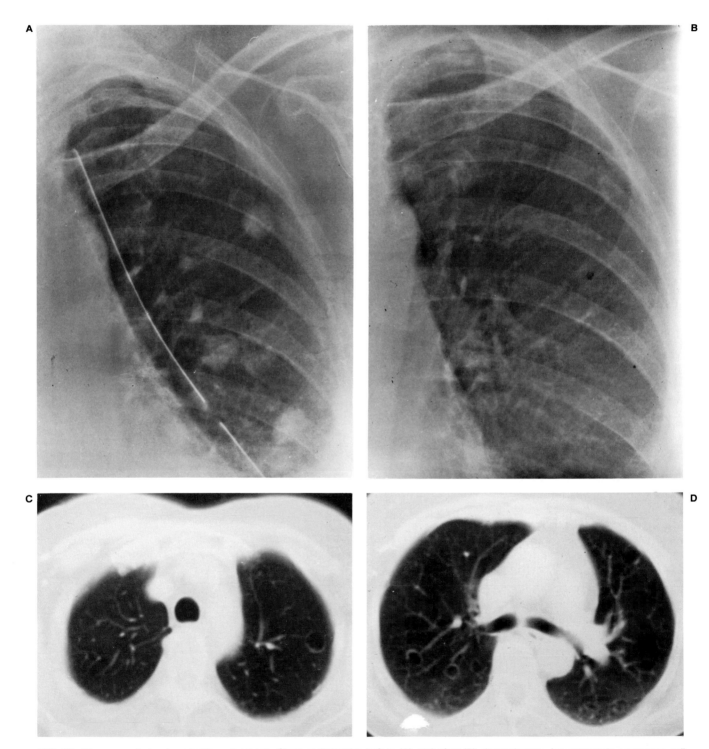

FIG. 31. Mass-vessel sign in necrotic metastases. Chest radiographs before (**A**) and after (**B**) chemotherapy for metastatic squamous cell carcinoma. Residual cavity is faintly seen in left upper lobe. Cavities are seen in left upper lobe (**C**) and lower lobes (**D**) with vessels directly connected to them. These cavities represent necrosed metastases.

not noted in any of the specimens with pulmonary edema, fibrosis, or in normal lungs. The authors concluded that the beaded septum sign on high-resolution computed tomography (HRCT) is highly suggestive of pulmonary metastases.

Although we are better able to differentiate metastatic lesions from other entities by location, shape, and relationship to nearby vessels and septa, it is not always possible to attain a high level of certainty. In such cases, biopsy of the lesion is an alternative if it would significantly alter management. In practice, however, needle biopsy of the many lesions often seen is not practical. Sequential CT examinations to assess tumor growth rate help resolve this problem. Indeed, the growth rate of a nodule is a reliable indicator of its nature. Nathan et al. (63) measured the doubling times of 177 malignant and 41 benign nodules. The longest doubling time for malignancy was 6–7 months. Lesions with doubling times of 18 months or more were invariably benign. Weiss and colleagues (64) found doubling times ranging between 1.8 and 10 months for malignancies. Active inflammatory lesions are prone to rapid changes in size that occur in less than one month. Such rapid evolution is unlikely in malignancies, except for metastases from very aggressive primary lesions such as choriocarcinomas or sarcomas. In patients with extrathoracic malignancies and questionable metastases, monitoring the growth rate over a 4–6 week period is desirable. Minimal to moderate growth or a decrease under specific chemotherapy is reliable evidence of the metastatic nature of these lesions (Fig. 31).

The Solitary Nodule in a Patient with a Known Malignancy

The discovery of a new, apparently solitary nodule when monitoring patients during or after therapy for an extrathoracic malignancy poses a different set of challenges. The possibility of a developing primary lung cancer rather than a solitary metastasis is, indeed, a real concern.

Cahan et al. (65) studied a series of 800 patients who presented with an apparently solitary pulmonary nodule a year or more after detection and treatment of an extrathoracic malignancy. Sixty-three percent proved to have a new primary lung tumor and fewer than 25% had a solitary metastasis. The likelihood of metastatic disease in these solitary nodules varied depending on the histology of the primary cancer. If the extrathoracic malignancy was a squamous cell carcinoma, the likelihood of a newly developing primary lung cancer was about 65%. If the extrathoracic malignancy was an adenocarcinoma, the likelihood of a new primary tumor was about 50%. For extrathoracic sarcomas, the likelihood was

much lower and a newly discovered solitary nodule was most likely to represent a metastatic lesion. Therefore, if no other lesions are present, a newly discovered solitary nodule in the context of a known extrathoracic malignancy should be considered a primary lung cancer until proven otherwise. CT, then, is indicated primarily to determine whether additional nodules are present in the thorax, which would make the diagnosis of metastatic disease much more likely. The high likelihood of additional lesions in these patients has been borne out in studies by Neifeld et al. (66). They discovered additional metastases at thoracotomy in 21% of patients with extrathoracic malignancies in whom a solitary nodule was found on whole lung tomography. If no other lesions are found, the nodule should be managed so as to reach a specific diagnosis as diligently as possible.

VASCULAR AND HEMATOGENOUS LESIONS

Increasing experience over the past few years has led to the realization that CT can demonstrate morphologic features that provide unique clues to the nature of focal lesions. One such feature is the demonstration of a connection between a focal process and adjacent vascular structures. As already discussed, for metastatic disease, this sign (which can only be reliably seen with CT), is of great value. Likewise, similar findings often provide the best evidence that a focal pulmonary process is of vascular or hematogenous origin.

Arteriovenous Malformation

Arteriovenous malformations (AVM) can be recognized by the demonstration of large feeding and draining vessels connected to the malformation (Fig. 32). The shape of these lesions can vary from round to ovoid to complex if associated with pulmonary sequestration. These lesions can be recognized with or without contrast injection because of their typical morphology. Rarely, thrombosis may lead to a lack of contrast enhancement. The radiologist should be aware of that possibility and not be swayed from the diagnosis of AVM even in the absence of contrast enhancement. As shown in Fig. 33, magnetic resonance (MR) may play a role in the investigation of pulmonary AVMs by noninvasively assessing the flow characteristics of these lesions before and after embolization therapy, if necessary (67).

Pulmonary Infarcts

Pulmonary infarcts typically present as wedge-shaped, peripheral, pleural-based densities on CT. Often, these

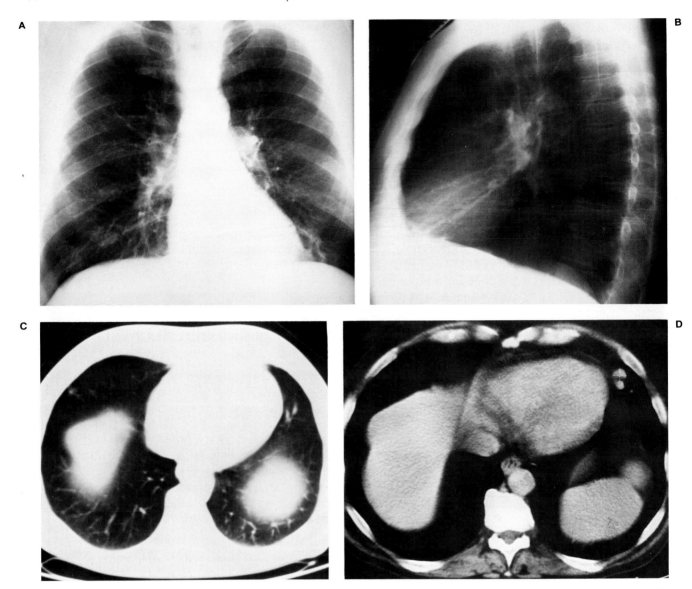

FIG. 32. Arteriovenous malformation. **A,B:** Posteroanterior and lateral chest radiographs show lesion in left anterior paracardiac region. Note prominent vessel leading to lesion. **C:** CT scan shows two prominent vessels in lingula. **D:** The malformation is depicted in paracardiac region of the lingula.

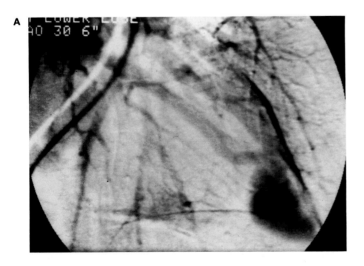

FIG. 33. Arteriovenous malformation (AVM) by MR. **A:** Angiogram demonstrates large AVM in left lower lobe. **B:** (opposite page) Spin-echo T1-weighted scan where AVM is barely visible (*arrow*) due to low signal of flowing blood and aerated lung. Thin rim of wall is seen. **C:** Gradient echo image demonstrates flow in AVM.

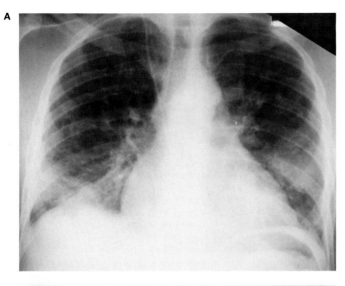

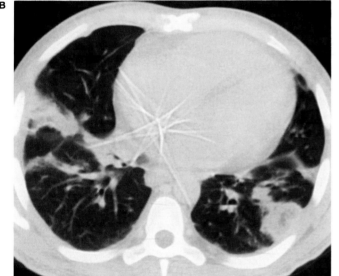

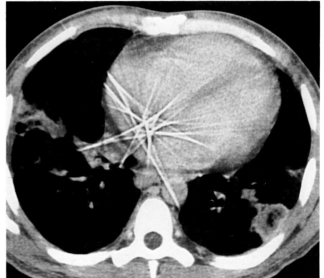

FIG. 34. Pulmonary infarcts. **A:** Chest radiograph demonstrating peripheral densities. **B,C:** CT scan demonstrates multiple pleural-based triangularly shaped densities with apices directed toward hila. Note lucencies within infarcts representing residual aerated lung. Note in (C) the rim of high density surrounding infarct in left lower lobe.

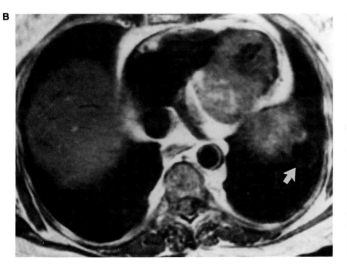

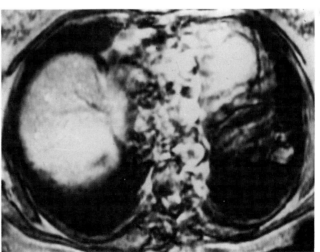

A

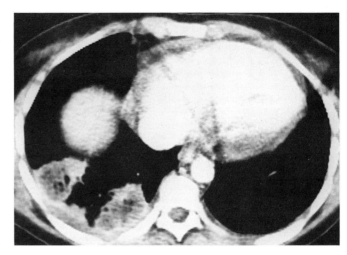

B

FIG. 35. Rim enhancement in pulmonary infarcts. **A,B:** Adjacent CT scans in case of pulmonary infarcts after bolus contrast injection. Note rim of enhancement at the edge of normal lung and infarct. Note also residual aerated lung in infarcts and typical pleural-based morphology.

wedge densities demonstrate a lucent center (Figs. 34 and 35). Correlative studies indicate that the central lucency is related to residual aerated lung (68). Another important finding is the presence of rim-enhancement of the infarct after contrast injection, probably reflecting the inflammatory response of the lung at the periphery of the infarct (Fig. 35). Later in the evolution of the infarct, central necrosis with cyst formation may be seen.

However, a wedge-shaped, pleural-based lesion is not diagnostic of pulmonary infarction. In a study by Ren et al. (68), radiologic/pathologic correlation was obtained in 83 postmortem lung specimens where subpleural wedge densities were seen. In 12 of these lungs, pulmonary infarcts were the cause of the subpleural wedge densities. But, in the 71 other cases, subpleural shadows were due to other processes such as hemorrhage, pneumonia, tumor, or focal edema. The authors found no significant difference in the incidence or appearance of wedge-shaped peripheral densities due to infarcts versus those due to other etiologies.

Others have suggested that a more specific diagnosis can be suggested if a vessel is demonstrated at the apex of the wedge density (60). In the study by Ren et al. (68), such an apical vascular connection was seen in 10 of 12 cases of infarct but rarely in wedge-shaped densities related to other processes. This would suggest that this vascular sign may be most helpful in diagnosing pulmonary infarcts. However, a potential pitfall is the possibility of misdiagnosis related to the appearance of a vascular connection due to partial volume averaging with an uninvolved adjacent vessel. Accordingly, to avoid this pitfall caution should be exercised, especially when thick-section scans are being interpreted. Preferably, thin-section scans (1.5–3 mm) should be used and analyzed in a sequential fashion.

Septic Emboli

Septic pulmonary emboli cause a wide spectrum of radiographic abnormalities. In 18 patients with documented pulmonary septic emboli, Kuhlman et al. (69) found peripheral nodules ranging from 0.5 to 3.5 cm in size in 83% of patients. Interestingly, in 67% of these cases, a vessel was seen to be connected to the abnormality (Figs. 36 and 37). The authors also pointed out the frequent finding of cavitation in half of the cases. As for pulmonary infarcts, septic emboli may appear as wedge-shaped, peripheral densities abutting the pleura in about 50% of the cases. However, in the remaining 50%, nodular or cavitary lesions were the rule. Air bronchograms could be seen within some nodules. A

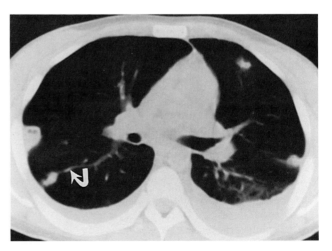

FIG. 36. Septic pulmonary emboli from infected indwelling catheter. Note combination of wedge-shaped as well as rounded densities with connection to vessels (*arrow*). (From Kuhlman et al., ref. 70, with permission.)

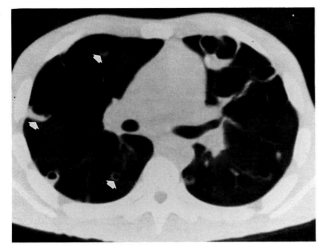 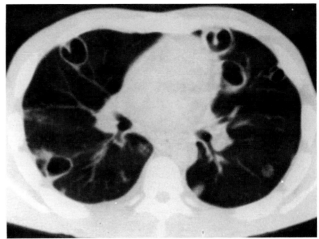

FIG. 37. Septic emboli from staphylococcus sepsis. **A,B:** Multiple cavitated necrosed nodules of various sizes are typical of this entity [*arrows* in (A)]. Note the frequent finding of vascular connection with the lesions. (From Kuhlman et al., ref. 70, with permission.)

similar study by Huang et al. (70) found clearly identifiable feeding vessels in association with septic embolic abscesses of the lung in 10 of 15 cases. Subpleural, wedge-shaped densities, with and without necrosis caused by septic infarcts, were shown in 11 of 15 cases (73%). The recognition of pulmonary septic emboli or infarct by CT has a significant clinical impact. Kuhlman et al. (69) noted that in 6 of 18 patients, CT was the first modality to suggest the diagnosis of septic emboli. In five cases the diagnosis was clinically unsuspected, and in eight patients CT enabled identification of more parenchymal lesions characteristic of septic emboli and more pleural involvement than was demonstrated on chest radiographs. In our opinion, CT should be extensively used in patients at high risk for infectious complications, namely, the immunocompromised individual with high fever and nondiagnostic chest radiographs or patients in whom chest radiographs demonstrate noncharacteristic abnormalities.

Other Vascular Lesions

The constellation of findings typical of vascular processes (the feeding vessel sign and wedge-shaped, pleural-based densities) is not unique to pulmonary infarcts and septic emboli. Indeed, the feeding vessel sign only indicates a connection between a vessel and a pathologic process. The wedge-shaped density is commonly observed in the lung whenever vascular compromise is present because the pulmonary circulation is of the terminal type. Thus, any vascular-based process such as metastatic disease or vasculitis may lead to the same combination of findings. Wegener's granulomatosis, for example, is often associated with cavitated nodules, many of which appear connected to adjacent vessels (Fig. 38).

Wegener's granulomatosis is a disease of unknown cause. It is generally considered a hypersensitivity disorder with granulomatous inflammation, small vessel vasculitis, and glomerulonephritis. A limited form of the disease, without renal involvement, also exists. The most common pulmonary parenchymal feature of the process is cavitary nodules that may be transient and recurrent.

Following chemotherapy, metastatic lesions can undergo necrosis. As a result, small pulmonary cavities which retain their initial connection to a branch of the pulmonary artery can be seen (Fig. 31). Other processes that primarily involve vessels may elicit an inflammatory response of such magnitude that different signs are observed. In pulmonary infarcts, a rim of contrast-en-

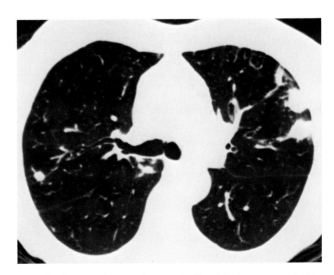

FIG. 38. Wegener's granulomatosis. Focal lesions connected to vessels can be seen in this entity. Note similarity to infarction and septic emboli. The mass-vessel sign, although helpful in pinpointing a vascular or hematogenous etiology, is not specific.

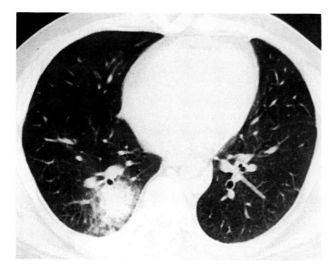

FIG. 39. Early invasive aspergillosis. Patient in leukopenic phase following bone marrow transplant. Note halo of intermediate density in the transition zone between the nodule and the normal lung. This sign is suggestive of infection by angiotropic organisms, the most common of which is *Aspergillus fumigatus*.

hanced tissue can often be seen at their periphery. This phenomenon is presumably due to the inflammatory reaction surrounding the infarcted tissue. These mechanisms lead also to better recognition of other specific entities, such as invasive pulmonary aspergillosis. Kuhlman et al. (71), studying bone marrow transplant patients, found that invasive pulmonary aspergillosis could often be recognized early in its course by the presence of a halo surrounding a focal pulmonary infiltrate (Fig.

39). These lesions, occurring during the leukopenia phase, strongly suggest the diagnosis. This helps institute effective and specific therapy earlier in the course of the disease.

The halo sign found around invasive aspergillosis is an interesting example of how closely CT can match the physiopathologic phenomena occurring in focal lung disease. Hruban et al. (72) undertook a radiologic-pathologic correlative study of focal invasive aspergillosis using postmortem fixed and air dried specimens. They showed that nodules from invasive aspergillosis corresponded to colonization of vascular structures by Aspergillus. The invasive aspergillotic lesion was seen to consist of a central, dense fungal ball colonizing a vessel which appeared surrounded by a rim of hemorrhagic infarction and coagulative necrosis. The thrombosed necrotic vessels associated with some of these nodules offer a clue to the pathogenesis of this sign. Aspergillus, unlike most other pathogens, is angiotropic and often invades blood vessels. The resulting micro-infarcts are usually spherical. The surrounding rim of hemorrhage is most probably a result of the destruction of this vessel. Later in the evolution of invasive aspergillosis, if the immune response is sufficient to control the disease, an air-crescent may develop between the aspergillotic nodule and the surrounding inflammatory reaction. This air-crescent sign is similar to that seen in cases of fungus ball colonizing pre-existing cavities (Fig. 40).

Most infectious causes of pulmonary disease—with the possible exceptions of Pseudomonas, Staphylococcus, and mucormycosis—are not angiocentric. Thus, in

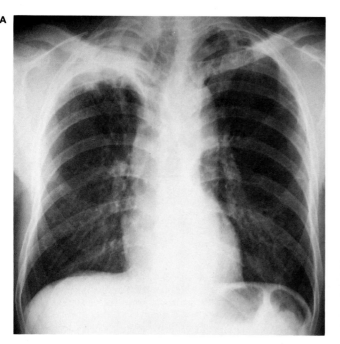

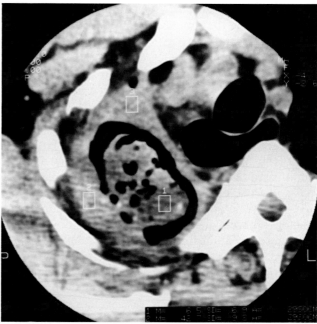

FIG. 40. Fungus ball with air-crescent sign. Patient with pre-existing chronic cavitation from healed tuberculosis. **A:** Chest radiograph demonstrates thin air crescent. **B:** With CT, fungus ball is seen in middle of tuberculous cavern.

the population at risk, the appearance of a target lesion with a surrounding halo due to coagulative necrosis and edema explains the observed high specificity of this sign.

NONVASCULAR FOCAL PULMONARY PROCESSES

In the absence of a vascular connection, typical appearances for other focal lung processes are few. A notable exception is the recognition of asbestos-related focal lung masses. Asbestos exposure is a predisposing condition to the development of bronchogenic carcinoma. Rounded atelectasis of the pulmonary parenchyma has also been well described. It is commonly observed in the same group of patients. Hence, noninvasive differentiation between benign and malignant masses in this context is important. Although the typical features of rounded atelectasis are easily recognizable on CT, atypical presentations are not uncommon (see Chapter 9). In our experience, a significant number of asbestos-exposed individuals present with apparent intrapulmonary focal masses that may be confused with lung cancer. Lynch et al. (73) found a 10% incidence of unsuspected intrapulmonary focal masses in a group of asbestos-exposed individuals. However only three of the 43 masses found in this group of 260 individuals were malignant.

Diagnostically, the most indicative CT features in intraparenchymal rounded atelectasis are: (a) contiguity to areas of diffuse pleural thickening; (b) a lentiform or wedge-shaped outline; (c) evidence of volume loss in the adjacent lung; and (d) the characteristic comet tail of vessels and bronchi sweeping into the margins of the mass (74,75) (see Chapter 9, Fig. 38). As originally described by Blesovsky (76), these masses represent areas of folded lung. The cause of these masses is unclear. Presumably, fibrous pleural effusions lead to infolding and atelectasis of a fixed segment of lung. With the resorption of the effusion, compensatory inflation of the surrounding lung may occur, displacing the atelectic area mimicking other intraparenchymal processes. In most cases, the atelectatic area will retain some form of connection to the pleura. Careful analysis of adjacent scans should establish such a connection (Fig. 41).

Solitary Bronchioloalveolar Cell Carcinoma

Bronchioloalveolar carcinoma is a histologically distinct variant of adenocarcinoma, representing an estimated 6–10% of primary lung cancers (77–79). Although it most often occurs as a small focal mass, its varied appearances include multi-nodular, pneumonic, and diffuse forms (see Chapter 8, Fig. 22). Its growth is characterized by a variable latency period. Some lesions remain dormant or grow slowly over years, and others form diffuse or multi-centric rapidly progressive forms. CT is helpful in differentiating solitary from diffuse bronchioloalveolar carcinoma (77). In a review of 30 cases, Kuhlman et al. (80) found several features that are often characteristic. These features include a peripheral or subpleural location, pseudo-cavitation, mixed attenuation, pleural tags, and irregular margins forming a star pattern (Fig. 42). These traits are reminiscent of similar findings with plain radiographs (78,79). Radiographic/pathologic correlations suggest that a pleural tag or star pattern may be the result of desmoplastic reactions surrounding the tumor, producing thickened fibrous strands radiating from the tumor. The frequent development of bronchioloalveolar carcinoma in pre-existing scars may also explain this pattern (81). Pseudo-cavita-

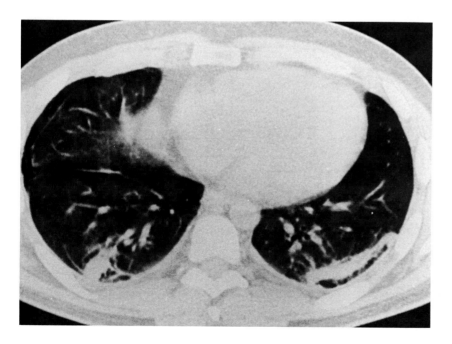

FIG. 41. Focal atelectasis secondary to asbestos exposure can simulate other intraparenchymal pathology when compensatory hyperinflation of the adjacent lung displaces the atelectatic region away from the pleura. Note thickening of the underlying pleura and displacement of bronchovascular structures toward lesions. (Compare with Fig. 42, Chapter 9.)

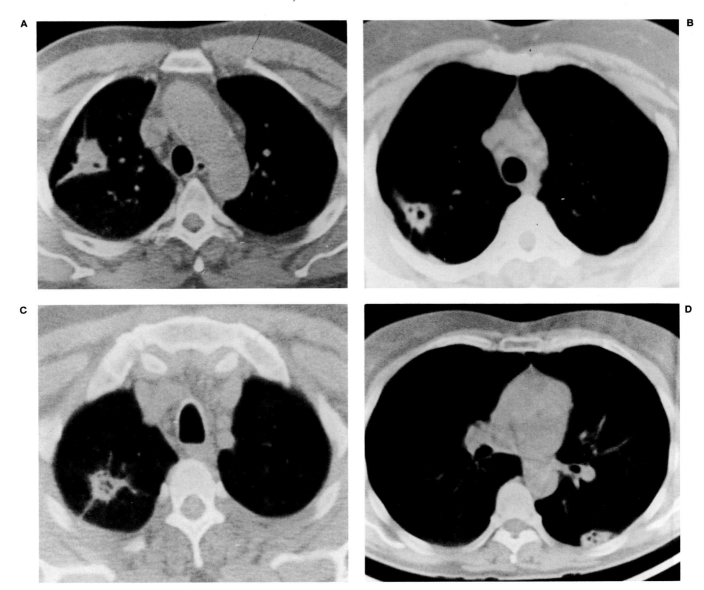

FIG. 42. A,B,C,D: Examples of solitary bronchioloalveolar cell carcinomas. Typical features include: peripheral, subpleural location; pseudocavitation with mixed attenuation representing residual air spaces; irregular margins often forming a star pattern; and pleural "tags" seen as parenchymal bands extending from the lesion to the visceral pleura. (From Kuhlman et al., ref. 80, with permission.)

tion or small oval areas of decreased attenuation appearing in or around a pulmonary mass reflects the propensity of this tumor to proliferate along the walls of the alveoli without disrupting overall lung architecture. Because bronchioles are preserved, there is no segmental atelectasis. Reactive fibrosis may cause dilatation of the surrounding intact air spaces, leading to the appearance of pseudo-cavitation or pseudobronchiectasis (see Chapter 3, Fig. 57). Focal emphysema or bronchiectasis can also be noted in proximity to these lesions. These findings are not highly specific, although several features suggest the diagnosis of bronchioloalveolar carcinoma.

Differential Diagnosis of Focal Infiltrates

The causes of focal pulmonary infiltrates are so numerous that a specific diagnosis based on their appearance is rarely possible. There are a few exceptions to this rule: some specific diagnoses can be suggested based on the distribution of the process. For example, in chronic eosinophilic pneumonia, focal areas of consolidation are predominantly peripheral even though this distribution is not always apparent on the radiograph. Accordingly, in the presence of focal peripheral infiltrates in association with eosinophilia, the distribution should be char-

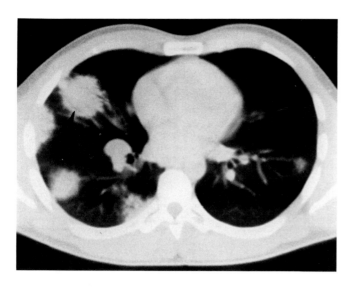

FIG. 43. Pulmonary sarcoidosis. Focal peripheral alveolar-type infiltrates with air bronchograms are typical of this entity (*arrow*).

acteristic enough to allow confident diagnosis. In sarcoidosis, focal areas of consolidation can also be seen, predominantly located at the periphery of the lung (Fig. 43; see also Chapter 8, Fig. 39). Typically, manifestations of sarcoidosis are in close proximity to bronchovascular structures. This bronchocentric distribution of the abnormalities seen in sarcoidosis is a clue to the nature of the process (82–84).

ROLE OF MR IN THE INVESTIGATION OF NODULAR LUNG DISEASE

Although blurring due to respiratory motion is a significant impediment, MR may have some unique but very limited advantages in the study of nodular parenchymal lesions. Because no signal is obtained from the lung parenchyma or pulmonary vessels, nodules are more easily recognized when they are located in the central regions of the lungs where no confusion between nodules and vessels occurs. In a comparison of MR and CT detection of pulmonary nodules, Müller et al. (85) showed that CT was superior for detecting nodules close to the diaphragm, chest wall, or other structures. MR, conversely, was better in the diagnosis of more central nodules because it allowed the distinction of a nodule from surrounding vessels. On CT, vessels and nodules may appear similar.

A drawback of MR is that fissures, lobar and segmental bronchi, and vessels are invisible or poorly seen. The exact location of a nodular process is thus difficult to determine. Although lower spatial resolution and respiratory motion are major impediments, high contrast between nodules and lung parenchyma can be achieved with MR, especially on T2-weighted sequences. Early attempts to use MR as a method to determine the nature of pulmonary nodules were unsuccessful. Gamsu et al. (86) performed a preliminary study of quantification by

MR of calcified pulmonary nodules. They found the problem to be extremely complex. In a few cases, MR was of value because of its ability to characterize tissues. In several patients, small hematomas have been accurately diagnosed because of the unique paramagnetic characteristics of subacute blood collections. But such cases are clinically uncommon. There is a theoretical possibility that MR could distinguish fibrotic nodules from more active inflammatory or malignant nodules. Fibrotic nodules exhibit a low signal intensity on T2-weighted scan, while malignant nodules show a high signal intensity. However, the inability to obtain scans at suspended respiration prevents accurate quantitation of signal intensities. Further research and improvements in MR technology have to occur before its role can be considered.

MR is, nevertheless, helpful in assessing vascular lesions in the thorax. The flow characteristics of arteriovenous malformations can easily be demonstrated by MR using flow-sensitive sequences (Fig. 33). It is helpful in the characterization of arterial or venous anomalies. MR demonstrates central pulmonary artery thrombosis or embolism without difficulty. However, peripheral pulmonary embolism remains an angiographic diagnosis despite the fact that lobar and segmental emboli can be seen with MR (87,88). Other pathologies, such as mucous plug or small masses, can simulate the appearance of pulmonary emboli with MR and thus limit its use. MR angiographic techniques, currently under development, may offer an alternative in the future. Very few specific focal lesions have been examined by MR. An exception is a study by Herold et al. (89) which evaluated invasive pulmonary aspergillosis. The authors found a typical target-like appearance and evidence of perilesional hemorrhage. These findings correspond well with the known pathologic correlates of lesions such as those described by Hruban et al. (72) (Fig. 44).

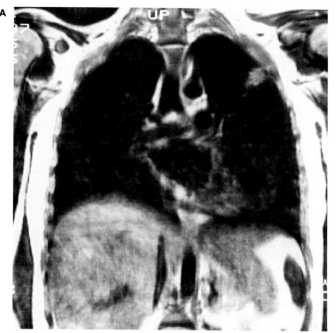
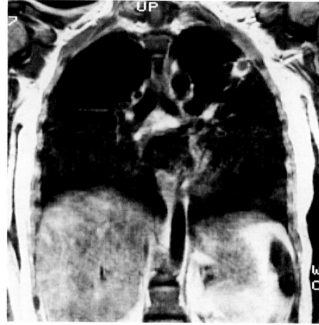

FIG. 44. Focal invasive pulmonary aspergillosis in an immunocompromised patient. **A:** T1-weighted coronal scan. **B:** T1-weighted scan post Gd-DTPA enhancement. Note target-like appearance of lesion with high signal intensity rim and nonenhancing center. (From Herold et al., ref. 89, with permission.)

REFERENCES

1. Theros EG. Caldwell lecture: varying manifestations of peripheral pulmonary neoplasms. A radiologic-pathologic correlative study. *AJR* 1977;128:893–914.
2. Stitik FP, Tockman MS. Radiographic screening in the early detection of lung cancer. *Radiol Clin North Am* 1978;16:347–366.
3. Keagy BA, Starck PJK, Murray GF, et al. Major pulmonary resection for suspected but unconfirmed malignancy. *Ann Thorac Surg* 1984;38:314–316.
4. Steele JD. The solitary pulmonary nodule: report of a cooperative study of resected asymptomatic solitary pulmonary nodules in males. *J Thorac Cardiovasc Surg* 1963;46:21–39.
5. Toomes H, Delphendah A, Milne HG, et al. The coin lesion of the lung. A review of 955 resected coin lesions. *Cancer* 1983;51:534–537.
6. Krudy AG, Doppman JL, Herdt JR. Failure to detect a 1.5 centimeter lung nodule by chest computed tomography. *J Comput Assist Tomogr* 1982;6:1178–1180.
7. Robinson PJ, Jones KR. Improved control of respiration during computed tomography by feedback monitoring. *J Comput Assist Tomogr* 1982;6:802–806.
8. Shaffer K, Pugatch RD. Small pulmonary nodules: dynamic CT with a single-breath technique. *Radiology* 1989;173:567–568.
9. Kalender W, Seissler W, Vock P. Single-breath-hold spiral volumetric CT by continuous patient translation and scanner rotation. *Radiology* 1989;173:414.
10. Cummings SR, Lillington GA, Richard RJ. Estimating the probability of malignancy in solitary pulmonary nodules. *Am Rev Respir Dis* 1986;134:449–452.
11. Higgins GA, Shields TW, Keehn RJ. The solitary pulmonary nodule. Ten year follow-up. Veterans Administration–Armed Forces cooperative study. *Arch Surg* 1975;110:570–575.
12. Zerhouni EA, Stitik FP, Siegelman SS, Naidich DP, et al. CT of the pulmonary nodule: a cooperative study. *Radiology* 1986;160:319–327.
13. Siegelman SS, Khouri NF, Leo FP, Fishman EK, Braverman RM, Zerhouni EA. Solitary pulmonary nodules: CT assessment. *Radiology* 1986;160:307–312.

14. Good CA. The solitary pulmonary nodule: a problem of management. *Radiol Clin North Am* 1963;1:429–437.
15. Good CA, Hood RT, McDonald JR. Significance of a solitary mass in the lung. *Am J Roentgenol Radium Ther Nucl Med* 1953;70:543–554.
16. O'Keefe ME Jr, Good CA, McDonald JR. Calcification in solitary nodules in the lung. *Am J Roentgenol Radium Ther Nucl Med* 1957;77:1023–1033.
17. Robbins SL. *Pathology,* 3rd ed. Philadelphia: WB Saunders, 1968:403–407.
18. Sagel SS, Stanley RJ, Evans RG. Early clinical experience with motionless whole-body computed tomography. *Radiology* 1976;119:321–330.
19. Jost RG, Sagel SS, Stanley RJ, Levitt RG. Computed tomography of the thorax. *Radiology* 1978;126:125–136.
20. Muhm JR, Brown LR, Crowe JK. Detection of pulmonary nodules by computed tomography. *AJR* 1977;128:267–270.
21. McLoud TC, Wittenberg J, Ferrucci JT. Computed tomography of the thorax and standard radiographic evaluation of the chest: a comparative study. *J Comput Assist Tomogr* 1979;3:170–180.
22. Raptopoulos V, Schellinger D, Katz S. Computed tomography of solitary pulmonary nodules: experience with scanning times longer than breatholding. *J Comput Assist Tomogr* 1978;2:55–60.
23. Siegelman SS, Zerhouni EA, Leo FP, Khouri NF, Stitik FP. CT of the solitary pulmonary nodule. *AJR* 1980;135:1–13.
24. Stark P, Wong V, Gold P. Solitary pulmonary granuloma with marked enhancement on dynamic CT scanning. *Radiology* 1988;28:489–490.
25. Godwin DJ, Speckman JM, Putman CE, Korobkin M, Breiman RS. CT densitometry: distinguishing benign from malignant pulmonary nodules. *Radiology* 1982;144:349–351.
26. McCullough EC. Factors affecting the use of quantitative information from a CT scanner. *Radiology* 1977;124:99–107.
27. Zerhouni EA, Spivey JF, Morgan RH, Leo FP, Stitik FP, Siegelman SS. Factors influencing quantitative CT measurements of solitary pulmonary nodules. *J Comput Assist Tomogr* 1982;6:1075–1087.
28. Rao SP, Alfidi RJ. The environmental density artifact: a beam hardening effect in computed tomography. *Radiology* 1981;141:223–227.

29. Cann CE. Quantitative CT applications: comparison of current scanners. *Radiology* 1987;162:257–261.
30. Levi C, Gray JE, McCullough EC, Hattery RR. The unreliability of CT numbers as absolute values. *AJR* 1982;139:443–447.
31. McCullough EC, Morin RL. CT number variability in thoracic geometry. *AJR* 1983;141:135–140.
32. Proto AV, Thomas SR. Pulmonary nodules studied by computed tomography. *Radiology* 1985;153:149–153.
33. Sagel SS. Lung, pleura, pericardium and chest wall. In: Lee JKT, Sagel SS, Stanley RJ, eds. *Computed body tomography.* New York: Raven Press, 1983;99–101.
34. Cann CE, Gamsu G, Birnberg FA, Webb WR. Quantification of calcium in solitary pulmonary nodules using single- and dual-energy CT. *Radiology* 1982;145:493–496.
35. Zerhouni EA, Boukadoum M, Siddiky MA, Newbold JM, et al. A standard phantom for quantitative CT analysis of pulmonary nodules. *Radiology* 1983;149:767–773.
36. Fullerton GD, White DR. Anthropomorphic test objects for CT scanners. *Radiology* 1979;133:217–227.
37. White DR, Martin RJ, Darlison R. Epoxy resin based tissue substitutes. *Br J Radiol* 1977;50:814–821.
38. Khan A, Herman PG, Stevens P, Graver M, Rojas K. Comparative evaluation of clinical history, chest radiographs, standard CT, thin-section CT, reference-phantom CT in the classification of solitary pulmonary nodule. *Radiology* 1986;161:204.
39. Huston J III, Muhm JR. Solitary pulmonary nodules: evaluation with a CT reference phantom. *Radiology* 1989;170:653–656.
40. Jones FA, Wiedemann HP, O'Donovan PB, Stoller JK. Computerized tomographic densitometry of the solitary pulmonary nodule using a nodule phantom. *Chest* 1989;96:779–783.
41. Ward HB, Pliego M, Diefenthal HC, Humphrey EW. The impact of phantom CT scanning on surgery for the solitary pulmonary nodule. *Surgery* 1989;106:734–739.
42. Shimizu T, Kono M, Watanabe H, Adachi S, Hasegawa M, Okuda K, Tanaka K, Kameda K, Hirota S, Sako M. CT evaluation in the diagnosis of pulmonary nodules using lung phantom. *Nippon-Igaku-Hoshasen-Gakkai-Zasshi* 1987;47(10):1251–1259.
43. DeGeer G, Gamsu G, Cann C, Webb WR. Evaluation of a chest phantom for CT nodule densitometry. *AJR* 1986;147(1):21–25.
44. Mahoney MC, Shipley RT, Corcoran HL, Dickson BA. CT demonstration of calcification in carcinoma of the lung. *AJR* 1990;154:255–258.
45. Goldstein MS, Rush M, Johnson P, Sprung CL. A calcified adenocarcinoma of the lung with very high CT numbers. *Radiology* 1984;150:785–786.
46. DeCaro LF, Paladugu R, Benfield JR, Lovisatti L, Pak H, Teplitz RL. Typical and atypical carcinoids within the pulmonary APUD tumor spectrum. *J Thorac Cardiovasc Surg* 1983;86:528–536.
47. Paladugu RR, Benfield JR, Pak HY, Ross RK, Teplitz RL. Bronchopulmonary Kulchitzky cell carcinomas: a new classification scheme for typical and atypical carcinoids. *Cancer* 1985;55:1303–1311.
48. Magid D, Siegelman SS, Eggleston JC, Fishman EK, Zerhouni EA. Pulmonary carcinoid tumors: CT assessment. *J Comput Assist Tomogr* 1989;13(2):244–247.
49. McCaughan BC, Martini N, Bains MS. Bronchial carcinoids: a review of 124 cases. *J Thorac Cardiovasc Surg* 1985;89:8–17.
50. Marks C, Marks M. Bronchial adenoma: a clinicopathologic study. *Chest* 1977;71:376–380.
51. Cooney T, Sweeney EC, Luke D. Pulmonary carcinoid tumours: a comparative regional study. *J Clin Pathol* 1979;32:1100–1109.
52. DeRooij PD, Meijer S, Calame J, Golding RP, Van Mourik JC, Stam J. Solitary hamartoma of the lung: is thoracotomy still mandatory? *Neth J Surg* 1988;40:145–148.
53. Siegelman SS, Khouri NF, Scott WW Jr, Leo FP, Hamper U-M, Fishman EK, Zerhouni EA. Pulmonary hamartoma: CT findings. *Radiology* 1986;160:313–317.
54. Gilbert HA, Kagan AR. Metastases: incidence, detection and evaluation without histologic confirmation. In: Weiss L, ed. *Fundamental aspects of metastasis.* Amsterdam:North-Holland Publishing, 1976.
55. Scholten ET, Kreel L. Distribution of lung metastases in the axial plane: a radiological-pathological study. *Radiol Clin (Basel)* 1977;46:248–265.
56. Crow J, Slavin G, Kreel L. Pulmonary metastasis: a pathologic and radiologic study. *Cancer* 1981;47:2595–2602.
57. Muhm JR, Brown LR, Crowe JK, Sheedy PF, Hattery RR, Stephens DH. Comparison of whole lung tomography and computed tomography for detecting pulmonary nodules. *AJR* 1978;131:981–984.
58. Schaner EG, Chang AE, Doppman JL, Conkle DM, Flye MW, Rosenberg SA. Comparison of computed and conventional whole lung tomography in detecting pulmonary nodules: a prospective radiologic-pathologic study. *AJR* 1978;131:154.
59. Gross BH, Glazer GM, Buchstein FL. Multiple pulmonary nodules detected by computed tomography: diagnostic implications. *JCAT* 1985;9:880.
60. Meziane MA, Hruban RH, Zerhouni EA, Wheeler PS, Khouri NF, et al. High resolution CT of the lung parenchyma with pathologic correlation. *Radiographics* 1988;8(1):27–54.
61. Milne ENC, Zerhouni EA. Blood supply of pulmonary metastases. *J Thorac Imag* 1987;2(4):15–23.
62. Ren H, Hruban RH, Kuhlman JE, Fishman EK, Wheeler PS, Zerhouni EA, Hutchins GM. Computed tomography of inflation-fixed lungs: the beaded septum sign of pulmonary metastasis. *JCAT* 1989;13:411–416.
63. Nathan MH, Collins VP, Adams RA. Differentiation of benign and malignant pulmonary nodules by growth rate. *Radiology* 1962;79:221–227.
64. Weiss W, Boucot KE, Cooper DA. Survival of men with peripheral lung cancer in relation to histologic characteristics and growth rate. *Am Rev Respir Dis* 1968;98:75–92.
65. Cahan WG, Shah JP, Castro ELB. Benign solitary lung lesions in patients with cancer. *Ann Surg* 1978;187:241–249.
66. Dinsmore BJ, Gefter WB, Hatabu H, Kressel HY. Pulmonary arteriovenous malformations diagnosis by gradient-refocused MR imaging. *J Comput Assist Tomogr* 1990;14:918–923.
67. Neifeld JP, Michaelis LC, Doppman JL. Suspected pulmonary metastases—correlation of chest X-ray, whole lung tomograms and operative findings. *Cancer* 1977;39:383–387.
68. Ren H, Kuhlman JE, Hruban RH, Fishman EK, Wheeler PS, Hurchins GM. CT of inflation-fixed lungs: wedge-shaped density and vascular sign in the diagnosis of infarction. *JCAT* 1990;14(1):82–86.
69. Kuhlman JE, Fishman EK, Teigen C. Pulmonary septic emboli: diagnosis with CT. *Radiology* 1990;174:211–213.
70. Huang RM, Naidich DP, Lubat E, Shcinella R, Garay SM, McCauley DI. Septic pulmonary emboli: CT radiographic correlation. *AJR* 1989;153:41–45.
71. Kuhlman JE, Fishman EK, Siegelman SS. Invasive pulmonary aspergillosis in acute leukemia: characteristic findings on CT, the CT halo sign and the role of CT in early diagnosis. *Radiology* 1985;157:611–614.
72. Hruban RH, Meziane MA, Zerhouni EA, Wheeler PS, Dumler JS, Hutchins GM. Radiologic/pathologic correlation of the CT halo sign in invasive pulmonary aspergillosis. *JCAT* 1987;11:534–536.
73. Lynch DA, Gamsu G, Ray CS, Aberle DR. Asbestos-related focal lung masses: manifestations on conventional and high-resolution CT scans. *Thorac Radiol* 1988;169:603–607.
74. McHugh K, Blaquiere RM. CT features of rounded atelectasis. *AJR* 1989;153(2):257–260.
75. Ren H, Hruban RH, Kuhlman JE, Fishman EK, Wheeler PS, Zerhouni EA, Hutchins GM. Computed tomography of rounded atelectasis. *J Comput Assist Tomogr* 1988;12(6):1031–1034.
76. Blesovsky A. The folded lung. *Br J Dis Chest* 1966;60:19–22.
77. Metzger RA, Mulhern CB, Arger PH, Coleman BG, Epstein DM, Gefter WB. CT differentiation of solitary from diffuse bronchioloalveolar carcinoma. *JCAT* 1981;5:830–833.
78. Edwards CW. Alveolar carcinoma: a review. *Thorax* 1984;39:166–174.
79. Shapiro R, Wilson GL, Yesner R, Shuman H. A useful roentgen sign in the diagnosis of localized bronchioloalveolar carcinoma. *AJR* 1971;114:516–524.
80. Kuhlman JE, Fishman EK, Kuhajda FP, Meziane MM, Khouri NF, Zerhouni EA, Siegelman SS. Solitary bronchioloalveolar carcinoma: CT criteria. *Radiology* 1988;167:379–382.

81. Berkmen YM. The many faces of bronchiolo-alveolar carcinoma. *Semin Roentgenol* 1977;12:207–214.

82. Lynch DA, Webb WR, Gamsu G, Stulbarg M, Golden J. Computed tomography in pulmonary sarcoidosis. *J Comput Assist Tomogr* 1989;13:405–410.

83. Müller NL, Kullnig P, Miller RR. The CT findings of pulmonary sarcoidosis: analysis of 25 patients. *AJR* 1989;152(6):1179–1182.

84. Hamper U-M, Fishman EK, Khouri NF, Johns CJ, Wang KP, Siegelman SS. Typical and atypical CT manifestations of pulmonary sarcoidosis. *J Comput Assist Tomogr* 1986;10(6):928–936.

85. Müller NL, Gamsu G, Webb WR. Pulmonary nodules: detection using magnetic resonance and computed tomography. *Radiology* 1985;155(3):687–690.

86. Gamsu G, deGeer G, Cann C, Müller N, Brito A. A preliminary study of MRI quantification of simulated calcified pulmonary nodules. *Invest Radiol* 1987;22(11):853–858.

87. Gamsu G, Hirji M, Moore EH, Webb WR, Brito A. Experimental pulmonary emboli detected using magnetic resonance. *Radiology* 1984;(153(2):467–470.

88. Moore EH, Gamsu G, Webb WR, Stulbarg MS. Pulmonary embolus: detection and follow-up using magnetic resonance. *Radiology* 1984;153(2):471–472.

89. Herold CJ, Kramer J, Sertl K, Kalhs P, Mallek R, Imhof H, Tscholakoff D. Invasive pulmonary aspergillosis: evaluation with MR imaging. *Radiology* 1989;173:717–721.

Chapter 8

Diffuse Lung Disease

Despite the well-established role of chest roentgenography to accurately and inexpensively display a wide range of parenchymal pathology, equally well-established limitations have been documented (1). Epler et al., in examining 458 patients with histologically confirmed infiltrative lung disease, showed that 44, or nearly 10%, had normal prebiopsy chest radiographs (Fig. 1) (2). Similar results have been reported by Gaensler and Carrington (3).

Abnormalities detected by chest radiographs are frequently nonspecific. Simple, precise, and consistent guidelines for recognizing the various patterns of diffuse lung disease seem difficult to define, probably due to variations inherently associated with the visual interpretation of nonfocal and complex abnormalities (Fig. 2). Utilizing a semi-quantitative approach based on a slight modification of the International Labour Office and Union Internationale Contre le Cancer (ILO/UC) classification, McLoud et al. found, in an evaluation of 365 cases of diffuse infiltrative lung disease proved with open-lung biopsy, that their first two radiologic diagnostic choices corresponded to the histologic diagnosis in only 50% of cases, improving to just 78% when the first three choices were included (4). Significantly, in this same study there was only 70% interobserver agreement as to the predominant type of opacity present or the degree of profusion.

By eliminating superimposition of structures and enhancing attenuation discrimination, computed tomography (CT) provides a direct visual window into the lungs. Although these advantages were appreciated early after the development of CT in the diagnosis of both focal and diffuse lung disease, technical limitations, including routine lack of access and 18-sec scan times, precluded widespread utilization (5–8). However, over the past several years with the development of rapid scan times (1–2 sec) and improved reconstruction algorithms, the role of CT has progressively changed. As first shown by Zerhouni et al., thin collimation (1.5 to 2-mm thick sections) and targeted reconstruction with a high spatial frequency (bone) algorithm—high-resolution computed tomography (HRCT)—can routinely provide remarkably detailed images of lung architecture (9). Resolution of structures of approximately 300μ has been reported (10).

In this chapter, the role of both routine chest radiography and CT in the evaluation of diffuse lung disease is reviewed; the role of CT in the evaluation of focal lung disease was considered in Chapter 7.

GENERAL PRINCIPLES AND METHODOLOGY

In no other portion of the chest is the diagnostic efficacy of CT so inextricably tied to scan technique as in the evaluation of diffuse lung disease. Variations in technique so alter the appearance of the lung that in select cases, accurate diagnosis may depend on the selection of appropriate scan parameters. As a consequence, accurate evaluation of diffuse lung disease requires that a variety of protocols that specifically reflect a wide range of clinical indications be established.

A detailed description of the HRCT technique is presented in Chapter 1. Optimally, this methodology re-

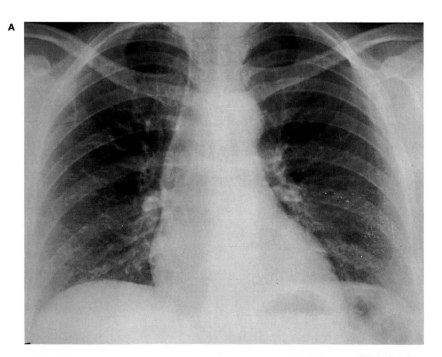

FIG. 1. Radiographically occult lung disease. A: Normal posteroanterior radiograph in a patient presenting with hemoptysis. B,C: Sequential 1.5-mm thick, target reconstructed CT sections through the mid and lower portions of the right lung, respectively. These show characteristic features of ground-glass opacification second to acute airspace consolidation. Note that there are numerous focal areas of increased lung density, within which normal anatomic structures can still be visualized (curved arrow in C). Note additionally that many of these densities are localized around core pulmonary arteries, identifiable as central dots within secondary pulmonary lobules (arrows in B and C). This distribution reflects the underlying anatomy as may be predicted in a patient clinically aspirating blood.

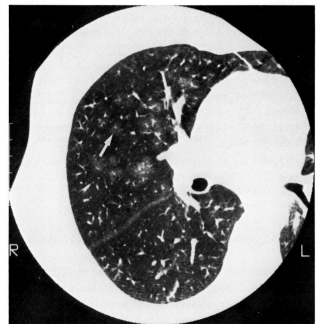

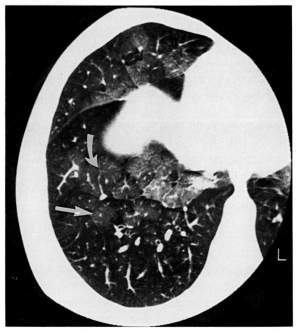

A

B

C,D

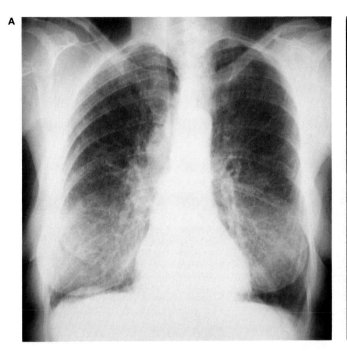
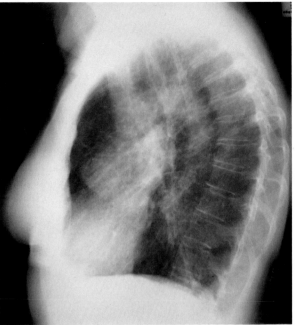
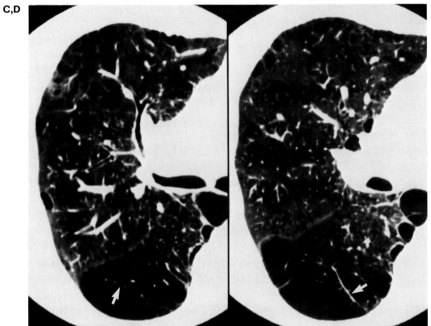

FIG. 2. "Dirty lung" emphysema. **A,B:** Posteroanterior and lateral radiographs show diffuse, ill-defined reticular densities throughout both lungs. **C,D:** Retrospectively targeted HRCT images of the right mid and lower lung fields, respectively, clearly reveal extensive emphysema without evidence of diffuse interstitial disease. The reticular lines seen on the chest radiographs are caused by the septa separating bullae, most easily identified laterally and posteriorly (*arrows*). In addition to peripheral bullae, discrete areas of markedly low tissue attenuation without clearly definable walls can be identified within the lung parenchyma, findings compatible with diffuse emphysematous disease. Note that the intervening lung parenchyma is normal and that intrapulmonary vessels are well-defined with smooth contours.

quires: (a) acquisition of thin, 1 to 3-mm thick sections; and (b) targeted reconstructions with fields-of-view (FOV's) restricted retrospectively to individual lungs utilizing a high spatial frequency (bone) algorithm. Although it has been reported that there is little difference between 1.5 and 3-mm thick sections in evaluating fine detail within the lung, in our experience thinner sections are always preferable (Fig. 3) (11). Routinely, images are acquired with the shortest possible scan time (generally 2 sec or less) using a 512 × 512 matrix, with mA typically varying between 140 and 170, depending on the

patient's size. It should be noted that considerable dose reduction, to as low as 10 mA, still allows acquisition of interpretable images of the lung parenchyma (see Chapter 1). The implications of this may be significant for the potential use of CT as a screening procedure, e.g., for populations at high risk for developing lung cancer (12).

Optimal technical parameters for individual images have been described (11,13) although, unfortunately, there is no general agreement as to what constitutes an acceptable high-resolution study (14). Individual reports

A,B

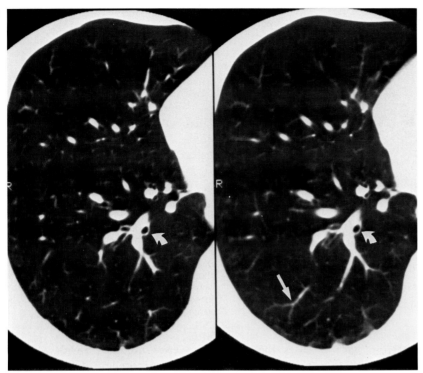

FIG. 3. HRCT: 1.5- vs. 3-mm thick sections. **A,B:** Retrospectively targeted HRCT section of the right mid lung, using 1.5- and 3-mm thick sections, respectively. The image obtained with 1.5-mm collimation is considerably sharper; compare, for example, the appearance of the major fissure in both A and B. Note, however, that an increase in resolution is accompanied by a decreased sense of overall parenchymal architecture. Although the sections are at identical levels, through the exact same basilar segmental bronchi (*curved arrows*), more peripherally, structures that are easily identified as branching vessels on the 3-mm thick section (*arrow* in B) cannot be identified as such on the 1.5-mm thick section (compare with A). Nonetheless, 1.5-mm thick sections should be preferred for HRCT.

differ strikingly in overall technique, especially in determining the number and levels of necessary scans, and the indications for both prone and supine images. In many institutions HRCT is performed without the routine use of retrospective target reconstructions.

As described in most reports, HRCT of the lung is usually performed in one of two fashions. In the first, high-resolution images are obtained as part of a routine CT examination. In this setting, a few additional images are obtained (generally one to three) either in select areas, following evaluation of an initial sequence of 8 to 10-mm thick sections to further define regions suspected or proven to be abnormal; or, alternatively, at specific, preselected levels, such as the aortic arch, carina, or just above the diaphragm. This approach requires little additional scan time, and may be of value in select cases by further defining the nature of focal abnormalities. Unfortunately, only a very limited portion of the lung is actually sampled with HRCT using this approach. As recently suggested by Zwirewich et al., in patients in whom diffuse lung disease is suspected, the initial sequence of 10-mm thick sections can be prospectively reconstructed using a bone algorithm; this has the effect of improving spatial visualization without cost in time (15).

A second method that has been described specifically emphasizes HRCT by using only thin sections from the outset. Images typically are obtained at preselected levels chosen to maximize evaluation of the different lung zones, frequently with the patient alternately supine and prone. Because this approach involves incomplete sampling of the airways, hila, mediastinum, and especially the lungs, this method is really only applicable to those select cases in which the specific clinical indication for the study is to exclude and/or further characterize diffuse parenchymal disease. Again, this approach is inherently limited in that only a small portion of the lung itself is actually sampled.

In our experience both approaches may be of diagnostic value, but the second approach is generally favorable. To maximize the effectiveness of HRCT, however, we emphasize acquisition of more than simply a few images obtained at preselected levels. Instead, our routine HRCT protocol for evaluating patients with known or suspected diffuse lung disease calls for 1.5-mm thick sections obtained every 10 mm from the thoracic inlet to the hemidiaphragms, prospectively reconstructed using a high spatial frequency (bone) algorithm. Select images may then be retrospectively targeted, as clinically indicated. Prone images are not routinely acquired, but are obtained in cases in which disease in dependent portions of the lungs needs to be excluded, as when evaluating patients with suspected asbestosis.

This approach allows more complete sampling of the lungs and permits far more precise characterization of the nature and extent of disease (16). In our experience, even with diffuse lung disease, focal alterations are the rule. These are easily missed when only a few random images are obtained. That this technique is likely to yield comparable or even higher diagnostic accuracy

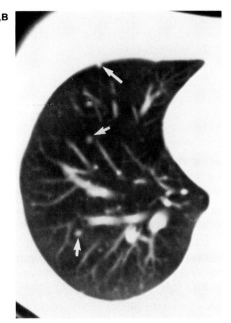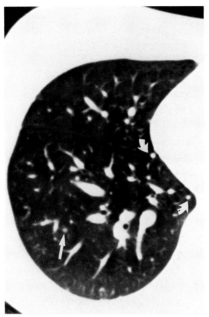

FIG. 4. Identifying pulmonary nodules: 10-mm vs. 1.5-mm thick section. **A,B:** Target reconstructed images through the right lower lobe at the exact same levels using 10-mm and 1.5-mm thick sections, respectively. In this case, identification of individual nodules is visually easier with 10-mm thick sections (*arrows*), although close scrutiny of the 1.5-mm thick section reveals the presence of nodules within the lungs. Some may even be seen to better advantage (*arrow* in B).

than routine CT studies using 10-mm thick sections has been documented (16,146). An important exception to this rule that "less is more" is in the evaluation of patients with suspected metastatic disease. In this setting, where the identification of even one nodule may be clinically significant, incomplete sampling is unacceptable; furthermore, nodules are easier to identify with 10-mm thick sections (Fig. 4). These considerations are less significant when imaging diseases are characterized by large numbers of nodules. As documented by Brauner et al., in patients with diffuse nodular diseases such as sarcoidosis, obtaining 1.5-mm sections every 10 mm throughout the lungs allowed identification of nodules in virtually all patients (146).

It should be emphasized that there are no predetermined "best" windows and levels for imaging the lung. Precise settings are often a matter of subjective preference. However, as a general guide, the window width should be set at twice the CT number range of the particular area of interest, while the window level should be set at the midpoint between the density of objects of interest. This generally corresponds to window widths between 1,800 and 2,000 HU, and window levels between −325 and −500 HU. In fact, as illustrated in this chapter, a wide range of settings is employed, depending on the particular nature of the pathology to be illustrated. Narrowing the window width enhances visual resolution. This may be particularly helpful when assessing focal increases and decreases in parenchymal density, as may be seen in patients with emphysema. Conversely, wide window widths are often more informative when the disease process occupies a large area and involves a wide range of tissue-density alterations, as may occur with complex pleural-parenchymal disease. In these

cases, the panoramic view afforded by a wide window width improves visual comprehension. Although rarely emphasized, it is worth noting that for the purposes of producing both slides and prints, images obtained with narrow windows are far easier to reproduce and display; this may, in part, explain the wide acceptance of narrower windows as "standard" (see Chapter 1 for a more detailed discussion).

DIFFUSE PULMONARY DISEASE— CT CLASSIFICATION

CT can be used to characterize lung disease in one of two fashions: (a) quantitatively, by measuring alterations in the density or attenuation coefficients of lung tissue, or (b) morphologically, by delineating alterations of parenchymal anatomy and relating these to documented pathologic abnormalities.

Quantitative Assessment

Considerable interest has been focused on the use of CT to obtain quantitative information concerning lung tissue density (17). CT lung density is a composite of pulmonary tissue, blood, extravascular water, and air, and is therefore inherently nonhomogeneous (5,7,18,19). Measurements may be obtained using either a whole-lung field method in which the entire volume of lung contained within a given section is analyzed or, alternatively, a sector method in which regions-of-interest (ROI's) are selected at specific sites, including both cortical and medullary lung (20).

Density gradients, primarily related to the influence

of gravity, are normally present between anterior, non-dependent and posterior, dependent portions of the parenchyma (Fig. 5) (5,17,18,21). These gradients are most pronounced in the lower lung zones as a result of both a decrease in the density of anterior lung and an increase in the density of posterior lung. These differences are accentuated still further when scans are obtained at end-expiratory lung volume (7). Additional gradients are measurable between cortical and medullary lung. As shown by Genereux, although precise methods for identification of these zones are lacking, cortico-medullary gradients remain positive regardless of whether they are measured anteriorly, laterally, or posteriorly (17). These findings suggest that physiological differences, such as blood flow regulation between the pulmonary medulla and cortex, may be measurable (22).

Unfortunately, and despite seemingly great potential, characterization of disease by density alterations has proven of far greater use in the assessment of focal rather than diffuse lung disease. Clinical use is hampered by numerous technical difficulties. Although attempts have been made to acquire density calculations by computer methods that automatically isolate the lungs, current methods remain laborious and time consuming (23,24,33,157,188). Additionally, there is tremendous overlap between various disease entities due to problems associated with partial volume averaging of the wide variety of different intrathoracic tissue densities (17). Problems also may be encountered in obtaining reproducible lung volumes, which is a critical factor in quantitative analysis. Although it has been suggested that this

problem may be solved by use of spirometrically controlled scanning, this technique remains experimental (25). As shown by Robinson and Kreel, there is a significant inverse correlation between lung volume and mean attenuation values of lung (7). This is important since there is considerable variation in lung expansion relative to midtidal volume not only during breath-holding in neutral respiration but even during breath-holding in deep inspiration.

Problems also are encountered with the use and reliability of absolute CT numbers. Although, as documented in a number of reports, total mean lung density actually varies only slightly (from between approximately −810 to −860 HUs), as shown by Levi et al., absolute density measurements vary widely when the same phantom is scanned on different machines, with significant fluctuations resulting from variations in kilovoltage, orientation, and positioning of patients within scanners, and the size of lesions and/or structures to be examined (26). These limitations have the effect of rendering absolute density determinations within the lung as ineffectual for the evaluation of most diffuse lung diseases; in fact, in most cases, quantification is no more accurate than simple visual inspection.

As a consequence, other investigators have emphasized the use of visual scoring systems, especially in the evaluation of emphysema (33–36,161). Using this approach, observers assess the extent of parenchymal damage by visually estimating the percentage of abnormal lung tissue.

To date, with varying degrees of success, CT densitometry has been used to evaluate normal lungs (27–32) as well as a wide range of abnormalities, both clinical and experimental, including emphysema (33–36), pulmonary edema (37–39), asbestos-related disease (40), and even patients undergoing bone marrow transplantation (41). In select cases in which patients present with unexplained dyspnea and a normal chest radiograph, it has been reported that CT densitometry has been helpful by documenting reversal of normal anteroposterior density gradients in patients with interstitial pneumonia (17). At present, continued evaluation of CT densitometry for assessing both the presence and/or extent of disease as well as possible patient management clearly warrants further investigation.

Morphologic Assessment

Basic HRCT Signs of Diffuse Lung Disease

The great wealth of information about HRCT scans necessitates an effective yet simple conceptual framework to classify basic signs and patterns of diffuse lung pathology. Unfortunately, no generally accepted standard criteria for HRCT interpretation have yet been de-

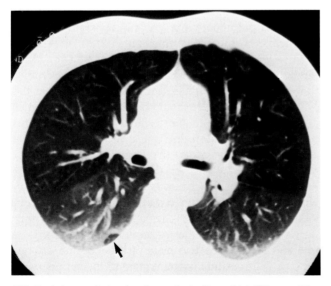

FIG. 5. Anteroposterior density gradients, 5-mm thick CT scan at the level of the bronchus intermedius in a patient with no known pulmonary disease. Anteroposterior density gradients are easily identified bilaterally. Note that at the right lung base, there is relative sparing of a subpleural secondary pulmonary lobule, possibly reflecting either focal shunting or emphysema (arrow).

veloped, despite the fact that clearly defined models of both lung structure and response to injury have been well described (42,43). In our experience, awareness that the lung has only a limited ability to respond to a wide range of injuries has led us to a step-by-step conceptualization and hence description of most of the basic signs of pulmonary disease seen on HRCT. As will be extensively illustrated, these basic signs can be used to analyze constellations of findings characteristic of specific disease entities.

Normal Adult Lung Structure: HRCT Evaluation

Detailed knowledge of normal lung anatomy serves as a necessary prerequisite to meaningful analysis of pathologic alterations. As discussed in Chapter 1, the lower limits of resolution achievable with current scanners, assuming optimal technique, is approximately 0.3 mm or 300 microns. *In vitro* CT evaluation of lungs in both animals and humans has documented that anatomic detail at the level of the secondary pulmonary lobule can be seen (10,44–47). On the basis of *in vitro* experiments performed on fixed and inflated lungs, Murata et al. have reported that normal septa, which measure 100 microns or more in thickness, can be resolved (10). In our experience, such a level of spatial resolution, even with the most advanced scanners, is not achievable *in vivo*. It is probable that this discrepancy is secondary to preparation methods artifactually increasing the thickness of septal structures which would otherwise not be visible by HRCT. A lower limit of 300 microns for effective resolution *in vivo* also explains why little additional information is gained when fields of view less than 15 cm are used (13), the diameter at which pixel size also measures about 300 microns (47). As a consequence, it is rarely necessary to use targeted reconstruction for imaging less than a single lung field; in fact, for most clinical applications, a field of view encompassing both lung fields simultaneously is usually satisfactory. It appears that most of the gain in detail achieved by using HRCT is largely attributable solely to the use of thin sections, especially when reconstructed prospectively with an edge-enhancing algorithm.

Awareness that the limit of resolution of HRCT is approximately 300 microns has profound implications as it determines what structures and pathologic processes can be actually expected to be visualized *in vivo*.

With inspiration, 80% of the lung volume represents air, 10% represents blood, and 10% represents tissue. Lung tissue is extremely delicate, the small mass of lung tissue being distributed over an enormous surface area equivalent to nearly the size of a tennis court (100 to 200 sq m). Thus, most of the lung appears featureless, identifiable as homogeneous gray "background" density. As the primary function of the lung is gas exchange, maintaining an extremely thin barrier between alveolar air and interstitial capillaries is essential. In fact, the thickness of alveolar walls normally measures approximately 20 to 30 microns and is therefore an order of magnitude below HRCT resolution.

These requirements necessitate a unique architectural design to ensure mechanical stability and to maintain open air spaces and capillaries to allow gas exchange. As previously described by Weibel (42), this is achieved by an organization characterized by central or core-supporting structures (bronchi and pulmonary arteries) and peripheral or "shell" elements (pleura and connective tissue septa). Between the core and shell structures lies the functional pulmonary parenchymal unit made up of alveolar sacs, acini, and lobules. A well-organized fiber network supports the alveolar wall structures, thus keeping capillaries and alveoli open for functional exchange. This fiber network connects the core and shell structures, ensuring the stability of the entire design. This core/shell arrangement of the lung is self-replicated from the largest lung units such as the lobes, to segments, lobules, and the smallest units, the acini.

The lung is maintained in a stable position within the chest by its hilar connections to which the central or core structures are ultimately attached. In brief, the bronchovascular structures form the "stems" upon which the functional parenchyma are distributed. The visceral pleura and its connective tissue extensions within the parenchyma form the envelope that maintains the structural integrity of the parenchymal elements (Fig. 6).

The major core structures include the pulmonary artery branches and the bronchi which characteristically run in a parallel fashion. Each bronchus is closely apposed to a pulmonary artery of similar diameter. Both are enclosed within a common connective tissue sheath, within which amorphous interstitial collagen, lymphatics, and small lymph nodes, ranging in size from 1 mm at the periphery of the lung to 5–10 mm near the hilum, can be found. It should be noted that lymphatics do not extend beyond the terminal bronchioles. This bronchoarterial relationship is strictly maintained all the way to the periphery, to the level of the respiratory bronchioles.

The major shell structure is the visceral pleura from which fibrous connective tissue septa emanate perpendicularly to penetrate the lung parenchyma. The pulmonary veins follow a course independent of the bronchial tree and lie between two pairs of bronchi and arteries (Fig. 6). This position is maintained to the periphery, as well, where veins are seen to run within connective septal structures wherever these are well defined. A rich pleural lymphatic system, also referred to as the superficial lymphatic network, drains the visceral pleura and courses within the interlobular septa in parallel with

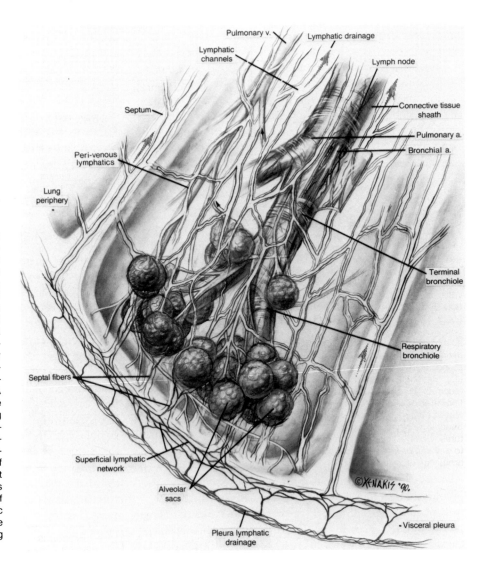

FIG. 6. The core-shell design of lung structure. A secondary lobule is represented to illustrate the architectural design of the lung. The central core supporting structures are composed of the terminal bronchiole and pulmonary artery, enclosed in a bronchovascular sheath. The bronchial artery runs in parallel to these structures within the connective tissue sheath. A deep lymphatic system located in close apposition to the core structures drains the interstitium. Note that lymphatics are not present around alveolar sacs. The shell structures are composed of the visceral pleura and septa extending from the visceral pleura into the lung substance. Within these peripheral structures run the pulmonary veins and the superficial lymphatic network that drains the pleura via septal lymphatics that are perivenous in location. A network of septal fibers is present in the shell structures and supports the lung parenchyma. Elastic fibers are also present in the connective tissue sheath surrounding the core structures. The functional units of the lung made up of collections of alveolar sacs are in effect suspended between the core structures and the shell structures via a network of interconnecting elastic fibers. This basic organization is self-replicated from the smallest to the largest functional lung unit.

septal veins; these ultimately lead to lymphatics and nodes within the hila. The normal visceral pleura varies in thickness between 200 and 300 microns, whereas septa are considerably more delicate, measuring between 100 and 150 microns. Importantly, at all levels the normal visceral pleura interfaces smoothly with the adjacent lung parenchyma.

Bronchi and pulmonary arteries divide by dichotomous branching. There are approximately 23 generations of dichotomous branching in airways, from the trachea to alveolar sacs (Fig. 7). There are 28 generations of pulmonary arterial branching. Since a bronchus is usually recognized only when its walls are visualized, it is not possible to resolve bronchi with a wall thickness of less than 300 microns. This corresponds to bronchi of about 1.5–2 mm in diameter, equivalent to between the seventh and ninth generation of airways. Rarely, smaller

bronchi approximately 1 mm in diameter can be recognized coursing perpendicularly within the plane of a very thin section by virtue of their lower density and their proximity to an adjacent pulmonary artery, even though their walls cannot be individually resolved.

As a consequence, normal bronchi cannot be visualized beyond a point midway between the hilum and the pleural surface, even on HRCT scans. On the other hand, blood vessels with diameters of 300 microns can be visualized, corresponding to 16th generation arteries at the level of the terminal and most proximal respiratory bronchioles (Fig. 8). Because vascular structures typically can be visualized to within a few mm of the pleural surfaces and can be followed to the level of the secondary pulmonary lobule (defined as parenchyma supplied by between three and five terminal bronchioles), the arterial tree is clearly the most useful land-

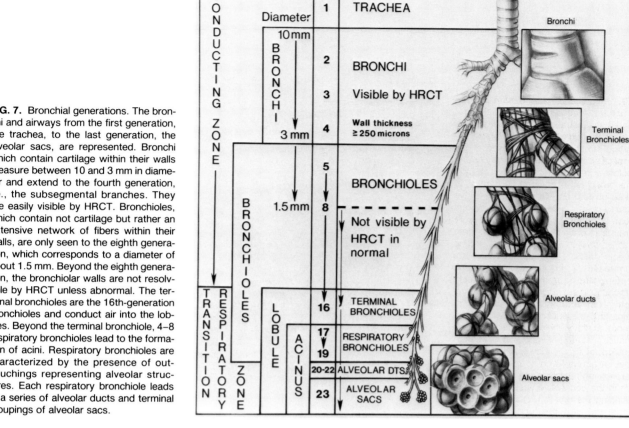

FIG. 7. Bronchial generations. The bronchi and airways from the first generation, the trachea, to the last generation, the alveolar sacs, are represented. Bronchi which contain cartilage within their walls measure between 10 and 3 mm in diameter and extend to the fourth generation, i.e., the subsegmental branches. They are easily visible by HRCT. Bronchioles, which contain not cartilage but rather an extensive network of fibers within their walls, are only seen to the eighth generation, which corresponds to a diameter of about 1.5 mm. Beyond the eighth generation, the bronchiolar walls are not resolvable by HRCT unless abnormal. The terminal bronchioles are the 16th-generation bronchioles and conduct air into the lobules. Beyond the terminal bronchiole, 4–8 respiratory bronchioles lead to the formation of acini. Respiratory bronchioles are characterized by the presence of outpouchings representing alveolar structures. Each respiratory bronchiole leads to a series of alveolar ducts and terminal groupings of alveolar sacs.

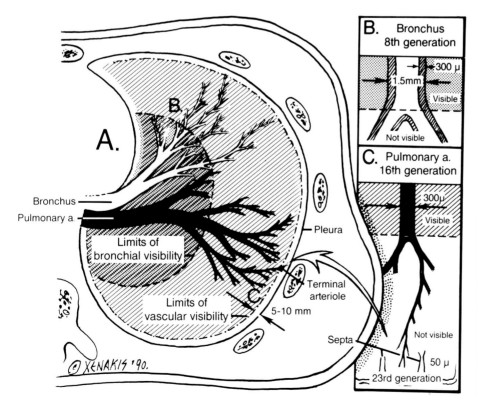

FIG. 8. Limits of visibility by HRCT. Bronchi and bronchioles are seen to the eighth generation, at which point their wall thickness is at the limit of HRCT's resolution. Pulmonary artery branches can be seen to the 16th generation extending from the hilum (A) which corresponds to 300μ vessels. In this figure we have represented the limits of bronchial visibility (B) which are usually at a point midway between the hilum and the pleural surface. The limits of vascular visibility (C) are much greater, reaching a point 5–10 mm from the visceral pleural surface.

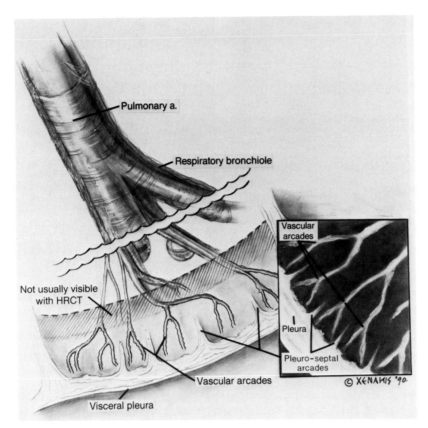

FIG. 9. Pleuro-septal and vascular arcades. Normally, the pulmonary artery at the center of secondary lobules is easily visualized along with its most proximal divisions only. Thus, pulmonary arteries are usually not visible with HRCT beyond a point 5–10 mm from the visceral pleural surface. Normal septal structures arising from the pleura are normally 100–150µ thick and are rarely visible *in vivo*. If septal veins or connective tissue within septa are thickened they may become visible, leading to the formation of so-called pleuro-septal arcades. These result from thickening of the "shell" structures made of the visceral pleura and septal connective tissue layers. They characteristically form right angles with the adjacent pleural surfaces. By comparison, if core lobular vessels become enlarged or their connective tissue sheaths are thickened, core vascular structures can be seen to extend almost to the visceral pleura. Core vessels form vascular arcades whose apices are directed toward the center of the lung, resulting in a characteristic V-shaped configuration.

mark for defining HRCT lung architecture. Characteristically, pulmonary arteries are seen to course through the center of this anatomical unit fanning into only a few branches.

When secondary lobules are sectioned tangentially, lobular core arteries form a characteristic appearance resembling a dot between 5 and 10 mm from the pleural surface, within the center of peripheral pleuro-septal arcades. Pleuro-septal arcades can be identified because they typically form right angles with the adjacent pleural surface (Figs. 9, 10). Less well appreciated, a second form of arcade may be identified: so-called vascular arcades. These represent peripheral branches of core pulmonary arteries that course in the same plane as the CT scan (Fig. 9). Unlike pleuro-septal arcades, vascular arcades may be recognized by their characteristic "V" shape as they approach the pleural surface (Fig. 9).

As noted by Murata et al. (10) and Webb et al. (46), identification of pleuro-septal arcades is very useful for recognizing lobular anatomy, especially when abnor-

mal, as may occur in patients with lymphangitic carcinomatosis (145). Typically, in normal lungs, secondary pulmonary lobules are only well-defined peripherally, in the anterior and lateral, nondependent portions of the upper and middle lung fields as well as along mediastinal borders. Most measure approximately 1 cm or less, although septa as long as 4 cm have been reported (46). As documented by Webb et al. in their evaluation of inflated lung specimens, an average of only four septa at least 1 cm in length extending to the pleura were visible over the anterior and lateral surfaces of the mid and upper lung zones, while an average of only two septa could be identified over the lateral and posterior lower lobes (46). Centrally, within the medullary portion of the lung, septa are often incomplete or nonexistent. It should be considered axiomatic, therefore, that visualization of lobular architecture, especially when easily identified throughout the lung periphery or when identifiable at all within the central portion of the lungs, is indicative of underlying interstitial disease.

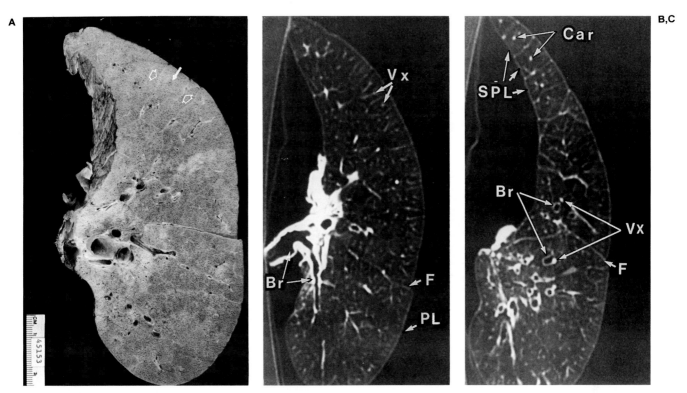

FIG. 10. A: Secondary pulmonary lobular anatomy. Inflated fixed lung section shows characteristic appearance of a subpleural secondary pulmonary lobule when oriented perpendicular to the plane of section. The secondary pulmonary lobule is defined as that portion of the lung subtended by three to five terminal bronchioles, and typically ranges from 1–2.5 cm in size. Peripherally, lobules are bordered by interlobular septa (*open arrows*) within which pulmonary veins and lymphatics are located; centrally, the lobule is defined by core structures, including bronchioles and accompanying branches of the pulmonary artery (*white arrow*). Note that in this section only a few well-defined peripheral and occasional central lobules can actually be identified. **B,C:** *In vitro* CT evaluation: 2-mm thick CT sections through the periphery of an inflated fixed lung specimen. A number of secondary lobules (SPL) can be identified, within which characteristic central arteries (Car) can be seen. F, fissure; PL, pleura; Br, central bronchi; Vx, vessels accompanying bronchi, presumably pulmonary artery branches. Note that within definable lobules, core or central bronchioles are too small to be visualized.

HRCT-Pathologic Correlation

In our opinion, interpretation of pathologic changes within the parenchyma identified with HRCT is most easily conceptualized by reference to basic defense and repair mechanisms of the lung. This process of injury and repair has been generically termed the *acute lung injury pattern,* a descriptive phrase for the predictable albeit nonspecific sequence of pathologic events following acute lung injury from a wide variety of causes, including infections, toxic fumes, drugs, radiation, and shock, among others (54–56). Depending on whether the basic injury is widespread or limited and whether the underlying etiology is known, patterns of acute lung injury may be further characterized as either diffuse alveolar damage (DAD), acute interstitial pneumonia (AIP), or bronchiolitis obliterans-organizing pneumonia (BOOP) (55). Of these designations, diffuse alveolar damage is most descriptive of the widest range of pathologic entities associated with acute lung injury. As a consequence, DAD serves as a convenient model on which to classify abnormalities identified by HRCT.

Acute and Subacute Lung Injury

The pulmonary interstitium is a complex structure of cells and extracellular matrix bounded by alveolar epithelial cells on one side and capillary endothelial cells on the other. The most important constituent of the interstitium is connective tissue which serves to provide the framework that maintains alveolar shape, preventing collapse of the alveoli during expiration and regulating

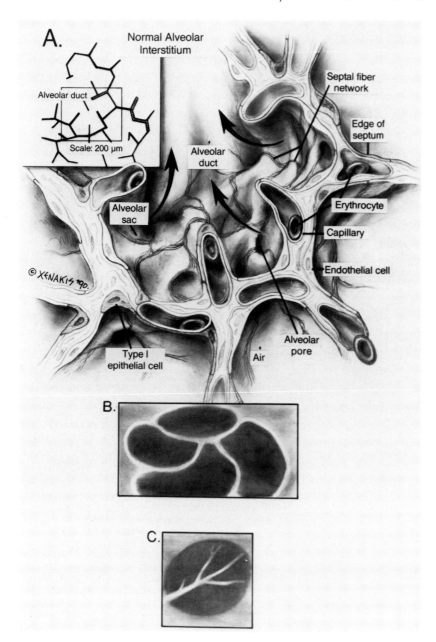

FIG. 11. The normal alveolar interstitium. **A:** The pulmonary interstitium is a very delicate structure designed to maintain a minimum distance between the blood capillaries and the air within the alveoli. The thickness of alveolar walls is approximately 20–30μ. The interstitium is made up of a framework of connective tissue into which multiple elastic fibers are connected (**A**). These fibers are designed to maintain alveolar shape and prevent collapse of the alveoli during expiration. Epithelial cells, mostly type I pneumocytes, cover the alveolar walls. Capillaries are in intimate contact with these epithelial cells, with no intervening interstitium seen on the capillary surface facing the alveolus. The connective tissue is made up of mostly extracellular matrix bounded by the alveolar and capillary endothelial cells. No lymphatics are found at the level of the alveolar interstitium. Normally, alveolar interstitium is not resolvable by HRCT. **B** represents a 1-mm HRCT section. Two to three alveolar sacs which are about 300μ in diameter may be contained within such a section. However, the alveolar walls are very thin (20–30μ) and form a very small proportion of the total thickness. Thus, as shown in **C,** normal alveolar interstitium will appear only as a featureless background density through which pulmonary vessels can easily be distinguished.

the movement of water, proteins, and cells within the alveolar walls (Fig. 11).

Although a large variety of agents can injure the lung parenchyma, the response of the lung to such injuries is limited. Typically, capillary endothelial cells and type 1 alveolar epithelial cells are the most vulnerable to injury. Damage can alter the permeability of these cells and cause them to swell and fragment. Leaks in the cellular lining of capillaries and/or alveoli then lead to intersti-

tial and alveolar edema. Depending on the type and severity of injury, this process can be self-limiting, although if sufficiently severe, the epithelial lining may be completely destroyed. The denuded underlying tissue becomes covered by a thick layer of fibrin and cell debris, filling the alveolar airspaces and appearing as hyaline membranes on histologic examination. Depending on the type of injury, inflammatory reaction with infiltration by inflammatory cells results in further

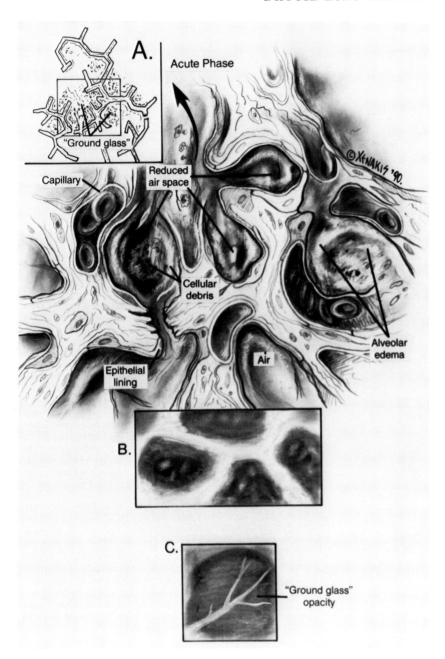

FIG. 12. A: Acute lung injury, acute phase (compare to Fig. 11). During the acute phase of the lung response to injury, type 1 pneumocytes are destroyed leading to swelling, increased accumulation of fluid, and cellular debris within the air spaces. Hyaline membranes can be formed at this stage, further reducing the available airspace. Within the interstitium, accumulation of fluid thickens the alveolar walls. Interstitial and alveolar edema are present. As shown in **A**, thickening of alveolar interstitium in addition to accumulation of fluid increases the proportion of waterlike substances and decreases the amount of airspace. In **B** (compare to Fig. 11) alveolar walls within an HRCT section are represented. These walls are much thicker and debris in the alveolar sacs is present. However, these events are not individually resolvable by HRCT. Nonetheless, the change in proportions between air and alveolar walls, and edema and alveolar fluids leads to an increase in background density which on the resulting CT image (**C**) is expressed as a "ground-glass" opacity.

filling of the airspaces and swelling of the interstitial structures. Necrotic debris subsequently is cleared through either the airways or the lymphatic system by macrophage action. The lymphatics distributed deeply around bronchovascular structures and superficially adjacent to the visceral pleura and contiguous lobular septa become engorged, leading to thickening of the walls of secondary pulmonary lobules as well as the connective tissue sheath surrounding bronchi and pulmonary arteries.

As illustrated in Fig. 12, changes occurring during the acute phase of injury reduce the amount of air in affected areas. Characteristically, these changes result in areas of ill-defined, homogeneously increased lung density, classically referred to as "ground-glass" opacification. In fact, pathologically, these areas of increased

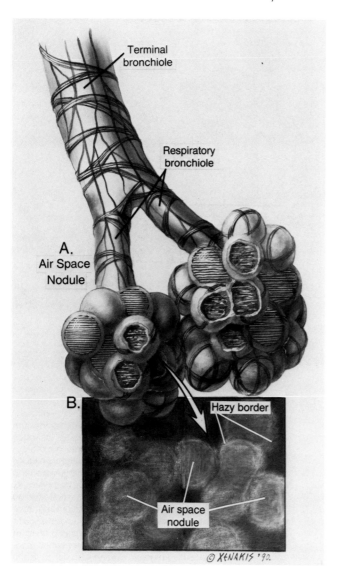

FIG. 13. Acute lung injury: airspace nodules. When pulmonary acini fill up with fluid they are large enough to be resolved by HRCT as ill-defined nodular structures or so-called "acinar" nodules (**A**). As air has been totally replaced by fluid the density of these nodules is greater than the ground-glass opacity seen in the early phase of diffuse alveolar damage (**B**). However, their borders can be hazy and coalesce with that of neighboring acinar nodules (**B**) (see also Figs. 1 and 20).

density are caused by a combination of inter-alveolar filling by debris and hyaline membranes, as well as interstitial swelling due to edema and inflammatory reaction. In the acute phases of pulmonary injury, visualization of these accompanying interstitial changes may occur when they are not totally obscured by accompanying ground-glass opacification.

Occasionally, nodular abnormalities predominate during the acute phase of lung injury (Fig. 13) (57,58). These so-called "acinar" nodules are characterized by ill-defined, hazy borders and presumably are the result of nonuniform involvement of secondary pulmonary lobules (Fig. 14). These may be seen in any patient with airspace pathology resulting from acute lung injury, including diseases that primarily affect distal bronchioles, alveolar ducts, and adjacent alveolar spaces, such as bronchiolitis obliterans-organizing pneumonia (55). The appearance of nodules that occur in the setting of acute inflammation is easily differentiated from nodules that are imaged at a time remote from any acute inflammatory disease. Typical "interstitial" nodules demonstrate sharply marginated borders and coalesce less commonly. Examined histologically, a sharp transition usually can be seen between aerated alveoli and nodules, accounting for their sharp demarcation. Whether such nodules represent foreign matter contained by a pre-

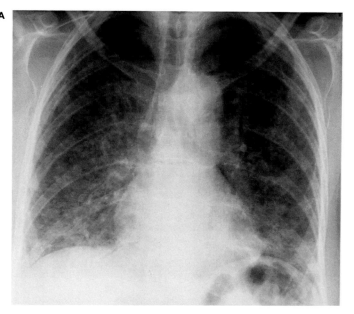

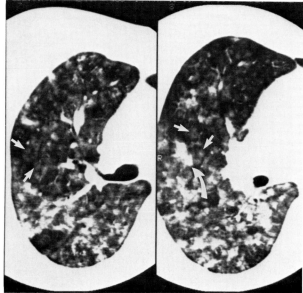

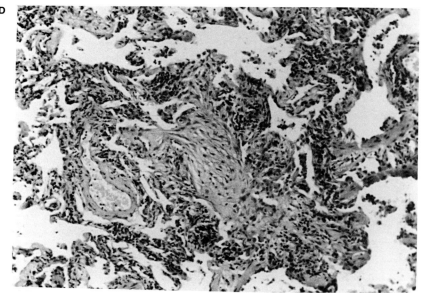

FIG. 14. Extrinsic allergic alveolitis–pigeon-breeder's lung. **A:** Posteroanterior radiograph shows ill-defined, predominantly nodular infiltrates in both lungs. **B,C:** Sequential 1.5-mm thick target reconstructed images through the right mid lung show a pattern of diffuse, poorly marginated nodules varying between 0.5 and 1 cm in size (*arrows* in B,C), a few of which have coalesced (*curved arrow* in C), an appearance characteristic of acute airspace disease. **D:** Histologic section obtained at open-lung biopsy shows characteristic pattern of an organizing alveolitis in this patient with subsequently verified pigeon-breeder's lung. It is significant that an earlier transbronchial biopsy obtained in the lateral basilar segment of the right lower lobe was interpreted as only showing interstitial fibrosis.

vious inflammatory response or established granulomata, they are easily distinguished by an absence of adjacent alveolar or interstitial fluid.

Within four to six days following injury, there is rapid proliferation of type 2 epithelial cells. These cells undergo extensive mitotic division and multiply in an attempt to cover the epithelial defect caused by destruction of type 1 cells. During this subacute phase, relative clearing of infiltrates and ground-glass opacities can be seen unmasking prominent septa and thickened bron-

chovascular sheaths secondary to edema, engorgement of lymphatics, and inflammatory cellular infiltration (Fig. 15).

Acute Lung Injury: Chronic Phase

Acute and subacute changes may lead to more chronic changes, although this is not invariable; complete healing without progression may occur at any phase. This so-called proliferative or organizing stage is

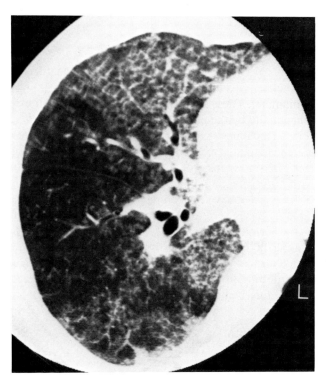

FIG. 15. Target reconstruction of a 1.5-mm thick section through the right mid lung in a patient with documented alveolar proteinosis, following therapy with bronchoalveolar lavage. Note that there is considerable reticulation identifiable, especially in the middle lobe, in addition to residual scattered foci of airspace consolidation. In this case, reticulation is secondary to prominent septa and thickened bronchovascular sheaths due to edema, engorgement of lymphatics, and inflammatory cellular infiltration. This appearance differs markedly from that seen in patients with acute alveolar proteinosis (compare with Fig. 21). (Case courtesy of Dr. Arfa Khan, Long Island Jewish Hospital, NY.)

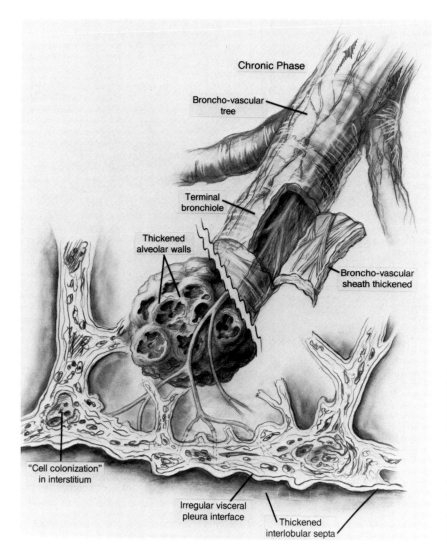

FIG. 16. Acute lung injury: chronic phase. At this organizing stage, cellular infiltration of the interstitium is noted with "colonization" by cells that are not native to the pulmonary interstitium. Chronic interstitial injury is thus expressed as thickening of the shell structures such as the visceral pleural as well as the intralobular septa. The bronchovascular connective tissue sheath is also thickened. Alveolar walls can be thickened and partially collapsed. On HRCT, irregular serration of the visceral pleural surfaces as well as that of the interface between bronchovascular structures and lung parenchyma can be noted. Numerous septal structures not normally seen can now be resolved by HRCT.

characterized by dense fibroblastic proliferation within both the interstitium and the alveolar spaces. Interstitial inflammatory infiltrates as well as hyaline membranes remain histologically prominent features. Residual alveolar infiltrate and debris ultimately may become incorporated within the alveolar walls themselves, resulting in still further thickening of the interstitium. Although characterized by fibrosis and interstitial thickening, even at this stage reversal of these pathologic processes is still possible (Fig. 16).

On HRCT, these findings are manifested by the following three features: (a) thickening of the visceral pleural surfaces; (b) irregular thickening of peripheral bronchi and vessels; and (c) identifiable interlobular septa (Fig. 17). Not infrequently, thickened interlobular septa are the first sign of chronic interstitial disease. This probably reflects the design of the lung's defenses, as these are geared toward rapid clearance of the insulting agent(s) as well as debris from the alveolar walls toward the septal or bronchovascular lymphatics to protect the functional capacity of the lung. Thus, secondary pulmonary lobular septa, which are thicker structures to begin with, are often the first reticular feature identified. This pattern is defined by "coarse" reticulation and is characterized especially in the central portions of the lungs by distinctive polyhedral elements between 15 and 25 mm in diameter. These are easily identifiable when sectioned tangentially by the presence of a core pulmonary artery (Fig. 17). Clinically, these findings are characteristically seen in patients with lymphangitic carcinomatosis; in fact, the purest form of this pattern occurs in patients with interstitial pulmonary edema.

With progressive thickening of the interstitial spaces, septa of varying sizes become recognizable. This results in the formation of a variety of reticular patterns, including both a "medium" reticular pattern, with elements measuring 5–10 mm in size, and a "fine" reticular pattern, with elements measuring 3–5 mm in size. During this evolution nodules may appear, typically localized to the junction points of the lines formed by reticulation. These variations primarily reflect the degree of underlying lung injury. When the nature or extent of injury is such that clearance mechanisms are overwhelmed or made inefficient, the result is finer and finer patterns of reticulation, as typically occurs in patients with miliary tuberculosis, for example.

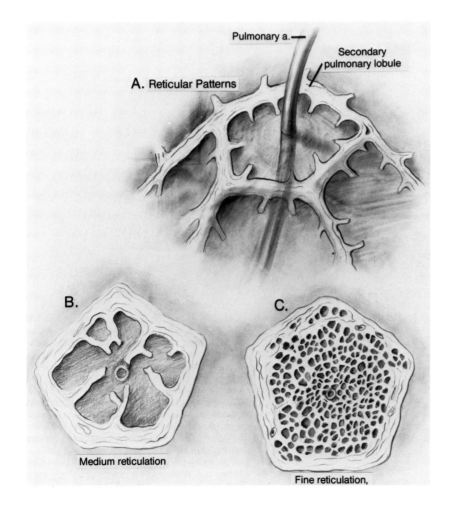

FIG. 17. Acute lung injury, chronic phase—reticular patterns. **A:** Secondary lobule pattern. Interlobular septa outlining secondary lobules are usually the first ones to appear thickened. This is probably due to more effective clearance of fluid from the alveolar walls toward lymphatics in the septal walls to preserve gas exchange, thus accumulation of fluids and cellular debris is more likely to first be noted in interlobular septa. **B:** With progressive thickening of the interstitial spaces, septa of varying sizes become recognizable. This results in the formation of a "medium" reticulation with elements measuring 5–10 mm in size. **C:** With more extensive interstitial involvement, fine reticular patterns with much smaller elements can then be noted (see also Fig. 15.)

Acute Lung Injury: End-Stage Disease

In the last stages of lung response to injury, alveolar structure is destroyed and the interstitium is no longer recognizable as a distinct entity (Fig. 18). Local collapse of alveoli with "fusion" of the interstitial connective tissue of adjacent alveoli results. In addition, healing by fibrosis leads to the formation of dense areas of collagen interspersed with regions of parenchymal destruction. Bronchi in such areas appear dilated and "tethered" secondary to this underlying destructive process involving the peribronchial connective tissue sheaths (Fig. 18). In areas of marked destruction of lung tissue, cystic areas rimmed with remnants of alveoli can be seen. Although the relative degree of fibrosis and resultant cystic and destructive change vary in each disease, the combination of these findings constitutes the hallmark of late phase lung disease (54–56).

Wherever fibrosis and scarring thicken structures within the resolution capabilities of HRCT, abnormal parenchymal features appear (Fig. 18). As defined with HRCT, marked degrees of fibrosis are characterized by the presence of very irregular, spikelike interfaces that can be seen along the visceral pleura and interlobular septa, in particular. The interface between bronchovascular structures and adjacent lung likewise appears distorted, irregular, and occasionally tethered. The number of visualized septa increases. Subpleural arcades become more prominent as do distal pulmonary arterial branches, which now can be seen extending peripherally almost to the visceral pleural surfaces. In addition, fibrotic fusion of alveolar walls with associated collapse if sufficiently extensive may lead to the development of small linear densities that do not correspond to identifiable vessels or septa. These so-called parenchymal bands can be located anywhere in the parenchyma. Although similar bands may result from other causes, including focal atelectasis that may occur especially in dependent portions of the lung thus simulating fibrosis, differentiation is easily accomplished by scanning patients in the prone position at deep inspiration.

Ultimately, the result of continued fibrosis and destruction is end-stage disease. Characteristically, this takes the form of cystic changes representing areas devoid of any residual alveolar tissue surrounded by collapsed remnants of interstitium (Fig. 19). These thick-walled cysts result in a classic honeycomb pattern which on HRCT is easily recognizable even when cysts measure less than 2–3 mm in size. Honeycombing is the most reliable HRCT sign of pulmonary fibrosis.

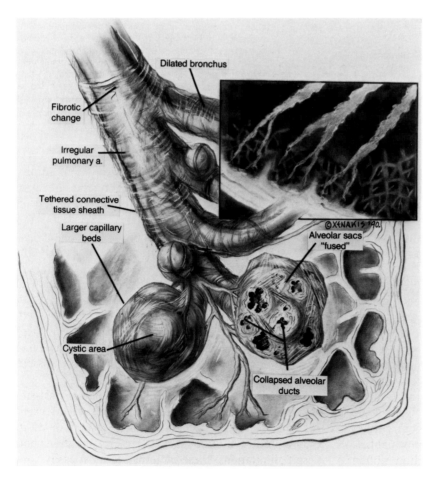

FIG. 18. Acute lung injury: Late-phase disease. In the late stages, formation of dense areas of collagen within the interstitium of the lung is seen. This leads to cystic dilation of bronchi as well as alveolar sacs. Bronchi may appear tethered. A combination of cystic areas rimmed with remnants of thickened alveoli leads to the formation of reticular patterns best seen in the subpleural regions of the lungs as illustrated (*top right insert*). As in Fig. 16, interfaces between visceral pleura and lung appear irregular. Interfaces between connective tissue sheaths surrounding bronchi and pulmonary arteries are also irregular. Vascular and pleural septal arcades are now apparent.

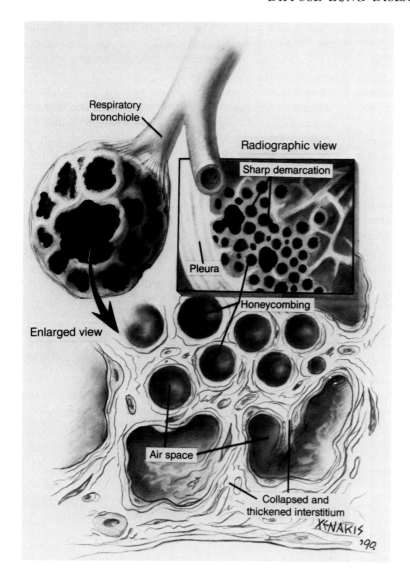

FIG. 19. Acute lung injury: late phase lung disease. Extensive destruction of residual alveolar airspaces with collapsed and thickened interstitium lead to honeycombing—the typical end result of the lung response. This pattern is nonspecific. At this stage, it is extremely difficult to determine the exact etiology of the process that led to pulmonary destruction. Thus, such areas should be avoided when guiding pulmonary biopsy for diffuse lung disease.

Morphologic Evaluation: Pattern Recognition in the Diagnosis of Specific Disease Entities

As described in the preceding sections, the basic signs of diffuse lung disease are easiest to understand in terms of the pathophysiologic mechanisms of lung injury and repair. Correlations between events at both gross and histologic levels and HRCT provide a conceptual framework for interpretation that is a far more accurate reflection of the true nature of underlying lung pathology than has been previously possible with plain chest radiography.

Traditionally, the key to radiologic diagnosis of diffuse lung disease has been pattern recognition (1). Unfortunately, while proponents of this approach claim that it represents the only rational means of radiologic evaluation given the great number of disease entities that are manifested by diffuse pulmonary abnormalities, critics have emphasized that pattern recognition is often misleading because so many diseases represent admixtures of patterns, and equally important, because radiologic-pathologic correlation frequently has been poor (3).

The most significant limitation of chest radiography is the two-dimensional representation of three-dimensional pathology. This problem is obviated with CT. Although the exact place of CT in the investigation of diffuse lung disease is still being actively evaluated, a significant body of work already has been published. Despite wide variation in descriptive terminology, these reports clearly document that CT can play a major role in redefining the basic patterns of diffuse lung disease (48–53).

On what constellation of findings should a CT classification of diffuse lung disease be based? As discussed previously, most parenchymal lung diseases manifest in only a limited number of patterns. In our judgment, despite limitations, these patterns are most easily conceptualized as resulting from basic processes of lung injury and repair. In this context, it is apparent that the classic distinctions of airspace or alveolar disease versus interstitial disease are somewhat arbitrary. In fact, in the early phases of both classic airspace and interstitial processes both airspaces and interstitium participate pathologically. Differentiation of airspace from interstitial processes, then, relates directly to the relative importance of each element in the lung's response to injury, usually easily determined with HRCT.

Additional key features may be disclosed by CT that significantly add to our understanding of the true nature of lung disease. These include more precise delineation of the underlying focal nature of many otherwise apparently diffuse lung diseases; differentiation between central and peripheral patterns of disease, including cortical versus medullary patterns of involvement; delineation of distinctly perivascular and peribronchial pulmonary

diseases; and direct visualization of abnormalities of vessels and airways themselves.

Despite the purposefully descriptive nature of this classification, in select diseases, radiographic-pathologic correlation is now sufficiently precise to accurately limit differential diagnosis to only a handful of specific diseases. For illustrative purposes, select entities will be discussed and analyzed independently.

Airspace Disease

The CT hallmark of acute airspace disease is poorly defined nodules. Similar to "acinar" nodules characteristic of airspace disease radiographically, these may be caused by a variety of pathologic processes, including: (a) aspiration of blood (Fig. 1), fluid, or especially infected material as occurs in patients with endobronchial spread of tuberculosis or other organisms (Fig. 20); (b)

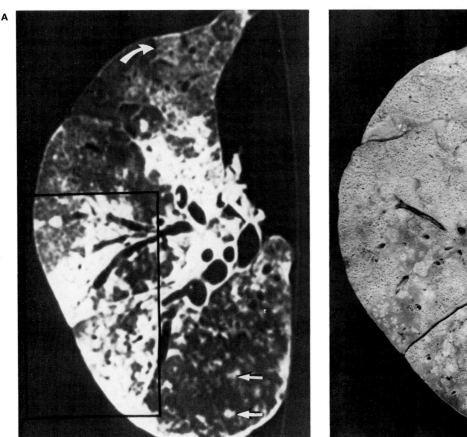
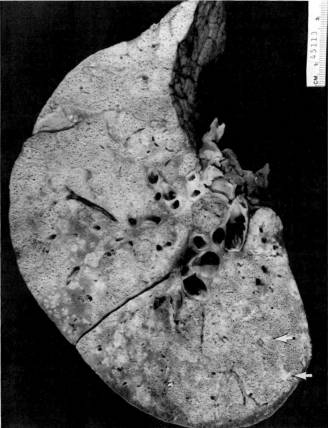

FIG. 20. Bronchopneumonia: CT-pathologic correlation. **A:** CT section through inflated fixed lung in a patient with documented Pseudomonas aeruginosa pneumonia shows numerous poorly marginated sublobular foci (*straight arrows,* A,B), as well as confluent opacities with air bronchograms and a geographic pattern of distribution. Additionally, poorly defined zones of homogenously increased ground-glass density can be identified (*curved arrow*). While frequently identifiable in patients with more characteristically interstitial disease, areas of ground-glass opacification may be identified in patients with purely airspace consolidation as well. **B:** Corresponding inflated fixed lung section.

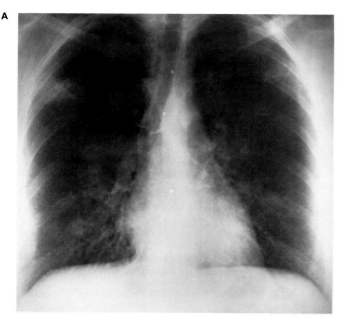

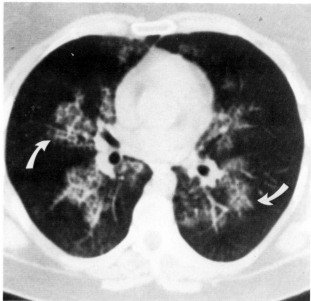

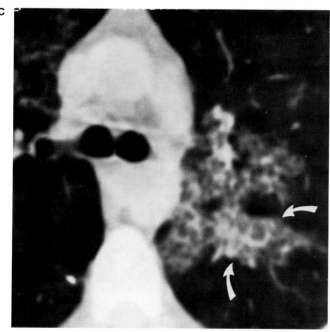

FIG. 21. Airspace consolidation—alveolar proteinosis. **A:** Posteroanterior radiograph in a patient with alveolar proteinosis documented by open-lung biopsy. Scattered foci of poorly defined parenchymal opacification are apparent: these appear to be focally confluent and are easiest to identify in the peripheral portions of the upper lobes. Abnormal densities can also be identified medially in the infrahilar zones. **B,C:** Section through the mid lung zone and an enlargement of a section through the carina, respectively. The predominant finding is that of airspace nodules, roughly uniform in size, largely restricted to the perihilar lung (*curved arrows*). Note that there is extremely sharp delineation between areas of normal and abnormal lung, similar in appearance to the pattern illustrated in Figs. 22 and 23. Although a variety of CT findings have been reported in patients with alveolar proteinosis, in this case the CT appearance mimics precisely those expected for a disease that characteristically is predominantly airspace in distribution. (Compare with Fig. 15.)

direct transudation of fluid or hemorrhage into the airspaces, as occurs in patients with pulmonary edema, as well as in patients with alveolar proteinosis (Fig. 21), idiopathic pulmonary hemosiderosis, and Goodpasture's syndrome; and (c) the presence of cells within airspaces, as occurs in patients with bronchioloalveolar cell carcinoma, parenchymal lymphoma, and leukemic infiltration of the lungs (Fig. 22) (57–69).

With progression, there is a tendency for airspace nodules to coalesce; this may lead to both air-bronchograms and even air-alveolograms. Typically, coalescence results in a geographic distribution of disease, including segmental and lobar patterns of involvement.

Not infrequently, despite the presence of consolidation, normal pulmonary vessels can be identified within involved portions of lung (70). Occasionally, sharp lines of demarcation between normal and abnormal areas of lung may be observed, appearing in many cases to correspond to anatomic boundaries between involved and uninvolved secondary pulmonary lobules. Although not pathognomonic (71), in our experience, this finding has most often been identified in patients with Pneumocystis carinii pneumonia (Fig. 23).

Experiments with inflated lungs scanned following intrabronchial injection of fluids reveal findings similar to those seen in patients with other forms of primary

A

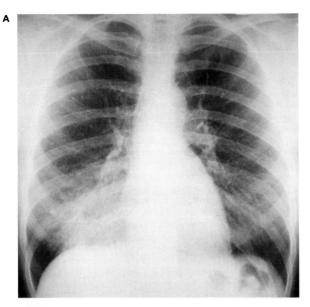

FIG. 22. Airspace consolidation—bronchioloalveolar cell carcinoma. A: Posteroanterior radiograph shows poorly marginated area of consolidation in the right lower lobe. The remainder of the chest appears normal. B: HRCT section through the right lower lobe shows features typical of airspace consolidation, including innumerable poorly defined nodules, as well as air-bronchograms (compare with Fig. 14). C: HRCT section through the left upper lobe. Discrete foci of airspace disease are present, in one of which there is a clearly definable air-bronchogram (*curved arrow*). Identification of contralateral disease is especially important in patients with documented bronchioloalveolar cell carcinoma for whom surgical resection is indicated when the disease is restricted to one lobe.

B

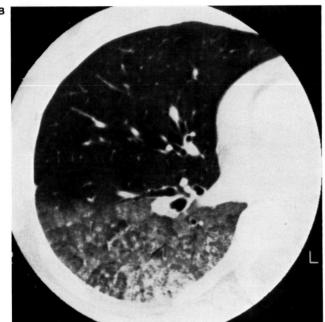

C

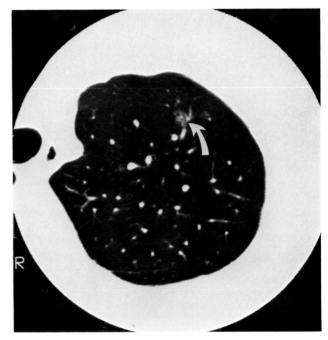

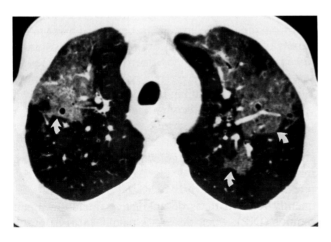

FIG. 23. Airspace consolidation with Pneumocystis carinii pneumonia (PCP). 1.5-mm thick CT section though the carina shows typical appearance of airspace consolidation in a patient with documented PCP. Note the geographic distribution of disease with sharp lines of demarcation separating normal from abnormal lung (*curved arrows*). Cystic changes, typical in patients with PCP, are easily identified within these foci of consolidated lung.

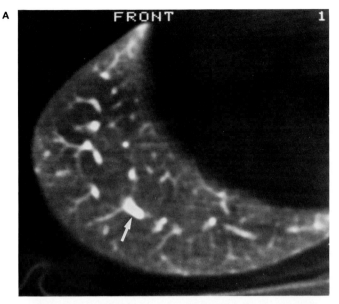

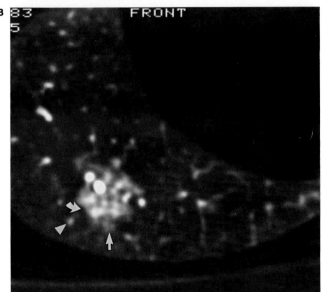
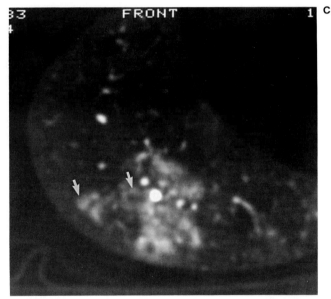

FIG. 24. Injected lung specimens: airspace disease. **A:** Enlargement of a 5-mm thick CT section through the tip of a catheter (*arrow*) inserted into the right lower lobe of an inflated normal lung prior to the injection of contrast. Branching vascular structures are easily identified, superimposed on a uniform gray background. Discrete airways cannot be visualized. **B,C:** Enlargements of sequential 5-mm thick sections obtained at and just below the same location shown in A following injection of 3 cc of dilute barium. Numerous poorly defined nodular densities can be defined around the tip of the catheter (*arrows*). When clustered these nodules create a quilt-like pattern that superficially mimics cystic lung disease. This bubbly appearance is due to residual normal aeration of portions of lung lying between and surrounded by airspace nodules. Note that in both B and C, the margins of a secondary pulmonary lobule can be seen, identifiable as straight lines demarcated by injected barium (*curved arrows*). A core pulmonary artery is now easily identified (*arrowhead* in B). This reinforces the basic principle that identification of pulmonary architectural detail is enhanced by the presence of pathology.

involvement of the airspaces (Fig. 24) (57). Coalescence due to diffusion of airspace nodules eventually leads to the formation of typical "alveolar" infiltrates. CT findings characteristic of airspace disease are summarized in Table 1.

Idiopathic Pulmonary Fibrosis

Idiopathic pulmonary fibrosis (IPF) is a specific disorder defined by a combination of clinical, morphologic, and radiologic features. It is characterized by diffuse inflammation confined largely but not exclusively to the pulmonary interstitium that in itself is nonspecific and may be the result of a number of diverse and apparently unrelated diseases, including: collagen-vascular diseases, scleroderma and rheumatoid arthritis in partic-

ular; pulmonary infections, including those caused by viruses, Chlamydia, and Mycoplasma, among others; drugs, especially chemotherapeutic agents; exposure to industrial inhalants, especially asbestos; as well as a wide variety of genetic, metabolic, or inflammatory disorders (54,55). Despite similarities, specific diagnoses may result from careful review of the patient's clinical history, laboratory data, including microscopic identification of either asbestos bodies or viral inclusions.

Histologically, IPF is associated with varying patterns of alveolar wall inflammation, intra-alveolar cellularity, and fibrosis (54,55). As noted, these findings in themselves are nonspecific: when disease is uniform with a preponderance of intra-alveolar cells, the process is frequently referred to as desquamative interstitial pneumonitis (DIP); when disease is patchy in distribution,

TABLE 1. *Airspace disease: CT features*

CT finding	Description/comment
Ground-glass opacification	Uniform increase in overall lung density due in part to pulmonary hypoinflation. May conform to lobular or sublobular anatomy.
Airspace nodules	Poorly marginated opacities up to 1 cm in size due to sublobular accumulation of fluid, blood, or cells.
Coalescence	Larger zones of increased density, usually resulting from confluence of nodules.
Air-bronchograms	Best visualized when the involved airway runs in the same plane as the CT section.
Geographic distribution	Central vs. peripheral; segmental vs. lobar. Airspace disease may be sharply marginated when delimited by lobular borders.

with more obvious alveolar wall inflammation, the same process is typically referred to as usual interstitial pneumonitis (UIP). Whether DIP and UIP are actually separate diseases or instead represent different ends of the spectrum of IPF is still a matter of dispute (54,55).

Typically, IPF occurs in middle-aged women without evidence of collagen vascular disease. The onset is generally insidious and follows a fairly relentless, downhill course with death usually resulting from progressive pulmonary insufficiency in only a few years. Radiologic manifestations reflect chronicity: early in the course of disease, diffuse ground-glass opacification is common; later, with the development of fibrosis, coarse reticulation predominates, with end-stage disease resulting in typical honeycombing.

CT findings in patients with IPF have been extensively reported (8,9,17,46–52,78–81). In addition to the finding of nonspecific, patchy areas of ground-glass opacification, IPF is characterized by a distinctive pattern of a reticular network of medium-sized, 6 to 10-mm elements largely restricted to the periphery of the lungs (Fig. 25). Initially this may take the form of linear, subpleural lines; with progression, reticulation can be seen extending into the central portions of the lungs (Fig. 26). As the severity of the disease increases still further, cystic spaces between 2–4 mm in size can be identified. In the final stages of disease, lung volume decreases markedly

and a characteristic pattern of honeycombing can be defined (Fig. 26). Detailed CT-pathologic correlation has confirmed that findings in all stages of disease precisely reflect architectural changes caused by pulmonary fibrosis as seen in both open lung and autopsy studies (Fig. 27) (47,78,80).

Not surprisingly, as compared with routine chest radiographs, most of these features are better delineated when the lungs are evaluated with CT, especially when 1.5-mm thick sections are acquired. As shown by Staples et al., in their study of 23 patients with UIP evaluated with both chest radiographs and CT, in all patients CT was clearly superior in defining the severity and extent of disease; in particular, CT disclosed honeycombing in 91% of cases as compared with only 30% identified prospectively by chest radiography (81).

Asbestosis

Asbestosis is defined as diffuse lung fibrosis due to asbestos exposure (55,82,83). The size, diameter, and shape of fibers determine their fate in the lung parenchyma. Longer fibers of 5 microns or more in diameter tend to be deposited in large airways from which clearance is relatively rapid through mucociliary action. Shorter fibers are more likely to be deposited in either the peripheral airways or, if extremely fine, the distal airspaces from which clearance is usually slower. These fibers are not likely to be ingested by the alveolar macrophages or, even less likely, the alveolar epithelial cells, and as a consequence may be transported into the interstitium of the lung with resultant formation of aggregates, usually at the level of the respiratory bronchioles. *In vitro* cell studies and research on animal models indicate that exposure to asbestos activates alveolar macrophages which in turn causes the release of chemotactic factors derived from neutrophils, as well as a protein factor similar to a collagenase inhibitor that disturbs the balance of collagen turnover in the lung. These result in fibrogenic changes within the interstitium (84,85).

Asbestosis characteristically occurs 15 to 20 years following exposure, with disease progressing even after exposure has ceased. Initially, asbestosis affects respiratory bronchioles with development of peribronchial fibrosis. Fibrosis subsequently spreads to replace the surrounding alveoli, and when severe, leads to solid areas of scarring that involve large portions of the lung, predominantly in the subpleural regions of the lower lobes. Although it has been suggested that peribronchiolar fibrosis is characteristic of early asbestosis, this finding is nonspecific per se, and may result from exposure to many types of mineral dust exposure (86). The development of diffuse interstitial fibrosis is held by most to be

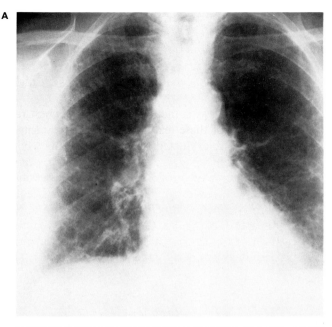

A

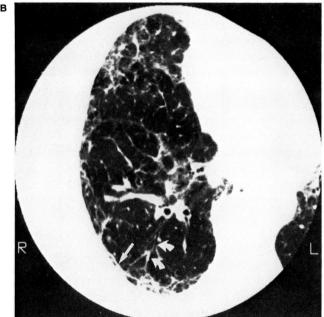

B

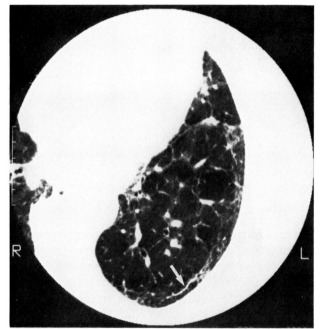

C

FIG. 25. Idiopathic pulmonary fibrosis. **A:** Posteroanterior radiograph shows a nonspecific pattern of increased linear densities especially prominent peripherally and inferiorly. **B,C:** HRCT images through the right and left lower lobes, respectively. A distinctive pattern of medium-sized reticular elements as well as subpleural lines (*arrow* in B) can be clearly seen, primarily involving the lung periphery, circumferentially. Changes consistent with early honeycombing are apparent along the mediastinal borders. Note that in this case, central secondary pulmonary lobules are easily identifiable (*curved arrows* in B), consistent with some degree of early central disease. Despite extensive changes within the perimeter of the lung, the lung-pleural interface is only minimally irregular and the configuration of both vessels and bronchi are still smooth (*arrow* in C).

dose-related: asbestosis generally occurs only in those patients with long-term, high-level exposure (83).

As pathologic evaluation is not usually obtained in individual cases, assessing pulmonary parenchymal fibrosis has necessitated the development of a constellation of clinical, functional, and radiographic findings to establish the diagnosis of asbestosis *in vivo.* As determined by the American Thoracic Society, the diagnosis can be inferred when there is a reliable history of non-trivial exposure to asbestos along with a combination of: (a) restrictive lung disease on pulmonary function testing as well as a diffusion abnormality; (b) the presence of rales at auscultation; and (c) abnormal chest radiographs. It has been suggested that among these, "the findings on the chest roentgenogram are the most important" (87).

Unfortunately, there are limitations to the value of radiographic interpretation in defining a population

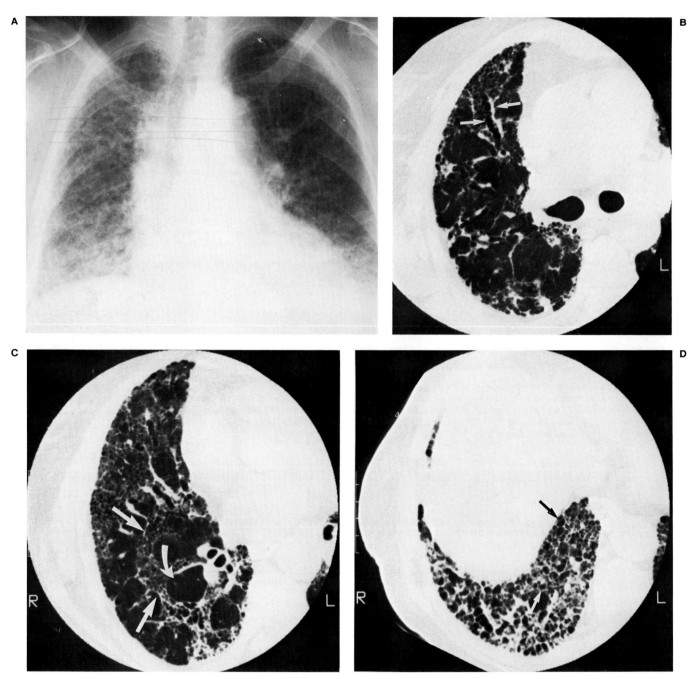

FIG. 26. Honeycomb lung—idiopathic interstitial fibrosis. **A:** Posteroanterior radiograph shows evidence of diffuse reticulation throughout both lungs in a pattern suggestive of honeycombing. **B,C,D:** Sequential, retrospectively targeted HRCT images through the right lung. These show a pattern of coarse reticulation with cystic spaces up to .05 cm in size which are easily identifiable (*arrows* in C). In portions of lung less severely involved, these areas of honeycombing can be seen to cut broad paths through the lung (*straight arrows* in C), in the process isolating relatively preserved, individual, secondary pulmonary lobules (*curved arrow* in C). The configuration of airways and vessels is now markedly irregular (*arrows* in B), and the pleural surfaces are more clearly irregular (compare with Fig. 25).

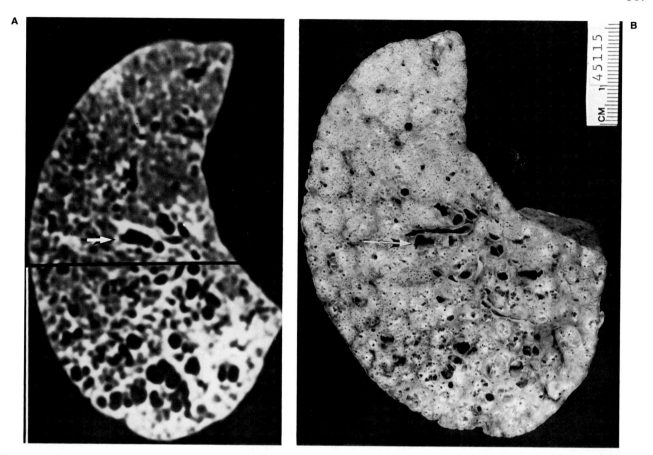

FIG. 27. Honeycomb lung: CT-pathologic correlation. **A:** CT section through an inflated fixed lung in a patient with end-stage idiopathic pulmonary fibrosis. A pattern of coarse reticulation with innumerable cysts, some as small as 2–4 mm in size, can be defined throughout the lungs (compare with Fig. 25). At this level, cysts are easily differentiated from dilated, thick-walled central airways (*arrows* in A and B); more peripherally, this differentiation may be more problematic. **B:** Corresponding inflated fixed lung specimen showing extensive honeycombing with numerous cysts in close association centrally with dilated central airways.

with asbestos-induced abnormalities (Fig. 28). In a review of 200 admission chest radiographs interpreted according to the ILO classification of diffuse lung disease, Epstein et al. found that 22 patients (11%) without occupational exposure had abnormalities that otherwise might have been interpreted as indicative of significant dust exposure (88). Additionally, radiographic-pathologic correlative studies have shown that interstitial fibrosis may be present despite normal appearing chest radiographs in up to 20% of patients (89,90). Rockoff and Schwartz, analyzing the limitations of the ILO classification in predicting histologically verified asbestosis, also found that chest radiographs can result in a 10–20% probability of a normal interpretation (91). Added to these difficulties are significant problems with interob-

server variability, specifically in the interpretation of opacities of mild profusion (92). Although the American Thoracic Society has specified as part of their definition of asbestosis and profusion (severity) of 1/1 or greater (87), as pointed out by Weill, it is unlikely that any one category will constitute a lower limit of abnormality that will prove diagnostic of asbestosis for all qualified readers (93).

The potential of CT to evaluate patients with documented exposure to asbestos has been noted by numerous investigators (94–107). Findings in patients with documented asbestos-related parenchymal fibrosis have been reported (97). In a prospective study of 29 patients with clinically documented asbestosis matched with 34 normal controls, Aberle et al. analyzed the following

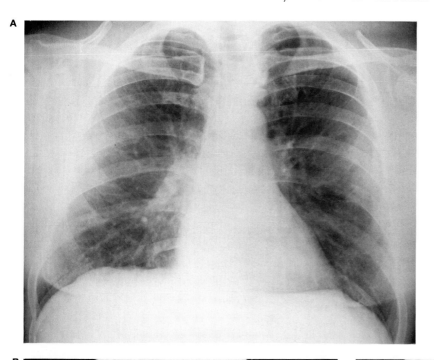

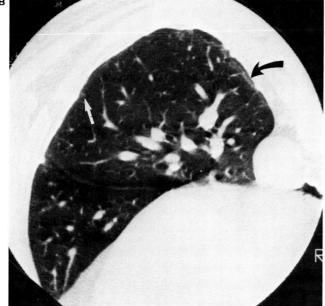

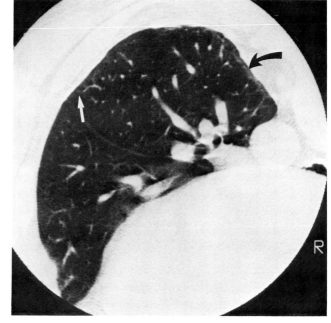

FIG. 28. Asbestosis. **A:** Posteroanterior radiograph shows minimal nodularity of the right hemidiaphragm. The lungs appear normal. **B,C:** Sequential 1.5-mm target reconstructed sections through the right lower lobe obtained with the patient in a prone position show subtle parenchymal changes consistent with asbestosis. In addition to pleural plaques, prominent intralobular septal lines and dots (*straight arrows* in B and C) are identifiable. These result in a prominent subpleural curvilinear line posteromedially (*curved arrows* in B and C).

HRCT signs: (a) thickened subpleural short septal (interlobular) and core (intralobular) lines, identifiable as either dots or single or branching lines of approximately 1–2 cm in length; (b) parenchymal bands, definable as course linear opacities extending through the lung, clearly separable from blood vessels, often extending at right angles to adjacent pleural surfaces; (c) curvilinear subpleural lines, defined as lying generally within 1 cm of the pleural surface parallel to the inner chest wall; (d) increased nondependent subpleural densities, identifiable as broad, featureless bands obscuring detail of the underlying parenchyma; and (e) honeycombing (Figs. 28–33) (97). These authors found a significant correlation between subpleural short lines, broad bands, and honeycombing in those patients with asbestosis as compared with controls, especially in combinations involving both lower lobes. Nondependent curvilinear lines per se were never seen in isolation but always occurred in conjunction with other CT manifestations, while increased density in itself was found to have little diagnostic value. Significantly, in this same study, HRCT performed in both supine and prone positions proved more sensitive than routine CT in the diagnosis of parenchymal disease (96% versus 83%, respectively) (97).

HRCT-pathologic correlation has been reported (102,103,106). Akira et al. obtained HRCT studies in seven inflated and fixed postmortem lungs in patients with documented asbestosis (106). These authors confirmed that thickened intralobular lines, in fact, do correlate with peribronchiolar fibrosis, and that subpleural curvilinear lines result from the arrangement of these structures along the inner chest wall. Furthermore, these authors also confirmed that parenchymal bands result from fibrosis extending along bronchovascular sheaths.

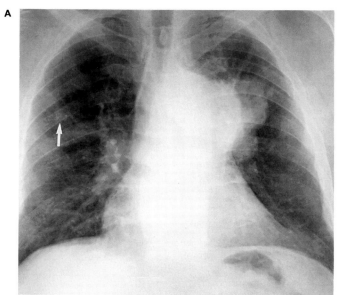

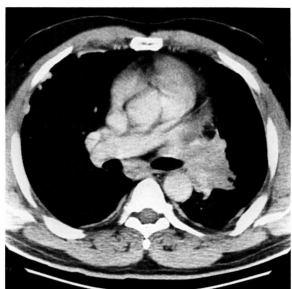

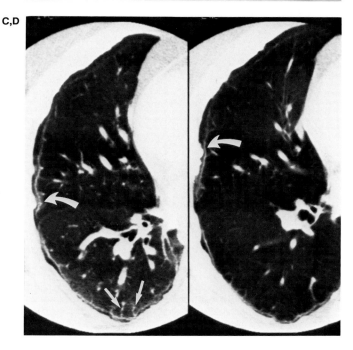

FIG. 29. Asbestosis. **A:** Posteroanterior radiograph shows a large mass in the left upper lobe and left hilum. Ill-defined contralateral densities can be seen as suggestive of pleural plaques (*arrow*). The lower lobes appear normal. **B:** Section through the left hilum and imaged with mediastinal windows shows a large tumor mass associated with subcarinal adenopathy. Bilateral pleural plaques are easily identifiable, characteristic of asbestos-related pleural disease. **C,D:** Sequential, retrospectively targeted HRCT sections through the right lower lobe show extensive, nearly circumferential subpleural curvilinear densities, associated with subtly thickened subpleural septal and core lines (*straight arrows* in C). Note that curvilinear lines can be seen both removed from as well as adjacent to pleural plaques (*curved arrows* in C and D).

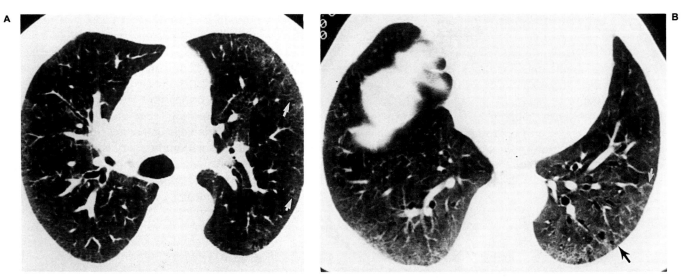

FIG. 30. Asbestosis. **A,B:** HRCT scans through the mid and lower lungs, respectively, in a patient whose chest radiograph was interpreted as showing a profusion of 1/0. Abnormalities clearly predominate in the subpleural lung, including thickened subpleural intralobular lines (*straight white arrows* in A and B). Additionally, peripheral branches of the pulmonary arteries appear to extend to the pleural surfaces, suggesting that there is thickening of the interstitium surrounding the core pulmonary arteries (*black arrows* in B). Note that the overall effect is a fine subpleural reticulation associated with very subtle cystic changes, indicative of early honeycombing.

The relationship between chest radiographic findings and HRCT has also been evaluated. Aberle et al. evaluated HRCT findings in 100 occupationally exposed individuals defined clinically as having asbestosis (98). The authors found that in 85% of patients with clinical asbestosis, HRCT scans were interpreted as consistent with a high probability of asbestosis, with low probability reported in only 4% of cases. Importantly, of 55 individuals without clinical evidence of asbestosis, HRCT studies were interpreted as highly suggestive of asbestosis in nearly one-third. Similar findings have been reported by Staples et al. (105). In this study of more than

400 asbestos-exposed workers with documented latency periods of at least 10 years, evaluated clinically, physiologically, and with HRCT, these authors found that in nearly one-third of patients, HRCT findings suggestive

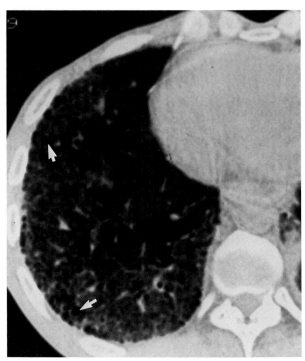

FIG. 32. Advanced asbestosis. Targeted reconstructed image of the right lower lobe in a patient with positive radiographic findings shows the typical peripheral, subpleural medium-type reticular changes. Early honeycombing is also present, associated with very small cystic spaces (*arrows*) within areas of interstitial thickening, findings typical of end-stage lung disease.

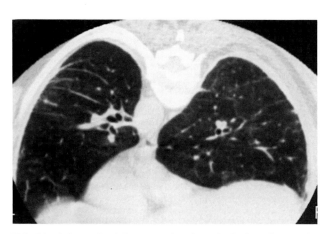

FIG. 31. Asbestosis. 1.5-mm section through the lung bases obtained with the patient in a prone position shows typical appearance of broad bands within both lower lobes (*arrows*). Note that on the left (corresponding to the right lower lobe), many of these bands have a curvilinear configuration. This finding presumably represents the earliest manifestation of incipient round atelectasis.

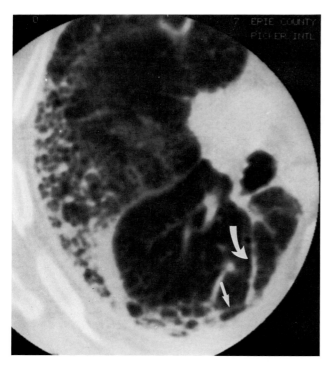

FIG. 33. Advanced asbestosis. HRCT section through the right lower lobe shows typical findings of subpleural honeycombing, associated with both subpleural curvilinear densities (*arrow*) and broad bands extending toward the pleural surfaces (*curved arrow*).

Most of the findings reported in patients with documented asbestosis have also been described in other diseases that result in diffuse pulmonary fibrosis. Indeed, no CT finding, alone or in combination, should be interpreted as pathognomonic of asbestosis (108). For example, subpleural linear densities initially thought to be diagnostic of asbestosis (110) now have been described in other diffuse infiltrative lung diseases, including UIP, as well as in patients with pulmonary congestion (111) and even in patients following lymphangiography, presumably reflecting involvement of subpleural lymphatic channels (112). Of course, given the wealth of data that has now been accumulated documenting the appearance of parenchymal fibrosis in particular, it has been argued that in patients with a history of documented nontrivial asbestos exposure, HRCT findings may be construed as significant indicators of asbestosis (109).

Another confusing issue that has been raised is the question of the effect of cigarette smoking on HRCT scans. To date, no significant correlation has been discovered (98,105), although the number of studies addressing this issue has been small. It is unlikely that cigarette smoking will limit HRCT evaluation of patients suspected of having asbestos-related diseases, but additional prospective studies are clearly required. Further assessment of normal variations within the lungs is also needed.

In a recent review of HRCT findings in 244 patients with infiltrative lung diseases and 29 healthy control subjects, Remy-Jardin et al. evaluated the frequency, profusion, and diagnostic value of identifying subpleural parenchymal micronodules (113). Defined as focal areas of increased attenuation less than 7 mm, these authors documented that while these were commonly present in patients with a variety of infiltrative lung diseases, especially those with coal workers' pneumoconiosis, they were also identified in 14% of controls.

In summary, it is apparent that there is considerable potential for the use of HRCT in the evaluation of patients with a history of significant exposure to asbestos. At present, in our judgment, the main indications for the use of HRCT include: (a) evaluation of patients with equivocal chest radiographs, especially those in whom the presence of pleural plaques makes definitive interpretation of underlying parenchymal disease difficult; and (b) evaluation of patients with clinical evidence of disease in whom chest radiographs are interpreted as normal. The role of HRCT to evaluate patients with classic radiograph evidence of diffuse lung disease is less clear. Given the greater contrast resolution of CT coupled with the ability of CT to provide unobstructed views of the pulmonary parenchyma, it can be anticipated that the role of CT to evaluate patients with suspected asbestos-related parenchymal disease will continue to grow. In this context, some effort toward

of asbestosis could be identified despite normal radiographic appearances. Furthermore, significant differences could be documented in both vital capacity and diffusing capacity between patients with normal scans and those with HRCT evidence of parenchymal abnormalities. These findings are especially interesting as it has been suggested that changes in both vital and diffusing capacity may actually precede chest radiographic abnormalities.

In addition to finding disease within the lungs of patients with normal chest radiographs, HRCT may be of value by excluding disease in otherwise equivocal cases. As documented by Friedman et al. in their analysis of chest radiographs and HRCT scans in 60 patients with clinically suspected asbestosis, the positive predictive values of well-performed chest radiographs compared with HRCT scans for documenting the presence of significant lung disease was 79% versus 100%, respectively (99). Most important, these authors concluded that HRCT is of greatest value in eliminating false-positive diagnoses of lung disease caused by obscuration of the underlying parenchyma by pleural plaques.

Despite these reports, the role of HRCT in evaluating patients suspected of having asbestosis remains controversial (108). Although HRCT has been shown to be more sensitive than routine chest radiography in detecting abnormalities within the lung, the specificity of HRCT findings, in particular, has been challenged.

standardization of HRCT interpretations ultimately will be necessary (114).

Silicosis

Silicosis occurs as a reaction to the inhalation of silica or silicon dioxide. Following chronic exposure, in pure form silicosis results in the formation of small, discrete, hyalinized nodules predominantly in the upper lobes. Nodules tend to localize around terminal bronchioles; microscopically they are extremely sharply defined, clearly separable from surrounding alveoli which may be either normal or showing evidence of emphysema (54,55). Similar lesions may develop in hilar lymph nodes, resulting in characteristic peripheral or "eggshell" calcifications. Other complications include infection with Mycobacterium tuberculosis, as well as development of rheumatoid nodules (Caplan's syndrome) in patients with rheumatoid arthritis. Rarely, following heavy exposure over a short period of time, an unusual reaction may develop that is histologically similar to pulmonary alveolar proteinosis.

The diagnosis of silicosis is generally made by correlating clinical history with characteristic plain radiographic findings, demonstrating either simple silicosis (characterized by multiple small opacities) or complicated silicosis (characterized by large coalescent pulmonary opacities resulting in so-called progressive massive fibrosis). According to the ILO 1980 international classification, small, rounded opacities typical of patients with silicosis are classified according to the diameter of the predominant lesion: type "p," up to 1.5 mm in size; type "q," 1.5–3 mm in size; and type "r," 3–10 mm in size (3).

CT studies of patients with silicosis have shown that, at least in patients with radiographic evidence of type "q" and "r" opacities, a characteristic appearance of sharply defined nodules can be identified, especially prominent in the posterior portions of the upper lobes and usually associated with focal hyperinflation and emphysema (Fig. 34) (49,50,72,73). Many of these nodules calcify and become identical in appearance to tuberculous and fungal granulomata.

Akira et al., in their study of 55 patients with a variety of pneumoconioses characterized by radiographic evidence of type "p" opacities, showed that when evaluated with HRCT these opacities appeared as tiny, binary branching structures; in 21 cases these were associated with nonperipheral, small areas of low attenuation with a central dot (74). In this same study, CT-pathologic correlation in two cases revealed that these tiny opacities and lucencies together corresponded histologically to irregular fibrosis centered around respiratory bronchioles and focal-dust emphysema, respectively. The significance of these findings to patients with documented silicosis has yet to be determined.

Surprisingly, as compared with plain radiographs, in two studies using 10-mm thick collimation, CT did not prove superior to routine chest radiography in the detection of nodules (Fig. 34) (72,73). However, in both studies CT was significantly more accurate in identifying patients with complicated silicosis due either to the presence of coalescence and large opacities or to emphysema. This latter finding may be especially significant. As shown by Bergin et al. in their study comparing CT scans with pulmonary function tests (PFT's) in 17 patients with documented silicosis, there was poor correlation between nodular profusion on both chest radiographs and CT and PFT's, but significant correlation was documented between the extent of emphysema shown by CT and both the FEV 1% predicted and the diffusing capacity (73).

Miliary Tuberculosis

The radiographic appearance of miliary nodules is well-known; the process by which tiny nodules theoretically below the threshold of radiographic visibility are detected is less clear, however. The summation mechanism of several nodules to make a larger visible one is generally invoked to answer this question. In the 1940s Resnick suggested that in such cases, individual shadows became visible only when not summed (75). More recent experiments by Heitzman, with implantation of subliminal lesions such as resected metastases and 3-mm polyethylene spheres into resected lung specimens, strongly indicate that alignment of subliminal structures parallel to the x-ray beam is the main factor in their visualization (43).

Regardless of the mechanism by which miliary nodules become visible radiographically, it is apparent that with CT discrete abnormalities can be visualized at a stage prior to that at which otherwise subliminal abnormalities become visible radiographically (76). Characterization of these changes occurs at the limits of cross-sectional spatial resolution. On routine HRCT sections, miliary nodules appear as a very fine, diffuse reticular network of 2 to 3-mm elements. Strikingly, using retrospective target reconstructions with limited FOV's, it is possible to resolve individual small nodules within lobular septa (Fig. 35). Additionally, the density of nodules present may have a pronounced anteroposterior gradient, especially when the lower lobes are imaged, presumably as a result of their hematogenous origin.

In addition to tuberculosis, numerous other diseases have been associated with a miliary pattern (48), including pulmonary alveolar microlithiasis (77) and even reports of reactions to methotrexate therapy (51). In our experience, especially in the AIDS population, miliary nodules are frequently the result of either disseminated

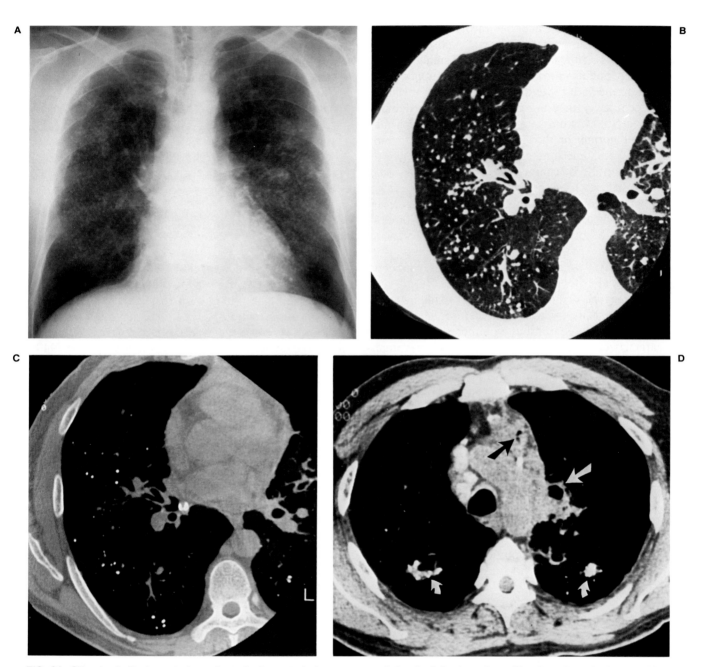

FIG. 34. Silicosis. **A:** Posteroanterior radiograph shows typical appearance of sharply defined small opacities throughout the lungs, with a suggestion of early coalescence in the upper lobes. **B,C:** HRCT section through the right lung imaged with wide and narrow windows, respectively. Innumerable well-defined small nodules are identifiable scattered randomly throughout the lung, many of which are calcified. Note that there is no evidence of fibrosis: the pleural margins and vessels are smooth. Emphysematous changes are apparent. **D:** Section at the level of the aortic arch shows calcified mediastinal nodes, as well as clearly definable cavities in both the left hilum and anterior mediastinum (*straight white and black arrows*). These cavities, which were not seen on plain radiographs, even retrospectively, proved to be tuberculous in a patient with documented silicotuberculosis. Note early progressive fibrosis in both upper lobes (*curved arrows*).

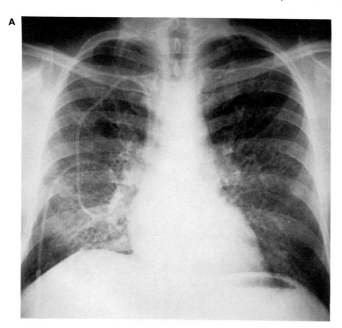

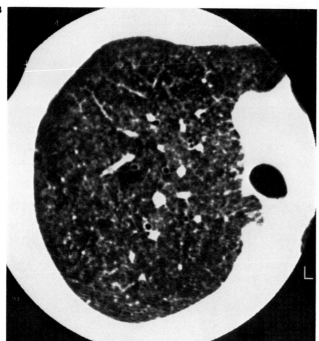

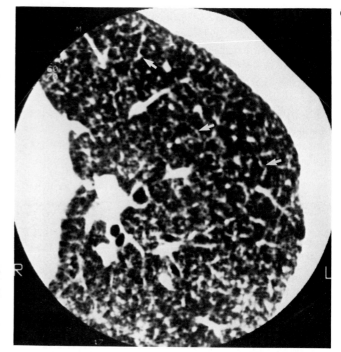

FIG. 35. Miliary disease. **A:** Posteroanterior radiograph shows pattern typical of miliary disease. **B:** Retrospectively targeted HRCT image of the right upper lobe shows innumerable widely scattered nodules, without obvious relation to lobular anatomy. **C:** Retrospectively targeted HRCT image through the lungs of another patient with transbronchial biopsy evidence of noncaseating granulomata, presumed to be secondary to sarcoidosis. In this case, spatial resolution has been maximized by using a small field of view. There is clear accentuation of reticular structures, with miliary-sized nodules clearly identifiable causing nodular thickening of lobular septa (*white arrows*) as a result of the presence of granulomata scattered throughout the interstitium.

histoplasmosis, or, in i.v. drug addicts, foreign body and/or talc granulomata.

Sarcoidosis

The spectrum of radiologic findings in patients with sarcoid has been exhaustively reviewed (43,115–119). Awareness that changes involving intrathoracic lymph nodes and the lung parenchyma can be sequential has led to a variety of staging classifications, usually divided into three groups: Stage 1, bilateral hilar adenopathy without evidence of pulmonary parenchymal disease;

Stage 2, bilateral lymphadenopathy with evidence of parenchymal infiltrates; and Stage 3, parenchymal infiltrates without hilar adenopathy (115,116). Parenchymal infiltrates typically are described radiographically as interstitial, with Stage 3 disease frequently described or equated with fibrosis.

Unfortunately, the usefulness of most radiographic staging systems is limited. Although, as shown by Siltzbach, this type of classification is of proven value in predicting prognosis, only poor correlation has been established between classic radiographic descriptions of parenchymal disease and most physiologic measurements of lung function (115–119). Correlation does improve when radiographs are interpreted utilizing a modification of the ILO system proposed by McLoud et al. (117), though there are limitations to routine utilization of this method. These problems are further complicated by the frequency of atypical manifestations which occur in approximately 25% of patients with sarcoidosis, reaching as many as 59% in elderly populations (120). Most significantly, as spontaneous resolution has been recorded for patients with classic Stage 2 and Stage 3 disease, pathologic inferences drawn from radiographic appearances clearly are also of limited value (54,55). Specifically, radiographic staging provides very little information regarding the relative degree of reversible inflammation in the form of alveolitis and granuloma formation as opposed to irreversible fibrosis (121,122). The need to determine the presence and extent of alveolitis has led to the increasingly widespread use of both bronchoalveolar lavage (BAL) and gallium-67 scanning (123–126); however, to date neither has proven sufficiently specific to play a significant role in routine clinical diagnosis (127,128).

Despite wide variability in the appearances of this truly protean disease, characteristic pathologic changes have been described within the lung in most patients with sarcoidosis (54,55,121). Anatomically, in cases with grossly recognizable disease, well-formed, noncaseating granulomata typically involve pulmonary lymphatics along the pleura, as well as centrally along bronchi and vessels (Figs. 36 and 37). This distinctive subpleural and especially peribronchovascular distribution is a significant morphologic hallmark of the disease, and helps to explain the high yield in establishing this diagnosis from routine transbronchial biopsies (3,43,54,55).

The CT findings in patients with sarcoid have been well-described and largely mimic the pathologic changes described above (Figs. 36–38) (6,8,9,17,48–52,129–139). Muller et al., in a study of 25 patients with biopsy-proved pulmonary sarcoidosis, including two with open-lung biopsies, found that in addition to hilar and mediastinal lymphadenopathy, typical CT findings included small and large nodules, often in association with irregular linear densities, distributed along bronchovascular sheaths (Fig. 37) (132). Occasionally this pattern mimicked that seen in patients with lymphangitic carcinomatosis. Similar findings have been reported by Lynch et al. utilizing HRCT to evaluate 15 patients with biopsy-proven sarcoidosis (135). HRCT features included small nodules, thickened interlobular septa, patchy focal increase in lung density, honeycombing, and central crowding of vessels and bronchi. Not surprisingly, nodular densities seen on CT correlated with the presence of granulomata histologically. Of potentially greater significance, in some cases the finding of patchy focal increased densities within the lung may be correlated with the presence of active alveolitis.

These findings have been further corroborated by Brauner et al. (137). Utilizing HRCT to evaluate 44 patients with histologically confirmed sarcoidosis, these

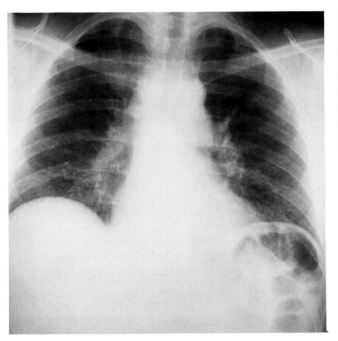
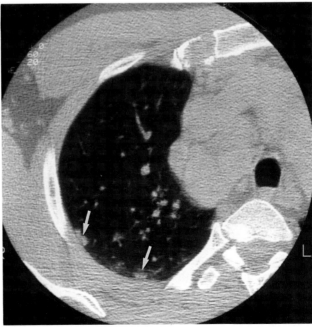

FIG. 36. Sarcoidosis. **A:** Posteroanterior radiograph shows roentgenographic evidence of Stage 1 sarcoidosis with marked mediastinal and bilateral hilar adenopathy, associated with clear lung fields. **B:** Target reconstructed 1.5-mm thick section through the right lung apex shows poorly defined, largely subpleural nodules (*straight arrows*) in association with more subtle central, perivascular densities (*arrows*). Massively enlarged mediastinal lymph nodes are also identifiable.

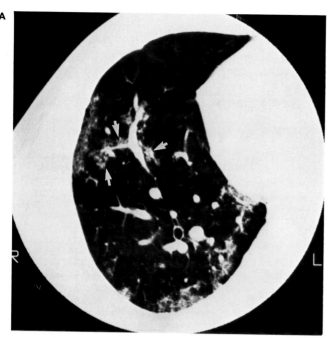
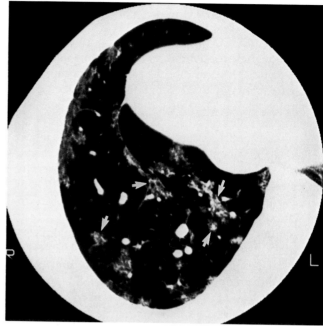

FIG. 37. Sarcoidosis. **A,B:** Retrospectively targeted HRCT sections through the right lower lobe in a patient with roentgenographic evidence of Stage 2 sarcoidosis (not shown) reveal a characteristic pattern of distinctly perivascular and peribronchial disease (*white arrows* in A and B) associated with scattered subpleural densities.

authors documented the nearly ubiquitous finding of both micro- and macronodular changes in all cases, frequently clustered around peripheral bronchovascular bundles. Nodules proved to be isolated in 19 cases, excavated in 3 cases, and associated with other lesions in 25 cases, including: irregular interfaces; linear networks; thickened pleural surfaces; ground-glass opacification;

lung distortion; traction bronchiectasis; and networks of large cavities, presumably secondary to fibrosis and scarring (Fig. 38). Nodular changes were identified in six cases with otherwise normal chest radiographs. Somewhat more surprisingly, in eight cases marked distortion of the lung was seen without identifiable fibrosis on corresponding chest radiographs. Significantly, in this series

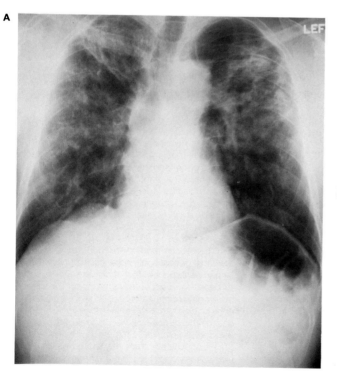
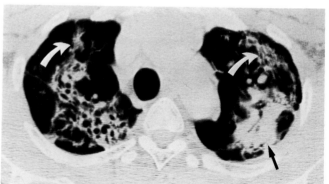

FIG. 38. Sarcoidosis. **A:** Posteroanterior radiograph in patient with roentgenographic evidence of Stage 3 sarcoidosis. Extensive upper lobe disease is apparent, with retraction of the hila bilaterally. **B:** Nontargeted HRCT section through the upper lobes shows a pattern of extensive fibrosis, with honeycombing especially prominent in the right upper lobe. The left upper lobe is also distorted: a conglomerate density is present (*straight arrow*), in this case stable over several years. In the periphery, despite extensive scanning, the pattern of disease remains distinctly peribronchial (*curved arrows*). Note subtle paratracheal adenopathy not apparent on the chest radiograph.

reticular opacities proved to be scant as compared with previous reports.

In our experience, although these findings are not pathognomonic, in the appropriate clinical setting, a specific CT diagnosis of sarcoidosis usually can be suggested.

Atypical patterns of disease have also been evaluated with CT (131,134). Rarely, sarcoid may be miliary (Fig. 35). More commonly, a pattern of poorly marginated nodular masses has been documented, the radiographic appearance of which has been traditionally called "alveolar sarcoid" (43,54,55,140). Although this manifes-

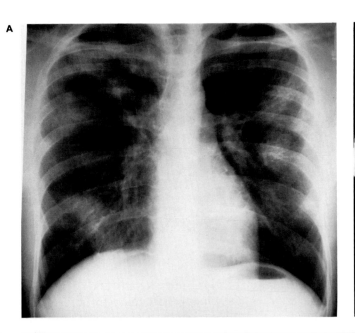

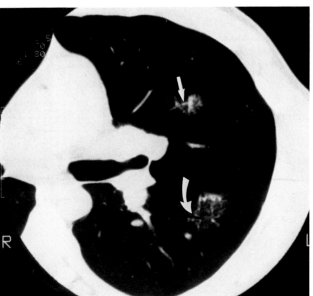

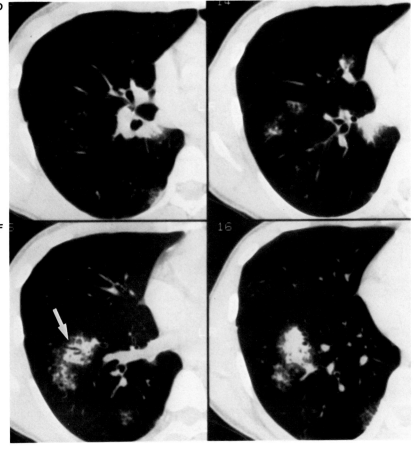

FIG. 39. Alveolar sarcoid—CT guided transbronchial biopsy. A: Posteroanterior radiograph shows ill-defined nodular masses scattered throughout the lungs, without evidence of mediastinal or hilar adenopathy. B: HRCT section through the left lung shows discrete foci of ill-defined, small nodular densities strikingly perivascular (*straight arrow*) and peribronchial (*curved arrow*) in distribution. C–F: Sequential HRCT sections through the right lower lobe in the same patient again show discrete perivascular and peribronchial foci of disease. Confluence of densities is apparent surrounding the proximal portion of the anterobasilar segmental bronchus of the right lower lobe (*arrow* in E). On the basis of these findings, fiberoptic bronchoscopy was performed with transbronchial biopsies obtained specifically from the anterobasilar segment; these confirmed the diagnosis of sarcoidosis. (Compare with Fig. 43, Chapter 7.)

tation has been considered by some to constitute a unique subset of the disease, evaluation with HRCT reveals the same pattern of peribronchovascular disease seen in routine cases of sarcoidosis (Fig. 39). Despite numerous descriptions in the literature, precise correlation between the radiographic pattern of alveolar sarcoid and pathologic findings remains unclear. Rarely, coalescence of nodules may result in a pattern similar to progressive massive fibrosis, as occurs in patients with complicated silicosis (129).

Lymphangitic Carcinomatosis

Pulmonary lymphangitic carcinomatosis refers to the spread of tumor within pulmonary lymphatics. In the majority of cases, the tumor origin is presumed to be hematogenous, with resultant thickening and infiltration of core bronchovascular bundles, the interlobular septa, and the subpleural interstitium. In approximately 25% of cases, lymphangitic carcinomatosis is secondary to retrograde spread of tumor from infiltrated and enlarged hilar nodes (43,54,55,141–144). In the vast majority of cases, lymphangitic carcinomatosis results from adenocarcinoma arising from the breast, lung, gastrointestinal tract, or prostate, or more rarely from an unknown primary.

Radiographic changes are usually described as interstitial, with diffuse, although occasionally unilateral, reticulation, prominent Kerley's A and B lines, and effusions (43,141–144). As noted, hilar adenopathy occurs in a significant minority of patients. Although these findings are highly suggestive, especially in the setting of

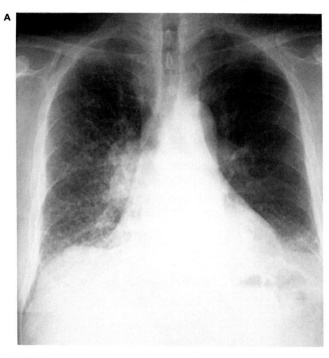

FIG. 40. Lymphangitic carcinomatosis. A: Posteroanterior radiograph shows asymmetric pulmonary infiltrates in the right lung associated with a mass in the superior segment of the right lower lobe. B–E: Sequential HRCT sections through the right lung confirm the presence of a mass in the superior segment of the right lower lobe (open arrow in C), associated with soft-tissue fullness within the right hilum. There is a diffuse increase in both medium and coarse reticular elements throughout the lung, including thickening of peripheral arcades (curved black arrows in B and C), markedly thickened central bronchial walls (curved white arrows in B,C,D), and most characteristic, prominent medium and coarse polyhedral reticular elements, frequently traceable along central bronchovascular pathways to hilar and mediastinal surfaces (black arrows in E), characteristic of thickened secondary pulmonary lobular septa (arrows in B–E). The appearance of these has been likened to "beaded septa."

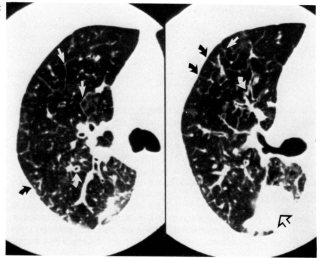

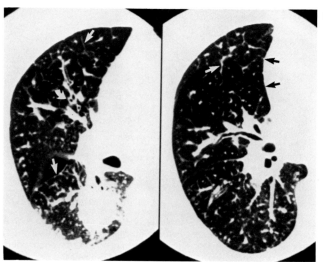

a known primary, the radiographic diagnosis of lymphangitic carcinomatosis may be problematic. In addition to a large differential of causes of interstitial disease in patients with known malignancies, in up to 50% of cases the radiograph may prove normal (43,142,144).

The CT findings in patients with lymphangitic carcinomatosis have been reviewed (9,17,46,47,49–52,145–148). Initial descriptions emphasized the finding of a large network of polyhedral reticular elements 15–25 mm in diameter, centered on a pulmonary artery, frequently traceable along central bronchovascular pathways to hilar and mediastinal surfaces, characteristic of thickened secondary lobular architecture (Figs. 40 and 41) (9). Stein et al., in a study of 12 patients with documented lymphangitic carcinomatosis evaluated with HRCT, also demonstrated findings consistent with infiltration of the interstitium, including thickening of peripheral arcades, a diffuse increase in linear and curvilinear structures throughout the lung, and distinctly polygonal structures, 1–2 cm in diameter, identifiable in 7 of 12 patients (145). Similar findings have been documented by Munk et al. in a retrospective study of 21 patients with proven lymphangitic carcinomatosis, including the finding of unevenly thickened bronchovascular bundles with a distinctly beaded or nodular appearance, as well as well-defined polygonal structures containing prominent central dots representing core bronchovascular structures in eight patients (146). It should be emphasized that in all these studies, detectability of disease was significantly augmented by CT when compared with routine radiography.

CT-pathologic correlation has been obtained in patients with pulmonary metastases. Ren et al. evaluated 32 postmortem inflated lungs with documented metastases (Fig. 42) (148). Multiple discrete nodules were found in the majority of cases, typically located in the periphery of the lung; in only 2 of 32 cases were solitary nodules discovered. In 30 (92%) of 32 cases, metastases were identified in the periphery, including both subpleural regions and the outer third of the lung. In addition to nodules, thickened septa were identified in the lung periphery in 22 (69%) of 32 cases, 19 of which proved to have a beaded appearance. When examined grossly, areas of beaded septal change identified on CT were found to correspond to nonuniform expansion of the septa by irregular tumor infiltration (Fig. 42). Histological examination showed nodules of neoplastic cells in the interalveolar capillaries and lymphatics as well as tumor in the septal interstitium around these vessels. Septal edema, fibrosis, and vascular dilatation could also be identified distal to points of tumor obstruction.

In summary, lymphangitic carcinomatosis may present a wide spectrum of CT findings depending on the degree of lymphatic infiltration. In its least severe form, simple prominence of subpleural septa and slight ill-definition of bronchovascular margins may be identified. As the disease progresses, tumor nodules enlarge and obstruct lymphatics causing edema and a desmoplastic reaction in septal structures, resulting in more typical polyhedral secondary lobular patterns. In still more advanced stages, sheaths of tumor cells invade the interstitium around bronchovascular structures and within sec-

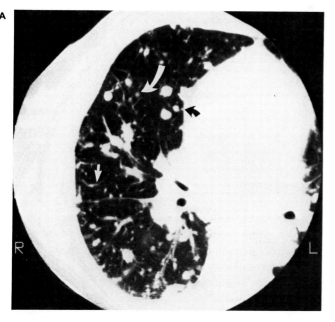
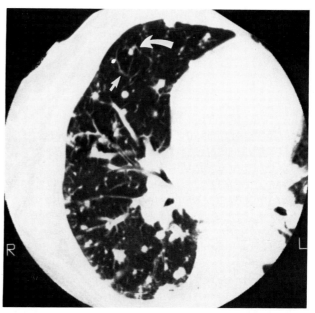

FIG. 41. Lymphangitic carcinomatosis. **A,B:** HRCT sections through the right lung in a patient with documented lymphangitic carcinomatosis. In addition to thickened bronchovascular bundles (*arrow* in A), thickened interlobular septa (*straight arrow* in B), thickened bronchial walls, and hilar adenopathy, numerous scattered, well-defined nodules are apparent, most associated with a distinct "feeding vessel" (*curved arrows* in A and B). This appearance is usually a manifestation of far-advanced disease.

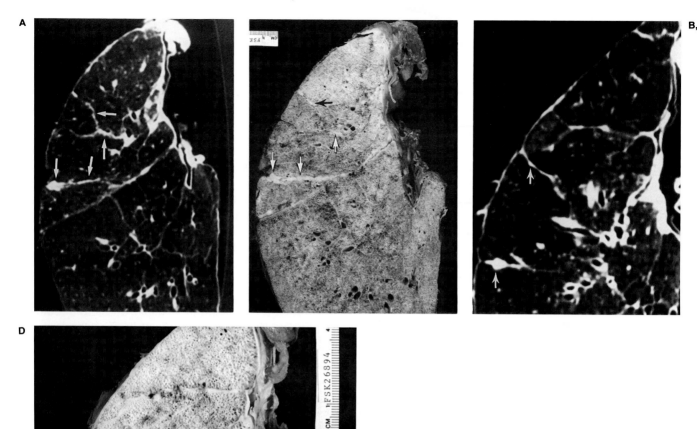

FIG. 42. Lymphangitic carcinomatosis: CT-pathologic correlation. **A,B:** CT section and corresponding inflated fixed lung specimen, respectively, in a patient with metastatic mediastinal germinoma. Coarse reticulation is apparent throughout the upper lobe, in particular. Note the characteristic "beaded chain" appearance of thickened secondary lobular septa (*arrows*). **C,D:** Enlargements of both CT and fixed inflated lung sections in the same patient show to better extent the "beaded chain" appearance of lymphangitic carcinomatosis. *Arrows* point to thickened interlobular septa infiltrated by tumor.

ondary lobules. This leads to a distinctly beaded appearance. Significantly, in Ren's study, no evidence of beaded septal change on HRCT could be found in the 148 control cases (148).

In our experience, a constellation of thickened and beaded interlobular septal lines associated with polygonal structures and prominent peripheral arcades in the clinical setting of known malignancy is essentially diagnostic of lymphangitic carcinomatosis. Although similar findings have been described in undocumented cases of viral pneumonia and, more importantly, have been reported to occur in patients with sarcoidosis, when identified in the appropriate clinical setting, these changes are in our judgment sufficiently characteristic in select cases to obviate the need for either transbronchial or open-lung biopsies (51).

Emphysema

As defined by the American Thoracic Society, emphysema represents an anatomic alteration of the lung characterized by an abnormal enlargement of the airspaces distal to the terminal, nonrespiratory bronchioles, accompanied by destructive changes of the alveolar walls (149). Although pulmonary functional abnormalities may be present, including an increase in total lung capacity (TLC), functional residual capacity (FRC), and residual volume (RV), and there may be a decrease in elastic recoil and maximal expiratory flow rates, these changes do not constitute part of emphysema's definition. Disease confirmation has required anatomic verification at either surgery or autopsy.

Emphysema usually is classified anatomically based

on changes within the pulmonary acinus, and includes: centriacinar (centrilobular) emphysema, if the primary focus of destruction centers on airspaces surrounding respiratory bronchioles, as typically occurs in smokers; panacinar emphysema, if airspaces are evenly destroyed throughout the acinus, as occurs in patients with alpha₁-antitrypsin deficiency; periacinar (paraseptal) emphysema, if there is selective involvement of the distal acini, which, when confluent, leads to the formation of blebs and bullae, with resultant spontaneous pneumothoraces, as occurs especially in younger patients; and irregular or paracicatricial emphysema, when destruction is random or is secondary to scarring, which may be focal, or may occur in association with diffuse cicatrizing lung diseases including tuberculosis, chronic sarcoidosis, and certain pneumoconioses, especially silicosis (150). It cannot be overstated that differentiation among these various forms of emphysema may be exceedingly difficult even for the pathologist, especially when more than one type is present at the same time, as occurs not infrequently.

Radiographic abnormalities in patients with emphysema have been well-documented: in most series the diagnosis is based on finding either avascular spaces within the lung; evidence of hyperinflation; and/or cardiovascular abnormalities, including a decrease in the caliber and number of vessels in the lung periphery, the so-called "arterial deficiency" pattern of emphysema (43,151–156).

Despite discrepancies in the reported significance of these signs, most radiographic-pathologic correlative studies have concluded that routine radiographs are of only limited utility and are an imprecise method of diagnosing emphysema. In the largest such study, Thurlbeck and Simon found that chest radiographs were positive in only 41% and 67% of cases shown to have moderate or severe emphysema, respectively, when graded pathologically (151). It should be noted that significantly different results have been reported by Sutinen et al. (152). Based on somewhat different radiographic criteria than that utilized by Thurlbeck and Simon, these authors concluded that when utilizing a

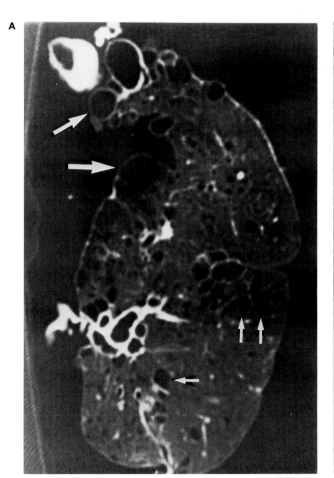
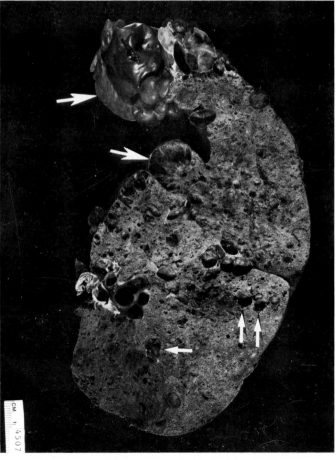

FIG. 43. Diffuse emphysema: CT-pathologic correlation. **A,B:** CT and corresponding fixed inflated lung specimen sections, respectively. Emphysematous disease is characterized by low-attenuation areas easily separable from surrounding normal parenchyma despite the absence of a clearly definable wall (*arrows* in A and B). These are easily differentiated from bronchiectasis because of the absence of associated pulmonary artery branches and definable wall thickness.

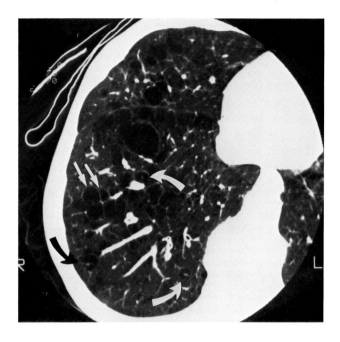

FIG. 44. Pulmonary emphysema. Retrospectively targeted HRCT section through the right lower lobe shows characteristic pattern of emphysema, definable as well-defined zones of diminished lung density, without definable walls. Instead, these spaces typically are delimited peripherally by interlobular veins which are particularly well seen along the course of large central veins (*straight arrows*). Occasionally when sectioned tangentially, central or core lobular vessels can be identified as well (*curved arrows*).

combination of varying signs, radiographs were reliable indicators of both the presence and absence of anatomically verified emphysema, especially when minimal grades of disease were considered positive.

Fueled in part by these inconsistencies, considerable interest has been focused on the potential role of CT in evaluating patients with emphysema (Fig. 2) (9,17,23,24,33–36,46,47,51,157–164). Characteristically, emphysema results in nonperipheral low-attenuation areas easily separable from surrounding normal parenchyma despite the absence of a clearly definable wall (Figs. 43–46). Using areas of low attenuation and vascular disruption as indicative of emphysema, Bergin et al., when correlating radiographic and pathologic

findings in 32 lungs obtained at surgery, assessed the accuracy of preoperative 10-mm thick CT scans both qualitatively and quantitatively as a method for diagnosing emphysema (159). In each case an emphysema grade was awarded pathologically and compared with a corresponding visual CT score; in all cases, significant correlation was found. Similar findings have been documented by Hruban et al. utilizing HRCT to evaluate 20 postmortem lung specimens (161).

It should be emphasized that the accuracy of CT for detecting emphysema may correlate with both scan technique and the methodology by which lungs are graded pathologically. Miller et al., in an evaluation of 38 patients undergoing surgical resections for lung

A

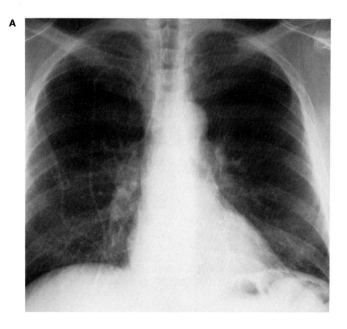

FIG. 45. Diffuse emphysema: CT-radiographic correlation. **A:** Posteroanterior radiograph shows classic appearance of arterial deficiency pattern of emphysema in both upper lobes. **B,C:** (opposite page) Sequential HRCT sections through the right upper lobe show characteristic pattern of geographic or zonal regions of diminished attenuation within which few if any pulmonary vessels can be found (*arrows* in B and C). These findings are characteristic of more advanced emphysema as compared with Figs. 43 and 44.

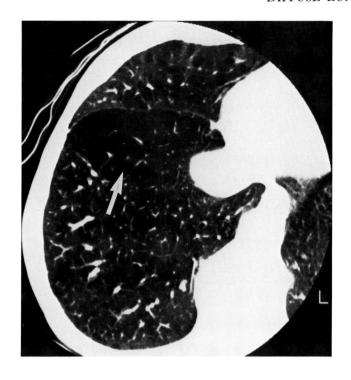

FIG. 46. Diffuse emphysema: differentiation from reticular lung disease. Target reconstructed 1.5-mm thick section through the right lower lobe shows diffuse emphysematous destruction of the lung, recognizable as regions of markedly low attenuation without definable walls. When extensive, emphysematous disease may take the configuration of secondary pulmonary lobules (*arrow*). Although this appearance superficially mimics diffuse reticular lung disease, differentiation is rarely problematic: unlike most reticular lung diseases, emphysema tends to be more central than peripheral. Additionally, despite their seeming prominence, interlobular septa are not actually thickened and there is no evidence of prominent or irregular bronchovascular markings. Diagnostic certainty is also enhanced by the finding of prominent central core lobular structures in otherwise destroyed secondary lobules (compare with Fig. 44).

cancer in whom CT scans were obtained preoperatively, found that when using a grid system instead of a panel of standards, the correlation between CT scores and pathologic scores were of a lower order of significance than previously reported (164). Of particular concern, CT was found to consistently underestimate the extent of both centriacinar and panacinar emphysema when lesions were less than 0.5 cm in diameter (164). These findings are at considerable variance with those reported by Kuwano et al. (36). These authors also evaluated a large number of patients undergoing thoracotomy in whom CT scans were obtained preoperatively. In this

B

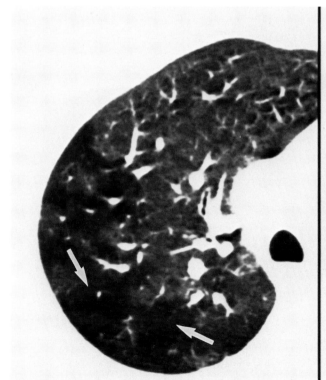

C

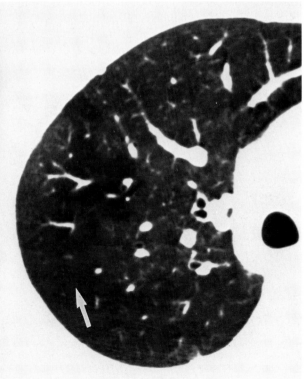

A
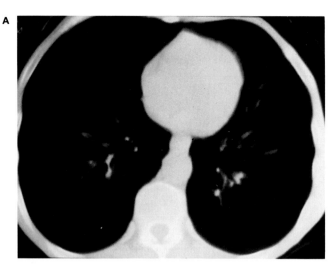
B
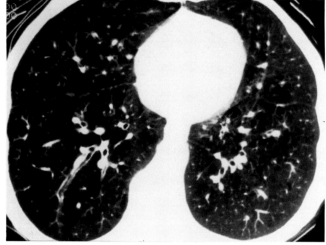

FIG. 47. Emphysema: 10-mm vs 1.5-mm sections. **A,B:** 10- and 1.5-mm thick sections, respectively, through the lower lobes in a patient with extensive emphysema. Although disease is obviously apparent on the thicker section, visualization of morphologic detail is considerably greater on the thinner section.

study, visual CT scores were compared to the pathology grade of emphysema as well as the so-called destructive index (DI) of lung specimens. CT scores at all levels of disease were found to correlate significantly with pathologic scores, leading these investigators to conclude that CT was of value in identifying even minor grades of emphysema. Although these differences undoubtedly relate in part to methods of pathologic grading, it should be noted that not all scans in the study reported by Muller et al. utilized thin (1.5 mm) sections, unlike Kuwano et al. (Fig. 47). The significance of these differences remains to be determined.

CT findings of bullous emphysema have also been described (Figs. 43 and 48) (165–170). Bullae are easily identified in most cases as peripheral zones of low density greater than at least a centimeter in diameter, frequently curvilinear in shape. When sufficiently large, these compress and distort the underlying parenchyma, sometimes into extremely bizarre configurations. Although large bullae are usually readily identified radiographically, identification is more difficult when there are multiple lesions, when bullae are centrally located, or when their edges do not lie tangential to the incident x-ray beam (Fig. 2).

In our experience, CT has proven beneficial in the early detection of emphysema, especially in select, high-risk populations, such as those with suspected alpha$_1$-antitrypsin deficiency or those who present with recur-

A
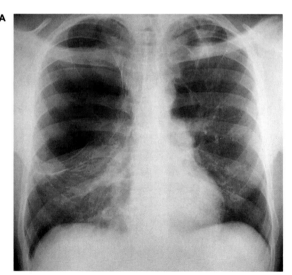
B
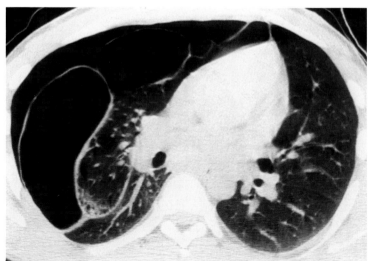

FIG. 48. Bullous emphysema: presurgical assessment. **A:** Posteroanterior radiograph shows extensive bullous emphysema involving both upper lung fields, more extensively on the right. **B:** Nontargeted HRCT section through the mid lung fields shows large bullae on the right side, causing considerable compression of the adjacent right upper lobe. Despite this, visualized lung is normal in appearance and without evidence of diffuse emphysematous change, supporting in this case operative intervention.

rent pneumothoraces, by detecting otherwise unsuspected blebs and bullae. In patients with alpha₁-antitrypsin deficiency, in particular, early diagnosis may be critical to prompt and effective therapy (171). Additionally, CT has been of value in the work-up of patients with otherwise unexplained respiratory symptomatology, especially those with so-called "increased markings" emphysema. Finally, CT has also proven to be helpful in the preoperative assessment of patients with potentially resectable bullae. As there is no consistent relationship between the presence of bullae and diffuse emphysema, CT can be used to assess or clarify the extent of associated lung disease.

Pulmonary Histiocytosis X

Also known as eosinophilic granuloma of the lung, pulmonary histiocytosis X is a granulomatous disorder of unknown etiology that typically affects young or middle-aged adults (54,55). In 60% of cases, disease is isolated to the lungs; however, 20% also have bone involvement, and another 20% have multi-visceral disease. Clinically, patients usually present with nonspe-

cific respiratory complaints; no consistent patterns of abnormality are shown on pulmonary function tests. Although up to 20% of patients present following a pneumothorax, as many as one-fifth are asymptomatic and are identified only because of abnormal chest radiographs (172,173). In most patients the course of the disease is surprisingly benign, with spontaneous resolution frequently occurring without therapy. Unfortunately, in a small percentage of patients, disease is progressive and leads to scarring and honeycombed lung.

Pathologically, pulmonary histiocytosis X is characterized by nodules and cysts (54,55). Histologically, the diagnosis is made by the presence of characteristic large histiocytes (Hx cells) that closely resemble Langerhans cells. Although necrosis is rarely identified, nodules frequently appear cavitated; small and large cysts may also be identified. Despite their common appearance, the etiology of these cavities and cysts is uncertain (Fig. 49).

Radiologically, pulmonary histiocytosis X most commonly causes a reticulonodular pattern primarily involving the mid and upper lung zones (172,173). Cysts and honeycombing have been reported in between 1% and 15% of cases. These findings significantly vary from

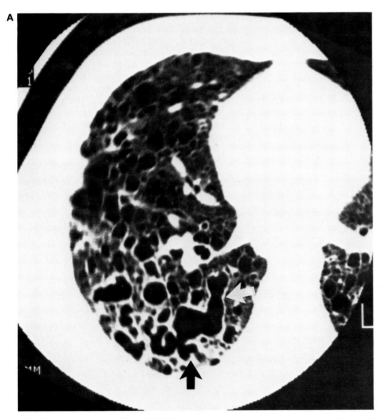
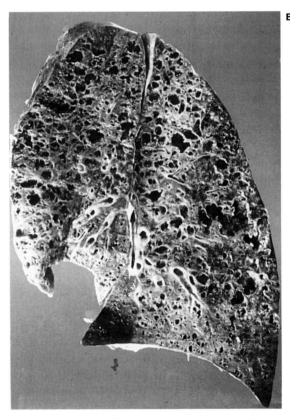

FIG. 49. Histiocytosis X. **A:** HRCT section through the right lung in a patient with documented histiocytosis X. Innumerable well-defined, uniformly thick-walled cysts are scattered throughout the lung, some in bizarre, branching patterns (*white arrow*) mimicking the appearance of bronchiectasis. Presumably this appearance is due to cyst fusion. Despite extensive disease, no obvious reticulation or fibrosis is apparent. **B:** Pathologic section from another patient with histiocytosis X showing multiple cysts throughout the lungs, frequently exhibiting unusual branching configurations. (Courtesy of Carlos R. R. de Carvalho, M.D., Universidade de São Paulo, Brazil).

the CT appearance of pulmonary histiocytosis X (Figs. 49 and 50). As documented by Moore et al. in their series of 17 patients with histologically documented disease, the predominant CT finding was the presence of cystic spaces, present in 12 patients (174). Differentiation from emphysema was usually possible due to the presence of identifiable walls; greater difficulty was experienced differentiating cysts from cavitating nodules and bronchiectasis, however, as both were occasionally present as well. Nodules, usually less than 5 mm in size, were also commonly present; as documented with HRCT, these frequently were distributed in the centers of secondary pulmonary lobules around small airways. Significantly, CT showed that many lesions that appeared reticular on plain radiographs were actually cysts. CT also showed clearly that the abundance of small nodules up to 5 mm in size was consistently underestimated on plain radiographs.

Nearly identical findings have been reported by Brauner et al. (175). In their series of 18 patients evaluated with HRCT, thin-walled cysts were found in all but one case. Other abnormalities, including nodules, cavitary nodules, and thick-walled cysts, were also present. By comparing abnormalities identified both early and late in the course of disease, the authors documented that a predictable pattern of progression from nodules, to cavitated nodules and thick-walled cysts, to thin-walled cysts with eventual confluence could be discerned. Although the exact mechanism of cyst formation remains unclear, in most cases the appearance of these in cross-section is strikingly characteristic (Figs. 49 and 50). Despite the appearance of extensive distortion

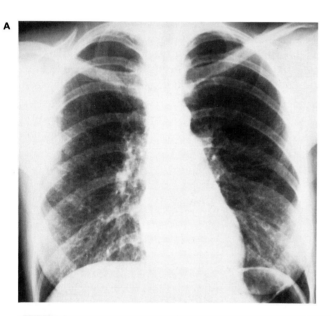

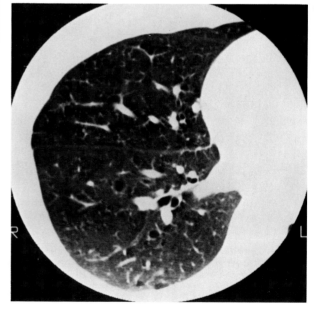

FIG. 50. Histiocytosis X: response to therapy. **A:** Posteroanterior radiograph shows diffuse increased markings interpreted by most observers as consistent with reticular, "interstitial" lung disease. **B:** Nontargeted HRCT section through the lower lobes shows a characteristic appearance of multiple well-defined cysts with uniformly thick walls, seemingly randomly distributed throughout the lungs (*straight arrow*). Many of the cysts are suggestive of dilated bronchi (*curved arrow*). Note the absence of diffuse reticulation within the lung. Transbronchial biopsy documented histiocytosis X. **C:** HRCT section through the right inferior pulmonary vein at precisely the same level as shown in B, following 6 months of medical therapy. Note that although some cysts are still present, they are smaller than seen previously. Significantly, a large number of cysts have disappeared altogether.

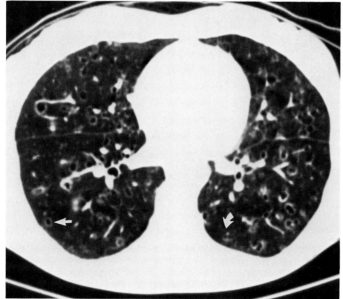

and destruction, as shown in Fig. 50, many of these changes, in fact, may be reversible.

Pulmonary Lymphangioleiomyomatosis

Lymphangioleiomyomatosis (LAM) is a rare disease characterized by the disorderly proliferation within the pulmonary interstitium of benign-appearing smooth muscle resulting in thickening of the walls of the lymphatics, blood vessels, and bronchioles, the lumens of which may become partially or completely occluded (54,55). The disease affects only women of child-bearing age. Typically patients present with progressive dyspnea and/or hemoptysis, with either recurrent pneumothoraces due to rupture of peripheral, dilated airspaces secondary to air-trapping from obstructed airways, or with chylous effusions secondary to dilated and obstructed lymphatics. Although clinical progression is usually characterized by progressive pulmonary insufficiency generally unresponsive to therapy, promising results have been obtained using hormonal therapy and/or oophorectomy (176).

Radiographically, the diagnosis is suggested when there is evidence of diffuse interstitial disease in the setting of normal or increased lung volume (Fig. 51). Interestingly, few reports emphasize cyst identification per se. As noted, pneumothoraces and effusions are common, especially as presenting abnormalities.

CT findings in patients with this disorder have been reported and are strikingly uniform in their descriptions (Figs. 51 and 52) (52,147,177–180). Innumerable thin-walled cysts can be identified, presumably the result of airspace ectasia secondary to progressive airway obstruction. When evaluated with HRCT, cysts typically vary in size from a few millimeters to up to 5 cm (179,182). Initially, only a few scattered cysts may be identifiable (Fig. 52). With progression, these become more uniformly distributed throughout the lungs (Fig. 50). Characteristically, intervening normal lung appears strikingly normal despite almost total replacement of lung tissue in cases with advanced disease. Nodularity, thickened interlobular septal lines, and vascular destruction are generally notable by their absence. Not surprisingly, similar CT findings have been reported to occur in patients with tuberous sclerosis (182). As compared with routine radiography, these changes have consistently been reported as easier to identify with CT (179,183).

In an evaluation of eight patients with documented lymphangioleiomyomatosis, Sherrier et al. (180) reported associated mediastinal and/or retrocrural lymphadenopathy in half of their cases. In our experience, the finding of nodular retrocrural densities in these patients should suggest also the possibility of dilatation of the thoracic duct. In these cases, differentiation may require that lymphangiography be performed.

In select cases, differentiation between lymphangioleiomyomatosis and pulmonary emphysema may present difficulties due to the seeming lack of an identifiable cyst wall in both disorders. However, uniform distribution throughout both lungs strongly favors the diagnosis of LAM. Identification of residual core lobular

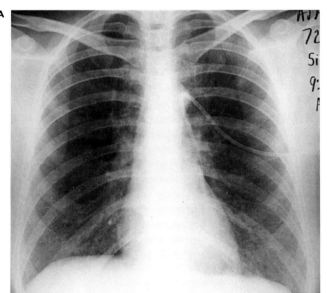
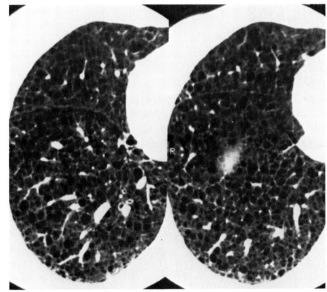

FIG. 51. Lymphangioleiomyomatosis (LAM). **A:** Posteroanterior radiograph shows only subtle suggestion of hyperaeration and a few scattered nonspecific reticular densities in this patient with open-lung biopsy-documented LAM. **B,C:** Sequential HRCT sections through the right lower lobe show diffuse cystic changes throughout the lungs. Although the appearance superficially mimics emphysema, note that the cysts are uniformly distributed throughout the lungs (compare with Figs. 44–46), and have thin but definable walls in the absence of obvious reticular or nodular disease.

A,B

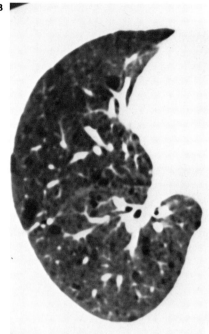 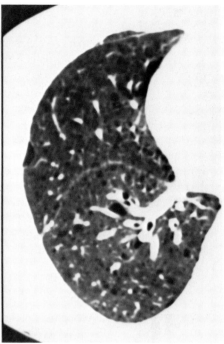

FIG. 52. Lymphangioleiomyomatosis (LAM). A,B: HRCT images through the right mid and lower lung fields, respectively, in a patient with documented LAM. Cysts of varying sizes can be seen scattered randomly throughout the parenchyma. Although there are considerably fewer cysts present as compared with the appearance in Figs. 51 B and C, their morphologic appearance is otherwise indistinguishable.

structures in the cyst centers, characteristic of emphysema, is also helpful in differentiating these conditions (Fig. 44). Differentiating lymphangioleiomyomatosis from pulmonary histiocytosis X also may prove problematic; identification of small nodules in the latter condition, however, is frequently valuable, as is clinical correlation (174,175).

Bronchiolitis Obliterans

Pure bronchiolitis obliterans is defined pathologically by the presence of granulation tissue within the lumen of bronchioles that have been destroyed by scarring (77). When associated with extension of disease into the distal airspaces, this process is referred to as bronchiolitis obliterans organizing pneumonia (BOOP) (Fig. 53) (55,245). Pure bronchiolitis obliterans itself is rare and is considered by some to be a separate entity, best described as obliterative bronchiolitis. Unlike patients with BOOP, in whom pulmonary function tests usually show a restrictive pattern and impaired gas exchange in the presence of a variety of different types of pulmonary infiltrates, obliterative bronchiolitis generally is characterized by severe air flow obstruction and distended lung fields without pulmonary infiltrates.

Bronchiolitis obliterans is associated with a variety of etiologies, resulting in the following classification: (a) toxic fume bronchiolitis obliterans, such as occurs following inhalation of gases such as nitrogen dioxide, sulfur dioxide, ammonia, phosgene, chlorine, and ozone; (b) postinfectious bronchiolitis obliterans, especially following Mycoplasma or viral infections; (c) bronchiolitis

obliterans associated with connective tissue disorders such as rheumatoid arthritis, including reaction to therapeutic drugs such as penicillamine; (d) localized bronchiolitis, occurring as a focal abnormality often incidentally detected radiographically as a focal density or nodule, often necessitating surgery; and (e) idiopathic bronchiolitis obliterans (245,246). BOOP may also be seen in association with bronchial obstruction, chronic aspiration, and following select drugs, including gold and amiodarone (55).

Obliterative bronchiolitis is associated with a variety of etiologies, including: (a) graft versus host disease following bone marrow transplantation; (b) chronic lung rejection in patients with heart-lung transplants; (c) collagen vascular diseases, especially rheumatoid arthritis; (d) drug reaction, particularly in association with gold and penicillamine; (e) viral infections, especially in childhood; (f) toxic inhalants; and rarely, (g) idiopathic. Of course, many of these same factors have been cited as etiologic in patients with BOOP (76).

In most cases, the etiology of BOOP is never established. As emphasized by Epler et al. (245), patients with idiopathic bronchiolitis present with a characteristic clinical syndrome. Typically these cases affect middle-aged patients who present with a chronic, nonproductive cough and low-grade constitutional symptoms. Pulmonary function tests usually show a restrictive pattern and impaired gas exchange.

BOOP causes no pathognomonic chest radiographic findings (246,248). Although nonspecific, as emphasized by McLoud et al. (246), radiographic changes do tend to reflect the nature and extent of the underlying

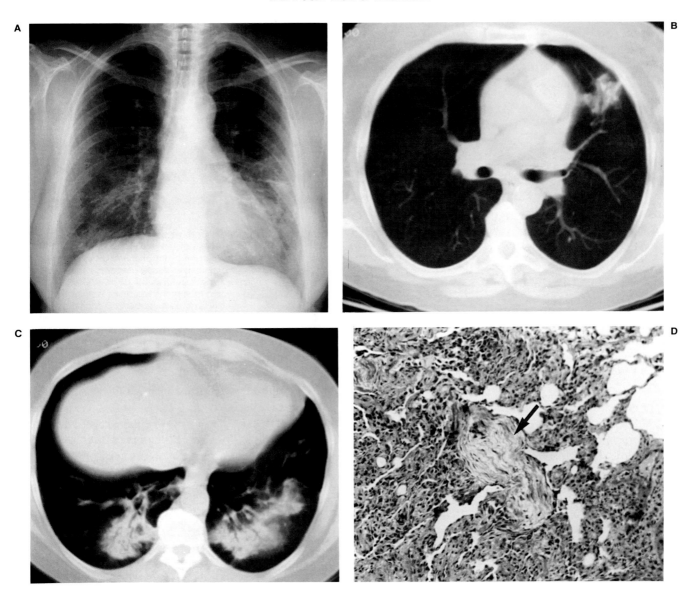

FIG. 53. Bronchiolitis obliterans organizing pneumonia (BOOP). **A:** Posteroanterior radiograph shows nonspecific findings of ill-defined, scattered areas of increased lung density throughout both lung fields. **B,C:** 10-mm thick sections through the upper and lower lobes, respectively, show the presence of otherwise nondescript foci of airspace consolidation, within which air-bronchograms are easily identified. Although this appearance is nonspecific and may result from inflammatory and/or neoplastic disease, the pattern of lung involvement is strikingly different from that seen in patients with usual interstitial pneumonitis (compare with Figs. 25–27). **D:** Histologic section obtained from an open-lung biopsy shows characteristic appearance of granulation tissue obstructing the lumen of peripheral airway (*black arrow*), with extension into adjacent alveoli.

pathology. Most patients present with bilateral ground-glass or airspace opacities, changes reflecting the presence of organizing pneumonias. When localized, bronchiolitis obliterans results in more discrete densities or nodules. Similar results have been reported by Muller et al. (249). In 10 of 14 patients with documented BOOP evaluated by these authors there were patchy areas of consolidation, while in seven cases discrete nodular opacities could be identified. These findings are believed to reflect localization of pathology to distal airways. In a recent analysis of 16 patients with documented bronchiolitis obliterans, Cordier et al. distinguished three distinct groups based in part on their radiographic pre-

sentations, including: group 1 patients with multiple, patchy migratory areas of pulmonary consolidation (four patients); group 2 patients with solitary abnormalities, presenting either as focal areas of consolidation and/or mass, necessitating surgical exploration (five patients); and group 3 patients presenting with diffuse interstitial lung disease (seven patients) (250).

The CT findings in patients with BOOP have been described, although only limited numbers of cases have been reported (249–252). Most frequently, CT shows scattered foci of airspace consolidation, identifiable as either ground-glass opacities or more commonly as focal areas of airspace consolidation with or without asso-

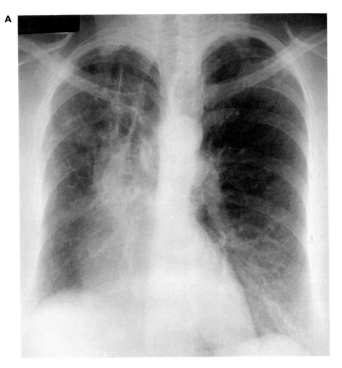

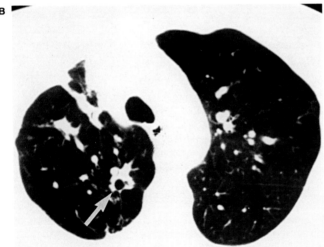

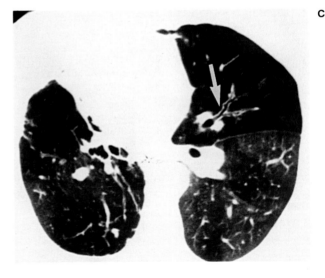

FIG. 54. Obliterative bronchiolitis (Swyer-James syndrome). **A:** Posteroanterior radiograph shows significant volume loss on the right side with ipsilateral shift of the heart and mediastinum. The right lung is slightly hyperlucent, associated with some attenuation of intraparenchymal vessels. The left lung appears normal. **B,C:** 1.5-mm thick sections through the carina and lower lobes, respectively, show diffuse emphysematous changes throughout both lungs, associated with dilated bronchi (*arrow* in B and C). Sections through the central airways showed no evidence of a central endobronchial lesion (not shown). Clinically asymptomatic, this patient did recall a history of childhood respiratory infections.

ciated air-bronchograms (Fig. 53). Although it has been suggested that the disease more often involves the periphery of the lung, it has been documented with CT that consolidation may occur anywhere within the parenchyma. In addition to patchy areas of airspace disease, in half of their cases, Muller et al. identified nodules, often well-defined and frequently peribronchovascular in distribution (251). The CT findings in patients with obliterative bronchiolitis (Swyer-James syndrome) also have been reported (Fig. 54) (253). Characteristic features include: (a) patency of the central bronchi; (b) diffuse emphysema, identifiable as a severe decrease in the density of involved lung segments which are atelectatic; and (c) bronchiectasis, frequently severe. Interestingly, despite the chest radiographic appearance of unilateral

involvement, otherwise unsuspected contralateral involvement appears to be common.

In most cases the CT appearance is entirely nonspecific; as reported by Muller et al. CT was of only marginal value in characterizing disease as compared with chest radiographs. One role yet to be addressed, however, is the potential for CT to help differentiate between patients with bronchiolitis obliterans and patients with UIP. Differentiation between these can be extremely problematic, as clinically and, more importantly, pathologically the two entities are frequently indistinguishable (246,248). This differentiation is all the more important because patients with BOOP, unlike most patients with UIP, frequently demonstrate a good clinical response to treatment with corticosteroids. This suggests that in equivocal cases, especially those presenting with diffuse lung infiltrates, CT should be obtained to further characterize radiologic abnormalities; in select cases, it may be anticipated that CT may also play a role in documenting early response to therapy.

DIFFUSE PULMONARY DISEASE: CLINICAL CORRELATIONS

Given the inherent advantages of CT to image the lungs, what indications are there for the use of CT in the evaluation of patients with either suspected or documented diffuse pulmonary disease? Accurate assessment of the role of CT requires answering the following questions:

1. To what extent does CT augment the diagnostic sensitivity and specificity of routine chest radiography?
2. How does CT compare with routine clinical measurements of lung function as determined by pulmonary function tests?
3. Is there a role for CT in assessing disease activity as compared with alternate techniques such as bronchoalveolar lavage (BAL), or gallium-67 citrate scanning?
4. How does CT compare with other modalities in predicting the accuracy of transbronchial versus openlung biopsies in the diagnosis of diffuse lung disease?

Comparison with Chest Radiography

Numerous reports have documented that CT is far more accurate than plain chest radiography in the detection and characterization of diffuse lung disease (16,48,52,59,66,81,99,131,133,135,137,145,175,180–184,254). Detailed evaluation of the diagnostic efficacy of CT versus that of plain radiography has been reported by Mathieson et al. (185). Using a modification of the ILO/UC classification and without prior knowledge of clinical or pathologic data, each observer assessed radiographs and CT scans by listing the three most likely diagnoses in order of probability, along with recorded degrees of confidence. The authors found that the highest level of confidence was reached in only 23% of radiographic but in 49% of CT interpretations, with the diagnosis confirmed in 77% and 93% of these confident interpretations ($p < .001$), respectively. Overall, on the basis of previous descriptions of the CT appearances of the most common infiltrative lung diseases, CT scans proved most accurate in the diagnosis of silicosis (93%), usual interstitial pneumonia (89%), lymphangitic carcinomatosis (85%), and sarcoidosis (77%) (186).

More recently, similar results have been reported by Schurawitzki et al. (254). These authors compared HRCT scans with chest radiographs in 23 patients with documented progressive systemic sclerosis. In 21 patients (91%), HRCT revealed findings of interstitial lung disease, including honeycombing in nearly one-third of cases, while chest radiographs were interpreted as showing interstitial lung disease in only nine patients (39%).

It should be emphasized that care must be taken in assessing reports comparing CT with chest radiography because of a natural tendency toward statistical bias in the selection of case material. To date, with few exceptions, most studies have been either limited in the number of patients studied, or excessively restricted in the range of pathologic entities examined. This may lead to false conclusions concerning the accuracy of both CT and chest radiography. Despite limitations in the design of some studies, the cumulative experience of most investigators has nonetheless confirmed overwhelmingly that CT is far superior to routine chest radiography in the detection and characterization of most diffuse lung diseases. Although the final role of CT vis-à-vis chest radiography remains to be established, it is apparent that the two modalities should be considered complementary, and that indications for the use of CT should continue to expand.

Correlation with Pulmonary Function Testing

Numerous reports have explored the relationship between CT findings, both quantitative and qualitative, and pulmonary function tests (PFTs) (23,24,33–36,73,81,105,133–135,162,174,181–184,187–189). In patients with emphysema, in particular, these attempts have met with varying although generally positive results (23,24,33–36,162,185–188).

Goddard et al., using a combination of both a visual grading system based on recognition of characteristic areas of low attenuation and vascular disruption and numerical analysis based on lung density measurements, found significant differences in the forced expiratory volume in 1 sec (FEV1), the forced expiratory volume in 1 sec/forced vital capacity (FEV1/FVC), and the single breath diffusing capacity for carbon monoxide (DLCO) between patients with high and low visual scores (33). Bergin et al., using a similar visual scoring system specifically correlating extent of disease with pulmonary function, also found significant but low correlation between the DLCO percent predicted, the FEV1 percent predicted, and the FEV1/FVC percent predicted in a study of 32 patients evaluated prior to surgery (159). On the basis of postsurgical pathologic correlation, CT scans proved to be a more sensitive and specific indicator of the presence and extent of emphysema than pulmonary function tests.

Similar findings also have been reported by Sanders et al. (187). In a study of 60 patients evaluated with both CT and PFTs, CT evidence of emphysema was found in

24 (69%) of 35 patients with normal pulmonary function tests, leading these authors, too, to conclude that CT may be more sensitive than PFTs in detecting mild grades of emphysema.

In an attempt to automate CT interpretation, Kinsella et al. have obtained good correlation between CT and pulmonary function tests using a computerized program to obtain density masks to outline pixels with attenuation values less than -910 HU. Quantitation of emphysema using density masks has been shown to correlate well with the pathologic extent of disease (23). In particular, these authors found a significant correlation between the extent of emphysema on CT and FEV1/FVC percent of predicted, functional residual capacity percent predicted, and Dsb percent predicted.

Despite these findings, the precise clinical role of CT in the evaluation of patients with emphysema is unclear. It has been suggested that because of its increased sensitivity in detecting emphysema as compared with routine pulmonary function tests, CT could be used for early screening of patients suspected of having alpha$_1$-antitrypsin deficiency (171,190). CT has been documented to be of value in the preoperative assessment of patients with localized bullous disease (166–170). CT may also prove helpful in defining the presence and assessing the extent of emphysema in patients with other pulmonary diseases, such as the pneumoconioses (189). Finally, in patients with otherwise unexplained clinical symptomatology, CT may also play a useful role (17). Although additional indications will no doubt develop, these must await further testing.

Correlation between CT scans and pulmonary function tests has been obtained in patients with a variety of other diseases including sarcoidosis, asbestosis, usual interstitial pneumonitis, lymphangioleiomyomatosis, and histiocytosis X. In general, these studies show significant correlation between the extent and severity of disease as shown by CT and functional abnormalities measured clinically, as, for example, the degree of dyspnea, as well as abnormalities documented by PFTs. The clinical significance of these findings is unclear. Positive correlation of this nature indicates the accuracy of CT to detect and to some extent quantify the presence of disease: it is, however, exceedingly unlikely that CT scans will ever replace pulmonary function tests in the evaluation of lung disease. Whether a role for CT will emerge as a correlative procedure to further assess pulmonary function remains to be documented.

Assessment of Disease Activity: The Significance of Ground-Glass Opacification

A potentially significant use of CT is the evaluation of disease activity in patients with established diffuse lung disease. Determining when and if to treat patients, especially with steroids, often proves to be a frustrating clinical dilemma. Attempts to correlate chest radiographic findings and disease activity have generally proved unrewarding (190). Presumably, the macroscopic information recorded on chest radiographs is a poor predictor, in itself, of physiologic function. Subjectivity in interpretation also presumably contributes to this inaccuracy (191). Despite advocacy by some of both gallium-67 and bronchoalveolar lavage, considerable controversy persists as to the value of these procedures (128,192). In patients with idiopathic pulmonary fibrosis, in particular, recent studies have shown a poor correlation between gallium-67 uptake and findings at bronchoalveolar lavage (193). More important still, it has also been shown that there is little correlation between disease activity as measured by gallium uptake and either response to treatment with corticosteroids or prognosis (194).

In principle, response to therapy in diseases such as sarcoidosis and usual interstitial pneumonitis is determined by the presence of active alveolitis. It is probable that this precedes and is probably instrumental in the evolution of diffuse scarring and fibrosis (121,122). Considerable speculation has centered on the potential of CT to diagnose disease activity by delineating focal areas of ground-glass opacification within the parenchyma (Fig. 55) (80,195). It is presumed that these correspond to areas of active alveolitis, although histologic verification is absent in most series. In fact, poorly demarcated, hazy densities within the lung probably result from a number of different processes defined as the accumulation of inflammatory cells in the interstitium and alveolar lumen. It is possible that these areas correspond to foci of alveolitis; however, in diseases such as sarcoidosis, these densities could result from widespread

FIG. 55. Idiopathic pulmonary fibrosis: correlation between disease activity and ground-glass opacification. **A:** Posteroanterior radiograph shows diffuse lung infiltrates, most prominent at the lung bases. **B:** 1.5-mm section through the lung bases shows typical appearance of pulmonary fibrosis with associated honeycombing. A few focal areas of ground-glass opacification can be identified (*arrows*). **C:** Corresponding Ga-67 scan shows faint diffuse uptake throughout the lungs, considerably less intense than the adjacent liver. At this time, an open-lung biopsy from the right lower lobe confirmed the diagnosis of idiopathic pulmonary fibrosis, and the patient was started on a course of steroids. **D:** Posteroanterior radiograph obtained 5 months after that shown in A. Although there clearly has been progression of disease, it is difficult to determine to what extent this reflects active, ongoing disease or progressive fibrosis. In the interval between radiographs the patient had stopped taking his medication. **E:** HRCT section through the right lower lobe at approximately the same level as in B. Ground-glass opacification is now far more prominent suggesting considerable alveolitis (compare with B). **F:** Corresponding Ga-67 scan shows intense bilateral uptake, consistent with extensive alveolitis.

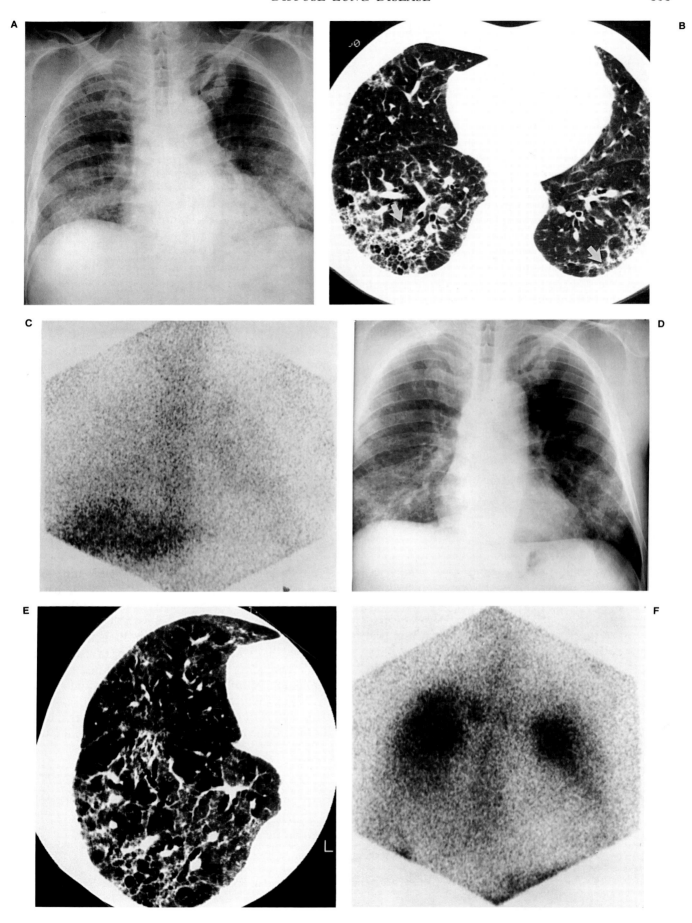

interstitial granulomata too small to be identified individually (135). Additionally, identical findings may result from focal alterations in either tissue perfusion or aeration, without the need to invoke primary tissue alterations (Fig. 56) (17). As described by Martin et al., a pattern of mosaic oligemia secondary to regional alterations in pulmonary blood flow, caused, for example, by central pulmonary emboli may result in remarkable differences in lung density, with areas of relative hyperperfusion simulating pulmonary infiltrates (196).

In a retrospective evaluation of 12 patients with idiopathic pulmonary fibrosis evaluated with both CT and open-lung biopsy, Muller et al. showed that patchy areas of increased lung density within the lung can, in fact, correlate pathologically with foci of alveolitis (80). Furthermore, using this finding, CT correctly identified all five patients with marked disease activity and five of seven patients with mild disease activity graded pathologically. Follow-up CT scans performed in one patient with a diagnosis of desquamative interstitial pneumonitis treated with steroids showed complete resolution of previously identified areas of patchy parenchymal densities. Significantly, of the four patients in this study with minimal or no disease activity identified on CT scans who received steroids, all showed progressive clinical and functional deterioration.

Confirmatory findings have been reported by others (135,136). Despite the absence of histologic verification, in most series the finding of ground-glass or hazy densities within the lung appears to correlate clinically with foci of active alveolitis. As reported by Lynch et al., in an HRCT study of 15 patients with documented sarcoidosis, in all five patients with positive Ga-67 scans, CT showed extensive areas of focal increased density to be the dominant CT finding within the lungs (135). Significantly, no correlation was found between CT scans and findings in patients with BAL. Bergin et al. also have shown a correlation between patchy areas of parenchymal disease on CT and activity as determined by Ga-67 scans (134). Again, no correlation could be found between CT appearances and disease activity as determined by BAL.

Another potential use of CT is to assess disease activity in patients undergoing treatment with a variety of antineoplastic and antiarrhythmic drugs. Of particular interest is the potential for CT to monitor drug-related lung damage, especially that resulting from bleomycin (184,197,198). Used to treat patients with a variety of tumors, including lymphomas and seminomatous and nonseminomatous germ cell tumors, bleomycin can result in extensive pulmonary toxicity, limiting the drug's use. Lung damage is reversible, however, provided that the diagnosis is made early and the drug is discontinued. As shown by Bellamy et al., in an evaluation of 100 patients treated with bleomycin evaluated with both plain radiographs and CT, lung damage was detected in

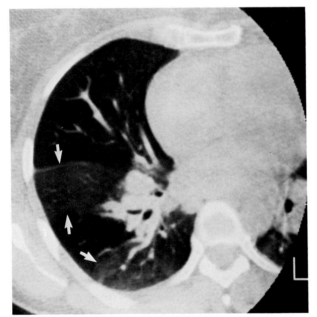 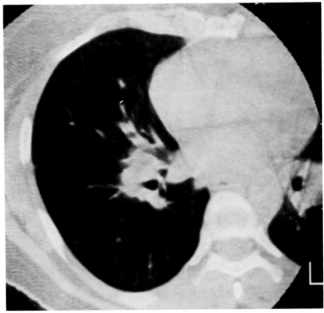

FIG. 56. Ground-glass opacification: sarcoidoisis. A: End-expiratory, HRCT section through the right lung in a patient with documented sarcoidosis. In addition to hilar adenopathy, regions of ground-glass opacification can be identified (arrows) in both the anterior basilar and posterior basilar segments. The appearance suggests active alveolitis. B: HRCT section obtained at the same level as A, following deep inspiration. Hilar adenopathy can again be appreciated. Significantly, previously identified areas of ground-glass opacification have disappeared; the right lower lobe appears normal. In this case, ground-glass opacification presumably was the result of decreased aeration within portions of the right lower lobe, probably due to central bronchial compression by enlarged hilar nodes. Note that the anterior basilar segmental bronchus is compressed in A. While the finding of ground-glass opacification suggests alveolitis in the appropriate clinical context, care must be taken not to overinterpret the significance of this finding.

38% of patients with CT as compared to only 15% detected by radiography (184). Although described by the authors as causing coarse reticular shadowing sometimes associated with nodularity on CT, review of the published images shows that ill-defined hazy densities are common, especially in the periphery of the lung. In the group of 19 patients assessed as having only minor lung damage, follow-up data was available in 16; of these, nine patients showed complete resolution of lung damage over a period of 2–8 months. Rimmer et al. have published nearly identical findings, including noting ill-defined opacities occurring predominantly in the subpleural regions as the primary CT manifestation of bleomycin toxicity (197).

CT-guided Lung Biopsy

In our experience, one of the main indications for the use of CT in evaluating diffuse pulmonary abnormalities is as a guide for transbronchial and open-lung biopsies (Figs. 2,14,39). The shortcomings of transbronchial biopsy (TBB) as a means for establishing the etiology of diffuse pulmonary disease have been well-documented. In a classic prospective study of 53 patients with diffuse lung disease, Wall et al. documented that TBB proved diagnostic in only 20 (38%) (199). In the remaining 33 cases, TBBs were interpreted as showing either normal lung, nonspecific abnormalities, interstitial pneumonia, or interstitial fibrosis. Open-lung biopsies in these same patients resulted in specific diagnoses in 92%. Significantly, these bore little if any relationship to the diagnoses originally established by TBB, suggesting that a TBB diagnosis of interstitial pneumonia, chronic inflammation, nonspecific reaction, or interstitial fibrosis, in particular, should be interpreted as unreliable. Furthermore, of those diseases accurately established by TBB, most proved to be due to either sarcoidosis or lymphangitic carcinomatosis, consistent with the fact that these entities preferentially involve peribronchial tissue and, as a consequence, are more accessible to TBB.

Recent improvements have led to an expanded role for the use of transbronchial biopsy in establishing specific histologic diagnoses, in particular histiocytosis X, pulmonary alveolar proteinosis, Goodpasture's syndrome, Wegener's granulomatosis, and eosinophilic granuloma (200). As summarized by Shure, however, controversy persists as to the overall accuracy of TBB in the diagnosis of diffuse pulmonary disease, especially in accurately categorizing a histologic diagnosis of either nonspecific pneumonitis or fibrosis. Although it has been reported that as many as 75% of patients with nonspecific TBBs subsequently can be shown to have benign clinical courses (201), as established by Wall et al., many

of these cases demonstrate significant diseases when evaluated by open-lung biopsy (199).

Even open-lung biopsy may be inaccurate if the disease process is not uniformly scattered throughout the lung. Although controversial, as documented by Newman et al., the common practice of routinely obtaining lingular biopsies may lead to nonspecific findings and therefore may not be a valid biopsy site when compared to biopsy material obtained simultaneously from two other lung segments (202).

The role of CT as a guide to fiberoptic bronchoscopy (FOB) has been addressed by numerous authors. As documented by Henschke et al., in a retrospective study of 46 patients with documented malignant disease evaluated with both routine 10-mm thick CT and FOB, CT proved positive in five cases in which visual findings at FOB were normal; in four of these five cases, a diagnosis of malignancy within the lung was subsequently established (203). More important, FOB proved diagnostic in 20 (69%) of 29 cases in which bronchial and peribronchial abnormalities were identified by CT, as compared with a positive diagnosis in only 5 (29%) of 17 cases in which CT was interpreted as negative. Nearly identical results have been reported comparing CT and FOB in the evaluation of peripheral nodules and masses using the predictive value of a positive CT-bronchus sign (204).

Other malignant diseases in which CT may be of aid to the bronchoscopist include lymphoma, alveolar cell carcinoma, and Kaposi's sarcoma (KS). Associated with characteristic endobronchial abnormalities, Kaposi's sarcoma may be particularly difficult to establish with routine transbronchial biopsies. It has been suggested that in select cases, CT findings of abnormal hilar densities extending into the adjacent lung along distinctly perivascular and peribronchial pathways may be helpful in establishing the diagnosis of intraparenchymal KS, even in the absence of histologic verification (Fig. 57) (241).

Similar findings have been reported in patients with nonneoplastic diseases. Hamper et al., in a retrospective evaluation of 36 cases of documented sarcoidosis that had proven to be diagnostic dilemmas, found that CT provided an essential road map for bronchoscopy in seven cases and further enabled choice of the most appropriate procedure to exclude an initial impression of malignancy in another six cases (131). In the most complete series reported to date, Mathieson et al. documented that HRCT, as compared with chest radiography, helped correctly predict whether transbronchial needle biopsy or open-lung biopsy was indicated in 87% of cases (versus 65% for radiography) (185). Significantly, in this series a transbronchial biopsy was considered to have been appropriately suggested only when the first choice diagnosis was correctly limited to either sarcoidosis or lymphangitic carcinomatosis, while an

A 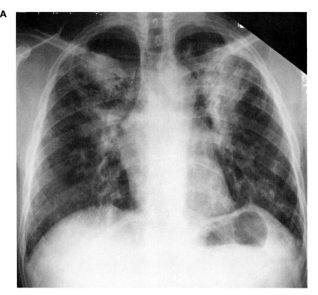 B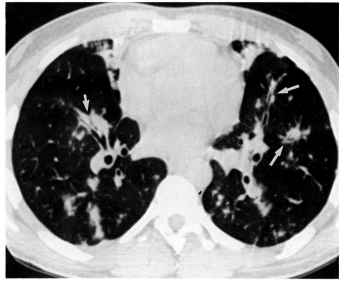

FIG. 57. CT-FOB correlation: Kaposi's sarcoma (KS). **A:** Posteroanterior radiograph shows scattered densities in both lungs, more prominent in the upper lung fields. **B:** HRCT scan through the lower lobes shows characteristic appearance of primarily peribronchial and perivascular infiltrates (*arrows*). In select cases, this appearance is sufficiently characteristic to allow a presumptive diagnosis of intrapulmonary KS.

open-lung biopsy was assumed to be the correct procedure when the first choice diagnosis avoided the erroneous inclusion of either of these two diseases. These guidelines clearly reflect the conclusions previously described by Wall et al. (201).

Based on these studies, it is our opinion that in cases for which TBB is planned specifically to evaluate patients with known or suspected diffuse lung disease, prior CT evaluation should be obtained. In patients with CT findings suggesting a probable high yield on TBB such as sarcoidosis, CT may be helpful by directing the bronchoscopist to optimal biopsy sites. In those cases in which findings at TBB are equivocal, such as interstitial pneumonia or interstitial fibrosis, CT can be of diagnostic value by suggesting the need for further tissue evaluation, obtained either by more precisely directed repeat TBB or from open-lung biopsy. Finally, in those cases in which CT indicates a probable low diagnostic yield, such as patients with CT findings of idiopathic pulmonary fibrosis, CT may play an invaluable role by suggesting preferential use of open-lung biopsy.

Of course, obvious exceptions include those cases in which the clinical indication strongly suggests infection, such as patients with AIDS in whom Pneumocystis carinii pneumonia is suspected or in patients with suspected miliary tuberculosis. Despite these exceptions, however, and occasionally even in problematic cases in which infection is suspected, by precise delineation of the extent, location, and appearance of pathology, CT can be beneficial in individual cases by helping to determine the most appropriate study to establish a diagnosis, or, in select cases, by obviating the need for additional studies.

MR

To date, the role of MR in the clinical evaluation of both diffuse and focal lung disease has been limited (205–216) due to a number of factors. Compared with other tissues, lung has relatively low water density, with tissue per unit volume measuring only approximately one-fifth that of solid organs, resulting in a low signal-to-noise ratio (206,217,218). Additionally, spatial resolution is diminished by a combination of respiratory and cardiac motion. Finally, susceptibility artifacts caused by innumerable air-water interfaces within the lung result in loss of signal, especially when gradient-refocused techniques are utilized. Despite these limitations, MR does have the potential to evolve into a powerful tool for the investigation of pulmonary disease because of markedly increased contrast resolution.

Experimental studies have documented that MR can be used to quantitate lung water content (219–226). Using animal models, close agreement has been documented between MR signal intensities and gravimetrically determined lung wet-to-dry weight ratios. Although determination of absolute lung water content has proven difficult *in vivo*, measurements of relative lung water changes have been shown to be proportional to true lung water content, and may prove to be a sensitive method for following the course of lung injury (206). Furthermore, using animal models, Schmidt et al. have shown documented differences in the MR characteristics of permeability versus hydrostatic pulmonary edema; to date, however, the pattern of distribution of edema has not proven sufficiently specific to provide reliable discrimination (224).

MR has been used to attempt to differentiate among various etiologies of parenchymal consolidation; so far, however, the results have been generally disappointing. Moore et al. in a study of 16 patients with known airspace diseases evaluated the potential of MR to differentiate among various etiologies and found considerable overlap in both T1 and T2 values, although one case of alveolar proteinosis was distinctive because of its especially low T1 value. It is likely that with greater experience a wide range of appearances will be documented for this entity as well (Fig. 58) (207). Similar attempts to differentiate pulmonary hemorrhage from edema have also proven equivocal (227). In distinction, a greater degree of success has been met in attempting to differentiate central obstructing masses from peripheral collapsed lung, especially utilizing T2-weighted sequences (see Chapters 1 and 4) (228).

Of considerably greater promise is the potential of MR to identify active interstitial lung disease. Investigating bleomycin-induced alveolitis and pulmonary fibrosis in 18 Lewis rats, Vitinski et al. found MR signal intensities to be markedly elevated in both disease states (208). Additionally, both T1 and T2 values of lungs with documented alveolitis and controls proved equivalent, although these values were significantly decreased in fibrotic lungs. Consistent differentiation between foci of active inflammation and fibrosis in the lung, however, has proven controversial (229–232).

McFadden et al., in a study of 34 patients with a variety of interstitial lung diseases, found a strong correlation between qualitative assessment of signal intensity within the lungs and clinical assessment of disease activity (210). In this study the most severely affected patients proved to have the greatest signal intensities, and follow-up examinations in 10 patients showed a decrease in image intensity in patients responding to treatment. Unfortunately, MR signal characteristics were of no use in differentiating patients who responded to therapy from those whose disease remained stable or worsened with therapy. Given the great diversity of diseases within the patient population and technical limitations of the study, these results must be seen as only provisional.

MR has documented that images of great anatomic clarity of within the lung parenchyma can be obtained (233,234). Using routine spin-echo (SE) techniques, remarkably precise anatomic detail can be seen on nonfixed, inflated, whole-lung specimens (Figs. 59 and 60). Attention also has been directed toward the potential of both routine SE and gradient-refocused techniques to evaluate pulmonary vasculature (235,236). Using dual 5-inch surface coils located on the anterior and posterior chest walls, Hatabu et al. evaluated both gradient-refocused sequences with breath-holding and SE sequences timed with diastole to visualize the lungs (235). In both instances, peripheral pulmonary vascular structures, including sixth- and seventh-order branches, could be identified, especially in portions of lung adjacent to the surface coils. Pursuing a different approach, Edelman et al. have produced high quality projection angiograms of the pulmonary arteries from a series of breath-held, two-dimensional, flow-compensated, gradient-echo images (236). More recently, Bergin and Pauli have reported the use of very short echo-time (TE) times (approximately 250 μs) to overcome problems related to magnetic susceptibility (*personal communication*). Preliminary results in volunteers appear to demonstrate details of the parenchyma previously not visualized. These

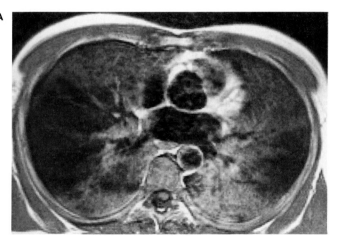
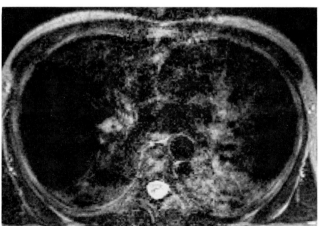

FIG. 58. Alveolar proteinosis: MR evaluation. **A,B:** T1- and T2-weighted images through the lung bases, respectively, in a patient with documented alveolar proteinosis. Although it has been suggested that little signal is present within the lungs on T1-weighted scans in patients with alveolar proteinosis, in this case considerable signal is present on both T1- and T2-weighted scans. This appearance is entirely nonspecific. (Courtesy of Dr. Arfa Khan, Long Island Jewish Hospital, NY.)

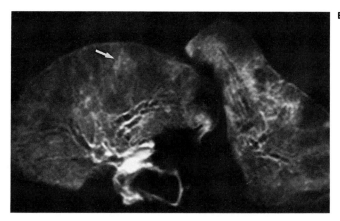

FIG. 59. Fixed-inflated lung specimens: CT/MR correlation. **A,B:** 1.5-mm thick CT section and corresponding 10-mm thick MR scan (TR = 500; TE = 30; four acquisitions) obtained at the same level in a patient with scattered foci of bronchopneumonia. Note that visualized anatomic structures are seen equally well, as are foci of pathology (*arrows* in A and B).

developments, if continued, promise to revolutionize magnetic resonance imaging of the pulmonary parenchyma.

CONCLUSIONS

The application of state-of-the-art CT to the investigation of diffuse lung disease has led to profound changes in our appreciation of pulmonary parenchymal

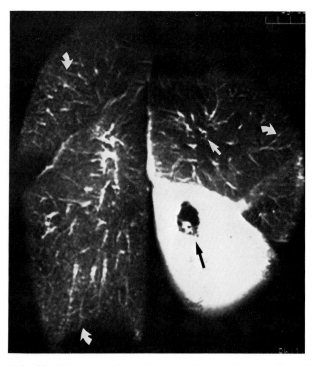

FIG. 60. Nonfixed, inflated lungs: MR evaluation. Routine T1-weighted, spin-echo 10-mm thick coronal section through nonfixed, inflated lungs. Note clear visualization of anatomic structures including identification of peripheral lobular structures (*curved arrows*). An obvious lung abscess is present within the left lower lobe (*straight arrow*).

pathology. This has necessitated a thorough re-examination of our concept of the imaging and diagnosis of diffuse lung diseases.

At least three separate levels of radiographic analysis are now possible. Although overlap is to be expected, each level represents a new magnitude or order of information, reflecting ever greater degrees of three-dimensional anatomic resolution (Tables 2 and 3).

The first level is occupied by routine chest radiography. Interpretation of abnormalities is governed by recognition of basic patterns of abnormality, as well as some estimate of the gross distribution and extent of disease (1). Specific classifications have evolved, from initial attempts to differentiate interstitial from alveolar disease, to a more generalized approach emphasizing purely descriptive terminology based on a semiquantitative modification of the ILO/UC classification (4). Although general agreement remains elusive, descriptive terms including reticular, nodular, reticulonodular, miliary, and honeycomb are well-accepted; other terms, such as alveolar, ground-glass, destructive, mottled, and vascular are generally less well-agreed upon. Characterization also includes distinguishing among predominantly upper, mid, and lower lung zones, and somewhat less accurately, distinguishing primarily peripheral from perihilar disease. As noted, both the advantages and limitations of this approach have been well-documented (1–4,43).

A second level of radiographic interpretation is occupied by routine, 8 to 10-mm section thoracic CT. By

TABLE 2. *Routine CT of the lung parenchyma: Indications*

Metastatic lung disease
Differentiation of pleural vs. parenchymal disease[a]
Lung cancer staging[a]
Airspace diseases
Bullous emphysema

[a] Preferably requiring i.v. contrast administration.

eliminating superimposition of shadows, CT has proven to be a more sensitive means for detecting parenchymal disease. Additionally, routine CT allows more precise characterization of abnormalities that are identified on routine chest radiographs, as well as more accurate delineation of the distribution of disease, including, in particular, differentiation between predominantly central versus peripheral patterns of involvement. Although similar information may be obtained in select cases from routine whole-lung tomography, given the ability of CT to more accurately evaluate the mediastinum, hila, pleura, and chest wall simultaneously, the utility of this technique should be considered extremely limited.

Routine thoracic CT has been proven especially valuable in the differentiation of pleural from parenchymal disease (237,238), including identification of patients with unsuspected asbestos-related pleural disease (94–105). It is also valuable in the diagnosis and characterization of airspace diseases (17,57–59,64) including identification of pulmonary infarcts (239), manifestations of pulmonary drug toxicity, including the effects of parenchymal irradiation (184,197,240,241), staging of lung cancer, including evaluation of pulmonary collapse and identification of contralateral disease, especially in patients with alveolar cell carcinoma (66), and identification of bullous lung disease (166–168) and other causes of both focal and diffuse lung density alterations, including pulmonary vascular disease (17,196). Most important, contiguously obtained 8 to 10-mm thick sections remain the most accurate way to assess the lungs for metastatic nodules (51,242,243). Considered together, these indications account for the majority of thoracic CTs in which evaluation of the lungs is of clinical significance.

Finally, a third, or still higher order of interpretation is achieved with use of HRCT. By minimizing slice thickness and accentuating spatial resolution using appropriate high frequency algorithms, HRCT represents a significant incremental advance in our ability to visualize and characterize diffuse parenchymal abnormalities (9,10,17,46–50,52,147,185). Because structures of approximately 300 microns are easily resolved, detailed and accurate assessment of otherwise nondescript abnormalities has become feasible. The result has been a significant expansion in our knowledge of the appearances of numerous lung diseases, including hematogenous and lymphangitic spread of tumor (145,146,148); fibrotic lung diseases, such as idiopathic interstitial fibrosis (78,80,81), and asbestosis (94–105), granulomatous diseases such as sarcoidosis and histiocytosis X (132–137,174,175), and cystic lung diseases, including centriacinar emphysema (158,161), and lymphangioleiomyomatosis (170), among others. As already extensively documented, despite individual variations, each of these diseases manifests a number of characteristic features, that when familiar result in a dramatic im-

TABLE 3. *HRCT of the lung parenchyma: Indications*

1. Evaluation of symptomatic patients with normal chest radiographs including patients presenting with: dyspnea, cough, hemoptysis, pain, or unexplained fever, especially in the immunocompromised patient.
2. Evaluation of diffuse parenchymal abnormalities, specifically as a means to further characterize underlying disease, as a guide for transbronchial or open-lung biopsy, or to determine disease activity, especially for the following diseases:

    lymphangitic carcinomatosis
    idiopathic pulmonary fibrosis[a]
    asbestosis[b]
    sarcoidosis[a]
    extrinsic allergic alveolitis[a]
    histiocytosis X
    lymphangioleiomyomatosis
    diffuse pulmonary emphysema
    miliary disease
    silicosis

[a] Includes both morphologic analysis and functional evaluation (alveolitis).
[b] Preferably requiring both supine and prone images.

provement in overall diagnostic specificity (52,185). Especially valuable has been the recognition that otherwise indeterminate densities identified radiographically or on routine CT may prove to be largely perivascular or peribronchial in distribution, such as occurs in sarcoidosis and even Kaposi's sarcoma (244).

Although the value of CT in assessing diffuse pulmonary disease has been firmly established, it is apparent that there is considerable confusion as to what constitutes an ideally performed study, especially when and how to utilize HRCT. In our experience, determining which technique to use depends primarily on the clinical indication. If the main purpose of the study is to differentiate pleural from parenchymal disease or rule out pulmonary metastases, as noted above, contiguous 8 to 10-mm thick sections should suffice (Table 2). When the clinical indication for CT is primarily to study diffuse, infiltrative lung disease, however, in our opinion, 1.5 to 2-mm thick sections obtained every 10 mm is the optimal approach.

When should target reconstructions be utilized? In our experience, in most cases, 1.5-mm thick images prospectively reconstructed using a bone algorithim alone are adequate for interpretation, without the need for routine target-reconstruction. The addition of targeting, however, does simplify visual interpretation, and in cases for which maximal spatial resolution is required, their use should be encouraged whenever possible. Resolution of this magnitude allows for detailed evaluation of the basic anatomic units of the lung, especially secondary pulmonary lobules. Although the true potential of this level of analysis has yet to be determined, it is already apparent that use of retrospective target reconstructions provides further distinguishing features in the evaluation of a number of the diseases for which routine HRCT is of value, including lymphangitic carcinomatosis, sarcoidosis, and miliary disease, as well as rarer diseases such as diffuse panbronchiolitis.

REFERENCES

1. Felson B. A new look at pattern recognition of diffuse pulmonary disease. *AJR* 1979;133:183–189.
2. Epler GR, McLoud TC, Gaensler EA, Mikus JP, Carrington CB. Normal chest roentgenograms in chronic diffuse infiltrative lung disease. *N Engl J Med* 1978;298:801–809.
3. Gaensler EA, Carrington CB. Open biopsy for chronic diffuse infiltrative lung disease: clinical, roentgenographic and physiological correlations in 502 patients. *Ann Thorac Surg* 1980;30:411–426.
4. McLoud TC, Carrington CB, Gaensler EA. Diffuse infiltrative lung disease: a new scheme for description. *Radiology* 1983;149:353–363.
5. Wegener OH, Koeppe P, Oeser H. Measurement of lung density by computed tomography. *J Comput Assist Tomogr* 1978;2:263–273.
6. Solomon A, Kreel L, McNicol M, Johnson N. Computed tomography in pulmonary sarcoidosis. *J Comput Assist Tomogr* 1979;3:754–758.
7. Robinson PJ, Kreel L. Pulmonary tissue attenuation with computed tomography: comparison of inspiration and expiration scans. *J Comput Assist Tomogr* 1979;3:740–748.
8. Kreel L. Computed tomography of interstitial pulmonary disease. *J Comput Assist Tomogr* 1982;6:181–199.
9. Zerhouni EA, Naidich DP, Stitik FP, Khouri NF, Siegelman SS. Computed tomography of the pulmonary parenchyma. 2. Interstitial disease. *J Thorac Imaging* 1985;1:54–64.
10. Murata K, Itoh H, Todo G, Kanaoka M, Noma S, Itoh T, et al. Centrilobar lesions of the lung: demonstration by high-resolution CT and pathologic correlation. *Radiology* 1986;161:641–645.
11. Murata K, Khan A, Rojas KA, Herman PG. Optimization of computed tomography technique to demonstrate the fine structure of the lung. *Invest Radiol* 1988;23:170–175.
12. Naidich DP, Marshall CH, Gribbin C, Arams RS, McCauley DI. Low-dose computed tomography (LDCT) of the lungs: preliminary observations. *Radiology (in press)*.
13. Mayo JR, Webb WR, Gould R, et al. High-resolution CT of the lungs: an optimal approach. *Radiology* 1987;163:507–510.
14. Naidich DP. Pulmonary parenchymal high-resolution CT: to be or not to be [editorial]. *Radiology* 1989;171:22–24.
15. Zwirewich CV, Terriff B, Muller NL. High-spatial frequency (bone) algorithm improves quality of standard CT of the thorax. *AJR* 1989;153:1169–1173.
16. Grenier P, Maurice F, Musset D, Menu Y, Nahum H. Bronchiectasis: assessment by thin-section CT. *Radiology* 1986;161:95–99.
17. Genereux GP. The Fleischner lecture: computed tomography of diffuse pulmonary disease. *J Thorac Imaging* 1989;4:50–87.
18. Rosenblum LJ, Mauceri RA, Wellenstein DE, Thomas FD, Bassano DA, Raasch BN, et al. Density patterns in the normal lung as determined by computed tomography. *Radiology* 1980;137:409–416.
19. Hedlund LW, Vock P, Effmann EL. Evaluating lung density by computed tomography. *Semin Respir Med* 1983;5:76–87.
20. Hedlund LW, Anderson RF, Goulding PL, Beck JW, Effmann EL, Putman CE. Two methods for isolating the lung area of a CT scan for density information. *Radiology* 1982;144:353–357.
21. Ball WS, Wicks JD, Mettler FA. Prone-supine change in organ position: CT demonstration. *AJR* 1980;135:815–820.
22. Vock P, Salzmann C. Comparison of computed tomographic lung density with haemodynamic data of the pulmonary circulation. *Clin Radiol* 1986;37:459–464.
23. Muller NL, Staples CA, Miller RR, Abboud RT. "Density mask": an objective method to quantitate emphysema using computed tomography. *Chest* 1988;94:782–787.
24. Kinsella M, Muller NL, Abboud RT, Morrison NJ, DyBuncio A. Quantitation of emphysema by computed tomography using a "density mask" program and correlation with pulmonary function tests. *Chest* 1990;97:315–321.
25. Kalender WA, Rienmuller R, Seissler W, Behr J, Welke M, Heninz Fichte D. Measurement of pulmonary parenchymal attenuation: use of spirometric gating with quantitative CT. *Radiology* 1990;175:265–268.
26. Levi C, Gray JE, McCullough EC, Hattery RR. The unreliability of CT numbers as absolute values. *AJR* 1982;139:443–447.
27. Gur D, Drayer BP, Borovetz HS, Griffith ZBP, Hardesty RL, Wolfson SK. Dynamic computed tomography of the lung: regional ventilation measurements. *J Comput Assist Tomogr* 1979;3:749–753.
28. Herbert DL, Gur D, Shabason L, Good WF, Rinaldo JE, Snyder JV, et al. Mapping of human local pulmonary ventilation by xenon enhanced computed tomography. *J Comput Assist Tomogr* 1982;6:1088–1093.
29. Gur D, Shabason L, Borovetz HS, Herbert DL, Reece GJ, Kennedy WH, Serago C. Regional pulmonary ventilation measurements by xenon enhanced dynamic computed tomography: an update. *J Comput Assist Tomogr* 1981;5:678–683.
30. Vock P, Malanowski D, Tschaeppeler H, Kirks DR, Hedlund LW, Effmann EL. Computed tomographic lung density in children. *Invest Radiol* 1987;22:627–631.
31. Fromson BH, Denison DM. Quantitative features in the computed tomography of healthy lungs. *Thorax* 1988;43:120–126.
32. Wollmer P, Albrechtsson U, Brauer K, Eriksson L, Jonson B, Tylen U. Measurement of pulmonary density by means of x-ray computerized tomography: relation to pulmonary mechanics in normal subjects. *Chest* 1986;90:387–391.
33. Goddard PR, Nicholson EM, Laszlo G, Watt I. Computed tomography in pulmonary emphysema. *Clin Radiol* 1982;33:379–387.
34. Gould GA, Macnee W, McLean A, Warren PM, Redpath A, Best JJK, Lamb D, Flenley DC. CT measurements of lung density in life can quantitate distal airspace enlargement—an essential defining feature of human emphysema. *Am Rev Respir Dis* 1988;137:380–392.
35. Biernacki W, Gould GA, Whyte KF, Fleney DC. Pulmonary hemodynamics, gas exchange, and the severity of emphysema as assessed by quantitative CT scan in chronic bronchitis and emphysema. *Am Rev Respir Dis* 1989;139:1509–1515.
36. Kuwano K, Marsyba K, Ikeda T, Murakami J, Araki A, Nishitani H, et al. The diagnosis of mild emphysema. Correlation of computed tomography and pathology score. *Am Rev Respir Dis* 1990;141:169–178.
37. Hedlund LW, Effmann EL, Bates WM, Beck JW, Goulding PL, Putman CE. Pulmonary edema: a CT study of regional changes in lung density following oleic acid injury. *J Comput Assist Tomogr* 1982;6:939–946.
38. Hedlund LW, Vock P, Effmann EL, Lischko MM, Putman CE. Hydrostatic pulmonary edema. An analysis of lung density changes by computed tomography. *Invest Radiol* 1984;19:254–262.
39. Hedlund LW, Vock P, Effmann EL, Putman CE. Morphology of oleic acid-induced lung injury. Observations from computed tomography, specimen radiography and histology. *Invest Radiol* 1985;20:2–8.
40. Wollmer P, Jakobsson K, Albin M, Albrechtsson U, Brauer K, Eriksson L, et al. Measurement of lung density by x-ray computed tomography. Relation to lung mechanics in workers exposed to asbestos cement. *Chest* 1987;91:865–869.
41. Lee JY, Shank B, Bonfiglio P, Reid A. CT analysis of lung density changes in patients undergoing total body irradiation prior to bone marrow transplantation. *J Comput Assist Tomogr* 1984;8:885–981.
42. Weibel ER. Looking into the lung: what can it tell us? *AJR* 1979;133:1021–1031.
43. Heitzman ER. *The lung: radiologic-pathologic correlations,* 2nd ed. St Louis: Mosby, 1984.
44. Todo G, Herman PG. High-resolution computed tomography of the pig lung. *Invest Radiol* 1986;21:689–696.
45. Coddington R, Mera SL, Goddard PR, Bradfield JWB. Patholog-

ical evaluation of computed tomography images of the lungs. *J Clin Pathol* 1982;35:536–540.

46. Webb WR, Stein MG, Finkbeiner WE, Im JG, Lynch D, Gamsu G. Normal and diseased isolated lungs: high-resolution CT. *Radiology* 1988;166:81–87.

47. Meziane MA, Hruban RH, Zerhouni EA, Wheeler PS, Khouri NG, Fishman EK, Hutchins GM, Siegelman SS. High resolution CT of the lung parenchyma with pathologic correlation. *Radiographics* 1988;8:27–54.

48. Nakata H, Kimoto T, Nakayama T, Kido M, Miyazaki N, Harada S. Diffuse peripheral lung disease: evaluation by high-resolution computed tomography. *Radiology* 1985;157:181–185.

49. Bergin C, Muller NL. CT in the diagnosis of interstitial lung disease. *AJR* 1985;145:505–510.

50. Bergin CJ, Muller NL. CT of interstitial lung disease: a diagnostic approach. *AJR* 1987;148:8–15.

51. Zerhouni EA. Computed tomography of the pulmonary parenchyma. An overview. *Chest* 1989;95:901–907.

52. Bergin CJ, Coblentz CL, Chiles C, Bell DY, Castellino RA. Chronic lung diseases: specific diagnosis by using CT. *AJR* 1989;152:1183–1188.

53. Swensen SJ, Aughenbaugh GL, Brown LR. High-resolution computed tomography of the lung. *Mayo Clin Proc* 1989;64:1284–1294.

54. Colby TV, Carrington CB. Infiltrative lung disease. In: Thurlbeck WM, ed. *Pulmonary pathology.* New York: Thieme, 1988.

55. Katzenstein AL, Askin FB. *Surgical pathology of non-neoplastic lung disease,* 2nd ed. Philadelphia: WB Saunders, 1990.

56. Genereux G. The end-stage lung. Pathogenesis, pathology and radiology. *Radiology* 1975;116:279–289.

57. Naidich DP, Zerhouni EA, Hutchins GM, Genieser NB, McCauley DI, Siegelman SS. Computed tomography of the pulmonary parenchyma. Part 1. Distal air-space disease. *J Thorac Imaging* 1985;1:39–53.

58. Genereux GP. CT of acute and chronic distal air space (alveolar) disease. *Semin Roentgenol* 1984;29:211–221.

59. Naidich DP, McCauley DI, Leitman BS, et al. Computed tomography of pulmonary tuberculosis. *Contemp Issues CT* 1984;4:175–217.

60. Recavarren S, Benton L, Gall EA. The pathology of acute alveolar diseases of the lung. *Semin Roentgenol* 1967;2:22–32.

61. Itoh H, Tokunaga S, Asamoto H, Furuta M, Funamoto Y, Kitaichi M, Torizuka K. Radiologic-pathologic correlations of small lung nodules with special reference to peribronchiolar nodules. *AJR* 1978;130:223–231.

62. Miki Y, Hatabu H, Takahashi M, Sadatoh N, Kuroda Y. Case report. Computed tomography of bronchiolitis obliterans. *J Comput Assist Tomogr* 1988;12:512–514.

63. Silver SF, Muller NL, Miller RR, Lefcoe MS. Hypersensitivity pneumonitis: evaluation with CT. *Radiology* 1989;173:441–445.

64. Godwin JD, Muller NL, Takasugi JE. Pulmonary alveolar proteinosis: CT findings. *Radiology* 1988;169:609–613.

65. Newell JD, Underwood GH, Russo DJ, Bruno PP, Wilkerson GR, Black ML. Computed tomographic appearance of pulmonary alveolar proteinosis in adults. *CT* 1984;8:21–29.

66. Metzger RA, Multhern CB, Arger PH, Coleman BG, Epstein DM, Gefter WB. CT differentiation of solitary from diffuse bronchioloalveolar carcinoma. *J Comput Assist Tomogr* 1981;5:830–833.

67. Akira M, Kitatani F, Yong-Sik L, Kita N, Yamamoto S, Higashihara T, et al. Diffuse panbronchiolitis: evaluation with high-resolution CT. *Radiology* 1988;168:433–438.

68. Onitsuka H, Onitsuka SI, Yokomizo Y, Matsuura K. Case report. Computed tomography of chronic eosinophilic pneumonia. *J Comput Assist Tomogr* 1983;7:1092–1094.

69. Mayo JR, Muller NL, Road J, Sisler J, Lillington G. Chronic eosinophilic pneumonia: CT findings in 6 cases. *AJR* 1989;153:727–730.

70. Bergin CJ, Wirth RL, Berry GJ, Castellino RA. Pneumocystis carinii pneumonia: CT and HRCT observations. *J Comput Assist Tomogr* 1990;14:756–759.

71. Kuhlman JE, Kavuru M, Fishman EK, Siegelman SS. Pneumocystis carinii pneumonia: spectrum of parenchymal CT findings. *Radiology* 1990;175:711–714.

72. Begin R, Bergeron D, Samson L, Boctor M, Cantin A. CT assessment of silicosis in exposed workers. *AJR* 1987;148:509–514.

73. Bergin CJ, Muller NL, Vedal S, Chan-Yeung M. CT in silicosis: correlation with plain films and pulmonary function tests. *AJR* 1986;146:477–483.

74. Akira M, Higashihara T, Yokoyama K, Yamamoto S, Nobuhiko N, Morimoto S, et al. Radiographic type p pneumoconiosis: high-resolution CT. *Radiology* 1989;171:117–123.

75. Resnick JEJ. Is a roentgenogram of fine structures a summation image or a real picture. *Acta Radiol* 1949;32:391–397.

76. Hauser H, Gurret JP. Miliary tuberculosis associated with adrenal enlargement: CT appearance. *J Comput Assist Tomogr* 1986;10:254–256.

77. Winzelberg GG, Boller M, Sachs M, Weinberg J. CT evaluation of pulmonary alveolar microlithiasis. *J Comput Assist Tomogr* 1984;8:1029–1031.

78. Muller NL, Miller RR, Webb WR, Evans KG, Ostrow DN. Fibrosing alveolitis: CT-pathologic correlation. *Radiology* 1986;160:585–588.

79. Millar AB, Fromson B, Strickland BA, Denison DM. Computed tomography based estimates of regional gas and tissue volume of the lung in supine subjects with chronic airflow limitation or fibrosing alveolitis. *Thorax* 1986;41:932–939.

80. Muller NL, Staples CA, Miller RR, Vedal S, Thurlbeck WM, Ostrow DN. Disease activity in idiopathic pulmonary fibrosis: CT and pathologic correlation. *Radiology* 1987;165:731–734.

81. Staples CA, Muller NL, Vedal S, Abboud R, Ostrow D, Miller RR. Usual interstitial pneumonia: correlation of CT with clinical, functional, and radiologic findings. *Radiology* 1987;162:377–381.

82. Craighead JE. The pathology of asbestos-associated disease of the lungs and pleural cavities: diagnostic criteria and proposed grading schema. Report of the Pneumoconiosis Committee of the College of American Pathologists and the National Institute for Occupational Safety and Health. *Arch Pathol Lab Med* 1982;106:544–596.

83. Churg A. Nonneoplastic diseases caused by asbestosis. In: Churg A, Green FHY, eds. *Pathology of occupational lung disease.* New York: Igaku-Shoin, 1988;213–277.

84. Becklate MR. Asbestos-related diseases of the lung and other organs: their epidemiology and implications for clinical practice. *Am Rev Respir Dis* 1976;114:187–227.

85. Crystal RG, Gadek JE, Ferrans VJ, Fulmer JD, Lune BR, Hunninghake TW. Interstitial lung disease: current concepts of pathogenesis, staging and therapy. *Am J Med* 1981;70:542–568.

86. Smith DD. What is asbestosis? *Chest* 1990;98:963–964.

87. American Thoracic Society. The diagnosis of non-malignant diseases related to asbestos. *Am Rev Respir Dis* 1986;134:363–368.

88. Epstein DM, Miller WT, Bresnitz EA, Levine MS, Gefter WB. Application of ILO classification to a population without industrial exposure: findings to be differentiated from pneumoconiosis. *AJR* 1984;142:53–58.

89. Gaensler EA, Carrington CB, Coutu RE, et al. Pathologic, physiologic, and radiologic correlations in the pneumoconioses. *Ann NY Acad Sci* 1972;200:574–607.

90. Kipen HM, Lilas R, Suzuki Y, et al. Pulmonary fibrosis in asbestos insulation workers with lung cancer: a radiological and histopathological evaluation. *Br J Ind Med* 1987;44:96–100.

91. Rockoff SD, Schwartz A. Roentgenographic underestimation of early asbestosis by International Labor Organization classification. Analysis of data and probabilities. *Chest* 1988;93:1088–1091.

92. Ducatman AM, Yang WN, Forman SA. 'B-readers' and asbestos medical surveillance. *J Occup Med* 1988;30:644–647.

93. Weill H. Diagnosis of asbestos-related disease [editorial]. *Chest* 1987;91:802–803.

94. Kreel L. Computed tomography in the evaluation of pulmonary asbestosis: preliminary experience with the EMI general purpose scanner. *Acta Radiol Diagn (Stockh)* 1976;17:405–412.

95. Katz D, Kreel L. Computed tomography in pulmonary asbestosis. *Clin Radiol* 1979;30:207–213.

96. Begin R, Boctor M, Bergeron D, et al. Radiographic assessment of pleuropulmonary disease in asbestos workers: posteroanterior, four view films, and computed tomograms of the thorax *Br J Ind Med* 1984;41:373–383.

97. Aberle DR, Gamsu G, Ray CS, Feuerstein IM. Asbestos-related pleural and parenchymal fibrosis: detection with high-resolution CT. *Radiology* 1988;166:729–734.

98. Aberle DR, Gamsu G, Ray CS. High resolution CT of benign asbestos-related diseases: clinical and radiographic correlation. *AJR* 1988;151:883–891.

99. Friedman AC, Fiel SB, Fisher MS, Radecki PD, Lev-Toaff AS, Caroline DF. Asbestos-related pleural disease and asbestosis: a comparison of CT and chest radiography. *AJR* 1988;150:269–275.

100. Slozewizc S, Reznek RH, Herdman M, et al. Role of computed tomography in evaluating asbestos related lung disease. *Br J Ind Med* 1989;46:777–781.

101. Sluis-Cremer GK, Hnizdo E. Progression of irregular opacities in asbestos miners. *Br J Ind Med* 1989;46:846–852.

102. Lynch DA, Gamsu G, Aberle DR, et al. Conventional and high resolution computed tomography in the diagnosis of asbestos-related diseases. *Radiographics* 1989;9:523–551.

103. Murata K, Khan A, Herman PG. Pulmonary parenchymal disease: evaluation with high-resolution CT. *Radiology* 1989;170:629–635.

104. Gamsu G, Aberle DR, Lynch D. Computed tomography in the diagnosis of asbestos-related thoracic disease. *J Thorac Imag* 1989;4:61–67.

105. Staples CA, Gamsu G, Ray CS, Webb WR. High resolution computed tomography and lung function in asbestos-exposed workers with normal chest radiographs. *Am Rev Respir Dis* 1989;139:1502–1508.

106. Akira M, Yamamoto S, Yokoyama K, Kita N, Morinaga K, Higashihara T, Kozuka T. Asbestosis: high-resolution CT–pathologic correlation. *Radiology* 1990;176:389–394.

107. Aberle DR, Balmes JR. Computed tomography of asbestos-related pulmonary parenchymal and pleural diseases. *Clin Chest Med (in press).*

108. McLoud TC. Editorial. The use of CT in the examination of asbestos-exposed persons. *Radiology* 1988;169:862–863.

109. Gamsu G. High resolution CT in the diagnosis of asbestos-related pleuroparenchymal disease [editorial]. *Am J Ind Med* 1989;16:115–117.

110. Yoshimura H, Hatakeyama M, Otsuji H, Maeda M, Ohishi H, Uchida H, et al. Pulmonary asbestosis: CT study of subpleural curvilinear shadow (*unpublished*).

111. Arai K, Takashima T, Matsui O, Kadoya M, Kamimura R. Transient subpleural curvilinear shadow caused by pulmonary congestion. *J Comput Assist Tomogr* 1990;14:87–88.

112. Pilate I, Marcelis S, Timmerman H, Beeckman P, Osteaux MJC. Pulmonary asbestosis: CT study of subpleural curvilinear shadow [letter to the editor]. *Radiology* 1987;164:584.

113. Remy-Jardin M, Beuscart R, Sault MC, Marquette CH, Remy J. Subpleural micronodules in diffuse infiltrative lung diseases: evaluation with thin-section CT scans. *Radiology* 1990;177:133–139.

114. Frazer HA. Imaging and the law. *Diagn Imaging* 1990;12:73–78.

115. Siltzbach LE. Sarcoidosis: clinical features and management. *Med Clin North Am* 1967;51:483–502.

116. DeRemee RA. The roentgenographic staging of sarcoidosis. Historic and contemporary perspectives. *Chest* 1983;83:128–133.

117. McLoud TC, Epler GR, Gaensler EA, Burke GW, Carrington CB. A radiographic classification for sarcoidosis. Physiologic correlation. *Invest Radiol* 1982;17:129–137.

118. Berkmen YM. Radiologic aspects of intrathoracic sarcoidosis. *Semin Roentgenol* 1985;20:356–375.

119. Ellis K, Renthal G. Pulmonary sarcoidosis: roentgenographic observations in course of disease. *AJR* 1982;88:1070–1083.

120. Rockoff SD, Rohatgi PK. Unusual manifestations of thoracic sarcoidosis. *AJR* 1985;144:513–528.

121. Thomas PD, Hunninghake GW. Current concepts of the pathogenesis of sarcoidosis. *Am Rev Respir Dis* 1987;135:747–760.

122. Keogh BA, Hunninghake GW, Line BR, Crustal RG. The alveolitis of pulmonary sarcoidosis. Evaluation of natural history and alveolitis-dependent changes in lung function. *Am Rev Respir Dis* 1983;128:256–265.

123. Fajman WA, Greenwald LV, Staton G, Check IJ, Pine J, Gilman M, et al. Assessing the activity of sarcoidosis: quantitative Gallium-67 citrate imaging. *AJR* 1984;142:683–688.

124. Johnson D, Johnson SM, Harris CC, Piantadosi CA, Blinder RA, Coleman RE. Ga-67 uptake in the lung in sarcoidosis. *Radiology* 1984;150:551–555.

125. Baughman RP, Fernandez M, Bosken CH, Mantil J, Hurtubise P. Comparison of gallium-67 scanning, bronchoalveolar lavage, and serum angiotensin-converting enzyme levels in pulmonary sarcoidosis. Predicting response to therapy. *Am Rev Respir Dis* 1984;129:676–681.

126. Abe S, Munakata M, Nishimura M, Tsuneta Y, Terai T, Nakano I, et al. Gallium-67 scintigraphy, bronchoalveolar lavage and pathologic changes in patients with pulmonary sarcoidosis. *Chest* 1984;85:650–655.

127. Turner-Warwick M, McAllister W, Lawrence R, Britten A, Haslam PL. Corticosteroid treatment in pulmonary sarcoidosis: do serial lavage lymphocyte counts, serum angiotensin converting enzyme measurements, and gallium-67 scans help management? *Thorax* 1986;41:903–913.

128. Whitcomb ME, Dixon GF. Gallium scanning, bronchoalveolar lavage, and the national debt [editorial]. *Chest* 1984;85:719–721.

129. Kuhlman JE, Fishman EK, Hamper UM, Knowles M, Siegelman SS. The computed tomographic spectrum of thoracic sarcoidosis. *Radiographics* 1989;9:449–466.

130. Henry DA, Kiser P, Scheer CE, Cho SR, Tisnado J. Multiple imaging evaluation of sarcoidosis. *Radiographics* 1986;6:75–95.

131. Hamper UM, Fishman EK, Khouri NF, Johns CJ, Wang KP, Siegelman SS. Typical and atypical CTY manifestations of pulmonary sarcoidosis. *J Comput Assist Tomogr* 1986;10:928–936.

132. Muller NL, Kullnig P, Miller RR. The CT findings of pulmonary sarcoidosis: analysis of 25 patients. *AJR* 1989;152:1179–1182.

133. Muller NL, Mawson JB, Mathieson JR, Abboud R, Ostrow DN, Champion P. Sarcoidosis: correlation of extent of disease at CT with clinical, functional, and radiographic findings. *Radiology* 1989;171:613–618.

134. Bergin CJ, Bell DY, Coblentz CL, Chiles C, Gamsu G, MacIntyre NR, et al. Sarcoidosis: correlation of pulmonary parenchymal pattern at CT with results of pulmonary function tests. *Radiology* 1989;171:619–624.

135. Lynch DA, Webb WR, Gamsu G, Stulbarg M, Golden J. Computed tomography in pulmonary sarcoidosis. *J Comput Assist Tomogr* 1989;13:405–410.

136. Klein JS, Webb WR, Gamsu G, et al. Hazy increased density in diffuse lung disease: high-resolution CT. *Radiology* 1989;173(P):140.

137. Brauner MW, Grenier P, Mompoint D, Lenoir S, de Cremoux H. Pulmonary sarcoidosis: evaluation with high-resolution CT. *Radiology* 1989;172:467–471.

138. Mendelson DS, Norton K, Cohen BA, Brown LK, Rabinowitz JG. Bronchial compression: an unusual manifestation of sarcoidosis. *J Comput Assist Tomogr* 1983;7:892–894.

139. Austin JHM. Pulmonary sarcoidosis: what are we learning from CT [editorial]? *Radiology* 1989;171:603–604.

140. Battesti JP, Saumon G, Valeyre D. et al. Pulmonary sarcoidosis with an alveolar radiographic pattern. *Thorax* 1982;37:448–452.

141. Janower ML, Blennerhasset JB. Lymphangitic spread of metastatic tumor to lung. *Radiology* 1971;101:267–273.

142. Trapnel DH. The radiological appearances of lymphangitic carcinomatosa of the lung. *Thorax* 1964;19:251–260.

143. Crow J, Slavin G, Kreel L. Pulmonary metastasis: a pathologic and radiologic study. *Cancer* 1981;47:2595–2602.

144. Goldsmith HS, Bailey HD, Callahan EL, Beattie ES Jr. Pulmonary metastases from breast carcinoma. *Arch Surg* 1967;94:483–488.

145. Stein MG, Mayo J, Muller N, Aberle DR, Webb WR, Gamsu G. Pulmonary lymphangitic spread of carcinoma: appearance on CT scans. *Radiology* 1987;162:371–375.

146. Munk PL, Muller NL, Miller RR, Ostrow DN. Pulmonary lymphangitic carcinomatosis: CT and pathologic findings. *Radiology* 1988;166:705–709.

147. Bergin C, Roggli V, Coblentz C, Chiles C. The secondary pulmo-

nary lobule: normal and abnormal CT appearances. *AJR* 1988;151:21–25.

148. Ren H, Hruban RH, Kuhlman JE, Fishman EK, Wheeler PS, Zerhouni EA, Hutchins GM. Computed tomography of inflation-fixed lungs: the beaded septum sign of pulmonary metastases. *J Comput Assist Tomogr* 1989;13:411–416.

149. American Thoracic Society. Chronic bronchitis, asthma, and pulmonary emphysema—a statement by the Committee on Diagnostic Standards for Nontuberculous Respiratory Diseases. *Am Rev Respir Dis* 1962;85:762–768.

150. Snider GL, Kleinerman J, Thurlbeck WM, Bengali ZH, et al. The definition of emphysema. Report of a National Heart, Lung, and Blood Institute, Division of Lung Diseases Workshop. *Am Rev Respir Dis* 1985;132:182–185.

151. Thurlbeck WM, Simon G. Radiographic appearance of the chest in emphysema. *AJR* 1978;130:429–440.

152. Sutinen S, Christoforidis AJ, Klugh GA, Pratt PC. Roentgenologic criteria for the recognition of nonsymptomatic pulmonary emphysema: correlation between roentgenologic findings and pulmonary pathology. *Am Rev Respir Dis* 1965;91:69–76.

153. Nicklaus TM, Stowell DW, Christiansen WR, Renzetti AD Jr. The accuracy of the roentgenologic diagnosis of chronic pulmonary emphysema. *Am Rev Respir Dis* 1966;93:889–900.

154. Laws JW, Heard BE. Emphysema and the chest film: a retrospective radiological and pathological study. *Br J Radiol* 1962;35:750–761.

155. Pratt PC. Role of conventional chest radiography in diagnosis and exclusion of emphysema. *Am J Med* 1987;82:998–1006.

156. Pratt PC. Radiographic appearance of the chest in emphysema. *Invest Radiol* 1987;22:927–929.

157. Hayhurst MD, Fleney DC, McLean A, Wightman AJA, MacNee W, Wright D, et al. Diagnosis of pulmonary emphysema by computerised tomography. *Lancet* 1984;2:320–322.

158. Foster WL, Pratt PC, Roggli VL, Godwin JD, Halvorsen RA, Putman CE. Centrilobar emphysema: CT-pathologic correlation. *Radiology* 1986;159:27–32.

159. Bergin C, Muller NL, Nichols DM, Lillington G, Hogg JC, Mullen B, et al. The diagnosis of emphysema. A computed tomographic-pathologic correlation. *Am Rev Respir Dis* 1986;133:541–546.

160. Bergin CJ, Muller NL, Miller RR. CT in the qualitative assessment of emphysema. *J Thorac Imaging* 1986;1:94–103.

161. Hruban RH, Meziane MA, Zerhouni EA, Khouri NF, Fishman EK, Wheeler PS, et al. High resolution computed tomography of inflation-fixed lungs. Pathologic-radiologic correlation of centrilobular emphysema. *Am Rev Respir Dis* 1987;136:935–940.

162. Kondoh Y, Taniguchi H, Yokoyama S, Taki F, Takagi K, Satake T. Emphysematous change in chronic asthma in relation to cigarette smoking. Assessment by computed tomography. *Chest* 1990;97:845–849.

163. Flanagan JJ, Flower CDR, Dixon AK. Compensatory emphysema shown by computed tomography. *Clin Radiol* 1982;33:553–554.

164. Miller RR, Muller NL, Vedal S, Morrison NJ, Staples CA. Limitations of computed tomography in the assessment of emphysema. *Am Rev Respir Dis* 1989;139:980–983.

165. Putman CE, Godwin JD, Silverman PM, Foster WL. CT of localized lucent lung lesions. *Semin Roentgenol* 1984;19:173–188.

166. Fiore D, Biondetti PR, Satori F, Calabro F. The role of computed tomography in the evaluation of bullous lung disease. *J Comput Assist Tomogr* 1982;6:105–108.

167. Morgan MDL, Stickland B. Computed tomography in the assessment of bullous lung disease. *Br J Dis Chest* 1984;78:10–25.

168. Carr DH, Pride NB. Computed tomography in the pre-operative assessment of bullous emphysema. *Clin Radiol* 1984;35:43–45.

169. Kobayashi H, Matsuoka R, Kitamura S, Tsunoda N, Saito K. Sjogrens syndrome with multiple bullae and pulmonary nodular amyloidosis. *Chest* 1988;94:438–440.

170. Gaensler EA, Jederlinic PJ, FitzGerald MX. Patient work-up for bullectomy. *J Thorac Imaging* 1986;1:75–93.

171. Wewers MD, Casolaro A, Sellers SE, Swayze SC, McPhaul KM, Wittes JT, Crystal RG. Replacement therapy for alpha-1-antitrypsin deficiency associated with emphysema. *N Engl J Med* 1987;316:1055–1062.

172. Lacronique J, Roth C, Battesti JP, Basset F, Chretien J. Chest radiological features of pulmonary histiocytosis X: a report based on 50 adult cases. *Thorax* 1982;37:104–109.

173. Friedman PJ, Liebow AA, Sokoloff J. Eosinophilic granulmona of lung: clinical aspects of primary pulmonary histiocytosis in the adult. *Medicine* 1981;60:385–396.

174. Moore ADA, Godwin JD, Muller NL, Naidich DP, Hammar SP, Buschman DL, et al. Pulmonary histiocytosis X: comparison of radiographic and CT findings. *Radiology* 1989;172:249–254.

175. Brauner MW, Grenier P, Mouelhi MM, Mompoint D, Lenoir S. Pulmonary histiocytosis X: evaluation with high-resolution CT. *Radiology* 1989;172:255–258.

176. Eliasson AH, Phillips YY, Tenholder MF. Treatment of lymphangioleiomyomatosis. A meta-analysis. *Chest* 1989;196:1352–1355.

177. Berger JL, Shaff MI. Case Report. Pulmonary lymphangioleiomyomatosis. *J Comput Assist Tomogr* 1981;5:565–567.

178. Merchant RN, Pearson MG, Rankin RN, Morgan WKC. Case report. Computerized tomography in the diagnosis of lymphangio-leiomyomatosis. *Am Rev Respir Dis* 1985;131:295–297.

179. Rappaport DC, Weisbrod GL, Herman SJ, Chamberlain DW. Pulmonary lympohangioleiomyomatosis: high-resolution CT findings in four cases. *AJR* 1989;152:961–964.

180. Sherrier RH, Chiles C, Roggli V. Pulmonary lymphangioleiomyomatosis: CT findings. *AJR* 1989;153:937–940.

181. Aberle DR, Hansell D, Brown K, Tashkin DP. Lymphangiomyomatosis: CT, chest radiographic, and functional correlations. *Radiology* 1990;176:381–387.

182. Lenoir S, Grenier P, Brauner MW, Fiija J, Remy-Jardin M, Revel D, Cordier JF. Pulmonary lymphangiomyomatosis and tuberous sclerosis: comparison of radiographic and thin-section CT findings. *Radiology* 1990;175:329–334.

183. Muller NL, Chiles C, Kullnig P. Pulmonary lymphangiomyomatosis: Correlation of CT with radiographic and functional findings. *Radiology* 1990;175:335–339.

184. Bellamy EA, Husband JE, Blaquiere RM, Law MR. Bleomycin-related lung damage: CT evidence. *Radiology* 1985;156:155–158.

185. Mathieson JR, Mayo JR, Staples CA, Muller NL. Chronic diffuse infiltrative lung disease: comparison of diagnostic accuracy of CT versus chest radiography. *Radiology* 1989;171:111–116.

186. Sider L, Dennis L, Smith LJ, Dunn MM. CT of the lung parenchyma and the pulmonary function test. *Chest* 1987;92:406–410.

187. Sanders C, Nath PH, Bailey WC. Detection of emphysema with computed tomography. Correlation with pulmonary function tests and chest radiography. *Invest Radiol* 1988;23:262–266.

188. Sakai F, Gamsu G, Im JG, Ray CS. Pulmonary function abnormalities in patients with CT-determined emphysema. *J Comput Assist Tomogr* 1987;11:963–968.

189. Begin R, Ostiguy G, Cantin A, Bergeron D. Lung function in silica-exposed workers. A relationship to disease severity assessed by CT scan. *Chest* 1988;94:539–545.

190. Nugent KM, Peterson MW, Jolles H, Monick MM, Hunninghake GW. Correlation of chest roentgenograms with pulmonary function and bronchoalveolar lavage in interstitial lung disease. *Chest* 1989;6:1224–1228.

191. Pottrratz ST, Martin WJ. Disparities in assessment of disease activity [editorial]. *Chest* 1989;6:1222–1223.

192. Helmers RA, Hunninghake GW. Bronchoalveolar lavage in the nonimmunocompromised patients. *Chest* 1989;96:1184–1190.

193. Scott-Miller K, Smith EA, Kinsella M, et al. Lung disease associated with progressive systemic sclerosis. Assessment of interlobar variation by bronchoalveolar lavage and comparison with noninvasive evaluation of disease activity. *Am Rev Respir Dis* 1990;141:301–306.

194. Pantin CF, Valind SO, Sweatman M, et al. Measures of the inflammatory response in cryptogenic fibrosing alveolitis. *Am Rev Respir Dis* 1990;138:1234–1241.

195. Vedal S, Welsh EV, Miller RR, Muller NL. Desquamative interstitial pneumonia. Computed tomographic findings before and after treatment with corticosteroids. *Chest* 1988;93:215–217.

196. Martin K, Sagel SS, Siegel BA. Case report. Mosaic oligemia simulating pulmonary infiltrates on CT. *AJR* 1986;147:670–673.

197. Rimmer MJ, Dixon AK, Flowqer CDR, Sikora K. Bleomycin lung: computed tomographic observations. *Br J Radiol* 1985;58:1041–1045.

198. Stein MG, Demarco T, Gamsu G, Finkbeiner W, Golden JA. Computed tomography: pathologic correlation in lung disease due to tocainide. *Am Rev Respir Dis* 1988;137:458–460.

199. Wall CP, Gaensler EA, Carrington CB, Hayes JA. Comparison of transbronchial and open biopsies in chronic infiltrative lung diseases. *Am Rev Respir Dis* 1981;123:280–285.

200. Shure D. Transbronchial biopsy and needle aspiration. *Chest* 1989;95:1130–1138.

201. Wilson RK, Rechner RE, Greenberg SD, Estrada R, Stevens PM. Clinical implications of a "non-specific" transbronchial biopsy. *Am J Med* 1978;65:252–256.

202. Newman SL, Michel RP, Wang NS. Lingular biopsy: is it representative? *Am Rev Respir Dis* 1985;132:1084–1086.

203. Henschke CI, Davis SD, Auh PR, Westcott J, Berkman YM, Kazam E. Detection of bronchial abnormalities: comparison of CT and bronchoscopy. *J Comput Assist Tomogr* 1987;11:432–435.

204. Naidich DP, Sussman R, Kutcher WL, Aranda CP, Garay SM, Ettenger NA. Solitary pulmonary nodules: CT-bronchoscopic correlation. *Chest* 1988;93:595–598.

205. Gamsu G, Sostman D. Magnetic resonance imaging of the thorax. *Am Rev Respir Dis* 1989;139:254–274.

206. Cutillo AG, Morris AH, Ailon DC, Durney CH. Clinical implications of nuclear magnetic resonance lung research. *Chest* 1989;96:643–652.

207. Moore EH, Webb WR, Muller N, Sollitto R. MRI of pulmonary airspace disease: experimental model and preliminary clinical results. *AJR* 1986;146:1123–1128.

208. Vitinski S, Pearson MG, Karlik SJ, Morgan WK, Carey LS, Perkins G, et al. Differentiation of parenchymal lung disorders with *in vitro* proton nuclear magnetic resonance. *Magn Reson Med* 1986;3:120–125.

209. Cohen MD, Scales RL, Eigen H, Scott P, Tepper R, Cory DA, Smith JA. Evaluation of pulmonary parenchymal disease by magnetic resonance imaging. *Br J Radiol* 1987;60:223–230.

210. McFadden RG, Carr TJ, Wood TE. Proton magnetic resonance imaging to stage activity of interstitial lung disease. *Chest* 1987;92:31–39.

211. Moss AA. Critical reviews. Proton magnetic resonance imaging to stage activity of interstitial lung disease. *Invest Radiol* 1988;23:648–649.

212. Naidich DP, Rumancik WM, Ettenger NA, Feiner HD, Hernanz-Schulman M, Spatz EM, et al. Congenital anomalies of the lungs in adults: MR diagnosis. *AJR* 1988;151:13–19.

213. Brasch RC, Gooding CA, Lallemand DP, Wesbey GE. Work in progress. Magnetic resonance imaging of the thorax in childhood. *Radiology* 1984;150:463–467.

214. Muller NL, Gamsu G, Webb WR. Pulmonary nodules: detection using magnetic resonance and computed tomography. *Radiology* 1985;155:687–690.

215. Gutierrez FR, Glazer HS, Levitt RG, Moran JF. Case report. NMR imaging of pulmonary arteriovenous fistulae. *J Comput Assist Tomogr* 1984;8:750–752.

216. Webb WR, Gamsu G, Golden JA, Crooks LE. Case report. Nuclear magnetic resonance imaging of pulmonary arteriovenous fistula: effect of flow. *J Comput Assist Tomogr* 1984;8:155–157.

217. Ailion DC, Case TA, Blatter DD, Morris AH, Cutillo AG, Durney CH, et al. Applications of NMR spin imaging to the study of lungs. *Bull Magn Reson* 1983;6:130–139.

218. Lallemand DP, Brasch RC, Gooding CA, Wesbey GE, Higgins CB. Abstract. NMR imaging of lung parenchyma. *Magn Reson Med* 1984;1:190–191.

219. Hayes CE, Case TA, Aillon DC, Morris AH, Cutillo A, Blackburn CW, et al. Lung water quantitation by nuclear magnetic resonance imaging. *Science* 1982;216:1313–1315.

220. Huber DJ, Adams DF. Abstract. Proton NMR of acute pulmonary edema and hemorrhage. *Invest Radiol* 1984;19:S21.

221. Skalina S, Kundel HL, Wolf G, Marshall B. The effect of pulmonary edema on proton nuclear magnetic resonance relaxation times. *Invest Radiol* 1984;19:7–9.

222. Cutillo AG, Morris AH, Blatter DD, Case TA, Ailion DC, Durney CH, Johnson SA. Determination of lung water content and distribution by nuclear magnetic resonance. *J Appl Physiol* 1984;57:583–588.

223. Wexler HR, Nicholson RL, Prato FS, Carey LS, Vinitski S, Reese L. Quantitation of lung water by nuclear magnetic resonance imaging. A preliminary study. *Invest Radiol* 1985;20:583–590.

224. Schmidt HC, McNamara MT, Brasch RC, Higgins CB. Assessment of severity of experimental pulmonary edema with MRI: effect of relaxation enhancement by Gd-DTPA. *Invest Radiol* 1985;20:687–692.

225. MacLennan FM, Foster MA, Smith FW, Crosher GA. Measurement of total lung water from nuclear magnetic resonance images. *Br J Radiol* 1986;59:553–560.

226. Schmidt HC, Tsay DG, Higgins CB. Pulmonary edema: an MR study of permeability and hydrostatic types in animals. *Radiology* 1986;158:297–302.

227. Huber DJ, Kobzik L, Solorzano C, Melanson G, Adams DF. Nuclear magnetic resonance spectroscopy of acute and evolving pulmonary hemorrhage: an *in vitro* study. *Invest Radiol* 1987;22:632–637.

228. Tobler J, Levitt RG, Glazer HS, Moran J, Crouch E, Evens RG. Differentiation of proximal bronchogenic carcinoma from postobstructive lobar collapse by magnetic resonance imaging. Comparison with computed tomography. *Invest Radiol* 1987;22:538–543.

229. Glazer HS, Lee JKT, Levitt RG, Emami B, Gronemeyer S, Murphy WA. Differentiation of radiation fibrosis from recurrent pulmonary neoplasm by magnetic resonance imaging. *AJR* 1984;143:729–730.

230. Inch WR, Prato FS, Butland TS, Frei JV. Use of nuclear magnetic resonance to monitor lung injury by x-irradiation: a preliminary study. *Respir Care* 1986;31:388–394.

231. Taylor C, Sostman HD, Gore JC, Smith GJW. Proton relaxation in bleomycin-induced lung injury. *Invest Radiol* 1987;22:621–626.

232. Shioya S, Haida M, Tsuji C, Ohta Y, Yamabayashi H, Fukuzaki M, et al. Acute and repair stage characteristics of magnetic resonance relaxation times in oxygen-induced pulmonary edema. *Magn Reson Med* 1988;8:450–459.

233. Johnston PW, MacLennan FM, Simpson JG, Smith FW. Nuclear magnetic resonance imaging of pulmonary infarction and oedema in excised cadaver lungs. *Magn Reson Imaging* 1985;3:157–161.

234. Naidich DP, Weinreb JC, Schinella R. Abstract. MR imaging of the pulmonary parenchyma: comparison with CT in evaluating cadaveric lung specimens. *Radiology* 1988;169(P):301.

235. Hatabu H, Gefter WB, Kressel HY, Axel L, Lenkinski RE. Work in progress. Pulmonary vasculature: high-resolution MR imaging. *Radiology* 1989;171:391–395.

236. Edelman RR, Wentz KU, Mattle H, Zhao B, Liu C, Kim D, Laub G. Projection arteriography and venography: initial clinical results with MR. *Radiology* 1989;172:351–357.

237. Pugatch RD, Faling LJ, Robbins AH, Snider GL. Differentiation of pleural and pulmonary lesions using computed tomography. *J Comput Assist Tomogr* 1978;2:601–606.

238. Stark DD, Federle MP, Goodman PC, Podrasky AE, Webb WR. Differentiating lung abscess and empyema: radiography and computed tomography. *AJR* 1983;141:163–167.

239. Huang RM, Naidich DP, Lubat E, Schinella R, Garay SM, McCauley DI. Septic pulmonary emboli: CT-radiographic correlation. *AJR* 1989;153:41–45.

240. Mah K, Poon PY, Dyk JV, Keane T, Majesky IV, Rideout DF. Assessment of acute radiation-induced pulmonary changes using computed tomography. *J Comput Assist Tomogr* 1986;10:736–743.

241. Ikezoe J, Takashima S, Morimoto S, Kadowaki K, Takeuchi N, Yamamoto T, et al. CT appearance of acute radiation-induced injury in the lung. *AJR* 1988;150:765–770.

242. Peuchot M, Libshitz HI. Pulmonary metastatic disease: radiologic-surgical correlation. *Radiology* 1987;164:719–722.

243. Gross BH, Glazer GM, Bookstein FL. Multiple pulmonary nod-

ules detected by computed tomography: diagnostic implications. *J Comput Assist Tomogr* 1987;2:15–23.

244. Naidich DP, Tarras M, Garay SM, Birnbaum B, Rybak BJ, Schinella R. Kaposi's sarcoma. CT-radiographic correlation. *Chest* 1989;96:723–728.

245. Epler GR, Colby TV, McLoud TC, Carrington CB, Gaensler EA. Bronchiolitis obliterans organizing pneumonia. *N Engl J Med* 1985;312:152–158.

246. McLoud TC, Epler GR, Colby TV, Gaensler EA, Carrington CB. Bronchiolitis obliterans. *Radiology* 1986;159:1–8.

247. Skeens JL, Fuhrman CR, Yousem SA. Bronchiolitis obliterans in heart-lung patients: radiologic findings in 11 patients. *AJR* 1989;153:253–256.

248. Gosink BB, Friedman PJ, Liebow SE, Myers JL, Katzenstein AL. Radiographic manifestations of bronchiolitis obliterans: roentgenographic-pathologic correlation. *AJR* 1973;117:816–832.

249. Muller NL, Guerry-Force ML, Staples CA, Wright JL, Wiggs B, Coppin C, Pare P, Hogg JC. Differential diagnosis of bronchiolitis obliterans with organizing pneumonia and usual interstitial pneumonia: clinical, functional, and radiologic findings. *Radiology* 1987;162:151–156.

250. Cordier JF, Loire R, Brune J. Idiopathic bronchiolitis obliterans organizing pneumonia. Definition of characteristic clinical profiles in a series of 16 patients. *Chest* 1989;96:999–1004.

251. Muller NL, Staples CA, Miller RR. Bronchiolitis obliterans organizing pneumonia: CT features in 14 patients. *AJR* 1990;154:983–987.

252. Miki Y, Hatabu H, Takahashi M, Sadatoh N, Kuroda Y. Case report. Computed tomography of bronchiolitis obliterans. *J Comput Assist Tomogr* 1988;12:512–514.

253. Marti-Bonmati L, Perales FR, Catala F, Mata JM, Calonge E. CT findings in Swyer-James syndrome. *Radiology* 1989;172:477–480.

254. Schurawitzki H, Stiglbauer R, Graninger W, Herold C, Polzleitner D, Burghuber OC, Tscholakoff D. Interstitial lung disease in progressive systemic sclerosis: high-resolution CT versus radiography. *Radiology* 1990;176:755–759.

Chapter 9

Pleura and Chest Wall

From the outset tremendous interest has focused on the use of computed tomography (CT) to augment routine chest radiography in the evaluation of diseases affecting both the pleura and chest wall (1,2). This reflects in part the wide range of pathology that affects these areas, as well as the accepted limitations of chest radiography, especially in the assessment of complex pleural and parenchymal disease. In this chapter, the value and limitations of CT in the assessment of diffuse and focal pleural disease and chest wall lesions will be discussed and illustrated. Potential applications of magnetic resonance (MR) also will be addressed.

CT TECHNIQUE

There is no standardized technique for the evaluation of the pleura and chest wall. Each case should be considered individually with regard to number of slices, section thickness, and use of intravenous contrast material.

Posteroanterior (PA) and lateral radiographs are always obtained prior to the CT study. For most cases, standard 10-mm thick sections are sufficient to evaluate most pleural diseases. Although the use of high-resolution techniques is usually unnecessary, thin sections may be advantageous in detecting asbestos-related pleural plaques (3,80). As will be extensively illustrated, the administration of intravenous contrast can play an indispensible role, especially in differentiating between pleural and parenchymal processes (4). In cases in which the major indication for CT is evaluation of complex pleuro-parenchymal disease, a bolus of i.v. contrast should be administered preferably using a power injector, with sections obtained using dynamic incrementation, when available. This technique allows optimal visualization of parenchymal vasculature during the phase of maximum pulmonary artery and vein enhancement. In select cases, this initial sequence can be augmented by obtaining delayed images through regions of interest; sections obtained a few minutes following the bolus administration of i.v. contrast may optimize visualization of the parenchyma, specifically when the lung is consolidated or collapsed (see Chapter 1).

If the disease process is localized, thorough examination of the entire chest may be unnecessary; in these cases, contiguous sections through the region of interest should be obtained, again preferably using bolus administration of i.v. contrast media.

PLEURAL DISEASE

CT is of greatest efficacy in (a) confirming the presence of a lesion; (b) determining its precise location and extent as either primarily pulmonary or pleural; and (c) further characterizing the nature of the pathology by means of attenuation coefficients.

FIG. 1. Schematic drawing of the cross-sectional appearance, typical and atypical, of extrapleural, pleural, and peripheral parenchymal lesions. Extrapleural lesions displace the overlying parietal and visceral pleura (a), resulting in an obtuse angle between the lesion and the chest wall. Associated chest wall pathology (for example, rib erosion) helps define the lesion as extrapleural. Pleural lesions generally remain confined between the layers of the pleura and cause obtuse angles between the lesion and the chest wall (b). Pleural lesions, however, may be pedunculated (c), in which case they may prolapse into the pulmonary parenchyma, resulting in acute angles between the lesion and the chest wall. Additionally, pleural fibrosis may result in fusion of the parietal and visceral pleura (d), leading to abnormal configurations of pleural lesions and/or loculation of pleural fluid. Parenchymal lesions, if subpleural, abut the pleura (e), resulting in acute angulation. If the pleura is infiltrated (f), the result is obtuse angulation with the chest wall. Clearly, while the mechanics vary, there is considerable overlap in the cross-sectional appearance of extrapleural, pleural, and parenchymal lesions. In practical terms, all peripheral soft-tissue lesions should be biopsied, regardless of site of origin.

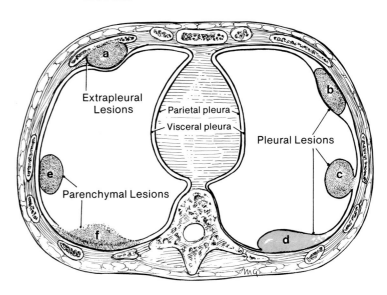

Localization

Peripheral lesions are generally classified as extrapleural, pleural, or parenchymal, and are usually characterized radiographically by the angle (either acute or obtuse) formed by the interface between the lesion and the adjacent pleura. Unfortunately, although CT is far superior to routine chest radiography in detecting the presence of pathology, there is considerable overlap in the cross-sectional appearance of these lesions, as shown in Fig. 1.

Extrapleural lesions usually displace the overlying parietal and visceral pleura, resulting in an obtuse angle between the lesion and the chest wall (Fig. 2). Associated changes, such as rib destruction or muscle infiltration,

help to confirm the site of origin as extrapleural, although these signs are often absent. Extrapleural lesions may prolapse into the adjacent lung resulting in acute angulation between the lesion and the chest wall; this is, however, uncommon.

Pleural lesions arising from the visceral or parietal pleura usually remain confined to the pleural space and have a configuration similar to that of extrapleural lesions. However, pedunculated pleural lesions, especially those arising from the visceral pleura, are an important exception (5,6). As shown in Fig. 1, these may prolapse or invaginate into the adjacent pulmonary parenchyma. If the lesion is small, the appearance will mimic a peripheral, subpleural parenchymal nodule; if the lesion is larger and broad-based, the appearance of a peduncu-

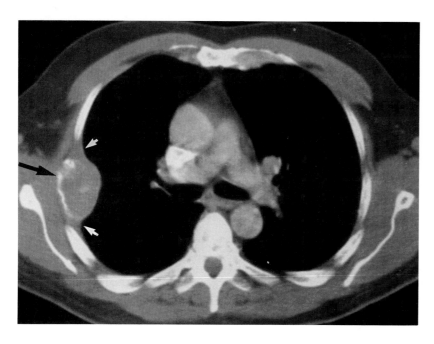

FIG. 2. Rib metastasis. CT section shows a lytic destructive rib lesion on the right side (*arrow*) associated with a large extraosseous soft-tissue component. Note obtuse angles between the lesion and the adjacent lung (*white arrows*).

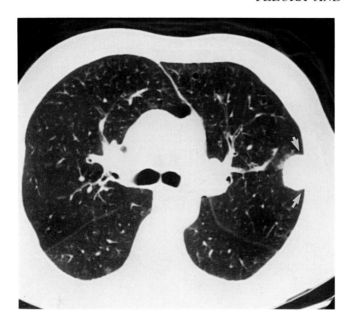

FIG. 3. Benign fibrous mesothelioma. Section through the left mid-lung shows a well-defined tumor mass on the left side, which at surgery proved to be a benign, pedunculated mesothelioma. Note acute angles between the lesion and adjacent lung, despite the pleural origin of this tumor (*arrows*).

lated pleural lesion may mimic larger intraparenchymal subpleural lesions (Fig. 3).

The cross-sectional appearance of pleural pathology, especially loculated pleural fluid collections, will also be affected by pleural adhesions along the lesion margins. Pleurodesis restricts the mobility of the pleural layers; the result may be acute angulation between the pleural lesion and/or fluid, and the adjacent chest wall (Fig. 1).

Pulmonary parenchymal lesions, when peripheral, may abut the pleura; this typically results in acute angulation between the lesion and the chest wall. However, if sufficiently large, parenchymal lesions may result in obtuse angles between the lesion and the chest wall, usually as the result of visceral and parietal pleural infiltration (Figs. 1 and 4) (7). It cannot be overemphasized that evaluation of peripheral lung lesions that only abut

pleural surfaces is extremely limited: the configuration of peripheral lung cancer in relation to the chest wall, for example, is of little use in determining whether or not there is histologic invasion of the pleura. As will be discussed in greater detail later, exclusion of tumor infiltration into the pleura or chest wall usually requires biopsy.

Another potential pitfall in differentiating parenchymal from pleural disease is the presence of fluid within pre-existing parenchymal cavities (8). As documented by Zinn et al., fluid within bullae may precisely mimic the appearance of a loculated pleural fluid collection. In fact, in select cases, differentiation may be possible only by reference to previous chest radiographs documenting the presence of prior bullous lung disease (Fig. 5).

It is apparent, therefore, that although the mechanics of pathology vary, the end result is that there may be

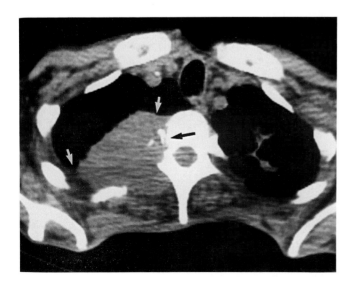

FIG. 4. Chest wall invasion: bronchogenic carcinoma. CT section through the lung apices shows a posterior lung mass on the right clearly invading both the chest wall and adjacent vertebral body (*straight arrow*). Note obtuse angles between the lesion and the adjacent lung (*white arrows*).

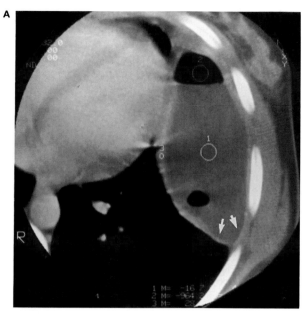
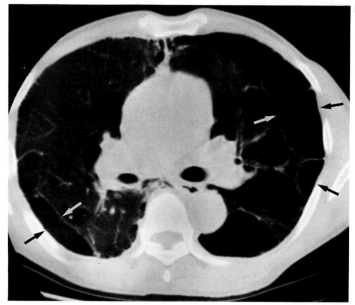

FIG. 5. A: Infected bulla. Enlargement of a CT section through the left midlung following a bolus of i.v. contrast media. A well-defined, smooth-walled, lenticular-shaped fluid collection is present on the left side, within which air can be identified. An enhancing membrane appears to surround the fluid collection (*arrows*) mimicking a split-pleura sign. Although this appearance suggests a loculated pleural fluid collection, at surgery this proved to be an infected bulla. **B:** CT section in a different patient showing characteristic appearance of numerous peripheral bullae (*arrows*). It is apparent that if any of these became fluid-filled, the appearance could precisely mimic that of loculated fluid within the pleural space (compare with A). (From Zinn et al., ref. 8, with permission.)

considerable overlap in the cross-sectional appearance of extrapleural, pleural, and peripheral subpleural parenchymal lesions (Fig. 1).

Tissue Density Characteristics

As compared with routine chest radiographs, a major value of CT is its ability to provide improved contrast resolution. This has proven to be immensely valuable in assessing pleural pathology, especially in detecting the presence of pleural fluid (9–12). Less commonly, CT may help in differentiating a pleural lipoma from a soft-tissue mass or cyst (Fig. 6) (13). Unfortunately, although CT is extremely accurate in detecting the presence of pleural fluid, CT densitometry is of no value in differentiating among the various etiologies of pleural effu-

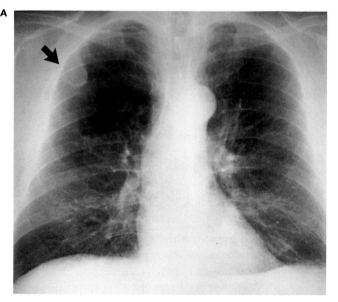
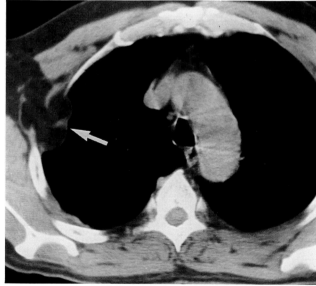

FIG. 6. Pleural/chest wall lipoma. **A:** Posteroanterior radiograph shows ill-defined soft-tissue density in the right upper lung field (*arrow*). Although suggestive of an extrapleural density, this appearance is nonspecific. **B:** CT section shows a lobular mass clearly composed of fat involving the chest wall and invaginating intrathoracically (*arrow*). This appearance is essentially pathognomonic of a lipoma.

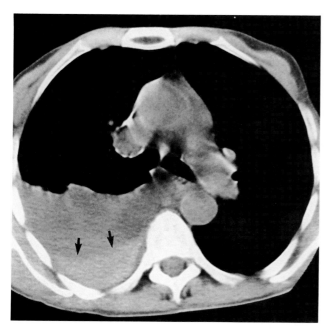

FIG. 7. Pleural hemorrhage. CT section shows a large right-sided pleural fluid collection within which there is a clear fluid-fluid level (*arrows*). The density within the dependent fluid collection measured within the range of acute hemorrhage, subsequently verified via thoracentesis.

sions. Specifically, CT numbers do not allow differentiation between transudative and exudative effusions, and cannot even be used reliably to detect chylous effusions (14–16). Rarely, in the setting of an acute bleed, CT may allow identification of hemorrhagic pleural effusions (Fig. 7). CT also easily detects the presence of even small pneumothoraces (Fig. 8). Similar limitations

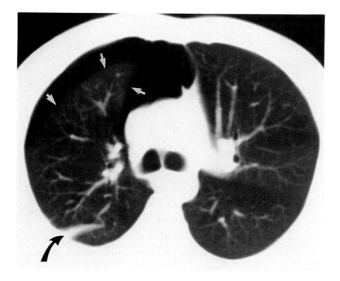

FIG. 8. Pneumothorax. CT section clearly shows an anterior pneumothorax on the right. A small quantity of fluid is present as well, loculated within the superior portion of the right major fissure (*curved arrow*). Note that although the lung is displaced posteriorly by air, the margin of the peripheral portions of the right upper lobe as well as its associated visceral pleura remains extremely smooth (*arrows*).

apply in the evaluation of soft-tissue masses, for which specific histologic diagnosis can be made only rarely. From a practical standpoint, any peripheral soft-tissue mass, regardless of its probable site of origin, should be biopsied.

PLEURAL FISSURES

The normal appearance on CT of both the pleural surfaces and pleural fissures has been described by numerous authors (3,17–23). In the series reported by Marks and Kuhns (17) utilizing 10-mm sections, pleural fissures could be identified in 84% of 23 consecutive CT scans, while in their report of 30 normal subjects also using 10-mm sections, Frija et al. (18) identified the fissures in 100% of cases.

Delineation of the pleural fissures is important because: (a) the fissures are major landmarks within the pulmonary parenchyma, allowing for accurate localization and staging of parenchymal disease; (b) lack of familiarity with the appearance of pleural fissures may lead to erroneous interpretations; and (c) accurate identification of loculated fluid within the fissures and differentiation between loculated fluid and parenchymal disease presupposes knowledge of the normal location and appearance of the fissures.

The appearance of the major fissures on CT using 10-mm sections is variable, depending on their axis relative to the plane of cross-section. Most often the major fissures can be identified as broad vascular bands within the pulmonary parenchyma (Fig. 9). They appear to be "avascular" because of diminished blood flow to the peripheral portions of the adjacent lung, especially the anterior portions of the lower lobes when patients are supine.

Occasionally the major fissures may be identified as linear structures, especially if the vertical axis of the major fissure is exactly perpendicular to the plane of the CT section (Fig. 9). Characteristically, the oblique fissures also appear as definable thin lines when imaged with 1.5-mm sections. Thin sections offer little diagnostically valuable information in most cases. In addition, potentially confusing motion artifacts have been described leading to the so-called "double-fissure" sign (24).

The oblique fissures may also appear as broad, dense bands on 10-mm sections, particularly when these are obtained through the uppermost portions of the fissures. Presumably, this appearance is due either to congestion and/or hypoinflation of the dependent portions of the upper lobes secondary to gravity. In support of this observation, this dense band appearance is more often seen when end-expiratory scans are obtained. Regardless of its cause, this appearance is a normal variant and should not be confused with pathology.

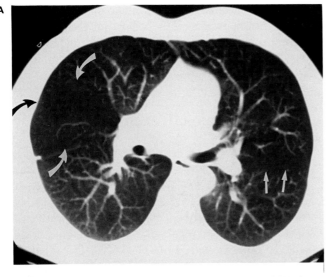

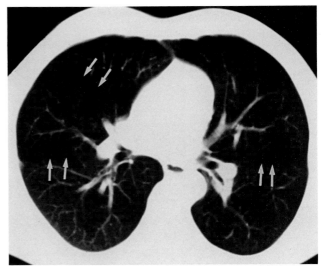

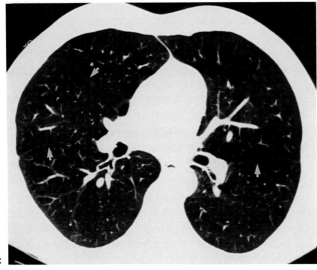

FIG. 9. Normal pleural fissures. **A,B:** 10-mm sections through the bronchus intermedius and origin of the middle lobe bronchus, respectively. The appearance on CT of the fissures is variable, depending on their axis relative to the plane of cross-section. As shown in A and B, the major fissures most often are identifiable as broad avascular bands within the pulmonary parenchyma (*straight arrows* in A and B). The minor fissure appears as a broad, triangular, or ovoid band in the anterior portion of the right lung typically located at the level of the bronchus intermedius (*curved arrows* in A). **C:** 1.5-mm thick section at the same level as shown in B. Note that using thin sections, the fissures now appear as sharply etched thin lines (*arrows*).

Unlike the major fissure, there is usually no significant variation in the appearance of the minor fissure when imaged with 10-mm sections. Characteristically, the minor fissure can be identified as a broad, frequently triangular, avascular band in the anterior portion of the right lung at the level of the bronchus intermedius (Fig. 9). Goodman et al. (19) labeled this the "right mid-lung window," and were able to identify this area of diminished vascularity in 92% of 50 patients. This appearance results from the minor fissure lying in approximately the same plane as the CT section.

The appearance of the minor fissure utilizing 1.5-mm thick sections has also been described (Fig. 10) (23–27). Berkman et al. evaluated the appearance of the minor fissure in 40 patients using 1.5-mm sections. These authors found that the minor fissure can be categorized into two major configurations (25). Depending on variations in the contour of the upper surface of the middle lobe, the minor fissure may appear either medial or lateral (Fig. 10). Furthermore, in 20% of cases the minor

fissure proved to be absent; of the remaining cases, the minor fissure proved to be incomplete in 72%. Similar findings using 1.5-mm sections have been reported by Frija et al. who also found that the minor fissure was incomplete in 76% of cases (26). Characteristically, it is the outer portion of the fissure that is incomplete. In addition to the appearances described by Berkman et al., these authors also described two additional appearances of the middle lobe, including the finding of a large opacity resulting from the CT section lying within the width of the fissure, and a circle or ring form occurring when the minor fissure is convex and oriented directly upward (Fig. 10).

Unlike the oblique fissure, familiarity with the appearance of the minor fissure using thin sections may help to differentiate the middle lobe from the right upper lobe (25,27). As emphasized by Otsuji et al., recognition of characteristic relationships between subsegmental bronchi and corresponding branches of the pulmonary artery allow confident differentiation between

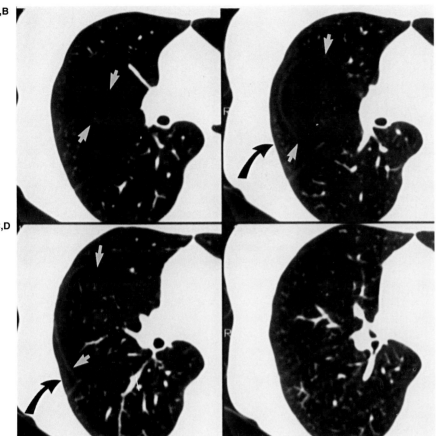
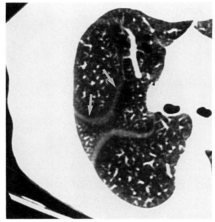

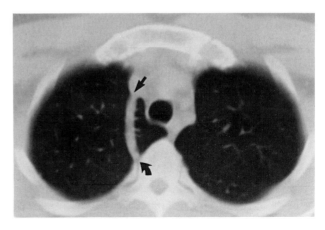

FIG. 10. Minor fissure: appearance on thin sections. **A–D:** Enlargements of sequential 1.5-mm sections through the right midlung beginning at the level of the bronchus intermedius. The minor fissure appears as a circular density that progressively enlarges until its lateral border meets the chest wall (*arrows* in A, B, and C). Note that peripherally, a portion of the anterior segment of the right upper lobe can be identified posterior and lateral to the middle lobe (*curved arrows* in B and C). **E:** 1.5-mm section in a different patient shows the middle lobe fissure to be more lateral than shown in A and B, a typical variant (*arrows*).

adjacent lobes (27). Similar observations have been made by Berkman et al. using visualization of the lowest tributary of the vein draining the anterior segment of the upper lobe. In these authors' experience, visualization of this vein allowed differentiation between the upper and middle lobe in 75% of their cases (25). Although of value in select cases, these distinctions require extremely detailed knowledge of subsegmental anatomy, which generally limits their application.

In addition to normal fissures and their variants, numerous accessory fissures also have been identified (28–31). Alterations in the normal appearance of the lung and mediastinum produced by an azygos lobe have been described (Fig. 11) (14). The azygos fissure limits the lateral margin of the azygos lobe, which frequently extends well behind the trachea and even behind the esophagus. The azygos fissure itself extends from the brachiocephalic vein anteriorly to a position beside the right posterolateral aspect of the T4 or T5 vertebral body, and is usually identifiable on CT as a thin, curved line. Other accessory fissures that have been described include: the left minor fissure, anatomically present in approximately 15% of normal lungs, separating the anterior segment of the left upper lobe from the lingula (Fig. 12) (30); a left azygos lobe, analogous to the more

typical right azygos lobe, in which there is a malpositioned left superior intercostal vein (31); the inferior accessory fissure, demarcating the medial basilar segment of the lower lobes (Fig. 13) (29); and the superior

FIG. 11. Azygos lobe. 10-mm section through the upper lobes shows characteristic appearance of an azygos fissure and lobe. Note that the fissure extends from the lateral border of the right brachiocephalic vein anteriorly (*straight arrow*) to the right superior intercostal vein, posteriorly (*curved arrow*).

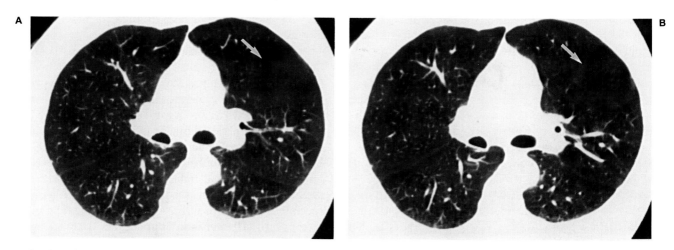

FIG. 12. Left minor fissure. **A,B:** Sequential sections through the left midlung show the presence of a left minor fissure, identifiable as a triangular area of decreased density (*arrows* in A and B), analogous to the appearance of the normal minor fissure (compare with Fig. 9A).

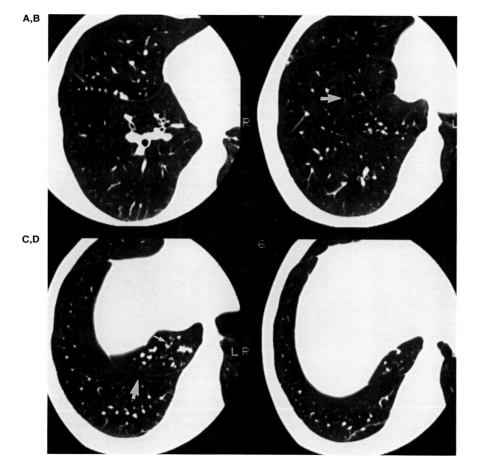

FIG. 13. Right inferior accessory fissure. **A–D:** Enlargements of sequential 1.5-mm sections through the right lung base show an accessory fissure identifiable as a thin curved line separating the medial basal segment of the right lower lobe from the remaining basilar segments (*arrows* in B and C). Note bronchiectasis limited only to the medial basal segment (*small arrow* in C).

accessory fissure, demarcating the superior segment from the remainder of the lower lobes (29). Identification of these accessory fissures rarely presents diagnostic difficulties: their recognition is of obvious benefit in identifying pathology related to the fissures (Fig. 13), including loculated interfissural fluid collections. Although identification of benign processes involving both normal and accessory fissures is generally straightforward, it is unfortunate that identification of transfissural extension of tumor is frequently more problematic, as will be discussed (32).

Another normal, frequently recognizable anatomic feature of the pleura is the inferior pulmonary ligaments (33–39). These ligaments represent reflections of the parietal pleura that extend from just below the inferior margins of the pulmonary hila caudally and posteriorly. The inferior margins of these ligaments are variable; in their most caudal extension they may assume a triangular configuration as they reflect onto the diaphragm (Fig. 14).

The CT appearance of these ligaments has been well-described (33–39). In a review of 100 CT studies using 10-mm sections, Cooper et al. identified at least one of these ligaments in 42% of cases (33). Using 10-mm sections, Rost and Proto could identify the left pulmonary ligament in 67% of cases, and the right inferior pulmo-

nary ligament in 37% of cases. Both ligaments were seen in only 27% of cases (34).

It should be emphasized that the inferior pulmonary ligaments need to be distinguished from the phrenic nerves which may run nearby (Figs. 14 and 15). As documented by Taylor et al., the left phrenic nerve generally can be identified as a 1 to 3-mm rounded structure lying adjacent to the pericardium. In this study, identification of the right phrenic nerve proved more difficult (37). Recently, the relationship between the right inferior pulmonary ligament and right phrenic nerve has been examined in detail by Berkman et al. (38). Using anatomic specimens, these authors have shown that the right inferior pulmonary ligament appears as a thin, high-attenuation line frequently identifiable above or at the level of the diaphragm, usually extending from the region of the esophagus. Although previous reports have suggested that the right inferior pulmonary ligament can be identified on CT as a thin line extending from the lateral margin of the inferior vena cava, Berkman et al. have shown that in fact this line represents the right phrenic nerve (Fig. 15) (38). Accurate identification of the inferior pulmonary ligaments is important as alterations in the normal appearance of these ligaments typically are produced by pleural effusions, pneumothoraces, and lobar collapse (35,39).

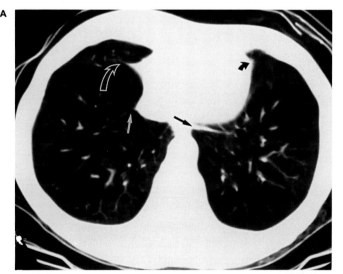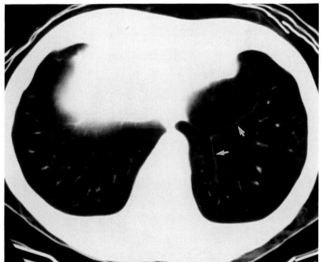

FIG. 14. Left inferior pulmonary ligament, left and right phrenic nerves. **A,B:** Sequential sections through the lung bases show characteristic appearance of the left inferior pulmonary ligament. This structure is identifiable as a broad band connected to the mediastinum just to the left of the esophagus (*black arrow* in A) prior to reflecting onto the diaphragm (*arrows* in B). The left phrenic nerve can just be identified in A, alongside the pericardium (*curved black arrow* in A). On the right side, the inferior pulmonary ligament must be differentiated from the phrenic nerves which lie adjacent to the inferior vena cava prior to reflecting onto the right hemidiaphragm (*straight white arrow* on right in A). In turn, the right phrenic nerve needs to be differentiated from the inferomedial portion of the right major fissure (*open curved white arrow* on right in A). As on the left side, the right inferior ligament generally lies adjacent to the esophagus, posterior to the inferior vena cava. In this case, the right inferior pulmonary ligament is not well seen.

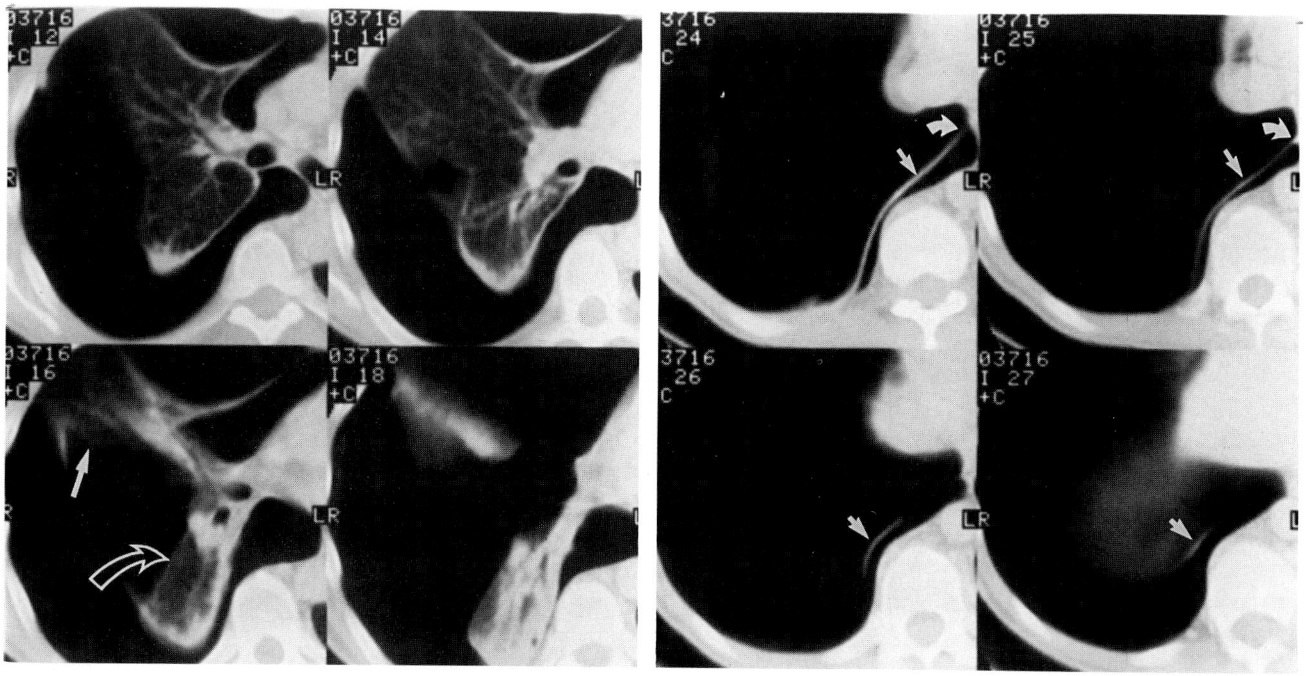

FIG. 15. Right inferior pulmonary ligament. **A–H.** Enlargements of sequential images through the right lower lung and inferior pulmonary ligament in a patient with a large right pneumothorax. The middle lobe (*arrow* in C) and right lower lobe (*curved arrow* in C) are collapsed. The right lower lobe is anchored inferiorly by the right inferior pulmonary ligament (*arrows* in E,F,G, and H). Note that medially, the inferior ligament is connected to the mediastinum behind the vena cava, in the vicinity of the esophagus (*curved arrows* in E and F).

PLEURAL FLUID: CT APPEARANCES

Free pleural fluid has a characteristic appearance when seen in cross-section. Fluid typically looks "meniscoid," occupying the posterior pleural space in patients scanned in the supine position (Fig. 16). As effusions increase in size, they conform to the natural boundaries of the pleura. Laterally, these boundaries are formed by the lateral chest wall and the lateral aspect of the oblique fissures, into which fluid may track; medially these boundaries are formed by the inferior pulmonary ligaments. In a surprising number of cases, small effusions may prove difficult to differentiate from pleural thickening and/or fibrosis. In these cases, scans obtained with the patient in the lateral decubitus position can be extremely helpful.

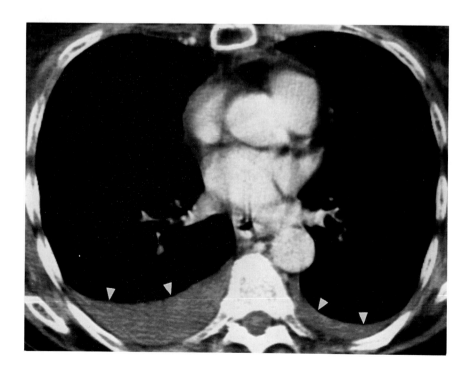

FIG. 16. Free-moving pleural fluid. CT section following bolus administration of i.v. contrast shows typical meniscoid appearance of free pleural fluid bilaterally (*arrowheads*). Note the lack of parietal and visceral pleural enhancement in this patient with transudative effusions.

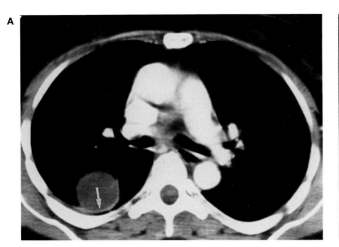
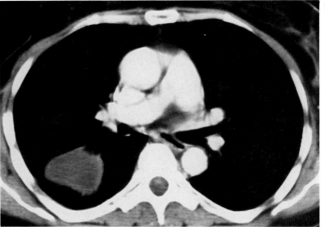

FIG. 17. Fissural pseudotumor: CT appearance. **A,B:** Sequential CT scans through the mid thorax show typical appearance of a loculated pseudotumor in the superior portion of the right major fissure. Characteristically, these conform to the expected position of the fissure, the posterior margin of which can be identified superiorly (*arrow* in A).

Fissural pseudo-tumors also are common and are usually secondary to congestive heart failure (40). Loculation of fluid within the fissures implies adherence of the pleural layers in the peripheral portions of the fissure, usually secondary to previous inflammatory disease. Identification of interlobar fluid is significant because its appearance on CT may be confused with that of an intrapulmonary lesion. The typical radiographic appearance of loculated fissural fluid has been described by Baron (40). Radiographically, fissural fluid usually is easily identified because: (a) the fluid collection lies in the expected region of the fissures; and (b) unless the fissure lies exactly perpendicular to the plane of the radiograph, the margins of the fluid collection appear hazy or poorly defined. These principles also apply to the appearance of fluid within fissures on CT (Figs. 17 and 18) (41). Fluid may collect in any portion of the fissures. If there is free communication between the lateral portion of the oblique fissure and the remainder of the pleural space, fluid will extend into the fissure and assume a characteristic triangular configuration with the apex pointing toward the hilum (Fig. 8).

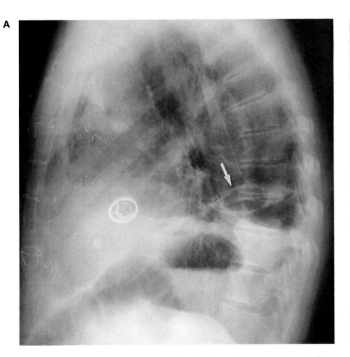
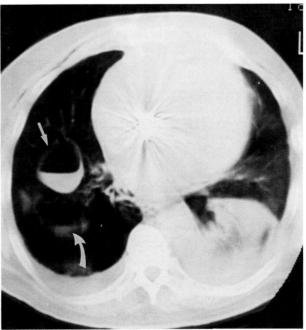

FIG. 18. Fissural pseudotumor: differentiation with parenchymal disease. **A:** Lateral chest radiograph shows an apparent cystic lesion (*arrow*) that is clearly intrafissural. **B:** CT scan through the lower lobes shows a well-defined cystic lesion with smooth walls and an air-fluid level (*straight arrow*). This appearance is characteristic of a loculated, intra-fissural hydropneumothorax. In addition, note a second air-filled level not as well defined posteriorly (*curved arrow*) also representing intra-fissural fluid. The apparent offset is due to the obliquity of the major fissure.

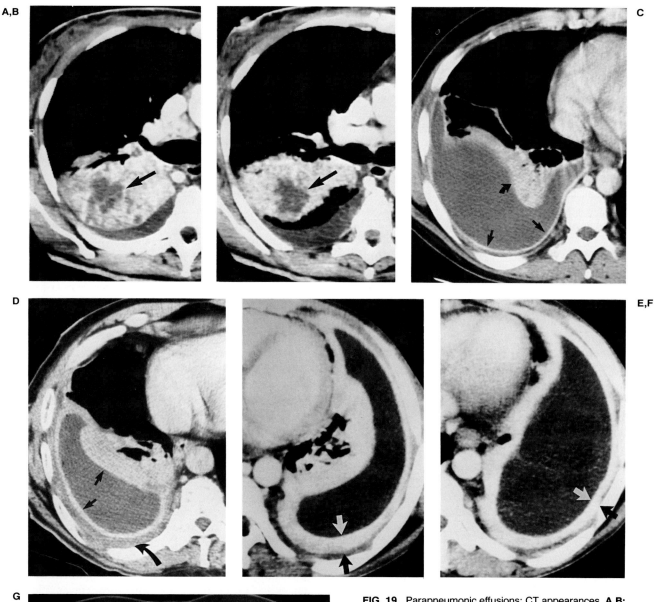

FIG. 19. Parapneumonic effusions: CT appearances. **A,B:** Exudative stage. Sequential contrast-enhanced CT scans through the right upper lobe show extensive consolidation throughout the posterior segment, within which poorly marginated areas of low density can be identified, compatible with the clinical diagnosis of a necrotizing pneumonia (*arrows* in A and B). Posteriorly, there is a moderate-sized, nonloculated pleural fluid collection. Note that there is no evidence of enhancing pleural membranes. Thoracentesis yielded clear pleural fluid without organisms. pH = 7.55; glucose = 76 mg/dL. protein = 2.4 g/dL, WBC = 2,000/mm^3, culture negative. **C:** Fibrinopurulent stage. Contrast-enhanced CT scan in a patient who had received antibiotics prior to admission. There is a moderate-sized right pleural effusion associated with volume loss and consolidation in the right lower lobe (*curved arrow*). The parietal pleura is slightly thickened and is clearly enhancing (*arrows*) (compare with A and B). Thoracentesis yielded clear pleural fluid without organisms. pH = 6.72; glucose = 22 mg/dL; pro-

The accuracy of CT to differentiate between pleural fluid and subdiaphragmatic fluid has been reviewed extensively (11,12). As will be discussed in far greater detail in Chapter 10, this differentiation is usually made on the basis of four specific CT criteria: (a) whether fluid appears central or peripheral to the line of the diaphragm, with pleural fluid lying outside; (b) displacement of the crura, indicative of pleural fluid; (c) the nature of the interface between fluid and the adjacent liver, with the liver-pleural fluid interface appearing indistinct; and (d) identification of the bare area of the liver, with pleural fluid identifiable medial to the bare area (42–44). Using these criteria, differentiation between ascites and pleural fluid should be possible in nearly all cases.

PARAPNEUMONIC EFFUSIONS/EMPYEMA

Infection within the pleural space most frequently follows primary infection in the lung from acute bacterial pneumonias, septic pulmonary emboli, and/or lung abscesses (45–47). Less frequently, infection may spread to the pleura from contiguous extrapulmonary sites, for example, from osteomyelitis of the spine, or infection in the subdiaphragmatic spaces, the liver, or the spleen. Additionally, pleural infection may be iatrogenic following needle aspiration and/or biopsy or thoracic surgery. The incidence of parapneumonic effusion is dependent to some degree on the infecting organism, ranging from about 10% for pneumonias caused by Streptococcus pneumoniae to over 50% for those caused by Staphylococcus pyogenes (46).

Regardless of the infecting organism, the natural history of empyemas may be predicted. Three stages in the development of empyema have been described, each of which is pathophysiologically and therapeutically distinct (48).

Stage 1: Exudative. In the exudative stage, generally an underlying pneumonic process causes inflammation of the visceral pleura. This results in the accumulation of thin, uninfected pleural fluid, probably secondary to increased capillary permeability, with resultant protein loss. A thoracentesis at this stage reveals sterile fluid, with a pH of >7.30, a glucose concentration > 60 mg/dL, and only a small number of polymorphonuclear leukocytes (PMNs) present (45–47). Such uncomplicated parapneumonic effusions resolve without drainage provided that the underlying cause of infection is adequately treated with appropriate antibiotics (Fig. 19) (45).

Stage 2: Fibrinopurulent. In this stage, large numbers of PMNs and bacteria accumulate in the pleural space, and sheets of fibrin are deposited over the visceral and parietal pleura. As a consequence, there is a progressive tendency toward fluid loculation; fluid resorption is impaired, presumably because of decreased lymphatic drainage (Fig. 19). If the underlying infection is not adequately treated, the pleural fluid becomes infected. Furthermore, there is a tendency for progressive thickening of the extrapleural subcostal tissues to develop as well, presumably secondary to spread of infection and edema to the adjacent chest wall tissues (Fig. 19).

A thoracentesis performed at this stage shows a tendency toward an increasing white blood cell count, decreasing glucose levels, and a decreased pH. Appropriate therapy is controversial. In most centers, complicated parapneumonic effusions are treated with immediate closed tube drainage based on the following findings: (a) gross pus; (b) organisms identified by gram staining; (c) pH < 7.10; and (d) glucose < 40 mg/dL (45–47). The results of a thoracentesis are usually considered indeterminate when the pH is between 7.10 and 7.29; in this setting, repeat thoracentesis within 24 to 48 hr is usually indicated.

It should be emphasized that the need for drainage of uninfected pleural fluid has been questioned (49,50). Berger and Morganroth retrospectively evaluated the clinical course of 62 patients with complicated parapneumonic effusions and found no significant differences in duration of hospitalization, fever, elevated

---

tein = 5.4 g/dL; LDH = 518 I.U.; WBC = 3,400/mm³ with 70% polymorphonuclear leukocytes. This patient was subsequently successfully treated with closed-tube drainage. **D:** Fibrinopurulent stage. Contrast-enhanced CT scan in a different patient than shown in A and B and C. A loculated pleural effusion is present on the right side compressing the adjacent right lower lobe. There is marked thickening of both the visceral and parietal pleura (*arrows*). In addition, there is considerable thickening of the extrapleural subcostal tissues, and increased attenuation of the extrapleural fat (*curved arrow*), presumably secondary to spread of infection and/or edema to the adjacent chest wall tissues. **E,F:** Organizing phase. Enlargements of sequential contrast-enhanced CT sections through the left lower thorax show a large, loculated pleural fluid collection causing compression atelectasis of the left lower lobe. Note that the pleural surfaces are markedly thickened (*arrows* in E and F). In this case there is only minimal distortion of the extrapleural soft tissues. These findings are compatible with a chronic empyema and with formation of an inelastic pleural peel. Pleural biopsy confirmed the presence of granulomas; pleural fluid culture confirmed the etiology as tuberculous. **G:** Late organizing stage. Non–contrast-enhanced CT scan in a patient with a history of prior tuberculous empyemas. There is extensive pleural calcification bilaterally, associated with expansion of the extrapleural fat (*arrows*). Despite the longstanding nature of these changes, note that there is a small pocket of residual loculated fluid in the right pleural space (*curved arrow*). This fluid represents a potential source of reactivation that can result in either a bronchopleural fistula or cold chest wall abscess (empyema necessitatis) developing even years following treatment.

blood counts, i.v. antibiotic therapy, or the time needed for roentgenographic resolution in those patients treated solely with antibiotics as compared with those treated with immediate pleural drainage (49). As will be discussed in greater detail later, there is also considerable controversy over the indications for closed versus open pleural drainage in patients with documented empyemas (50–52).

Stage 3: Organizing. In this stage, there is an ingrowth of fibroblasts along the fibrin sheets lining the visceral and parietal pleura. The end result is pleural fibrosis, which acts as an inelastic membrane trapping the adjacent lung (45,46). Progression from the fibrinopurulent to the organizing stage may be quite rapid, occasionally occurring in the course of therapy with closed pleural tube drainage. In most cases, however, the organizing phase typically occurs within two to three weeks after initial pleural fluid formation. Eventually, especially if the infection is inadequately treated, the pleura may calcify, appearing initially as small, punctate foci involving both the visceral and parietal pleura, eventually progressing to form a calcified rind of pleura (Fig. 19). Clinically, this most often occurs from tuberculous empyema, and it was particularly common in the past following pneumothorax therapy. Whatever the etiology, with the formation of a fibrothorax there is contraction of the involved hemithorax and an expansion of the extrapleural fat. The underlying lung can no longer expand, necessitating decortication. Expansion of the extrapleural fat is especially characteristic, and may be accompanied by periosteal changes in the adjacent ribs.

As documented by Schmitt et al., despite extensive pleural calcification, residual pleural fluid may be identified in a surprisingly high percentage of cases, especially when evaluated by CT (Fig. 19) (53). In their study of 140 patients with calcification of both the parietal and visceral pleura, these authors showed persistent pleural effusions in 22 (15%) of cases. This finding is especially important given the propensity for residual infection to result in either a bronchopleural fistula or chest wall infection (empyema necessitatis) (54). Similar findings have been reported for tuberculous empyemas (55,56).

The radiologic evaluation of complex pleuroparenchymal disease is limited. Although chest radiographs can identify the presence of free pleural fluid, identifying loculated fluid is frequently problematic. Furthermore, although radiographic signs for differentiating abscesses from empyemas have been described, they are usually contingent on the presence of air, usually secondary to communication with adjacent airways (57).

CT Evaluation of Complex Pleuro-parenchymal Disease

CT has been documented to be of considerable value in assessing all aspects of complex pleuro-parenchymal disease (58–63). In our experience, CT has been of greatest value in: (a) differentiation of pleural from parenchymal disease; (b) characterization of underlying parenchymal disease, including identification of necrotizing pneumonias, lung abscesses, and pulmonary infarcts; (c) characterization of pleural fluid as either free or loculated, as well as characterization of the appearance of the pleural membranes themselves; and (d) assessment and guidance of therapy.

It cannot be overemphasized that optimal evaluation of complex pleuro-parenchymal disease requires the use of a bolus of intravenous contrast media. Besides allowing precise localization of fluid collections, intravenous contrast media may enhance both pleural membranes, especially when inflamed, and adjacent lung tissue. In most cases in which there is suppurative lung disease, characteristic patterns of enhancement may be identified, allowing more precise determination of the nature and extent of underlying lung disease.

Differentiation of Pleural from Parenchymal Disease

The role of CT in differentiating pleural from parenchymal disease has been well established (58–62). Stark

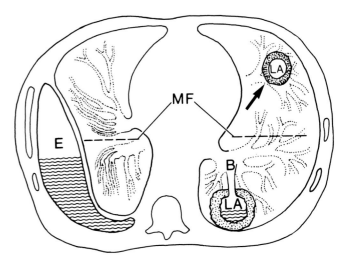

FIG. 20. CT differentiation between empyema and lung abscess. Empyemas (E) typically appear lenticular in shape with a smooth wall, conform to the shape of the chest wall, and, if sufficiently large, cause compression of the adjacent lung with displacement of vessels and airways. Unlike infected bullae, empyemas may extend past the margins of the adjacent major fissure (MF). In distinction, lung abscesses (LA) lie within the substance of the lung. Initially, lung abscesses are smooth walled, and prior to communication either with an airway or the pleural space, contain no air (*arrow*). At this stage, administration of i.v. contrast may be invaluable due to marked enhancement of the abscess wall. Later, after communication with an adjacent bronchus (B), abscesses become thick walled and irregular. Even at this stage, however, abscesses generally cause little displacement of surrounding structures within the lung. Although as drawn lung abscesses appear to form acute angles with the adjacent pleura and chest wall, in fact, in our experience, absence of this sign is unreliable.

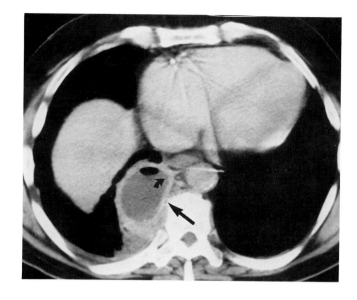

FIG. 21. Lung abscess vs. empyema: limitation in CT diagnosis. Contrast-enhanced CT section through the lower lobes shows a well-defined, smooth-walled fluid collection with a small air-fluid level within marginating the posterior mediastinum on the right (*arrow*). Despite the suggestion of a "split-pleura" sign (*curved arrow*) and the appearance of oblique angles along the margins of this lesion, at surgery this proved to be a thick-walled lung abscess associated with adjacent pleural thickening but without evidence of an empyema.

et al. reported a retrospective review of 70 inflammatory thoracic lesions where CT alone was able to differentiate lung abscesses from empyemas in 100% of cases (61). In these authors' experience, lung abscesses characteristically appear spherical with an irregularly thick wall and cause little compression of the adjacent pulmonary parenchyma. By comparison, empyemas are usually lenticular with a smooth wall, conform to the shape of the chest wall, and, if sufficiently large, cause compression of the adjacent lung. Unfortunately, not all cases fall into such easily classifiable subgroups: in our experience, in a small but significant percentage of cases, even using strict CT criteria, differentiation between lung abscesses and empyemas may be difficult (Figs. 20–22). In select cases, of course, both lung abscesses and empyemas may co-exist, further complicating interpretation (Fig. 22). In fact, this differentiation may even prove difficult at surgery. In addition to occasional cases

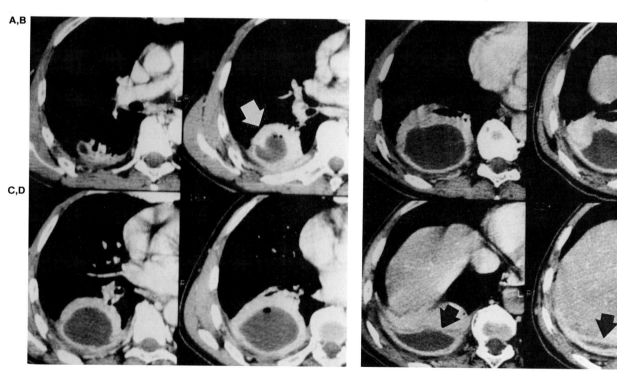

FIG. 22. CT differentiation: lung abscess vs. empyema. **A–H:** Enlargements of sequential contrast-enhanced CT sections through the right lung show findings suggestive of both a lung abscess and an empyema. A smooth-walled, lobular fluid collection is clearly present within the lung (*arrow* in B), corresponding to a lung abscess. However, inferiorly, the shape of this fluid collection becomes increasingly lenticular, assuming an unequivocally pleural configuration at the lung base (*arrows* in G and H). In this case, a lung abscess presumably has communicated with the pleural space resulting in a co-existent empyema. It is apparent that in select cases, differentiation between these entities with CT may be extremely difficult.

in which empyemas and lung abscesses appear to share similar characteristics, fluid within pre-existing pulmonary cavities also may pose problems. As documented by Zinn et al., even the split-pleura sign may be mislead-

ing, as fluid within a bulla may have an identical appearance (Fig. 5) (8). As noted previously, in difficult cases administration of a bolus of i.v. contrast medium may be of value in complicated cases (Fig. 23) (4,61).

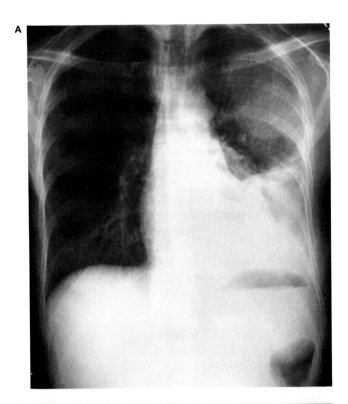

FIG. 23. Pleural vs. parenchymal disease: the role of i.v. contrast enhancement. **A:** Posteroanterior radiograph shows nonspecific increased density throughout the left lung field, especially inferiorly. On the basis of this radiograph it is difficult to differentiate pleural from parenchymal disease. **B,C:** Sequential non–contrast-enhanced CT sections through the lower lung fields show diffuse densities within the left hemithorax. Again, differentiation between pleural and parenchymal disease is difficult. **D,E:** Sequential CT sections through the lower lung fields at precisely the same levels as shown in B and C, following a bolus of i.v. contrast media. Two separate loculated pleural fluid collections are now easily identified (*arrows in D and E*). It is apparent that i.v. contrast administration dramatically improves identification of loculated fluid collections, allowing more precise therapeutic intervention.

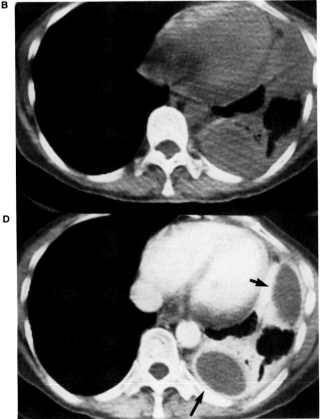
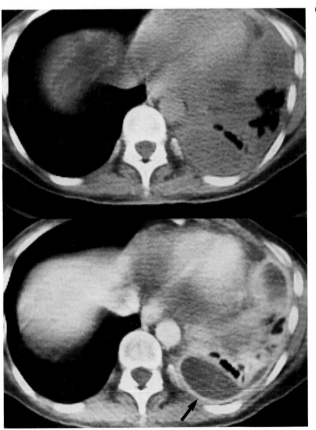

Characterization of Underlying Parenchymal Disease

In addition to differentiating pleural from parenchymal pathology, CT offers a unique opportunity to characterize lung disease. Given the spectrum of potential parenchymal causes of parapneumonic effusions, identification of the underlying disease process may have both prognostic and therapeutic value.

In our experience, CT has been most useful in identifying lung abscesses. Lung abscesses are part of a spectrum of pulmonary suppurative processes characterized by necrosis and cavitation, most commonly associated with Staphylococcus aureus, Pseudomonas aeruginosa, Klebsiella pneumoniae, and anaerobes (64). The most common pathogenic mechanisms in their development are aspiration of oral flora, necrosis within an antecedent pneumonia, bronchial obstruction, septic emboli, and penetrating trauma. The necrosis and cavitation that frequently are associated with these infections tend to take several forms. Development of multiple small areas of necrosis and/or cavitation within a larger area of necrosis is generally termed necrotizing pneumonitis

(64). By comparison, a lung abscess is characterized by a dominant focus of suppuration surrounded by a containing wall composed of well-vascularized fibrous and granulation tissue (Fig. 20), characteristically supplied by hypertrophied bronchial arteries. This accounts for the association between lung abscesses and hemoptysis. Initially self-contained, with time communication is eventually established with nearby airways or the adjacent pleural space into which the abscess contents are expelled. Rarely, these infections lead to pulmonary gangrene characterized by still more extensive necrosis with resultant sloughing of lung tissue. As previously discussed, all these manifestations of pulmonary suppuration are frequently accompanied by parapneumonic effusions or empyema.

Each of these forms of suppurative lung disease have characteristic CT appearances. Lung abscesses are easily recognized as homogeneous areas of low density surrounded by a markedly enhancing wall usually associated with a smooth inner contour (Fig. 24). Due to the presence of hypertrophied bronchial arteries, the wall of most lung abscesses tends to be extremely hypervascular

A,B

C,D

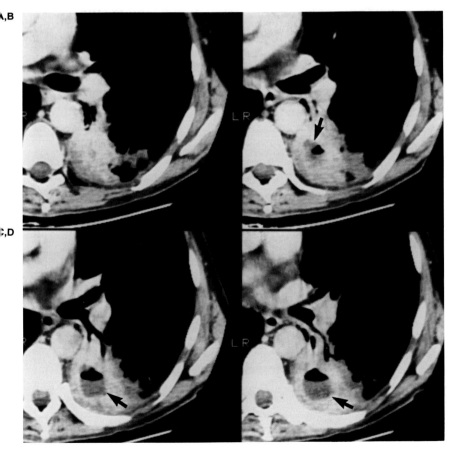

FIG. 24. Lung abscess: CT evaluation. **A–D.** Enlargements of sequential contrast-enhanced scans through the left lower lobe in a patient with a documented lung abscess. Although commonly thought of as isolated parenchymal lesions, in fact, lung abscesses typically begin in areas of consolidated lung as discrete, well-defined, smooth-walled lesions that only later become irregular in shape following communication with either adjacent airways or the pleural space. In this case, a lung abscess is easily identified as a sharply marginated area of fluid with a markedly enhancing wall within a consolidated and collapsed left lower lobe (*arrows* in B,C, and D).

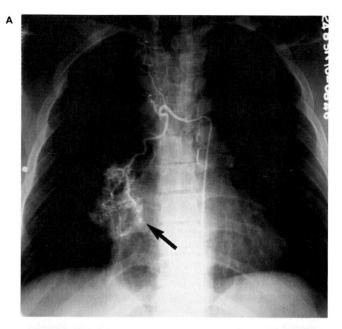

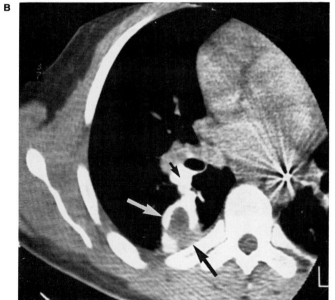

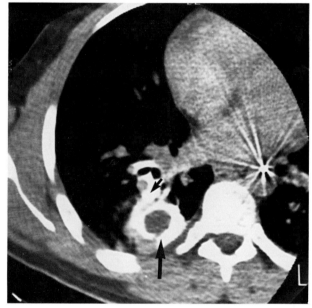

FIG. 25. Lung abscess: CT demonstration of hypertrophied bronchial arteries. **A:** Posteroanterior radiograph obtained following catheterization of the right bronchial artery. A focal area of hypermia can be identified on the right, associated with considerable hypertrophy of the distal bronchial arteries (*arrow*). **B,C:** Enlargements of sequential sections through the right lower lobe in the same patient. In this case, CT scans were obtained with the catheter still in place within the right bronchial artery, using a slow drip infusion of i.v. contrast media. Hypertrophied bronchial arteries can be identified within the right hilum (*small arrows* in B and C) leading to a well-defined, smooth-walled fluid collection in the right lower lobe (*large arrow*). Note that the wall of this lesion is dramatically enhancing, consistent with a bronchial arterial blood supply. Surgically documented lung abscess.

(Fig. 25). For this reason, optimal evaluation of lung abscesses is accomplished using a bolus injection of i.v. contrast, optimally timed to coincide with the early arterial phase of enhancement (Fig. 26). Following communication with the pleural space or adjacent airways, lung abscesses cavitate; at this time their walls become thick and irregular (Fig. 27). In contrast, necrotizing pneumonitis is characterized by multiple, poorly defined foci of low density, unassociated with enhancing margins (Fig. 28). When extensive, this appearance merges with pulmonary gangrene (Fig. 29). Although in typical cases

differentiation between patients with lung abscesses and necrotizing pneumonitis is not associated with significant differences in therapy, this differentiation is of importance in those cases for which percutaneous drainage of lung abscesses may be considered (65). CT may also be valuable in detecting complications that may occur within abscesses, including the presence of intracavitary fungus balls (see Fig. 40, Chapter 7). It should be noted that although cavitary lung neoplasms may mimic the appearance of a lung abscess, in most cases there is only minimal enhancement of the tumor wall as compared

A

B

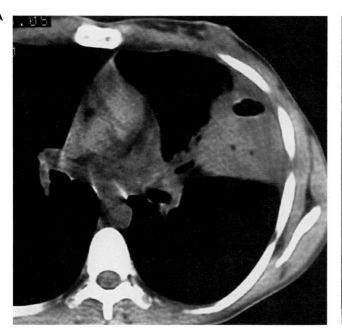
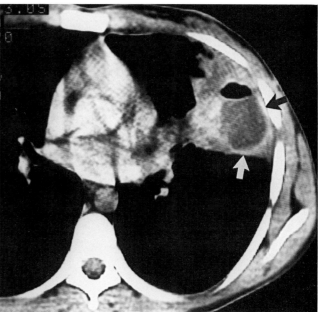

FIG. 26. Lung abscess: the value of contrast enhancement. **A,B:** Enlargements of identical CT sections obtained pre and postadministration of a bolus of i.v. contrast media, respectively. Prior to contrast administration, increased density is apparent in the lingula within which an air-fluid level can be identified. Following contrast administration, a well-defined, sharply marginated fluid collection can be identified with a markedly enhancing wall (*arrows*). This constellation of CT findings is characteristic of lung abscesses.

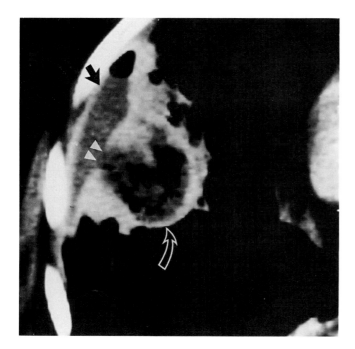

FIG. 27. Lung abscess: communication with the pleural space. Enlargement of a contrast-enhanced CT section through the right mid-lung shows a typical lung abscess (*curved arrow*). In this case, the abscess is beginning to communicate with the adjacent pleural space (*arrowheads*), within which a small, loculated pleural fluid collection is beginning to form (*straight arrow*). Note the presence of air within both the pleural fluid collection and the abscess. (Case courtesy of Peter Nardi, M.D., Brooklyn, NY.)

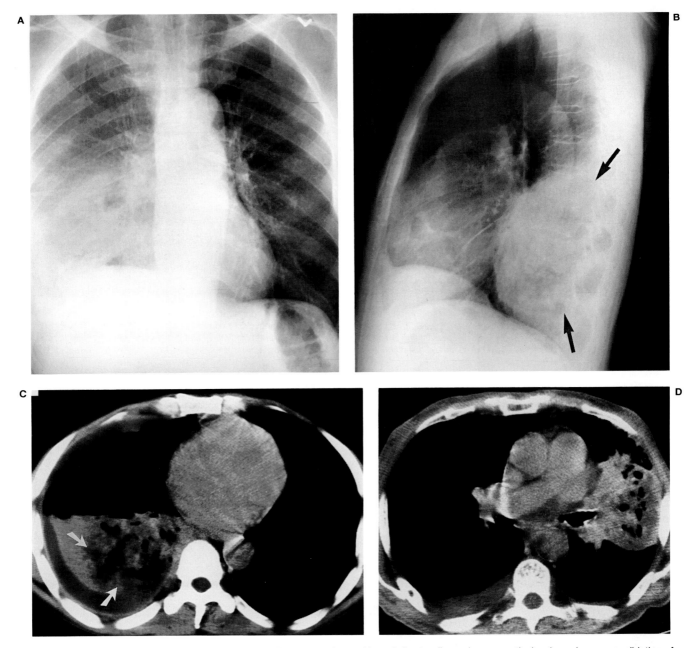

FIG. 28. Necrotizing pneumonitis: CT evaluation. **A,B:** Posteroanterior and lateral chest radiographs, respectively, show dense consolidation of the right lower lung. The appearance on the lateral film suggests the possibility of a loculated pleural fluid collection or empyema (*arrows*). **C:** Contrast-enhanced CT section through the right lower lung field shows extensive consolidation of the entire right lower lobe, associated with a moderate-sized pleural fluid collection. As compared with lung abscesses, necrotizing pneumonias appear as poorly marginated areas of low density and pockets of air without a well-defined enhancing membrane (*arrows*). **D:** Contrast-enhanced CT section in another patient with a proven necrotizing pneumonia. This appearance is identical to that shown in C. Differentiation between abscesses and necrotizing pneumonias may have therapeutic implications, especially for those cases in which percutaneous drainage of lung abscesses may be considered.

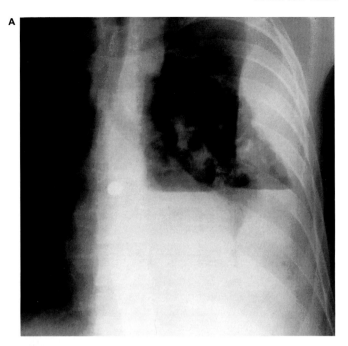

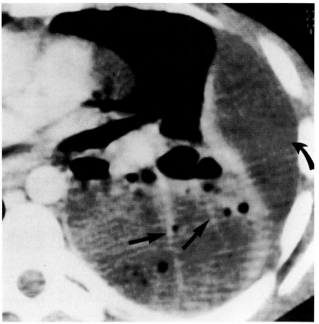

FIG. 29. Pulmonary gangrene. **A:** Posteroanterior radiograph shows apparent cavitation throughout the left lung associated with a large air-fluid level, and evidence of loculated pleural fluid, superiorly. **B:** Enlargement of a contrast-enhanced CT section through the left midlung shows that the entire left lower lobe has liquefied. Note that a few remaining vessels can be identified (*arrows*) confirming that this in fact represents lung tissue. In addition, there is an associated loculated pleural fluid collection on the left (*curved arrow*). Extensive necrosis of the entire left lower lobe was subsequently documented at surgery.

with lung abscesses, especially in squamous cell carcinomas (66). Finally, in select cases, in our experience it is even possible to identify pulmonary infarcts, identifiable as peripheral, poorly marginated, triangular areas of low density with the base oriented against the pleura (Fig. 30). Obviously, identification of pulmonary infarcts distinct from routine lung abscesses or pneumonias has clear diagnostic implications.

Characterization of Pleural Pathology

Although there are no pathognomonic CT signs to diagnose empyema, some degree of correlation has been noted between CT appearances and the nature of the underlying pleural fluid. In a retrospective evaluation of 48 patients with pleural effusions who had a sono-

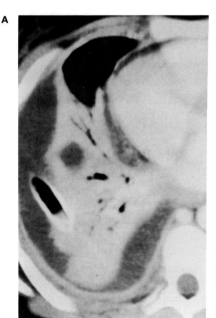

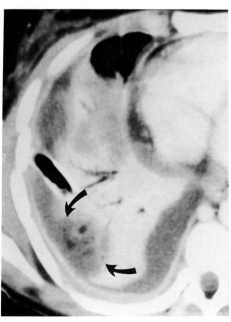

FIG. 30. Pulmonary infarct. **A,B:** Enlargements of contrast-enhanced CT sections through the right lung base show extensive consolidation and volume loss within the right middle and lower lobes associated with a loculated pleural fluid collection. A pleural tube is present as well. Note that within the right lower lobe a peripheral, triangular area of low density can be identified (*arrows*), with the base oriented against the visceral pleura. This appearance should suggest the possibility of pulmonary infarction, in this case subsequently confirmed by pulmonary angiography (not shown).

graphically directed thoracentesis, Himmelman and Callen found a significant correlation between pleural fluid loculation and exudative pleural fluid chemistries. In addition, patients with loculated effusions tended to have larger effusions, longer hospitalizations, and more frequently required tube drainage (67). Seven of nine empyemas (78%) and ten of 28 exudates (36%) were loculated. In 30% of cases pleural fluid loculation was identified only by CT or sonography. Lung cavitation was seen in 10% of cases, while pleural gas was identified by CT in 8%. None of these findings was noted in any patient with a transudative effusion.

More recently, empyemas have been correlated with the appearance of the parietal pleura following a bolus of i.v. contrast media. In a retrospective analysis of 35 patients with documented thoracic empyema, 30 patients with malignant pleural effusions, and 20 patients with transudative effusions, Waite et al. found that enhancement of the parietal pleura was present in 96% of 25 patients with empyema who underwent contrast-enhanced CT scans, while 86% showed thickening of the parietal pleura, 60% showed thickening of the extrapleural subcostal tissues, and 35% showed increased attenuation of the extrapleural fat (68). Identification of expansion and edema of this fat usually is easily recognized in patients with empyema (Fig. 19). In distinction, none of these findings were present in the 20 patients with transudative effusions. Although 27% of patients with malignant effusions showed findings similar to those with empyemas, many of these patients were evaluated following sclerotherapy. Furthermore, in this same study, some degree of correlation was also noted between both the thickness of the parietal pleura and the extent of pleural enhancement with the stage of empyema. Of 14 patients with complicated late Stage 2 parapneumonic effusions, the thickness of the parietal pleura and extrapleural tissues averaged 3 and 3.5 mm, respectively, while in eight patients requiring decortication, the average thickness of these layers was 4 and 4.5 mm, respectively (68). It should be emphasized that Himmelman and Callen reported pleural enhancement in only 2% of their cases, although these authors fail to specify their method of contrast administration (67).

Although the thickness of the parietal pleura appears to correlate with the stage of empyema, there is little correlation between this appearance and the ability to predict which patients ultimately will require decortication. In a prospective study of serial CT scans in 10 patients following radiologic catheter drainage of empyemas, Neff et al. found that although the pleura was noticeably thickened four weeks following catheter removal in all patients, at 12 weeks the pleura was essentially normal in four patients, and showed only minimal or mild residual pleural thickening in the remainder (69).

Assessment and Guidance of Therapy

CT is of proven efficacy for assessing the response of patients to therapy. By identifying areas of loculated fluid, CT can be used to guide the appropriate placement of chest tubes (Fig. 23). Although similar information may be obtained from a sinogram performed at the time of thoracentesis, sinograms do not provide any information concerning the nature of underlying parenchymal disease or associated chest wall pathology. Additionally, sinograms are of little value in disclosing the presence of multiple loculations, as frequently occurs in larger effusions. In patients with chest tubes CT can be especially valuable by disclosing chest tubes inadvertently placed within the major fissures or within the lungs, as well as those inadequately positioned to ensure proper drainage (Fig. 31) (70,71). CT can help detect more serious complications of chest tube placement, including significant chest wall hemorrhage (Fig. 32). As documented by Stark et al., in a study of 26 patients with tube thoracostomies for treatment of empyema, malpositioned tubes were identified on frontal radiographs in only one of 21 patients while all were identified by CT (70). In addition to assessing the adequacy of chest tube placement, CT has also been proven effective in identifying residual changes caused by previous pleural tubes. CT may play an especially important role in the evaluation of patients who have undergone surgical therapy including thoracoplasties (Fig. 33), open drainage procedures including Eloesser window thoracostomies (Fig. 34), and even findings in patients who have been treated with oleothoraces and/or plombage (72–74).

Recently, considerable attention has been focused on radiologically guided percutaneous catheter drainage (PCD) of pleural fluid collections and pneumothoraces in both untreated and previously treated patients (75–80). Typically, these procedures are performed utilizing fluoroscopy, ultrasound, or CT, with comparable results (Fig. 35). Merriam et al. using a combination of imaging modalities retrospectively reviewed the outcome of percutaneous catheter drainage of pleural fluid collections in 18 patients, including 16 patients with documented empyemas, nine of whom had previous unsuccessful surgical chest tube drainage (77). Twelve (80%) of 15 patients who had an adequate trial of guided drainage were cured. VanSonnenberg et al. reported similar results using both CT and ultrasound to drain 17 patients in whom previous conventional chest tube drainage had proven unsuccessful; in this study 15 (88%) of patients were successfully drained, averting the need for open drainage (76). Using fluoroscopic guidance, Westcott successfully drained 11 of 12 patients with documented empyemas; in five of these patients, PCD was used as the sole means of drainage (75). Although most

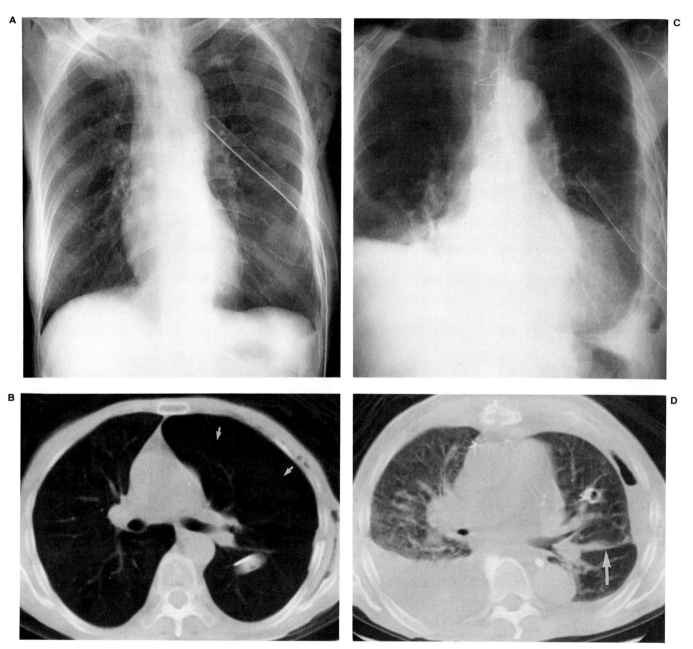

FIG. 31. Malpositioned chest tubes: CT evaluation. **A:** Posteroanterior radiograph shows a chest tube on the left side in a patient presenting with a pneumothorax. The presence of subcutaneous air limits evaluation of the adequacy of therapy. No definite residual pneumothorax can be seen. **B:** CT section through the mid thorax shows a moderate residual anterior pneumothorax (*arrows*). The pleural tube is malpositioned within the major fissure. **C:** Posteroanterior radiograph in a different patient than in A and B. Bilateral effusions are present: air can be identified in the pleural space on the left, a pleural tube is present on the left side as well. **D:** CT section in the same patient as in C. The left pleural tube is malpositioned within the lung parenchyma. Note that there is fluid in the left major fissure (*arrow*) confirming that the pleural tube is within the lung. Despite this, there is no evidence of either associated hemorrhage or apparent pulmonary laceration (compare with B).

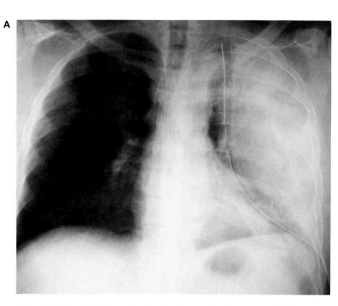
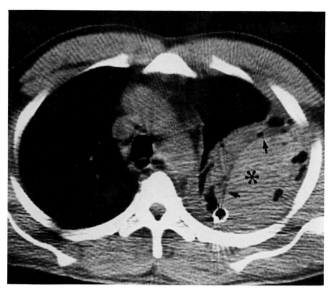

FIG. 32. Complication of closed chest tube placement: CT evaluation. **A:** Posteroanterior radiograph obtained shortly after placement of a left-sided chest tube shows nonspecific increased density on the left, suggestive of a loculated pleural fluid collection. **B:** Non–contrast-enhanced CT section shows that the pleural tube is displaced medially by a large, high density, extrapleural fluid collection compressing and displacing the adjacent lung and pleura (*arrows*), consistent with extrapleural hemorrhage. At surgery these findings were confirmed to be secondary to traumatic injury to an intercostal artery that presumably occurred at the time of chest tube insertion.

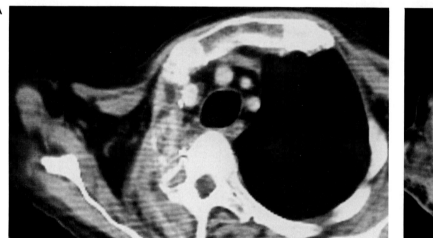
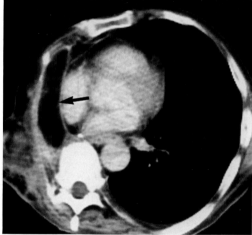

FIG. 33. Postsurgical assessment: thoracoplasty. **A,B:** Contrast-enhanced CT sections through the upper and lower chest, respectively, in a patient status-post a thoracoplasty for tuberculous empyema. The entire right hemithorax is deformed, following surgical resection of numerous ribs and collapse of the ipsilateral hemithorax. Note that there has been a marked expansion of the extrapleural fat (*arrow* in B).

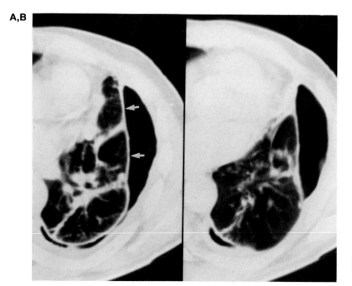
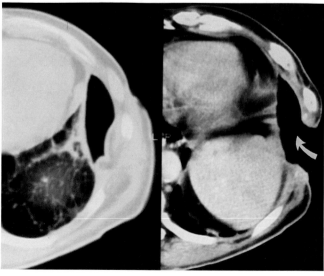

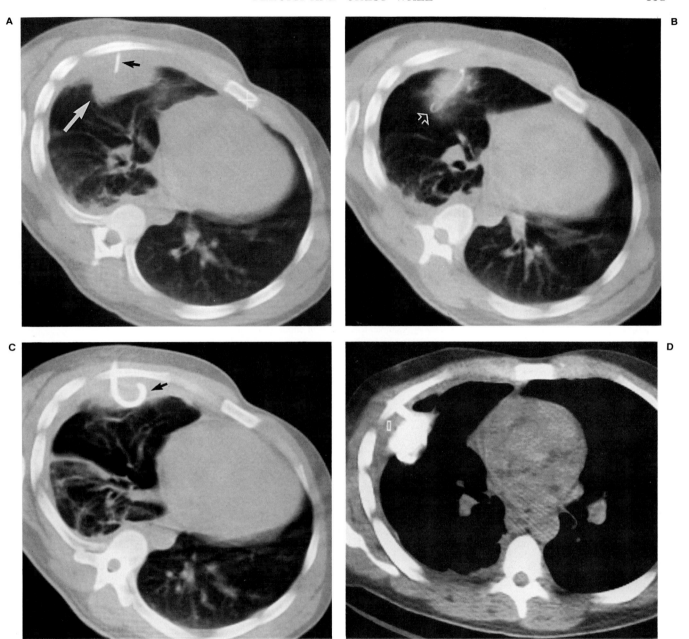

FIG. 35. CT-guided chest tube placement. **A:** CT section in a patient previously treated with a rib resection and open chest tube placement for an empyema. A moderate-sized, residual, loculated fluid collection is present within the lateral aspect of the minor fissure (*arrow*). Note that the patient has been placed in a slightly oblique position: the tip of a 22-gauge needle can be seen within the loculated fluid (*small arrow*). **B:** Section obtained at approximately the same level as A, following withdrawal of about 50 cc of pleural fluid. A guidewire is now present within the minor fissure (*arrow*). **C:** Section at the same level as A and B, following placement of a catheter (*arrow*) within the minor fissure and withdrawal of the guidewire. **D:** Section at the same level as A,B, and C, following installation of approximately 10 cc of contrast material to confirm that the tube is in fact in the minor fissure.

FIG. 34. Postsurgical assessment: Eloesser window thoracostomy. **A–C:** Sequential enlargements of sections through the lower right lung in a patient status-post Eloesser window thoracostomy. The purpose of this procedure is to provide open drainage of chronic empyemas. Note that the visceral pleura is markedly thickened (*arrows* in A). Despite open communication through the chest wall, the left lung has not collapsed. **D:** Section obtained slightly more caudal than C, imaged with a narrow window confirming that there is open communication with the pleural space (*curved arrow*).

A 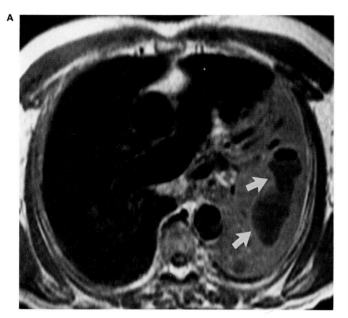 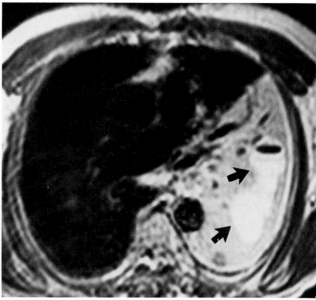 B

FIG. 36. Lung abscess: MR evaluation. **A,B:** T1- and T2-weighted MR scans, respectively, through the mid thorax shows extensive consolidation throughout the entire left lung. A well-defined, smooth-walled, fluid-filled cavity can be identified within which there is a discrete air-fluid level (*arrows* in A and B). A central mass is also present, obliterating the left lower lobe bronchus and significantly narrowing the left upper lobe bronchus. In this case, MR clearly discloses the presence of a lung abscess developing distal to a central obstructing lesion.

investigators advocate the use of closed pleural drainage in the initial management of complicated parapneumonic effusions, it should be noted that the use of closed drainage of empyemas is controversial (49–52). In a series of 70 patients with thoracic empyemas, closed tube thoracostomy was successful in only 35% of cases, while rib resection proved curative in 91% (50). Hood has argued that closed pleural drainage should be attempted only if the pleural process is less than 3 days duration; otherwise, patients should be treated with a rib resection with tube drainage (51).

In the absence of definitive data, it is apparent that the procedure of choice will remain a matter of individual physician's preference. This applies to the choice of imaging modality used to direct PCD as well. Ultrasonic guidance has the advantage of being relatively inexpensive and portable, allowing studies to be performed even in intensive care units. Unfortunately, ultrasound is far more operator-dependent than CT. Furthermore, despite claims to the contrary, CT is far more accurate in detecting underlying lung pathology, as well as in identifying multiple areas of loculation, especially when these are paramediastinal. Additionally, CT is not limited by bandages, drains, or tubes. Finally, it should be noted that in select cases, especially in those for whom there is a contraindication for the use of i.v. contrast

media, magnetic resonance (MR) may be of value in differentiating pleural from parenchymal pathology, as well as detecting lung abscesses (Fig. 36).

ASBESTOS-RELATED PLEURAL DISEASE

Benign pleural manifestations of asbestos exposure include: (a) circumscribed pleural plaques, (b) benign exudative effusions, and (c) diffuse pleural fibrosis. Although these may be associated with underlying parenchymal abnormalities, they frequently occur independently (81). Of these, CT has proven most valuable in identifying pleural plaques and diffuse pleural thickening (82–89). The subject of CT findings in asbestosis is covered in detail in Chapter 8.

Circumscribed Pleural Plaques

Pleural plaques are the most common benign pleural manifestations of asbestos exposure (Figs. 37 and 38). They occur after a latency period of between 20 and 30 years and generally are asymptomatic. Presumably the result of parietal pleural irritation caused by asbestos fibers protruding from the visceral pleural surface, plaques appear as discrete, elevated, sharply defined foci

→

FIG. 38. Asbestos-related pleural disease: pleural plaques. **A:** Posteroanterior radiograph initially interpreted as showing multiple discrete pulmonary nodules, a common indication for obtaining CT (*arrows*). **B:** CT section through the great vessels shows calcified and noncalcified plaques bilaterally. In this case, many of these have a more nodular configuration than that shown in Fig. 37. Several appear to have prolapsed into the adjacent lung (*arrows*), accounting for the radiographic appearance of lung nodules.

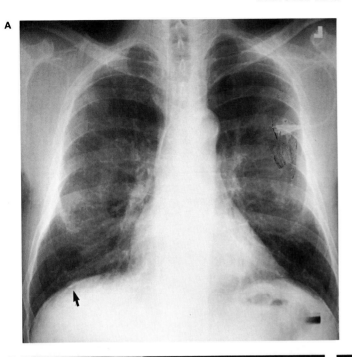

FIG. 37. Asbestos-related pleural disease: pleural plaques. **A:** Posteroanterior radiograph shows typical appearance of asbestos-related pleural plaques, associated with diaphragmatic calcifications (*arrow*), **B,C:** CT sections through the mid and lower chest, respectively, show characteristic appearances of both calcified and noncalcified pleural plaques, as well as punctate calcifications along the diaphragm (*arrow* in C).

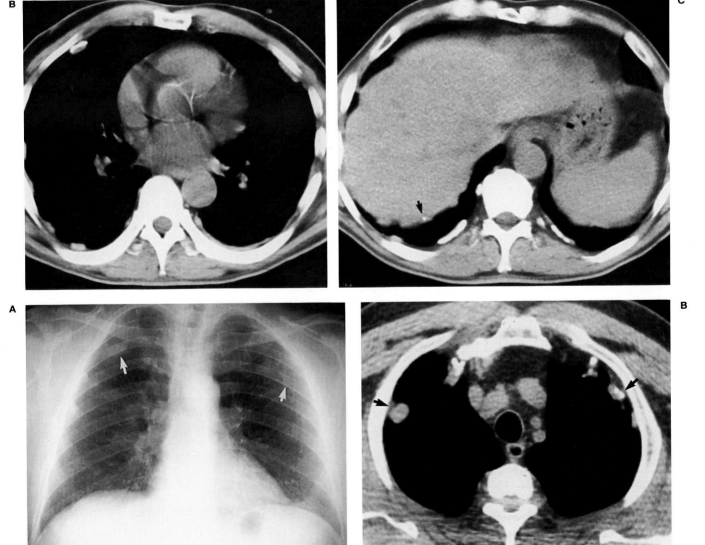

of pleural thickening up to 15-mm thick (85,90). Although typically found posterolaterally along the inferior costal margins as well as along the diaphragm, rarely plaques may involve the visceral pleura within fissures (91). Characteristically bilateral, some have observed a distinct unilateral, left-sided predominance (92). Calcifications occur in approximately 10% of plaques (89). These may appear punctate, linear, or occasionally "cake-like," especially when located along the diaphragmatic surfaces. Less commonly, calcified plaques may be pedunculated, in which case they may be mistaken for intraparenchymal nodules (Fig. 38). Histologically, plaques are composed of predominantly acellular bundles of collagen usually described as having an undulating or "basketweave" configuration (81,93,94). Although plaques have been attributed to other causes including previous empyema and hemothorax, correlation between the presence of bilateral plaques and asbestos-exposure is sufficiently high to warrant defining them as markers of previous dust exposure. A history of asbestos exposure can be elicited in greater than 80% of individuals with pleural plaques (81,93,94). Pleural plaques are always benign.

Benign Exudative Effusions

Benign exudative effusions generally occur considerably earlier than other pleural manifestations of asbestos-related pleural disease, usually occurring within 10 to 20 years following exposure. They may be unilateral or bilateral, and recur in up to 30% of patients. As these effusions are usually nondescript and self-limited, their true incidence is difficult to determine. Epler et al. have reported identifying 35 cases (3.1%) of benign asbestos effusion among a survey group of 1,135 asbestos-exposed workers (95). Although the relationship between benign exudative effusions and the subsequent development of malignancy is unclear, it is unlikely that they represent a significant risk factor for mesothelioma (44). Nonetheless, as noted by Gefter et al., extra caution is probably warranted in those individuals with histories of asbestos exposure in whom a benign exudative effusion is identified (96).

Diffuse Pleural Thickening

In addition to pleural plaques and benign exudative effusions, diffuse pleural thickening may also result from asbestos exposure (Fig. 39). Unfortunately, radiographic differentiation between these entities may be problematic. McLoud et al. have defined diffuse pleural thickening as a smooth, noninterrupted pleural density extending over at least one-fourth of the chest wall, with or without costophrenic angle obliteration (90). Unlike pleural plaques, diffuse pleural fibrosis presumably in-

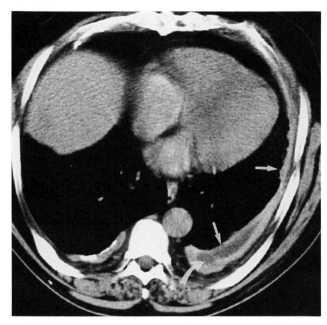

FIG. 39. Asbestos-related pleural disease: diffuse pleural fibrosis. Enlargement of a CT section through the left lung base shows a markedly thickened pleural rind, associated with marked expansion of the extrapleural fat (arrows). In addition, there is a small, residual pleural fluid collection identifiable as well (curved arrow). The presence of residual fluid suggests the possibility of a mesothelioma; however, pleural aspiration and biopsy showed only dense fibrosis and noninfected non-malignant fluid. It is probable that with CT, small, residual pleural fluid collections will be recognized more commonly in patients with asbestos-related pleural fibrosis.

volves both the visceral and parietal pleural surfaces (Fig. 39). The exact mechanism by which this occurs is controversial. It has been postulated that diffuse fibrosis results from an extension of underlying parenchymal disease to involve the adjacent visceral pleura (97). The frequency with which this occurs has been challenged, however. As documented by McLoud et al., in a study of 185 individuals with diffuse pleural thickening, this radiographic appearance proved to be the residue of a prior benign asbestos effusion in 31% of cases, and the result of confluent pleural plaques in 25%. Only 10% of cases in this study with diffuse pleural fibrosis proved to have underlying diffuse parenchymal fibrosis with extension to the visceral and parietal pleura (90). Differentiation between pleural plaques and diffuse pleural thickening is important, as the latter may be associated with significant alterations in pulmonary function (90,98,99).

CT Evaluation of Benign Asbestos-Related Pleural Disease

As early as the late 1970s Kreel and Katz showed CT to be significantly more sensitive than plain radiographs in the detection of asbestos-related pleural disease

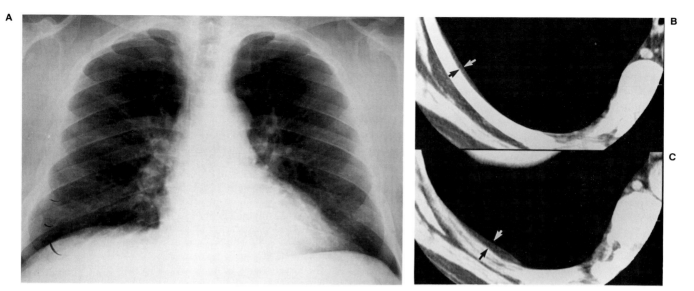

FIG. 40. Prominent extrapleural fat: CT evaluation. **A:** Outside posteroanterior radiograph interpreted as showing pleural plaques (*marks* on right) in a patient with documented exposure to asbestos. **B,C:** Enlargements of sequential CT scans obtained at the same level as in A shows the presence of prominent extrapleural fat pads (*arrows* in B and C), without evidence of pleural plaques or fibrosis.

(1,82,83). In their series of 36 patients with known asbestos exposure, 27 (75%) individuals were found to have abnormal pleural thickening on CT, whereas 24 (66%) individuals had abnormalities detected on chest radiographs (83). In this same series, CT was 50% more sensitive in detecting pleural calcifications than were conventional radiographs.

It is apparent that there is a significant advantage to visualizing the pleural surfaces without superimposition of densities. Not only does CT allow a more precise

assessment of the extent of pleural disease, but in a significant percentage of cases, CT can clarify otherwise indeterminate chest radiographic findings (84,85,100). As documented by Sargent et al., in a study of 30 patients with known asbestos exposure in whom radiographic interpretations were equivocal for the presence of pleural plaques, in 14 cases (48%), CT confirmed that the changes were due to increased amounts of subpleural fat (Fig. 40) (101). Similar findings have been reported by Friedman et al. (88). In a study of 60 indi-

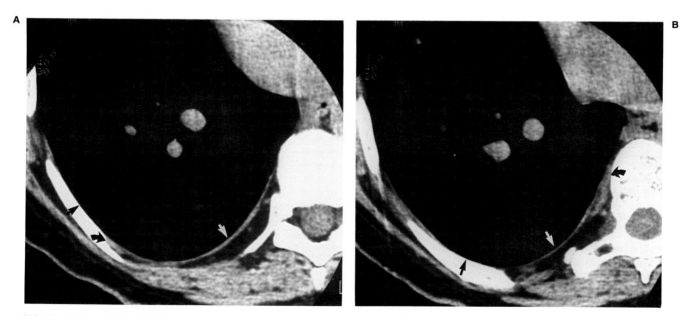

FIG. 41. High-resolution CT of the costal pleura. **A,B:** Enlargements of sequential 1.5-mm sections through the right lower lobe. A thin line can be identified as marginated by lung anteriorly and fat posteriorly. It has been shown that this line represents both the visceral and parietal pleura. Note that this pleural line cannot be visualized adjacent to ribs (*black arrows* in A and B). Furthermore, care must be taken not to confuse the presence of intercostal vessels with masses, or, more important, as evidence of pleural thickening when these lie adjacent to the pleural surfaces (*curved arrows* in A and B).

A

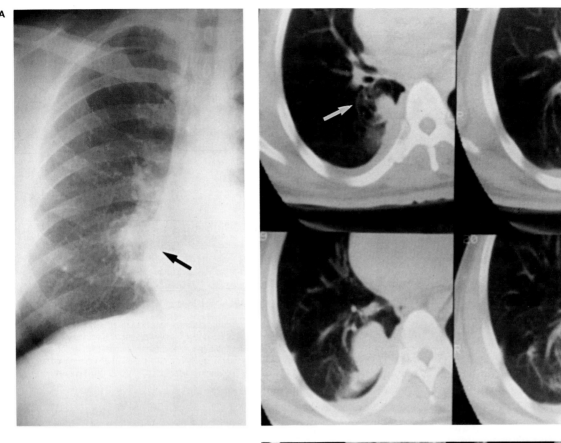

B,C

D,E

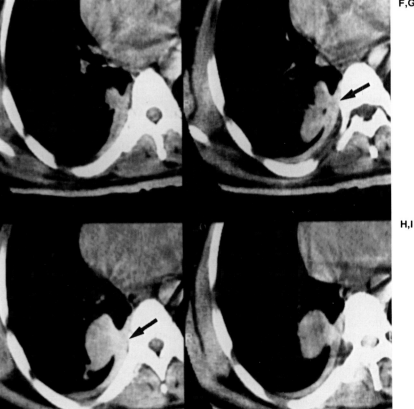

F,G

H,I

FIG. 42. Round atelectasis: CT/MR correlations. **A:** Posteroanterior radiograph shows ill-defined right lower lobe density (*arrow*) indistinguishable from lung cancer. **B–E:** Enlargement of sequential CT sections through the right lower lobe shows characteristic appearance of round atelectasis, presenting as a focal mass adjacent to an area of marked pleural thickening, associated with focal lung distortion. Note that along the superior margin of this lesion the adjacent vessels have a curvilinear appearance, the so-called "comet sign" (*arrow* in B). **F–I:** Identical CT sections as in B–E, imaged with narrow windows. Note that there is considerable pleural thickening which is most prominent adjacent to the mass (*arrow* in G and H).

J 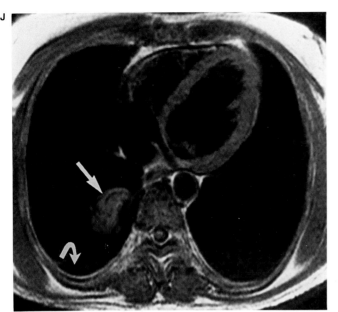 K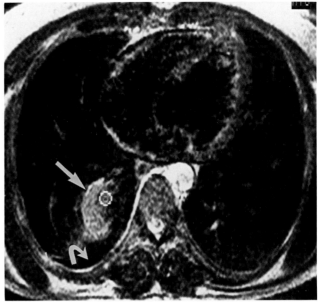

FIG. 42. *(Continued)* **J,K:** T1- and T2-weighted images, respectively, show a complex mass of intermediate signal intensity within the right lower lobe on both T1- and T2-weighted images *(arrows)*. Contrary to opinion, foci of round atelectasis do not represent areas of parenchymal fibrosis, but instead, infolded lung. It is therefore not surprising that considerable signal can be identified within these lesions, especially on T2-weighted scans. In distinction, note that the adjacent pleura, composed as it is of dense, mature fibrous tissue, generates no signal at all *(curved arrows in J and K)*. Potentially, in equivocal cases, MR may be of value by confirming that the pleural thickening seen on CT does not represent tumor infiltration.

viduals with histories of occupational exposure to asbestos comparing the value of high-resolution CT (HRCT) scans to routine radiographs for diagnosing pleural abnormalities, these authors showed the positive predictive value of chest radiographs to be 79% compared with a positive predictive value of 100% for HRCT. Out of eight cases, false positive chest radiographs proved to be secondary to extra subpleural fat in seven, and a prominent intercostal muscle in one.

The role of HRCT in the evaluation of benign asbestos-related pleural disease has also been evaluated by Aberle et al. In a study of 29 subjects with histories of occupational exposure to asbestos, these authors showed that pleural thickening was identified in 100% of cases using HRCT compared with 93% using routine 10-mm thick CT sections (86). In addition to identifying pleural plaques, CT can be of value by disclosing diffuse pleural fibrosis. Gamsu et al. have suggested a useful CT definition of diffuse thickening: a continuous sheet of increased density at least 5-cm broad, 8 to 10-cm long, and more than 3-mm thick (89). It should be emphasized that care must be taken in assessing pleural thickness, especially when using HRCT. As shown by Im et al., in normal patients, identification of the usually pencil-thin line of the normal pleural surfaces may be obscured, especially in the paravertebral regions, because of a normal increase in the amount of extrapleural soft tissue due to the incorporation of adjacent intercostal vessels (Fig. 41) (3). As a consequence, the diagnosis with HRCT of diffuse pleural thickening requires that abnormalities be identified at several levels, preferably identifiable in other than just the paraspinal region.

The appearance of diffuse pleural thickening generally is easily differentiated from mesothelioma. Rabinowitz et al., however, have drawn attention to a variant of asbestos-related pleural fibrosis that closely mimics the appearance of malignant mesothelioma (102). In their series of 40 patients with known asbestos exposure, seven had a diffusely thickened, nodular pleura, indistinguishable from malignant mesotheliomas. None of these patients, however, had evidence of malignant transformation detected by multiple biopsies or by surgery. The significance of this type of fibrosis has yet to be established, as long-term follow-up studies of these patients was not undertaken.

Round Atelectasis

Referred to by a variety of terms including folded lung, atelectatic pseudo-tumor, shrinking pleuritis, and pleuroma, rounded atelectasis, as it is now described, is yet another manifestation of asbestos-related parenchymal and pleural disease (103). First described in this century, round atelectasis has been recognized with increasing frequency over the last 10 years (85,89).

Radiologically, round atelectasis usually presents as an incidental finding on routine chest radiographs (104,105). A distinct preponderance in men has been identified. Typically, conventional radiographs reveal a sharply defined pleural-based mass, ranging between 2 and 7 cm in size, usually located posteriorly in the lower lobes adjacent to an area of pleural thickening (Fig. 42) (see also Fig. 41, Chapter 7). Air-bronchograms may be present within. Characteristically, the mass is associated with vessels and bronchi that have a curvilinear appearance, coursing like a "comet tail" toward the hilum. These findings are often associated with focal volume loss and/or hyperlucency of adjacent lung segments.

CT findings in round atelectasis have been extensively reviewed (87,89,106–111). The major CT sign is a rounded or wedge-shaped peripheral lung mass forming an acute angle with the adjacent pleura which is almost invariably focally thickened and scarred (Fig. 42). Additionally, both vessels and bronchi can be identified curving toward the mass, creating a "comet tail" appearance analogous to that seen on routine chest radiographs. Minor signs include focal emphysema, punctate areas of calcification, and uniform enhancement following administration of i.v. contrast media. Unfortunately, hypervascular lesions have been described in patients with asbestos-related pleural disease and lung cancers (112,113). Other tumors, albeit exceedingly rare, also have been described in association with asbestos-related pleural disease (114,115).

Histologically, round atelectasis occurs adjacent to areas of both parietal and visceral pleural fibrosis (103). Round atelectasis probably results from at least one of two mechanisms. As hypothesized by Blesovsky, atelectasis probably results as a consequence of asbestos-induced pleural fibrosis (116). In support of this explanation, extensive fibrotic changes involving the adjacent visceral pleura have been verified pathologically (103,110). Alternatively, it is also likely that in some cases round atelectasis results from compression of the lung caused by a pleural effusion causing infolding and distortion of the adjacent lung (117). Interestingly, parenchymal changes have been reported to resolve following decortication (103). Although generally associated with asbestos-related pleural disease, in fact, round atelectasis may result from any process that causes extensive focal pleural fibrosis. In an evaluation of 74 patients with rounded atelectasis evaluated by Hillerdal, 64 patients gave a prior history of asbestos exposure (118). Of the remaining 10 cases, two occurred following trauma and four occurred after a pleural exudate. Round atelectasis also has been described in association with histoplasmosis (119).

In addition to the typical appearances described above, several variant forms of round atelectasis have been described. In patients with extensive pleural fibrosis, in particular, a pattern of single or multiple fibrous strands within the lung radiating toward a focal area of pleural thickening has been described in the absence of a definable parenchymal mass. These so-called "crow's feet" have been interpreted by some as the earliest manifestation of round atelectasis (Fig. 43) (see also Fig. 31, Chapter 8) (120). As noted by Lynch et al., other benign lesions also occur in association with asbestos-exposure, including benign pleural-based masses, intra-

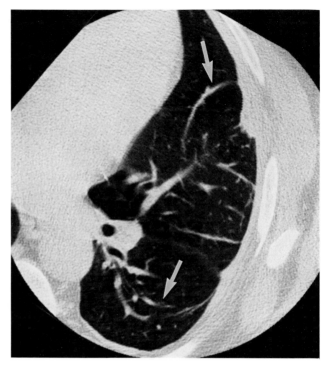

FIG. 43. Round atelectasis: early recognition by CT. High-resolution CT scan shows multiple curvilinear strands within the left lower lobe, all oriented toward approximately the same places along the pleura, both superiorly and inferiorly, which is only minimally thickened. These so-called "crow's feet" have been described as the earliest sign of developing round atelectasis (*arrows*).

fissural pleural plaques, and masslike fibrotic sheets, especially adjacent to the hemidiaphragms (121). These authors have calculated that CT will detect asymptomatic benign masses in up to 10% of individuals with histories of significant exposure to asbestos (89).

In most cases, especially when there is a history of prior asbestos-exposure, the CT appearance of round atelectasis is sufficiently characteristic to obviate the need for histologic verification. Recently, MR has been used to evaluate a case of round atelectasis (Fig. 45) (122). In our experience, we have found no consistent pattern of signal intensity within areas of rounded atelectasis; however, MR may disclose the densely fibrotic nature of the adjacent pleural thickening, eliminating possible confusion with tumor infiltration into the pleura. Of course, in those cases that are either clinically or radiographically equivocal, confirmation of the true nature of these masses may require biopsy.

MALIGNANT PLEURAL DISEASE

Evaluation of patients with suspected pleural malignancy represents an important practical use of CT. This is largely a reflection of the frequency of malignant pleural disease. Leff et al. have noted that approximately 25% of all pleural effusions in older patients in the general hospital setting are malignant in origin (123). In their series of 96 patients with carcinomatous involvement of the pleura, Chernow and Sahn showed that an effusion provided the basis for the first diagnosis of cancer in 44 of 96 patients (46%) (124).

Carcinoma of the lung is the most common cause of pleural malignancy, constituting between 35% and 50% of cases in most series. Breast cancer is also common, in some series equaling the incidence of lung cancer as a cause of malignant effusions. In approximately 7% of cases, the primary tumor site is unknown at the time of initial diagnosis; these frequently prove to be adenocarcinomas of "unknown origin" (46). Most unilateral malignant effusions are the result of pulmonary arterial tumor emboli seeding the visceral pleura with subsequent spread to the ipsilateral parietal pleura (Fig. 44) (125). In distinction, bilateral malignant pleural effusions generally result from tumor spread to the liver, with subsequent hematogenous seeding. Pleural fluid may also accumulate in patients without direct pleural invasion. Mechanisms that have been proposed to account for paramalignant effusions include: (a) tumor obstruction of both central lymphatics and airways, with resultant pneumonia or atelectasis; (b) systemic effects of the disseminated tumor; and (c) results of radiation or drug therapy (46).

The definitive diagnosis of malignant pleural disease usually requires pleural fluid cytology, pleural biopsy, or even exploratory thoracotomy (126,127). In a review of recent literature, Sahn documented that the diagnostic yield from pleural fluid cytology was 66% and from pleural biopsy was 46% (46). Combining procedures resulted in a 73% diagnostic yield. That a diagnosis of pleural malignancy may be elusive has been shown by

Ryan et al. who emphasized that pleural effusions caused by malignancy may go undiagnosed even with careful examination of the pleura, lungs, and mediastinum at thoracotomy (128). In their retrospective study of the outcome of 51 patients with pleural effusions of indeterminate cause at thoracotomy, 25% were found later to have malignant pleural disease.

Malignant effusions usually imply a poor prognosis, although long-term survival has been reported, particularly in patients with metastatic breast carcinoma (46). In addition to radiation and chemotherapy, specific therapies that have been used to control malignant effusions include repeated thoracentesis; tube thoracostomy, with or without the use of sclerosant agents; and pleurectomy (129). Although controversial, in most centers, malignant effusions are treated initially by tube thoracostomy. Sclerosant agents that have been evaluated include tetracycline, bleomycin, quinacrine, and talc, among others (46,47,129). As shown by Martini et al., in patients in whom initial tube thoracostomy is unsuccessful, pleurectomy may be effective; unfortunately, this procedure results in considerable morbidity and mortality (130).

Bronchogenic Carcinoma

As previously noted, bronchogenic carcinoma is the most frequent cause of a malignant pleural effusion, especially adenocarcinoma. As discussed in detail in Chapter 6, evidence of pleura involvement significantly

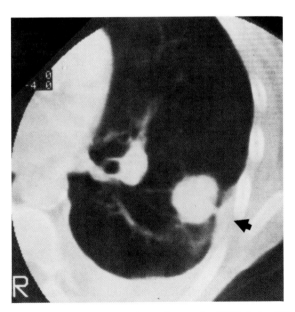

FIG. 45. Peripheral bronchogenic carcinoma: the CT "tail sign." Enlargement of a section through the left lower lobe shows that the tumor has extended peripherally by means of the perivascular sheaths and lymphatics to the adjacent pleura, which is markedly thickened (*arrow*). A small pleural fluid collection is present as well. Unfortunately, this appearance is nonspecific and does not necessarily imply tumor extension to the pleura.

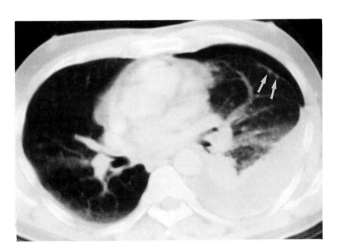

FIG. 44. Pleural metastases: CT correlation. CT section through the mid thorax in a patient shows a moderate-sized left pleural effusion, following thoracentesis. A small anterior pneumothorax is present. Note that several small peripheral nodules can be identified involving the visceral pleural surface (*arrows*), which is particularly well seen due to the pneumothorax. Most metastatic malignant effusions are the result of pulmonary arterial tumor emboli seeding the visceral pleura (compare with Fig. 8).

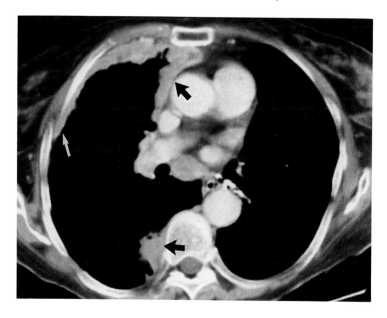

FIG. 46. Pleural seeding: CT evaluation. Contrast-enhanced CT section through the mid thorax shows nodular thickened pleura in a patient with biopsy-proved adenocarcinoma of the lung. Note that pleural involvement is discontinuous, with foci of tumor infiltration (*arrows*) clearly separated by apparently normal intervening pleura. Enlarged subcarinal nodes are present as well.

alters the staging, prognosis, and therapy of these tumors. The pathways by which the pleura becomes involved with tumor have been described by Heitzman et al. (131). Tumor may extend to the pleura secondary to reversal of the centripetal flow of lymph (commonly caused by primary central tumors) or tumorous involvement of hilar nodes. Central venous obstruction also may be present. Alternatively, peripheral tumors may directly invade the adjacent pleura, either by tumor growth along peripheral perivascular-lymphatic sheaths (Fig. 45) or by direct invasion of the adjacent pleura with subsequent pleural seeding (Fig. 46) (see also Figs. 3–6, Chapter 6). Evidence of pleural seeding may be discovered in sites far removed from the primary tumor, including the mediastinal pleura. Interestingly, tumor

may involve the pleura without producing pleural fluid; these tumors may also involve the chest wall.

Unfortunately, assessment of pleural involvement is limited when tumors, both peripheral and central, abut the pleura but do not appear to directly invade either the chest wall or mediastinum (Fig. 45) (132–137). CT is also limited in assessing patients with superior sulcus tumors because of the limitations of cross-sectional imaging through the lung apices (Fig. 47). Even high-resolution CT offers little improvement; definitive evaluation usually still requires pleural biopsy (Fig. 48). Another problem is encountered in evaluating patients with central endobronchial lesions with secondary obstructive pneumonitis and/or apparent lobar collapse: differentiation of infiltrate from tumor may be difficult.

A 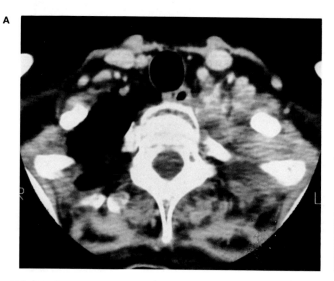   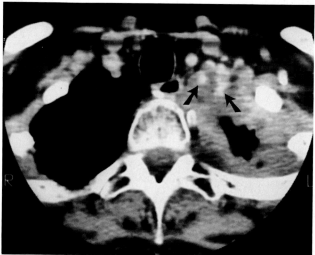 B

FIG. 47. Superior sulcus tumor: CT evaluation. **A,B:** Sequential contrast-enhanced CT sections through the left lung apex show diffuse infiltration of the pleura as well as the adjacent soft-tissue structures of the neck. Encasement of vessels by tumor is especially well visualized in B (*arrows*). Although in this case CT clearly depicts the extent of tumor, evaluation of apical tumors in general can be problematic with CT.

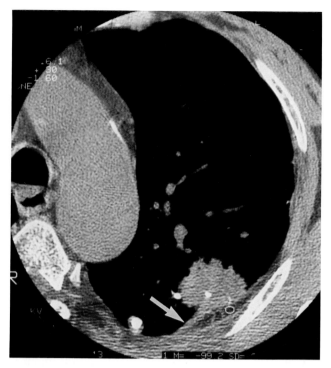

FIG. 48. Peripheral lung cancer: evaluation with high-resolution CT. Retrospective target reconstruction of the left lung in a patient with a peripheral lung cancer associated with apparent pleural thickening on posteroanterior and lateral chest radiographs (not shown). The mass clearly abuts the pleura which is thickened (*arrow*). There is considerable expansion of the extrapleural fat adjacent to the mass, suggesting that there is no gross chest wall involvement. These findings were confirmed at surgery.

Recent evidence suggests that in these cases MR may be more accurate than CT, especially in predicting parietal pleural and chest wall involvement (Fig. 49) (see also Figs. 17–19, Chapter 6) (138–143).

Mesothelioma

Malignant pleural mesothelioma is a rare neoplasm representing less than 5% of pleural malignancies (46,144–146). The association between malignant mesotheliomas and asbestos exposure is well documented (46,146). Unlike the association between asbestos and bronchogenic carcinoma, the development of malignant mesotheliomas does not appear to be dose related: tumors have been documented after only relatively trivial environmental or household exposure. It is probably for this reason that malignant mesotheliomas are frequently identified in patients without evidence of either pleural plaques or pleuropulmonary fibrosis (85). The risk of mesothelioma is related to the type of fiber to which patients are exposed: crocidolite poses a far greater risk for development of a mesothelioma than either amosite or chrysolite (46,146). The latency period for the development of malignant mesothelioma is long, generally between 20 and 30 years. Approximately 80% of mesotheliomas are pleural while 20% are peritoneal (146).

The diagnosis of mesothelioma is especially difficult

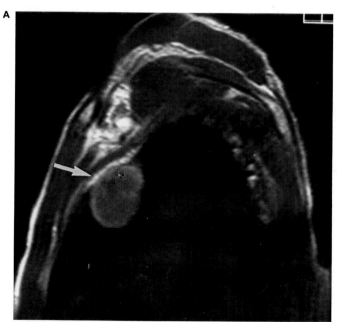
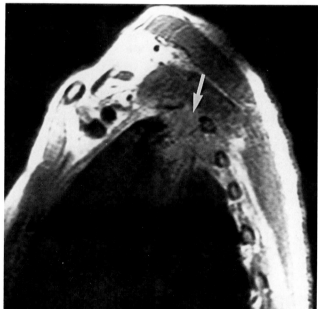

FIG. 49. Peripheral lung cancers: MR evaluation. **A:** T1-weighted sagittal MR image shows a peripheral tumor that abuts the pleural surface. Note that there is complete preservation of the extrapleural fat adjacent to the tumor (*arrow*), indicating that the chest wall is not grossly infiltrated by tumor. **B:** T1-weighted sagittal image in a different patient with a superior sulcus tumor. In this case, tumor has clearly invaded the adjacent chest wall, obliterating the normal extrapleural fat planes (*arrow*). Although CT is superior to MR in evaluating bony pathology, because of its greater contrast resolution, MR has proven more valuable than CT in detecting tumor infiltration into the soft tissues of the chest wall, especially infiltration into chest wall fat and adjacent muscles.

to make cytologically: as a consequence, diagnosis usually necessitates thoracotomy (46,146). Differentiation between mesothelioma and adenocarcinoma may be difficult with routine light microscopy, and definitive diagnosis often requires electron microscopy and/or immunohistochemistry. Histologically, three forms of diffuse malignant mesothelioma have been recognized: epithelial, mixed, and sarcomatous (144). Although the best prognosis has been reported with epithelial tumors, median survival for most patients, regardless of cell type, is typically only between 6 and 12 months.

Characteristically, mesotheliomas grow by contiguous spread throughout the pleura, including the mediastinal pleural surfaces and the fissures (Figs. 50 and 51). Not infrequently, spread occurs into the chest wall and the hemidiaphragms (Figs. 52 and 53); less frequently, mesotheliomas may metastasize hematogenously to mediastinal lymph nodes, as well as to the contralateral lung (46,146). Based on these spread patterns, Butchart et al. have proposed the following staging system (147):

Stage 1. Tumor confined within the ipsilateral parietal pleura, including adjacent pericardium and diaphragm.

Stage 2. Tumor invasion of the chest wall or mediastinum and/or mediastinal lymph node involvement.

Stage 3. Tumor penetration of the diaphragm with peritoneal involvement and/or involvement of the contralateral pleura, or extrathoracic lymph node metastases.

Stage 4. Distant hematogenous metastases.

Therapeutically, two surgical approaches have been utilized: extrapleural pneumonectomy and pleurectomy with irradiation. Of these, the latter has proven more popular due to a lower morbidity rate and better survival (145).

The appearance on CT of both benign and malignant mesotheliomas has been well-described (Figs. 50–53) (85,89,148–159). The main value of CT is in: (a) precisely delineating the intra- and extrathoracic extent of

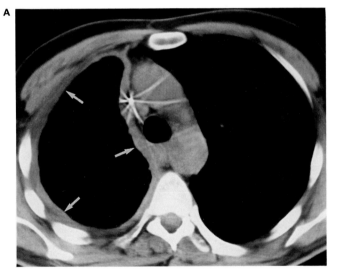

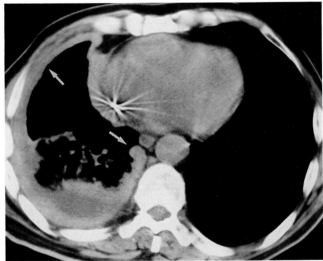

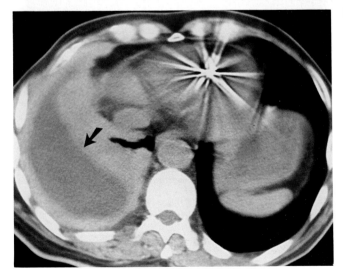

FIG. 50. Malignant mesothelioma: CT evaluation. A–C: Sequential CT scans through the lungs show typical appearance of a circumferential rind of thickened, nodular pleura (*arrows* in A and B) associated with loculated fluid (*arrow* in C). Additionally, there is some loss of volume with shift of the mediastinum to the right, best seen in A. Note the absence of contralateral pleural plaques or fibrosis, a frequent finding in patients with malignant mesotheliomas.

A

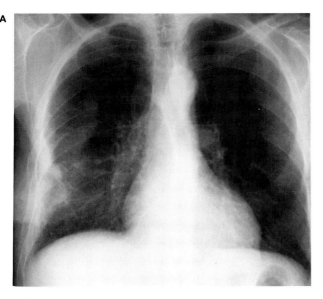

B

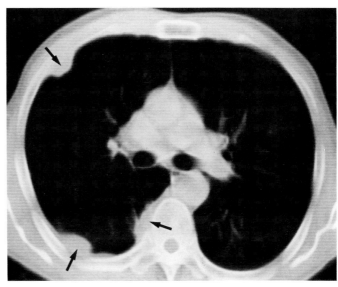

FIG. 51. Malignant mesothelioma: CT evaluation. **A:** Posteroanterior radiograph shows nodular appearing pleura inferiorly on the right without evidence of a pleural effusion. **B:** CT scan at the level of the carina shows focal areas of pleural nodularity (*arrows*), between which the pleura appears normal. This appearance is nonspecific and can be seen in patients with pleural seeding from bronchogenic carcinomas as well (compare with Fig. 46).

disease; (b) determining the best therapeutic approach; and (c) monitoring the results of therapy. Characteristically, mesothelioma permeates the pleural space, causing the pleura to become markedly thickened, irregular, and nodular (Figs. 50 and 51). The tumor often encircles the lung, which may then become entrapped. Effusions are present in up to 80% of cases. Ancillary findings

include mediastinal and hilar lymphadenopathy and pulmonary nodules, which have been reported to be present in up to 60% of cases (89). In a recent review of 50 cases of documented diffuse malignant mesothelioma, Kawashima and Libshitz found 92% of cases had pleural thickening, 86% had thickening of the pleural surfaces of the interlobar fissures, 74% had pleural effu-

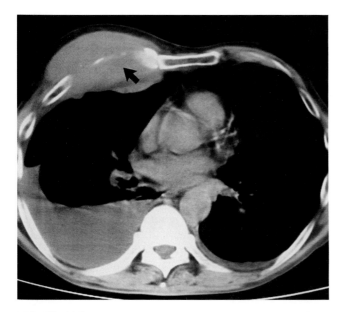

FIG. 52. Malignant mesothelioma: chest wall invasion. CT scan through the mid thorax in a patient who presented with a palpable chest wall mass and radiographic evidence of a large effusion associated with rib destruction (not shown). A large chest wall mass is apparent (*arrow*) and is associated with destruction of a rib. No other masses were identified. This appearance is nonspecific and initially suggested either a rib metastasis or a primary bone malignancy. Malignant mesothelioma was biopsy-proved. (Case courtesy of Dr. Norman Ettenger, Manhattan V.A. Hospital, NY.)

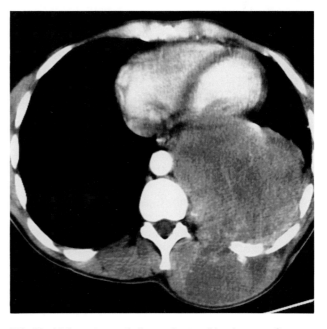

FIG. 53. Malignant mesothelioma: chest wall involvement. Contrast-enhanced CT scan shows extensive tumor involving the left lower lobe, ribs, and chest wall. This appearance is nonspecific, and initially suggested a primary lung cancer with secondary chest wall invasion. Malignant mesothelioma was biopsy-proved.

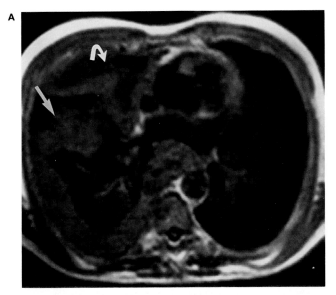

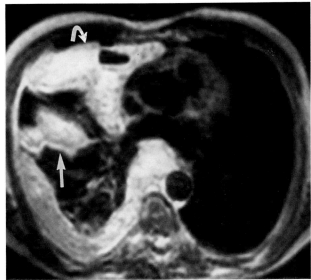

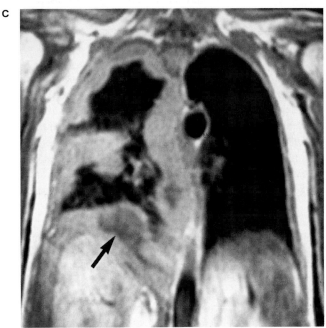

FIG. 54. Malignant mesothelioma: MR evaluation. **A,B:** T1- and T2-weighted images, respectively, through the lower chest in a patient with documented malignant mesothelioma. The pleura is circumferentially thickened and nodular, with evidence of tumor infiltration into the major fissure (*arrows* in A and B). In addition, a focal area of loculated fluid can be identified anteriorly within which a small air-fluid level can be seen (*curved arrows* in A and B). **C:** Coronal T1-weighted image shows to better advantage the full extent of tumor, from the lung apex to the diaphragms, including the fissures. Note the presence of another area of loculated fluid inferiorly (*arrow*).

sions, but only 20% had evidence of pleural calcifications (157). It should be emphasized that malignant mesotheliomas rarely may present as more localized masses, making CT distinction from benign fibrous mesotheliomas more difficult. It should also be noted that there are no CT-specific signs for mesothelioma: almost any malignancy involving the pleura can simulate the appearance of a mesothelioma (160,161).

Alexander et al. have shown that plain radiographs, compared with CT, frequently underestimate the disease extent (151). CT disclosed unexpected areas of involvement in each of their five cases. Extension into the contralateral chest was demonstrated in two cases, and extension into the abdomen and chest wall were each shown in one case. Unfortunately, although CT is superior to plain radiography, CT may underestimate the

true extent of disease. In an evaluation of 20 patients with malignant mesothelioma evaluated with CT prior to therapy, CT failed to diagnose chest wall invasion in nine patients, mediastinal lymph node involvement in four patients, transdiaphragmatic extent in four patients and peritoneal studding and distant metastases in one patient (156). However, it is important to note that in this same series used to evaluate the effects of therapy, in six of eight cases CT disclosed the presence of recurrent disease from one to eight months prior to the onset of symptoms.

Metastatic Disease

Pleural metastases, apart from those due to bronchogenic carcinoma, occur most frequently from primary

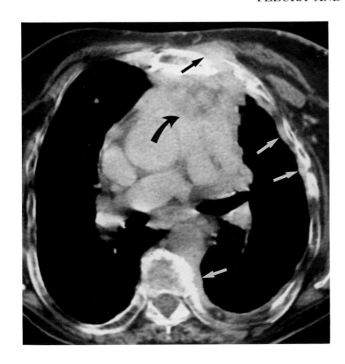

FIG. 55. Malignant thymoma. CT section through the mid thorax shows a large inhomogeneous anterior mediastinal mass (*curved arrow*) clearly infiltrating the anterior chest wall (*straight black arrow*). Note that the pleura is markedly nodular, secondary to both direct tumor infiltration and pleural seeding with distant implants (*white arrows*). Malignant thymoma was biopsy-proved.

neoplasms of the breast, gastrointestinal tract (including pancreas), kidneys, and ovaries (Figs. 44 and 46) (46,124,125). Malignant thymoma also frequently involves the pleura, usually by contiguous invasion. Malignant thymomas may also cause pleural seeding resulting in the development of discrete pleural masses often at a distance far removed from tumor within the anterior mediastinum (Fig. 55; see also Fig. 86, Chapter 2) (162,163).

In patients with metastatic disease, pleural effusions may develop for a variety of reasons. These include increased permeability of the capillaries supplying tumor

implants, as well as increased capillary permeability due to pleuritis associated with obstructive pneumonitis if present; direct tumor erosion of pleural blood and lymphatic vessels; and decreased removal of pleural fluid due to mediastinal lymph node infiltration (46).

The same wide variation in the appearance on CT described for mesotheliomas may be seen with metastatic pleural disease (Figs. 44, 46, 55, 56). Pleural metastases may cause marked thickening and nodularity of the pleura associated with only a small quantity of pleural fluid; alternatively, pleural metastases may cause large pleural effusions in which the foci of malignancy

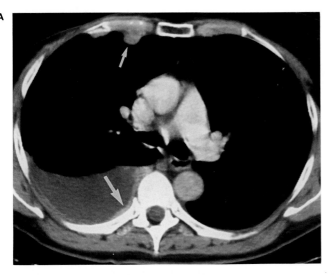
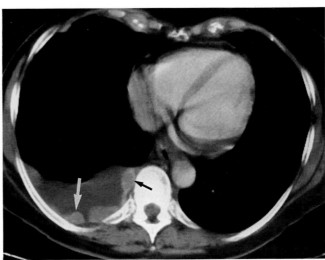

FIG. 56. Pleural metastases: breast cancer. **A,B:** Contrast-enhanced CT scans through the carina and the lower lobes in a patient status-post a right mastectomy. In addition to a moderate-sized right pleural effusion, enlarged internal mammary lymph nodes can be identified on the right (*small arrow*). The pleural surface is nodular and thickened superiorly (*large arrow* in A). Inferiorly, discrete pleural masses can be seen easily separable from the surrounding effusion (*arrows* in B). Metastatic breast cancer was biopsy-proved.

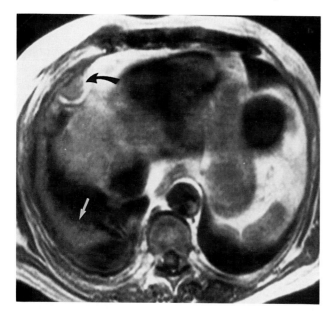

FIG. 57. Pleural metastases: MR evaluation. T1-weighted section in a patient with radiographic evidence of a nonspecific right-sided effusion (not shown). A pleural effusion is apparent on the right side compressing the adjacent right lower lobe (*arrow*). Additionally, there is an enlarged anterior mediastinal lymph node embedded in fat (*curved arrow*), strongly suggesting malignant disease. Adenocarcinoma of the pleura was documented.

are difficult to identify. Similar findings can be seen using MR (Figs. 54 and 57).

Not infrequently, pleural biopsy will reveal adenocarcinoma of the pleura of unknown primary (Fig. 46). Many of these are presumed to be secondary to primary adenocarcinomas of the lung, although the primary tumor may be obscured by the extensive pleural disease.

Pleural Lymphoma

It has been estimated that approximately 10% of malignant pleural effusions are the result of lymphoma (46). Pleural effusions are more likely to occur in non-Hodgkin's lymphomas (NHL) than with Hodgkin's disease (HD), and are more likely to occur in patients with extensive disease (164,165). Although distinctly uncommon at the time of initial diagnosis, up to 30% of patients with Hodgkin's disease may eventually develop effusions (166). In patients with lymphoma, pleural effusions result from a variety of causes including: (a) impaired lymphatic drainage due to obstruction of hilar and mediastinal lymph nodes; (b) obstruction of the thoracic duct, frequently associated with a chylous effusion;

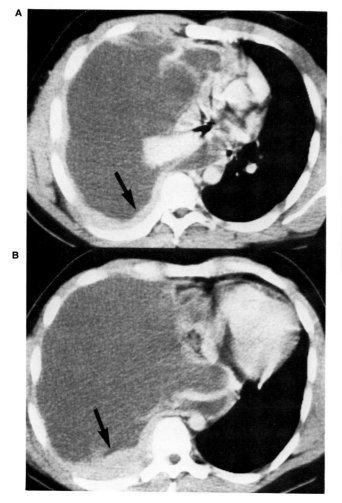

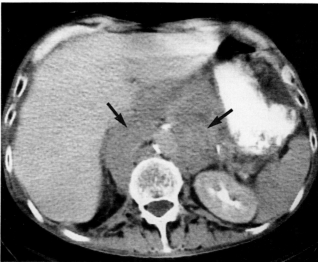

FIG. 58. Pleural lymphoma. **A,B:** Contrast-enhanced CT scans through the mid and lower thorax, respectively, show a massive right-sided pleural effusion, with shift of the heart and mediastinum to the left. Pleural fluid can be seen crossing the midline to lie anterior to the descending aorta. There is considerable thickening of the posterior pleural surfaces, suggesting a mantle or plaque of tumor, involving both the pleura and extrapleural spaces (*arrows* in A and B). **C:** CT section through the upper abdomen shows extensive retroperitoneal lymphadenopathy surrounding the aorta (*arrows*). Non-Hodgkin's lymphoma was biopsy-proved.

and (c) direct pleural infiltration as a result of involvement of adjacent ribs with subsequent extension through the chest wall and pleura, or secondary to involvement of the adjacent lung (46,47).

As documented by Stolberg et al., lymphoma frequently causes subpleural deposits of tumor in the form of either nodules or plaques (Fig. 58) (167). Similar observations have been made by others (168). In a retrospective radiographic review of 112 nonselected patients with documented histiocytic lymphoma, Burgener and Hamlin showed that pleural involvement was present in 18% of cases, including four cases with localized pleural plaques (169). More recently, Shuman and Libshitz have documented a role for CT in detecting pleural involvement (170). In a series of 71 patients with both

documented HD (n = 47) and NHL (n = 24) evaluated by CT, these authors showed solid pleural manifestations in 31%. Although this most probably does not represent a typical population of patients, as pointed out by the authors themselves, it is apparent that documentation of the presence of pleural disease can be of particular benefit in the development of appropriate treatment strategies, both following initial diagnosis and as a means for follow-up (171).

Postpneumonectomy Space

As first shown by Biondetti et al., CT is especially efficacious in evaluating the postpneumonectomy space (Fig. 59) (172). As documented by these authors, a range

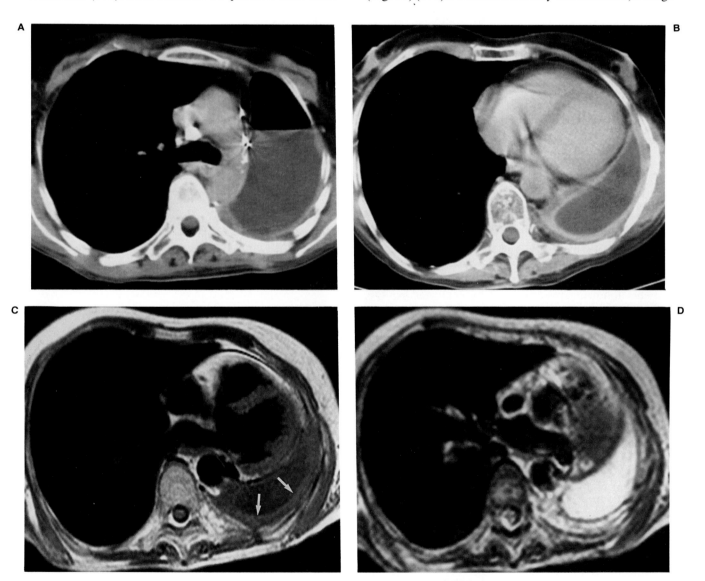

FIG. 59. Postpneumonectomy space: CT/MR correlations. **A,B:** Contrast-enhanced CT scans through the carina and lower lobes, respectively, show typical appearance following a recent pneumonectomy in a patient with lung cancer. A large air-fluid level can be seen in A. The pleural surfaces appear smooth, without evidence of focal masses or nodules. **C,D:** T1- and T2-weighted images, respectively, obtained at the same level through the lower chest in the same patient as shown in A and B, several months later. The pneumonectomy space is now entirely filled with fluid. The pleural surfaces are smooth without evidence of nodules or masses. Note that the pleural surfaces are most easily evaluated on the T1-weighted scans (*arrows* in C).

A 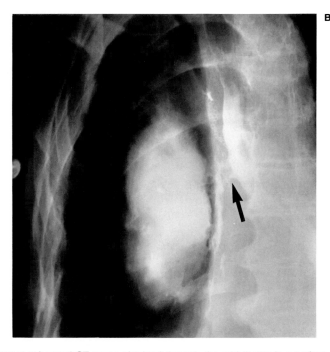 B

FIG. 60. Postpneumonectomy space empyema: CT evaluation. A: Contrast-enhanced CT scans obtained through the mid thorax in a patient status-post a right-sided pneumonectomy years prior for treatment of bronchiectasis. An air-fluid level is present within the pneumonectomy space, consistent with a fistula. Sections at the level of the carina and right main-stem bronchus show no evidence of airway pathology (not shown). Increased soft-tissue density is apparent in the region of the esophagus, which is difficult to identify (*straight arrow*). There is also a suggestion of a potential communication with the pneumonectomy space at this level (*curved arrow*). Note that the fluid level within the pneumonectomy space has extremely high density (*open arrow* in B). B: Coned-down view from an esophagram showing fistulous communication between the esophagus (*arrow*) and the pneumonectomy space.

of normal postoperative appearances may be anticipated, consequent to rotation and ipsilateral displacement of mediastinal and hilar structures, as well as hyperaeration of the contralateral lung. In their series of 22 patients following pneumonectomy evaluated by CT, residual fluid was present in 13 (60%) of 22 cases, even years following surgery, while in 9 (40%) of 22 cases, CT showed the postpneumonectomy space to be completely obliterated (172). Tumor recurrence can be identified in most cases as mediastinal or hilar masses or, less commonly, as discrete peripheral masses projecting into the lower-density fluid within the pneumonectomy space (173,174).

In addition to demonstrating a normal postoperative appearance as well as recurrent tumor, CT can be of value by showing other complications, including the development of an empyema within the postpneumonectomy space (Fig. 60) (175). As shown by Shepard et al., CT may also be valuable in diagnosing the so-called "right pneumonectomy syndrome" (176). In this condition, sometimes years following surgery, patients develop symptoms of dyspnea and recurrent pulmonary infections in the left lung due to compression of the distal trachea and/or left main-stem bronchus due to the marked shift of the mediastinum to the right side.

Recently, MR has been used to evaluate the postpneumonectomy space (Fig. 59) (177). Not surprisingly,

the main advantage of MR is nonreliance on the use of intravenous contrast administration to delineate hilar and mediastinal structures from recurrent tumor masses (see Fig. 25, Chapter 6).

Malignant Pleural Disease: Overview

Due to its unobstructed view of the pleural space coupled with its ability to differentiate between fluid and soft-tissue densities, CT represents an important method for evaluating patients with suspected malignant pleural disease. As discussed, numerous articles have documented the appearance of pleural tumors, both benign and malignant (13,129–139,141,148–163,168,178,179). Specific CT signs that have been described for both primary and metastatic disease include: (a) circumferential thickening of the pleura; and (b) focal and/or diffuse nodularity of the pleura. Recently, Leung et al. in an evaluation of 74 patients with proved diffuse pleural disease, including 39 cases of pleural malignancy, showed CT findings to be highly specific (180). Using the criteria of circumferential pleural thickening, nodular pleural thickening, parietal pleural thickening greater than 1 cm, and mediastinal pleural thickening alone or in combination, CT correctly diagnosed pleural malignancy in 28 of 39 cases (sensitivity = 72%; specificity = 83%). Significantly, in this series, circumferential pleural thickening proved to be 100% specific in predicting malignant pleural disease. It is apparent that CT represents an important adjunct to routine chest radiography in the evaluation of patients with suspected malignant effusions. Although specific histologic diagnosis may be impossible, as documented by Leung et al., the appearance of malignant pleural disease is sufficiently characteristic to suggest the diagnosis, especially in those cases where establishing the diagnosis by conventional means, including pleuroscopy and thoracotomy, proves difficult (180).

THE CHEST WALL

Computed tomography plays an important role in the evaluation of patients with chest wall pathology (181–183). In an evaluation of 49 patients, Leitman et al. (55) found that compared with routine radiographs, CT provided additional information in two-thirds of cases, frequently detecting unsuspected bone, lung, pleural, and mediastinal pathology (183). In one-third of these cases, treatment was altered or the surgical approach was modified based on CT findings. Equally important, CT may play an indispensible role by excluding significant pathology. In the series reported by Leitman

et al. of those patients referred for evaluation because of palpable chest wall "masses," CT proved these apparent masses to be related to minimal scoliosis in three patients, asymmetry of the scapulae in one, and asymmetry of the anterior chest wall muscles and costal cartilages in three other patients (183).

The Sternum

The sternum and sternoclavicular joints are difficult to evaluate with plain radiographs, mainly because overlying structures are difficult to exclude from view on frontal and oblique projections. The sternoclavicular joints are angled obliquely, making their visualization particularly difficult. The potential role of CT to image the sternum has long been appreciated (185). Several reports have outlined in detail the normal appearance of the sternum and its articulations, including normal variants (Fig. 61) (185–189). With the patient's arms held above the head, the proximal portions of the clavicles have a steep obliquity and will appear in cross-section as elongated or oval structures. The sternal notch is easily defined between the clavicular heads. The manubrium is the widest part of the sternum and forms the anterior wall of the superior mediastinum. Superiorly, the middle part of the superior border of the manubrium is

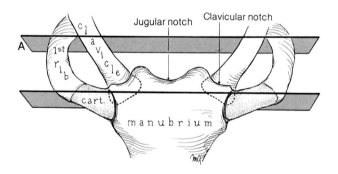

FIG. 61. A: Schematic drawing of the manubrium and sternoclavicular joints. Characteristic levels are labeled A and B. The sternoclavicular joints are posterior structures. **B:** Section at the level of the sternal notch, imaged with bone window settings. **C:** Section through the sternoclavicular joints. The clavicular heads articulate with the manubrium (M) posteriorly. The costal cartilage of the first ribs articulates with the sternum anteroinferiorly. Cl, proximal clavicles; cart 1, first costo-chondral junction.

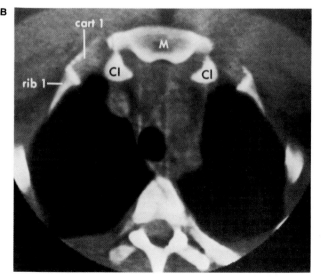

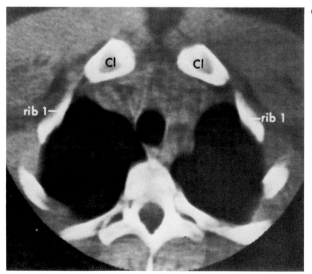

rounded; this portion is called the jugular notch. To each side of the jugular notch, posteriorly, an indentation in the manubrium can be identified; these are the clavicular notches, which represent the sternal part of the sternoclavicular joints. Sequential scans through the clavicular notches show close approximation of the sternum with the clavicular heads. Just below this, and somewhat more laterally, a rough projection in the contour of the manubrium can be defined, representing the point of articulation between the sternum and the first costal cartilage.

The value of CT in assessing lesions of the sternoclavicular joints and sternum has been repeatedly documented (Figs. 62–65) (190–199). In their series of 17 patients with sternoclavicular abnormalities evaluated by CT, Destouet et al. demonstrated pathology better, or

provided additional diagnostic information in the majority of cases (185). These included six cases of sternoclavicular joint dislocation, two cases of nonspecific synovitis and osteoarthritis, and two cases of osteomyelitis.

In our experience, CT has proven especially valuable: (a) in assessing the sternum following sternotomy, both to rule out postoperative infections and to evaluate the use of rotated pectoral flaps following sternal debridement (Figs. 62 and 63) (187,188,190–193), (b) to assess the sternum and sternoclavicular joints, especially in intravenous drug addicts, to rule out infection, including associated mediastinitis (Fig. 64) (185,187,188,190, 198,199,200); (c) to evaluate posttraumatic abnormalities (Fig. 65) (185,190,195,196); and (d) to evaluate patients in whom there is a clinical suspicion of a possible

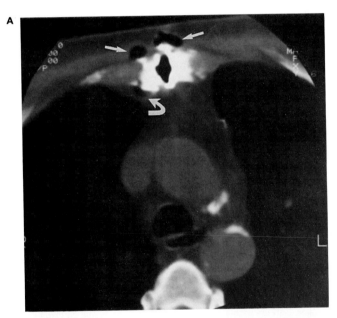

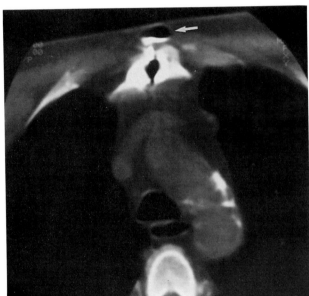

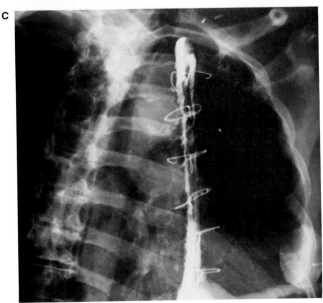

FIG. 62. Poststernotomy infection: CT sinogram. **A,B:** Enlargements of sequential CT sections through the sternum in a patient status-post sternotomy. This study was performed following injection of dilute contrast media into a catheter left in place following surgery. A space can be seen between the two halves of the sternum filled with contrast; additionally, pockets of air and contrast can be identified anteriorly in the chest wall (*arrows* in A and B) as well as posteriorly, adjacent to the sternum (*curved arrow* in A). Note that there is no evidence of a significant fluid collection or contrast within the anterior mediastinum. **C:** Corresponding sinogram. Note that CT is far more precise in delineating the exact number and locations of fluid collections.

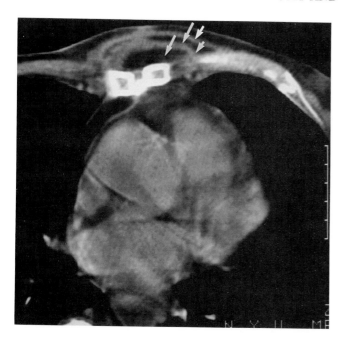

FIG. 63. Pectoral flaps: CT evaluation. Enlargement of a CT scan in a patient status-post sternotomy requiring bilateral pectoral flaps following sternal debridement. Concentric rings of alternating density (*short arrows*) and lucency (*long arrows*) can be identified anterior to the sternum, corresponding to attenuated muscle and fat, respectively. This appearance is pathognomonic and should not be confused with chest wall pathology. (From Leitman et al., ref. 193, with permission.)

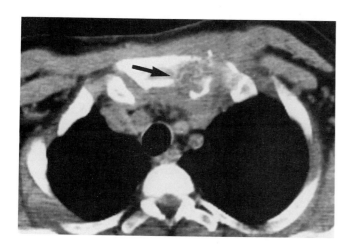

FIG. 64. Sternoclavicular osteomyelitis. CT section through the sternoclavicular joints shows lytic destruction of the lateral aspect of the sternum (*arrow*) as well as the distal clavicle, associated with considerable soft-tissue thickening in a known i.v. drug addict. Needle aspiration was positive for Staphylococcal infection.

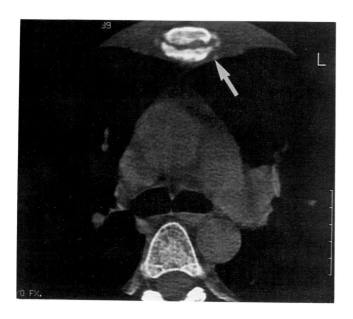

FIG. 65. Sternal fracture. Enlargement of a CT section through the sternum showing transverse fracture (*arrow*).

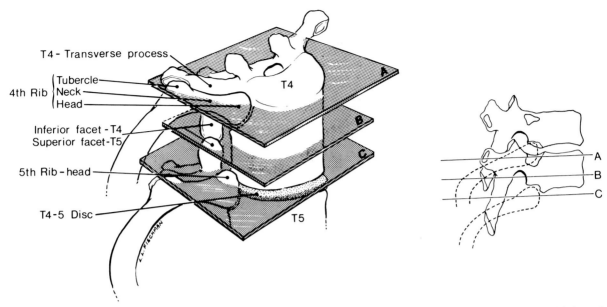

T4 - Transverse process
Tubercle
4th Rib { Neck
Head
Inferior facet - T4
Superior facet - T5
5th Rib - head
T4 - 5 Disc
T4
T5
A
B
C

FIG. 66. Diagram of costovertebral articulations at T4 and T5, with a sagittal schematic representation of the corresponding axial planes in A,B, and C. (From Bhalla et al., ref. 206, with permission.)

sternal lesion, especially in patients with known breast cancer, as well as to evaluate sternal pathology following irradiation (181,184,185,188,190,194).

The Ribs

A wide variety of lesions affecting the ribs and costal cartilages have been identified with CT (181,183,184, 190,201–205). Although the value of CT to assess rib pathology is somewhat limited because of the oblique configuration of the ribs as they traverse the CT scan plane, as recently documented by Bhalla et al., it is possible to accurately localize pathology to particular ribs, provided detailed knowledge of the CT appearance of the costovertebral and costotransverse articulations as well as the relationship of the clavicle to the first rib (206). This anatomy is illustrated in Figs. 66 and 67. Briefly, the heads of the first, tenth, eleventh, and twelfth ribs articulate only with the body of the corresponding vertebra, while the heads of the second to ninth ribs articulate with the articular facet on the lateral aspect of the body of the corresponding vertebra, the intervening disc, and the demifacet on the vertebral body above. The first 10 ribs also articulate with their corresponding transverse processes. The intervening space between the neck of the rib and the transverse process is called the costotransverse foramen. Although only a short segment of each rib is visualized on an axial CT image because of the caudal slope of the ribs, the

head and neck of a rib are usually in the same horizontal plane as the pedicle and the transverse process of the corresponding vertebra. Knowledge of these relationships allows individual ribs to be identified in most cases. As outlined by Bhalla et al., this involves the following steps (Fig. 68):

1. Identify the first rib. The first rib is most easily identified on the axial image showing the middle third of the clavicle.
2. Identify the next two or three ribs on the same section by counting posteriorly along the rib cage.
3. Proceed sequentially through the remaining images, concentrating on the costovertebral articulations. Each subsequent and numerically higher thoracic vertebra and the corresponding rib are enumerated.
4. Localize individual rib or pleural lesions by sequentially enumerating the ribs along the rib cage proceeding anteriorly from the spine. Each successive rib encountered represents the numerically preceding rib.

In a retrospective review of 12 cases with documented rib pathology, Bhalla et al. successfully localized 21 lesions, including 17 costal and 5 thoracic spine lesions, using this approach (206). Familiarity with the normal appearance of the ribs clearly facilitates recognition of pathology, including normal variants such as cervical ribs and the rare anomaly of an intrathoracic rib (206–208).

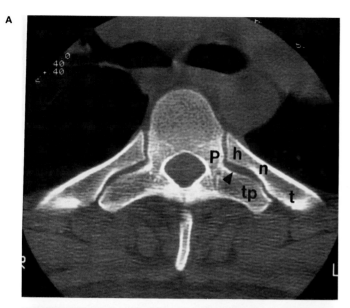

A

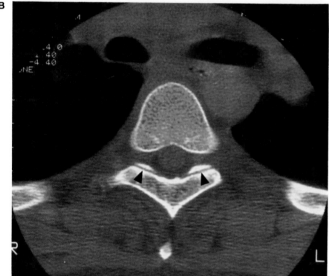

B

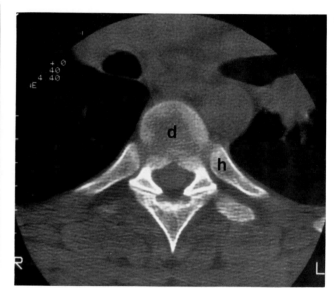

C

FIG. 67. Representative axial CT images through the planes indicated in Fig. 66. **A:** Through plane A: head (h), neck (n), and tubercle (t) of the left fourth rib; transverse process (tp) and pedice (P) of the T4 vertebra: costotransverse foramen (*arrowhead*). **B:** Through plane B: T4–T5 facet joints (*arrowheads*). **C:** Through plane C: T4–5 disk space (d), head of left fifth rib (h). Note partial volume effect of corresponding pedicle and the transverse process. (From Bhalla et al., ref. 206, with permission.)

Chest Wall and Axilla

Detailed evaluation of the soft tissue structures of the chest wall requires thorough familiarity with normal cross-sectional anatomy (209). Anatomic relationships in the region of the axilla are especially important given the significance of this area for identifying chest wall neoplasia, especially manifestations of breast cancer and lymphoma, as well as identifying lesions that affect the brachial plexus. Sequential cross-sectional anatomic illustrations of the axilla are shown in detail in Figs. 69 to 71. As described by Fishman et al., the axilla is a pyramidal-shaped space between the upper arm and the chest wall, with the apex directed superiorly and the base directed downward (210). The boundaries of the axilla include: (a) an anterior wall formed by the pectoralis major and minor, subclavius muscles, the clavipectoral facia, and the suspensory ligament of the axilla; (b) a posterior wall, formed by the subscapularis, latissimus

A

B

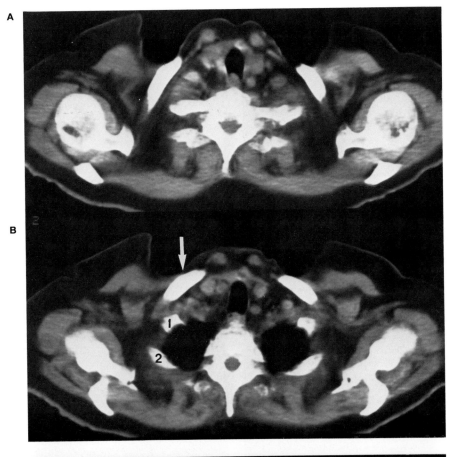

C

D

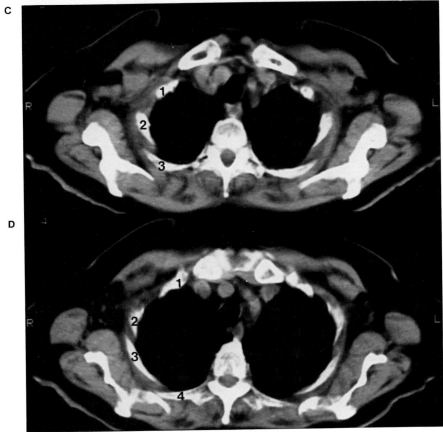

FIG. 68. *Continues on next page.*

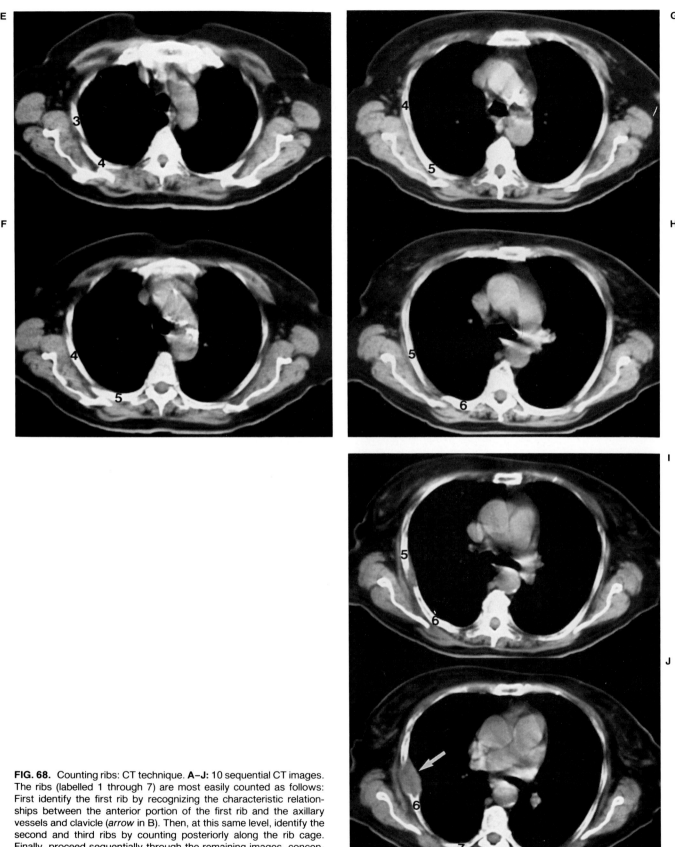

FIG. 68. Counting ribs: CT technique. **A–J:** 10 sequential CT images. The ribs (labelled 1 through 7) are most easily counted as follows: First identify the first rib by recognizing the characteristic relationships between the anterior portion of the first rib and the axillary vessels and clavicle (*arrow* in B). Then, at this same level, identify the second and third ribs by counting posteriorly along the rib cage. Finally, proceed sequentially through the remaining images, concentrating on the costovertebral articulations. In this case, a lytic lesion can be identified in the sixth rib on the right (*arrow* in J).

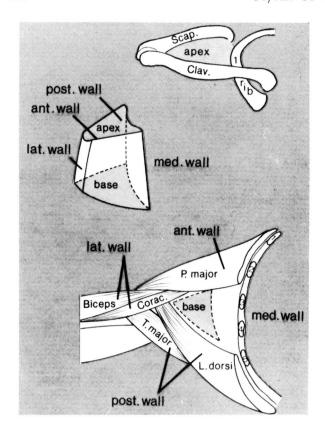

FIG. 69. The boundaries of the axilla. Lat. wall, lateral wall; ant. wall, anterior wall; P. major, pectoralis major; med. wall, medial wall; L. dorsi, latissimus dorsi; post. wall, posterior wall; T. major, teres major; Cora c., coracobrachialis. (From Fishman et al., ref. 210, with permission.)

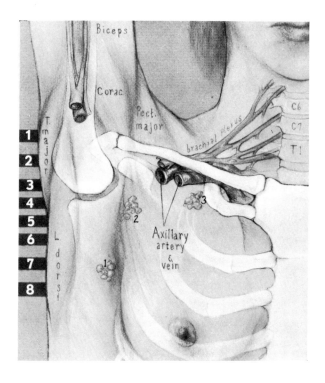

FIG. 70. The structures of the normal axilla, with corresponding characteristic transaxial segments labelled 1 to 8. Corac., coracobrachialis; Pect. major, pectoralis major; L. dorsi, latissimus dorsi; T. major, teres major. (From Fishman et al., ref. 210, with permission.)

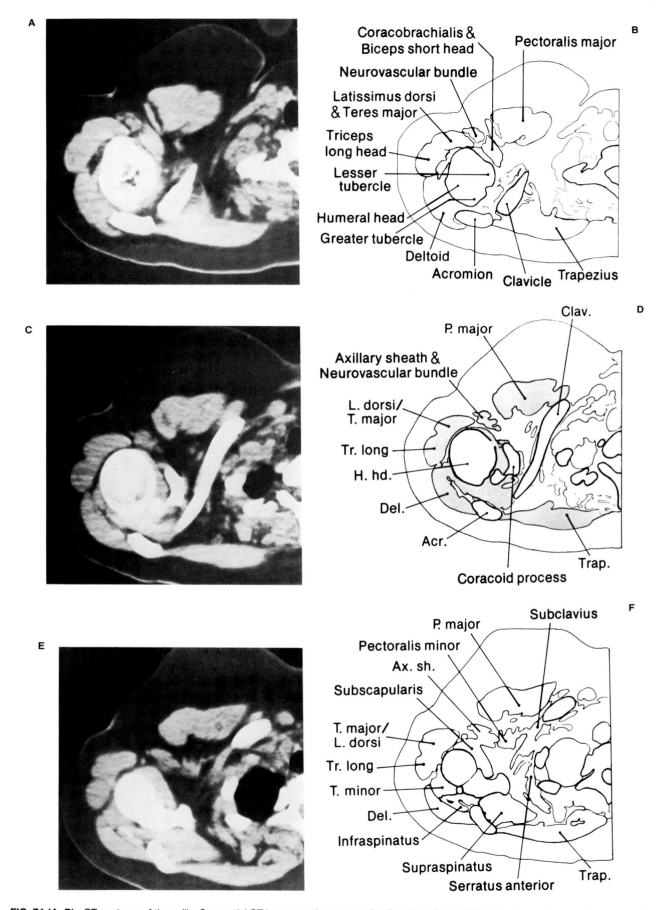

FIG. 71 (A–P). CT anatomy of the axilla. Sequential CT images and corresponding line through the axilla, from above-downward, corresponding to the 8 planes identified in Fig. 70. **A,B** correspond to level 1, Fig. 70; **C,D** correspond to level 2, Fig. 70. **E,F** correspond to level 3, Fig. 70.

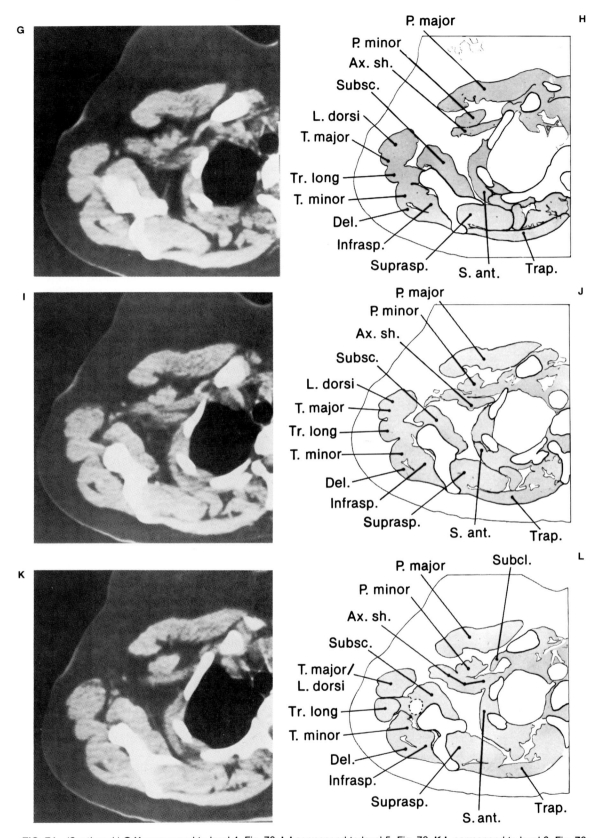

FIG. 71. *(Continued)* **G,H** correspond to level 4, Fig. 70; **I,J** correspond to level 5, Fig. 70; **K,L** correspond to level 6, Fig. 70;

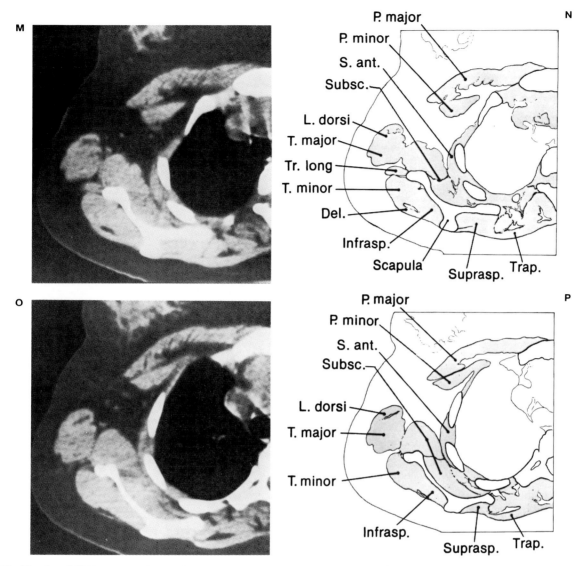

FIG. 71. *(Continued)* **M,N** correspond to level 7, Fig. 70, **O,P** correspond to level 8, Fig. 70. (From Fishman et al., ref. 210, with permission.)

dorsi, and teres major muscles; (c) a medial wall, formed by the first through the fifth ribs, their intercostal spaces, and the serratus anterior muscle; (d) a lateral wall, formed by the humerus and the coracobrachial and biceps brachii muscles; (e) an apex formed by the clavicle and upper border of the scapula and outer border of the first rib; and finally, (f) a base formed by the anterior and posterior axillary folds, the serratus anterior muscle, and the chest wall. Important landmarks within the axilla include the axillary artery and vein and the cords of the brachial plexus, all of which are enclosed in a connective tissue sheath, the axillary sheath. Of these only the artery and vein can be identified as discrete structures: the axillary vein courses cephalad and lies successively on the anterior, medial, and inferior sides of the axillary artery. With the arm raised, characteristically the vein tends to lie anterior to the artery throughout its

course. In addition to these structures, numerous lymph node chains are also present within the axilla. Although variably described, these usually include: (a) nodes located between the inferolateral margin of the pectoralis minor muscle and the latissimus dorsi muscle; (b) nodes located behind the pectoralis muscle in the axilla; and (c) nodes located between the superomedial margin of the pectoralis muscle and the thoracic inlet (210,211). Additional nodes identifiable by CT include interpectoral lymph nodes, normally seen only as small dots in the interpectoral fat (212).

Knowledge of the axilla and remaining chest wall anatomy has proven clinically useful in assessing patients with breast cancer, especially following radiation and/or surgery (Figs. 72 and 73) (181,190,214–219). The appearance of the normal postoperative chest wall after mastectomy as well as the CT appearance of tumor

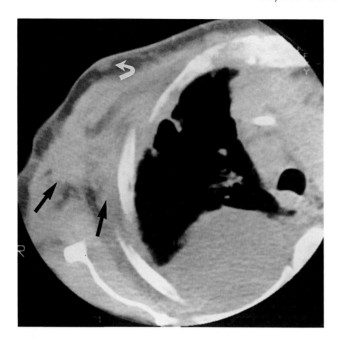

FIG. 72. Recurrent breast cancer. Enlargement of a CT section through the right axilla in a patient status-post a right mastectomy. A poorly marginated soft-tissue mass can be identified within the axilla (*arrows*) associated with subcutaneous nodules (*curved arrow*). In addition, nodular tumor implants can be associated with a large pleural effusion; mediastinal lymphadenopathy is present as well.

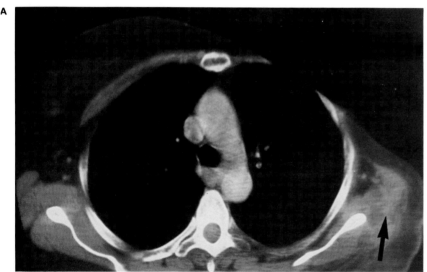

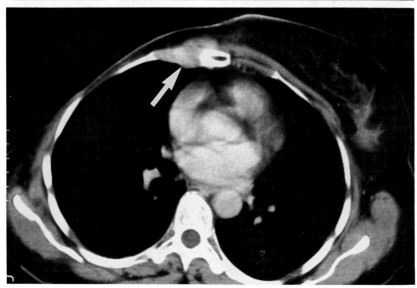

FIG. 73. Recurrent breast cancer: chest wall evaluation. **A:** CT scan in a patient status-post left mastectomy shows an ill-defined soft-tissue mass anterior to the scapula (*arrow*). Recurrent breast cancer was biopsy-proved. **B:** CT scan in another patient following a left mastectomy. A poorly defined soft-tissue mass can be identified just to the right of the sternum (*arrow*). Recurrent breast cancer was biopsy-proved.

recurrence have been well described by Shea et al. (216,217). As shown by these authors, in a study of 19 patients suspected of tumor recurrence following mastectomy, CT allowed identification of tumor recurrence in all 15 cases in whom recurrence was biopsy-proved. Similar results have been previously reported by Gouliamos et al. (181). In an evaluation of 64 patients following mastectomies for breast cancer, these authors found that 21 of these patients had axillary adenopathy, 11 of whom had metastatic disease subsequently verified histologically, while 9 showed internal mammary node enlargement, and 6 had local chest wall recurrence. As shown by Lindfors et al., CT can detect foci of tumor recurrence unsuspected on physical examination (215). In their study of 42 patients with local and/or regional recurrence of breast cancer, of 33 patients with clinical evidence of chest wall recurrence, 16 patients (49%) had areas of disease identified by CT that were clinically unsuspected. Despite these reports and in our experience, in the absence of unequivocal tumor mass or extensive adenopathy, differentiation between postoperative changes and tumor recurrence can be problematic. In these cases we advise either follow-up CT scans or biopsy, depending on the specific clinical setting.

In addition to breast cancer, a wide variety of diseases, both benign and neoplastic, may result in the development of axillary or chest wall adenopathy or masses (181,183,190,220–227). These generally are nonspecific and frequently require biopsy (Figs. 74–76). In exceptional cases, CT can provide specific tissue diagnoses. In patients with chest wall lipomas, for example, CT may play an invaluable role by excluding more significant pathology, especially in patients with previously documented malignancies (Fig. 6) (13,223–225). CT can also be of specific value in identifying patients with chest wall abscesses, especially those associated with tuberculosis (Fig. 77) (54–56,183,228). CT also has proven to be of diagnostic aid in detecting chest wall infiltration in patients with actinomycosis (Fig. 78) (190,229–231).

As previously discussed, considerable interest has focused on the role of CT in detecting neoplastic infiltration of the chest wall, especially in patients with lung cancer (Figs. 4 and 47) (132–136). The value of CT in detecting other infiltrating lesions, including mesothelioma (Figs. 52 and 53) (151–158) and lymphoma (45,164,168,170,171) have also been described. In general, CT is only effective in patients with relatively extensive tumor, as has been emphasized previously, CT is considerably less accurate in assessing patients with only minimal or subtle chest wall infiltration. In distinction, CT is especially sensitive in detecting chest wall collaterals that may develop in patients with central tumors causing superior vena caval obstruction (Fig. 79) (232–235). In general, these are easily distinguished from the transient thoracic venous collaterals that may be seen normally in occasional patients following the bolus administration of i.v. contrast (236).

Finally, CT may play an important role in assessing

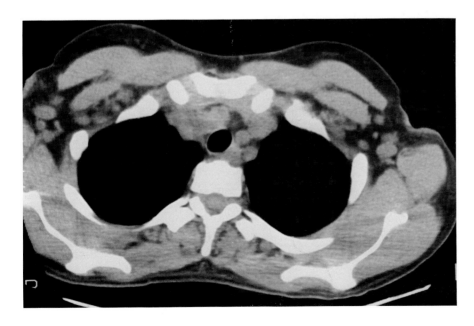

FIG. 74. Axillary adenopathy. CT scan through the axilla shows typical appearance of nonspecific bilateral axillary adenopathy. Hodgkin's disease was biospy-proved.

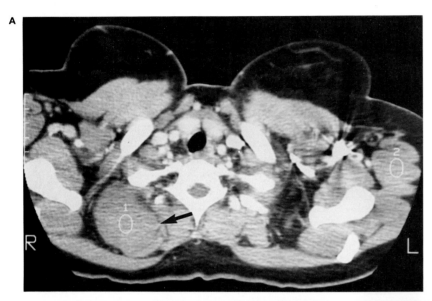

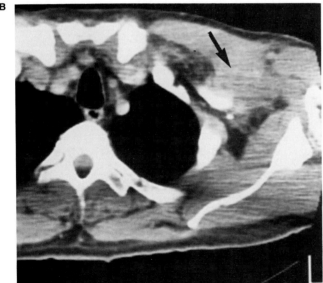

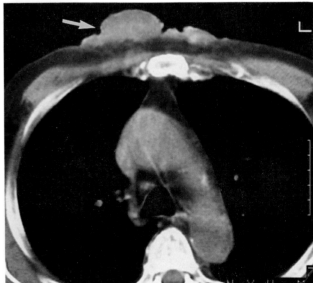

FIG. 75. Soft-tissue masses in the chest wall and axilla: CT appearances. **A:** CT scan at the level of the thoracic inlet shows a well-defined soft-tissue mass posteriorly (*arrow*). Benign desmoid tumor was biopsy-proved. **B:** CT scan through the left axilla shows enlarged axillary lymph nodes and/or masses associated with a loss of the normal facial planes within the axilla (compare with the normal contralateral side). Melanoma was biopsy-proved. **C:** Enlargement of a CT scan through the anterior mid thorax shows a lobular exophytic soft-tissue mass involving the skin, sparing the immediate subcutaneous fat (*arrow*). Basal cell carcinoma was biopsy-proved. These cases have in common the presence of nonspecific soft-tissue masses in either the chest wall or axilla. Although CT allows precise localization of these tumors in most cases, CT rarely obviates the need for biopsy.

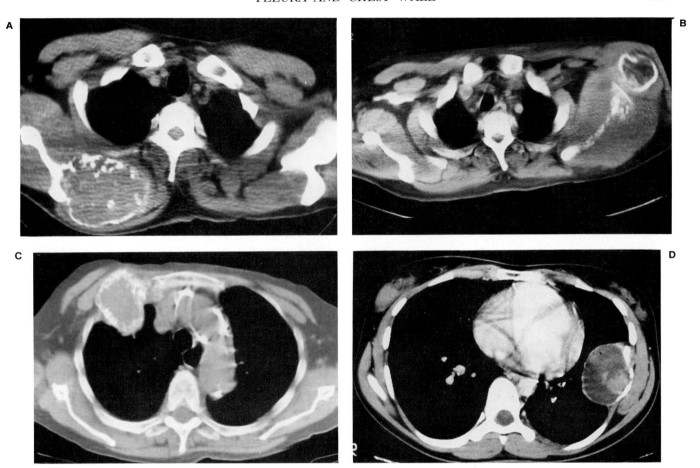

FIG. 76. Bony lesions of the thorax: CT scans in four different patients showing a variety of bony chest wall lesions. As with soft-tissue masses, the CT appearance of these lesions is rarely specific. **A:** Chondrosarcoma of the right scapula. **B:** Ewings sarcoma of the left scapula. **C:** Hemangioma arising within a rib. **D:** Aneurysmal bone cyst within a rib.

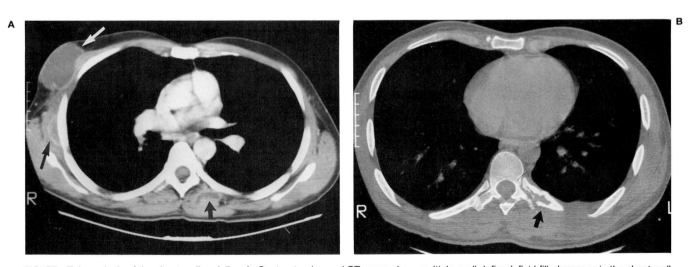

FIG. 77. Tuberculosis of the chest wall and ribs. **A:** Contrast-enhanced CT scans show multiple, well-defined, fluid-filled masses in the chest wall bilaterally, associated with markedly enhancing rims (*arrows*). **B:** CT scan at a lower level than in A, imaged with bone windows. There is lytic destruction of the posterior portion of the ninth rib on the left (*arrow*). At a higher level, a lytic lesion involving a solitary thoracic vertebra was identified as well (not shown). Aspiration of the chest wall fluid confirmed extensive chest wall and osseous tuberculosis.

A

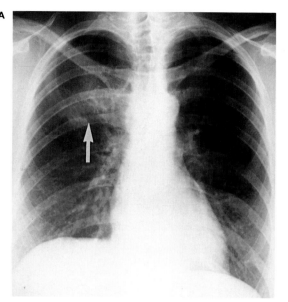

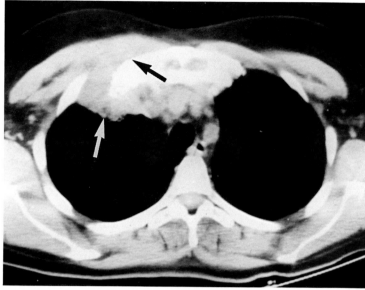

B

FIG. 78. Actinomycosis. **A:** Posteroanterior radiograph shows a poorly defined, nonspecific area of increased density on the right (*arrow*). **B:** CT scan through the sternum shows increased soft-tissue density (*arrows*) involving the chest wall, corresponding to the ill-defined density seen on the PA radiograph. Actinomycosis was biopsy-proved. (Case courtesy of Robert Maissel, M.D., Queens, NY.)

patients with trauma, including iatrogenic causes such as in-dwelling chest wall catheters, chest tubes, and pacemakers, as well as postsurgical changes (237–247). CT specifically detects unsuspected small pneumothoraces and/or hemothoraces, especially following rib fractures, and identifies sternoclavicular dislocation and sternal fractures, including retrosternal hematomas, injuries involving the thoracic spine, scapular injuries, and pulmonary lacerations and contusions (245). As docu-

mented by Tocino et al., CT frequently detects small, incidental pneumothoraces following head trauma, a finding that can be important in patients requiring mechanical ventilation (239). Similar findings have been reported following abdominal trauma (238). As documented by Mirvis et al., CT may also be of value in assessing patients with multi-system trauma to identify possible thoracic sources of infection, including both lung abscesses and empyemas (243). CT also can play a

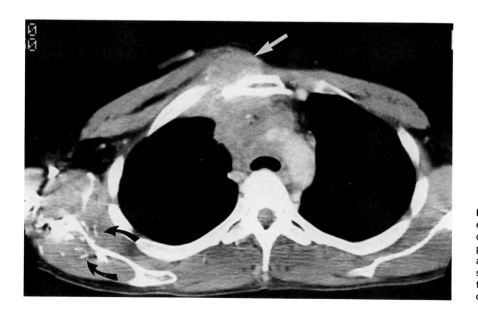

FIG. 79. Chest wall collaterals. Contrast-enhanced CT section shows innumerable chest wall collaterals on the right side in a patient with extensive mediastinal tumor associated with superior vena caval obstruction (*curved arrows*). Note that the tumor is also invading the chest wall anteriorly (*straight arrow*).

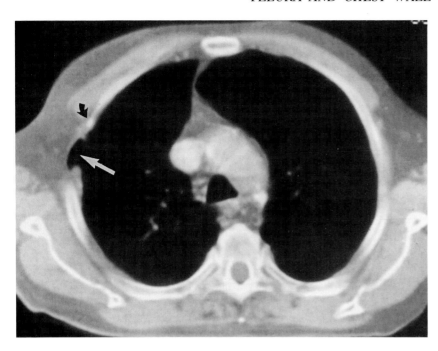

FIG. 80. Posttraumatic lung herniation. CT scan through the mid thorax shows focal herniation of lung into the chest wall (*arrow*) adjacent to a healed rib fracture (*curved arrow*). (From Bhalla et al., ref. 249, with permission.)

role in evaluating late sequelae of trauma, including the finding of post-traumatic lung herniation (Fig. 80) (248,249).

MR EVALUATION OF THE PLEURA AND CHEST WALL

Compared with other usages, little has been written concerning the use of MR to evaluate pleural disease. Although some correlations have been found both *in vitro* and *in vivo* between MR signal intensities and pleural fluid composition, MR has not yet proven to be a reliable means for differentiating among various etiologies of pleural effusions (250–253). In a study of 22 patients with pleural effusions from a variety of etiologies evaluated by MR, Davis et al. have shown apparently consistent quantitative and qualitative relationships between the MR signal characteristics of transudative versus exudative effusions (253). Using a triple spin-echo multi-slice sequence, these authors found that as indicated by relative signal intensity ratios, effective T2 relaxation times, and/or qualitative visual assessment, complex exudates (infected or malignant) were always brighter than simple exudates, which in turn were always brighter than transudates, regardless of which echo was evaluated (253). Furthermore, MR proved of additional value by clearly differentiating between free and loculated effusions, as well as identifying co-existent underlying lung disease. Despite these findings, however, no clear clinical role for the use of MR in evaluating pleural fluid collections has yet emerged. MR has also been used to evaluate patients with malignant

mesotheliomas of both the pleura and pericardium (Fig. 54). Although MR clearly delineates the extent of tumor, and also allows differentiation between pleural tumor and fluid, the role for MR in assessing malignant effusions has yet to be firmly established (Fig. 57) (254,255).

If the role of MR is limited in the evaluation of pleural disease, a considerably more convincing argument can be made for the use of MR in the evaluation of chest wall pathology (Fig. 49). The main advantages of MR for evaluating the chest wall are multi-planar imaging and increased contrast resolution. This may have implications for those patients for whom surgery is planned, in order to better delineate the disease extent (Fig. 81).

To date, the most important application of MR has been in evaluating chest wall invasion in patients with lung cancer (Fig. 47) (see also Figs. 17–19, Chapter 6). As previously discussed, CT is of only limited use in assessing parietal pleural and chest wall invasion. By comparison, MR has proven significantly more accurate in assessing tumor infiltration, especially in patients with superior sulcus tumors (138–143). In a study of 31 patients evaluated with both thin-section CT scans and MR, Heelan et al. showed that MR was 94% accurate in detecting tumor invasion into the chest wall as compared with 63% accuracy for CT (139). In these authors' opinion, the improved accuracy of MR appeared to be related primarily to improved visualization of anatomy obtained with coronal and saggital images. In a study of 10 patients with superior sulcus tumors evaluated with MR, McLoud et al. also showed MR to be of value in detecting chest wall and mediastinal invasion. MR proved to be particularly sensitive for detecting tumor

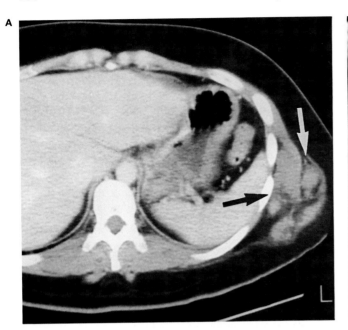
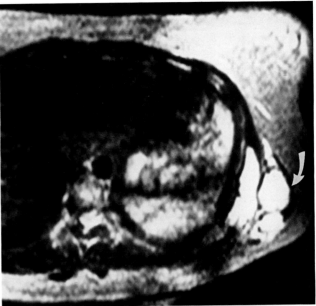

FIG. 81. Chest wall hemangioma: CT/MR correlations. **A:** Contrast-enhanced CT scan through the upper abdomen shows complex nodular masses in the chest wall on the left (*arrows*). On the basis of this scan, precise delineation of the hemangiomas from adjacent chest wall structures is difficult. **B:** T2-weighted scan at a slightly different level than shown in A. Numerous hemangiomas are identifiable as masses of extremely high signal intensity (*arrow*). Compared with CT, these lesions are somewhat easier to identify with MR, simplifying presurgical evaluation.

infiltration into the soft tissues of the chest wall due to marked differences in the signal intensity of tumor as compared to both fat and muscle on T2-weighted sequences in particular. Unfortunately, in this same series, MR failed to identify subsequently confirmed rib destruction in five patients due to poor visualization of cortical bone (140). Recently, MR has also been proven more sensitive than CT in detecting chest wall involvement by malignant lymphoma (256). In a study of 28 patients examined with both CT and MR, Bergin et al. showed that while CT detected chest wall invasion in seven sites in four patients, MR showed chest wall lesions in 14 cites in seven patients (45).

MR has also been used to evaluate a variety of other chest wall masses, both benign and malignant, including lipomatous lesions and soft-tissue hemangiomas (Fig. 81), and even abnormalities involving the sternum and clavicles (257–260). Although MR has been shown to help identify chest wall infections, MR is less accurate in detecting osteomyelitis compared with CT (261).

Finally, a number of reports have confirmed that MR may be useful in the evaluation of both the brachial plexus and the supraclavicular region (262–266). The advantages of multi-planar imaging for these regions is apparent, especially as compared with CT. As shown by Rapoport et al., in an evaluation of 32 patients with symptoms referable to the brachial plexus, in 6 of the 12 cases of neoplasia in which CT scans were also obtained, MR showed more extensive disease in all (264). In the remaining 6 cases, findings were sufficiently characteristic on MR to obviate the need for additional imaging

studies altogether. Additionally, MR provided definitive diagnoses in three cases of trauma. Similar findings have been reported by Castagno and Shuman (263).

CONCLUSION

Computed tomography plays a valuable role in assessment of patients with a wide variety of diseases of the pleura and chest wall. Despite limitations, CT frequently provides precise anatomic localization of lesions of the pleura and chest wall. CT is especially valuable in differentiating pleural from parenchymal disease, especially in patients with complex pleuro-parenchymal pathology. Additionally, the ability of CT to differentiate among various tissue densities in select cases can allow precise histologic characterization of lesions such as pleural lipomas or hemorrhagic effusions. Even in those cases in which a precise histologic diagnosis is impossible, CT can still play a vital role, for example, by aiding in the diagnosis of malignant pleural effusions by identifying otherwise undetectable subpleural nodules, or focal areas of nodular or irregular pleural thickening. CT may also play an important role in monitoring therapy, both for neoplastic and nonneoplastic diseases. In select cases, CT can be used to guide needle placement for tissue biopsy or direct placement of pleural tubes.

In comparison, the role of MR in evaluating pleural disease is presently still limited, although MR may be useful in differentiating pleural from parenchymal disease. MR has proven of greater value in assessing the chest wall, especially in patients with peripheral or apical lung tumors. The brachial plexus, in particular, appears to be easily assessed with MR. It may be anticipated that with further refinement, MR will play an increasingly important role in patients with pleural and chest wall disease.

REFERENCES

1. Kreel L. Computed tomography of the lung and pleura. *Semin Roentgenol* 1978;13:213–225.
2. Pugatch RD, Faling IJ, Robbins AH, Snider GL. Differentiation of pleural and pulmonary lesions using computed tomography. *J Comput Assist Tomogr* 1978;2:601–606.
3. Im JG, Webb WR, Rosen AW, Gamsu G. Costal pleura: appearances at high-resolution CT. *Radiology* 1989;171:125–131.
4. Bressler EL, Francis IR, Glazer GM, Gross BH. Bolus contrast medium enhancement for distinguishing pleural from parenchymal lung disease: CT features. *J Comput Assist Tomogr* 1987;11:436–440.
5. Berne AS, Heitzman ER. The roentgenographic signs of pedunculated pleural tumors. *AJR* 1962;87:892–895.
6. Lewis MI, Horak DA, Yellin A, Rotter A, Belman MJ, Benfield JR. The case of the moving intrathoracic mass. *Chest* 1985;88:897–898.
7. Williford ME, Hidalgo H, Putman CE, Korobkin M, Ram PC. Computed tomography of pleural disease. *AJR* 1983;140:909–914.
8. Zinn WL, Naidich DP, Whelan CA, Litt AW, McCauley DI, Ettenger NA. Fluid within preexisting air-spaces: a potential pitfall in the CT differentiation of pleural from parenchymal disease. *J Comput Assist Tomogr* 1987;11:441–448.
9. Rassch BN, Carsky EW, Lane EJ, O'Callaghan JP, Heitzman ER. Pictorial essay. Pleural effusion: explanation of some typical appearances. *AJR* 1982;139:899–904.
10. Maffessanti M, Tommasi M, Pelegrini P. Computed tomography of free pleural effusions. *Eur J Radiol* 1987;7:87–90.
11. Griffin DJ, Gross BH, McCracken S, Glazer GM. Observations on CT differentiation of pleural and peritoneal fluid. *J Comput Assist Tomogr* 1984;8:24–28.
12. Federle MP, Mark AS, Guillaumin ES. CT of subpulmonic pleural effusions and atelectasis: criteria for differentiation from subphrenic fluid. *AJR* 1986;146:685–689.
13. Epler GR, McLoud TC, Munn CS, Colby TV. Pleural lipoma. Diagnosis by computed tomography. *Chest* 1986;90:265–268.
14. Levi C, Gray JE, McCullough E, Hattery RR. The unreliability of CT numbers as absolute values. *AJR* 1982;139:443–447.
15. Vock P, Effmann EL, Hedlund LW, Lischko MM, Putman CE. Analysis of the density of pleural fluid analogs by computed tomography. *Invest Radiol* 1984;19:10–15.
16. Rawkin RN, Raval B, Finley R. Case report. Primary chylopericardium: combined lymphangiographic and CT diagnosis. *J Comput Assist Tomogr* 1980;4:869–870.
17. Marks BW, Kuhns IR. Identification of the pleural fissures with computed tomography. *Radiology* 1982;143:139–141.
18. Friga J, Schmit P, Katz M, Vadrot D, Laval-Jeantet M. Computed tomography of the pleural fissures: normal anatomy. *J Comput Assist Tomogr* 1982;6:1069–1074.
19. Goodman LR, Golkow RS, Steiner RM, Teplick SK, Haskin ME, Himmelstein E, Teplick JG. The right mid-lung window. *Radiology* 1982;143:135–138.
20. Proto AV, Ball JB. Computed tomography of the major and minor fissures. *AJR* 1983;140:439–448.
21. Genereux GP. The posterior pleural reflections. *AJR* 1983;141:141–149.
22. Proto AV, Ball JB. The superolateral major fissures. *AJR* 1983;140:431–437.
23. Chasen MH, McCarthy MJ, Gilliland JD, Floyd JL. Concepts in computed tomography of the thorax. *Radiographics* 1986;6:793–832.
24. Mayo JR, Muller NL, Henkelman RM. The double-fissure sign: a motion artifact on thin-section CT scans. *Radiology* 1987;165:580–581.
25. Berkman YM, Auh YH, Davis SD, Kazam E. Anatomy of the minor fissure: evaluation with thin-section CT. *Radiology* 1989;170:647–651.
26. Frija J, Yana C, Laval-Jeantet M. Letter to the editor. Anatomy of the minor fissure: evaluation with thin-section CT. *Radiology* 1989;173:571–572.
27. Otsuji H, Hatakeyama M, Kitamura I, Yoshimura H, Iweasaki S, Ohishi H, Uchida H, Kitamura S, Narita N. Right upper lobe versus right middle lobe: differentiation with thin-section high-resolution CT. *Radiology* 1989;172:653–656.
28. Speckman JM, Gamsu G, Webb WR. Alterations in CT mediastinal anatomy produced by an azygos lobe. *AJR* 1981;137:47–50.
29. Godwin JD, Tarver RD. Accessory fissures of the lung. *AJR* 1985;144:39–47.
30. Austin JHM. The left minor fissure. *Radiology* 1986;161:433–436.
31. Takasugi JE, Godwin JD. Left azygos lobe. *Radiology* 1989;171:133–134.
32. Quint LE, Glazer GM, Orringer MB. Central lung masses: prediction with CT if need for pneumonectomy versus lobectomy. *Radiology* 1987;165:735–738.
33. Cooper C, Moss AA, Buy J-N, Stark DD. CT appearance of the normal inferior pulmonary ligament. *AJR* 1983;141:237–240.
34. Rost RC Jr, Proto AV. Inferior pulmonary ligament: computed tomographic appearance. *Radiology* 1983;148:479–483.
35. Godwin JD, Vock P, Osborn DR. CT of the pulmonary ligament. *AJR* 1983;141:231–236.
36. Rabinowitz JG, Cohen BA, Mendelson DS. The pulmonary ligament. *Radiol Clin North Am* 1984;22:659–672.
37. Taylor GA, Fishman EK, Kramer SS, Siegelman SS. CT demonstration of the phrenic nerve. *J Comput Assist Tomogr* 1983;7:411–414.
38. Berkmen YM, Davis SD, Kazam E, Auh YH, Yankelevitz D, Girgis FG. Right phrenic nerve: anatomy, CT appearance, and differentiation from the pulmonary ligament. *Radiology* 1989;173:43–46.
39. Godwin JD, Merten DF, Baker ME. Paramediastinal pneumatocele: alternative explanations to gas in the pulmonary ligament. *AJR* 1985;145:525–530.
40. Baron MG. Radiologic notes in cardiology: interlobar effusion. *Circulation* 1971;44:475–483.
41. Pecorari A, Weisbrod GL. Computed tomography of psuedotumoral pleural fluid collections in the azygoesophageal recess. *J Comput Assist Tomogr* 1989;13:803–805.
42. Griffin DJ, Gross BH, McCracken S, Glazer GM. Observations on CT differentiation of pleural and peritoneal fluid. *J Comput Assist Tomogr* 1984;8:24–28.
43. Halvorsen RA, Fedyshin PJ, Korobkin M, Thompson WM. CT differentiation of pleural effusion from ascites. An evaluation of four signs using blinded analysis of 52 cases. *Invest Radiol* 1986;21:391–395.
44. Halvorsen RA, Fedyshin PJ, Korobkin M, Foster WL Jr, Thompson WM. Ascites or pleural effusion? CT differentiation: four useful criteria. *Radiographics* 1986;6:135–149.
45. Light RW. Management of parapneumonic effusions. *Chest* 1976;70:3–4.
46. Sahn SA. The pleura. *Am Rev Resp Dis* 1988;138:184–234.
47. Miller KS, Sahn S. Chest tubes. Indications, technique, management and complications. *Chest* 1987;91:258–264.
48. American Thoracic Society Subcommittee on Surgery. Management of non-tuberculous empyema. *Am Rev Resp Dis* 1962;85:935.
49. Berger HA, Morganroth ML. Immediate drainage is not required for all patients with complicated parapneumonic effusions. *Chest* 1990;97:731–735.
50. Orringer MB. Thoracic empyema—back to basics. *Chest* 1988;93:901–902.
51. Hood RM. *Surgical diseases of the pleura and chest wall*. Philadelphia: WB Saunders, 1987;95.
52. Hoover EL, Hsu H-K, Ross MJ, Gross AM, Webb H, Ketosugbo A, Finch P. Reappraisal of empyema thoracis. Surgical interven-

tion when the duration of illness is unknown. *Chest* 1986;90:511–515.

53. Schmitt WGH, Hubener KH, Rucker HC. Pleural calcification with persistent effusion. *Radiology* 1983;149:633–638.

54. Bhatt GM, Austin HM. Case report. CT demonstration of empyema necessitatis. *J Comput Assist Tomogr* 1985;9:1108–1109.

55. Peterson MW, Austin JHM, Yip AC, McManus RP, Jaretzki A. Case report. CT findings in transdiaphragmatic empyema necessitatis due to tuberculosis. *J Comput Assist Tomogr* 1987;11:704–706.

56. Hulnick D, Naidich DP, McCauley DI. CT of pleural tuberculosis. *Radiology* 1983;149:759–765.

57. Friedman PJ, Hellekant CAG. Radiologic recognition of bronchopleural fistula. *Radiology* 1977;124:289–295.

58. Baber CEJ, Hedlund LW, Oddson TA, Putman CE. Differentiating empyemas and peripheral pulmonary abscesses. The value of computed tomography. *Radiology* 1980;135:755–758.

59. Shin M, Ho K-J. Computed tomographic characteristics of pleural empyema. *J Comput Tomogr* 1983;7:179–182.

60. Williford ME, Godwin JD. Computed tomography of lung abscess and empyema. *Radiol Clin North Am* 1983;21:575–583.

61. Stark D, Federle MP, Goodman PC, Podrasky AE, Webb WR. Differentiating lung abscess and empyema: radiography and computed tomography. *AJR* 1983;141:163–167.

62. Peters ME, Gould HR, McCarthy TM. Identification of a bronchopleural fistula by computerized tomography—a case report. *J Comput Tomogr* 1983;7:267–270.

63. Naidich DP. Radiologic evaluation of pleural disease. In: Hood RM. *Surgical diseases of the pleura and chest wall.* Philadelphia: WB Saunders, 1986;95.

64. Bartlett JG. Anaerobic bacterial pneumonitis. *Am Rev Respir Dis* 1979;119:19–23.

65. Robinson Baker R. The treatment of lung abscess. Current concepts [Editorial]. *Chest* 1985;87:709–710.

66. Viamonte M Jr, Parks RE, Smoak WM. Guided catheterization of the bronchial arteries. Part 2. Pulmonary and mediastinal neoplasms. *Radiology* 1965;85:205–230.

67. Himmelman RB, Callen PW. The prognostic value of loculations in parapneumonic pleural effusions. *Chest* 1986;90:852–856.

68. Waite RJ, Carbonneau RJ, Balikian JP, Umali CB, Pezzella AT, Nash G. Parietal pleural changes in empyema: appearances at CT. *Radiology* 1990;175:145–150.

69. Neff CC, vanSonnenberg E, Lawson EX, Patton AS. CT followup of empyemas: pleural peels resolve after percutaneous catheter drainage. *Radiology* 1990;176:195–197.

70. Stark DD, Federle MP, Goodman PC. CT and radiographic assessment of tube thoracostomy. *AJR* 1983;141:253–258.

71. Webb WR, LaBerge JM. Radiographic recognition of chest tube malposition in the major fissure. *Chest* 1984;85:81–83.

72. Panicek DM, Randall PA, Witanowski LS, Raasch BN, Heitzman ER. Chest tube tracks. *Radiographics* 1987;7:321–342.

73. Shapiro MP, Gale ME, Daly BD. Eloesser window thoracostomy for treatment of empyema: radiographic appearance. *AJR* 1988;150:549–552.

74. Mullin DM, Rodan BA, Bean WJ, Gocke TM, Feng TS. Computed tomography of oleothorax. *CT* 1987;10:197–199.

75. Westcott J. Percutaneous catheter drainage of pleural effusion and empyema. *AJR* 1985;144:1189–1193.

76. vanSonnenberg E, Nakamoto SK, Mueller PR, et al. CT- and ultrasound-guided catheter drainage of empyemas after chesttube failure. *Radiology* 1984;151:349–353.

77. Merriam MA, Cronan JJ, Dorfman GS, Lambiase RE, Haas RA. Radiographically guided percutaneous catheter drainage of pleural fluid collections. *AJR* 1988;151:1113–1116.

78. Hunnam GR, Flower CDR. Radiologically guided percutaneous catheter drainage of empyemas. *Clin Radiol* 1988;39:121–126.

79. Moulton JS, Moore PT, Mencici RA. Treatment of loculated pleural effusions with transcatheter intracavitary urokinase. *AJR* 1989;153:941–945.

80. Reinhold C, Illescase FF, Atri M, Bret PM. Treatment of pleural effusions and pneumothorax with catheters placed percutaneously under imaging guidance. *AJR* 1989;152:1189–1191.

81. Sison RF, Hruban RH, Moore GW, Kuhlman JE, Wheeler PS, Hutchins GM. Pulmonary disease associated with pleural "asbestos" plaques. *Chest* 1989;95:835.

82. Kreel L. Computer tomography in the evaluation of pulmonary asbestosis: preliminary experiences with the EMI general purpose scanner. *Acta Radiol [Diagn] (Stockh)* 1976;17:4.

83. Katz D, Kreel L. Computed tomography in pulmonary asbestosis. *Clin Radiol* 1979;30:207–213.

84. Gefter WB, Epstein DM, Miller WT. Radiographic evaluation of asbestos-related chest disorders. *CRC Crit Rev Diagn Imaging* 1984;21:133–181.

85. Aberle DR, Balmes JR. Computed tomography of asbestos-related pulmonary parenchymal and pleural diseases. *Clin Chest Med.* 1991. [In press].

86. Aberle DR, Gamsu G, Ray CS, Feuerstein IM. Asbestos-related pleural and parenchymal fibrosis: detection with high-resolution CT. *Radiology* 1988;166:729–734.

87. Aberle DR, Gamsu G, Ray CS. High-resolution CT of benign asbestos-related diseases: clinical and radiologic correlation. *AJR* 1988;151:883–891.

88. Friedman AC, Fiel SB, Fisher MS, Radecki PD, Lev-Toaff AS, Caroline DF. Asbestos-related pleural disease and asbestosis: a comparison of CT and chest radiography. *AJR* 1988;150:269–275.

89. Gamsu G, Aberle DR, Lynch D. Computed tomography in the diagnosis of asbestos-related thoracic disease. *J Thorac Imag* 1989;4:61–67.

90. McLoud TC, Woods BO, Carrington CB, Epler GR, Gaensler EA. Diffuse pleural thickening in an asbestos-exposed population: prevalence and causes. *AJR* 1985;144:9–18.

91. Rupp SB, Jolles H. Calcified plaque in the superior portion of the major fissure. An unusual manifestation of asbestos exposure. *Chest* 1989;96:1436–1437.

92. Withers BF, Ducatman AM, Yang WN. Roentgenographic evidence for predominant left-sided location of unilateral pleural plaques. *Chest* 1984;95:262–264.

93. Craighead JE, Abraham JL, Churg A, et al. The pathology of asbestos-associated diseases of the lungs and pleural cavities: diagnostic criteria and proposed grading schema. *Arch Pathol Lab Med* 1982;106:544–596.

94. Churg A. Asbestos fibers and pleural plaques in a general autopsy population. *Am J Pathol* 1982;109:88–96.

95. Epler GR, McLoud TC, Gaensler EA. Prevalence and incidence of benign asbestos pleural effusion in a working population. *JAMA* 1982;247:617–622.

96. Gefter WB, Conant EF. Issues and controversies in the plain-film diagnosis of asbestos-related disorders in the chest. *J Thorac Imag* 1988;3:11–28.

97. Becklake MR. State of the art: asbestos-related disease of the lung and other organs: their epidemiology and implications for clinical practice. *Am Rev Respir Dis* 1976;114:187–227.

98. Jones RN, McLoud T, Rockoff SD. The radiographic pleural abnormalities in asbestos exposure: relationship to physiologic abnormalities. *J Thorac Imag* 1988;3:57–66.

99. Schwartz DA, Fuortes LJ, Galvin JR, Burmeister LF, Schmidt LE, et al. Asbestos-induced pleural fibrosis and impaired lung function. *Am Rev Respir Dis* 1990;141:321–326.

100. Begin R, Boctor M, Bergeron D, et al. Radiographic assessment of pleuropulmonary disease in asbestos workers: posteroanterior, four viewfilms, and computed tomograms of the thorax. *Br J Ind Med* 1984;41:373–383.

101. Sargent EN, Boswell WD Jr, Ralls PW, Markovitz A. Subpleural fat pads in patients exposed to asbestosis: distinction from noncalcified pleural plaques. *Radiology* 1984;152:273–277.

102. Rabinowitz JG, Efremidis SC, Cohen B, Dan S, Efremidis A, Chakinian AP, Teirstein AS. A comparative study of mesothelioma and asbestosis using computed tomography and conventional chest radiography. *Radiology* 1982;144:453–460.

103. Menzies R, Fraser R. Round atelectasis. Pathologic and pathogenetic features. *Am J Surg Pathol* 1987;11:674–681.

104. Schneider H, Felson B, Gonzalez L. Rounded atelectasis. *AJR* 1980;134:225–232.

105. Mintzer RA, Gore RM, Vogelzang RL, Holz S. Rounded atelectasis and its association with asbestos-induced pleural disease. *Radiology* 1981;139:567–570.

106. Tylen U, Nilsson U. Computed tomography in pulmonary pseudotumors and their relation to asbestos exposure. *J Comput Assist Tomogr* 1982;6:229–237.

107. Glass TA, Armstrong P, Minor GR, Dyer RB. Computed tomographic features of round atelectasis. *J Comput Tomogr* 1983;7:183–185.

108. Doyle T, Lawler G. CT features of rounded atelectasis of the lung. *AJR* 1984;143:225–228.

109. McHugh K, Blaquiere RM. CT features of rounded atelectasis. *AJR* 1989;153:257–260.

110. Ren H, Hruban RH, Kuhlman JE, Fishman EK, Wheeler PS, Zerhouni EA, Hutchins GM. Case report. Computed tomography of rounded atelectasis. *J Comput Assist Tomogr* 1989;12:1031–1034.

111. Lynch DA, Gamsu G, Aberle DR. Conventional and high resolution computed tomography in the diagnosis of asbestos-related diseases. *Radiographics* 1989;9:523–551.

112. Taylor PM. Dynamic contrast enhancement of asbestos-related pulmonary pseudotumors. *Br J Radiol* 1988;61:1070–1072.

113. Coleman BG, Epstein DM, Arger PH, Miller WT. Case report. CT features of an unusual hypervascular lung carcinoma complicating chronic asbestosis related pleural disease. *J Comput Assist Tomogr* 1985;9:554–557.

114. Sinner WWN. Pleuroma—a cancer mimicking atelectatic pseudotumor of the lung. *Fortschr Geb Rontgenst Nuklarmed Erganzungsband* 1980;133:578–585.

115. Reifsnyder AC, Smith HJ, Mullhollan TJ, Lee EL. Case report. Malignant fibrous histiocytoma of the lung in a patient with a history of asbestos exposure. *AJR* 1990;154:65–66.

116. Blesovsky A. The folded lung. *Br J Dis Chest* 1966;60:19–22.

117. Hanke R, Kretzschmar R. Rounded atelectasis. *Semin Roentgenol* 1980;15:174–182.

118. Hillerdal G. Rounded atelectasis. Clinical experience with 74 patients. *Chest* 1989;95:836–841.

119. Stancato-Pasik A, Mendelson DS, Marom Z. Case report. Rounded atelectasis caused by histoplasmosis. *AJR* 1990;155:275–276.

120. Hillerdal G. Asbestos-related pleural disease. *Semin Respir Med* 1987;9:65–74.

121. Lynch DA, Ferrsci MB, Gamsu G et al. Asbestos-related focal lung masses: manifestations on conventional and high-resolution CT scans. *Radiology* 1988;169:603–607.

122. Verschakelen JA, Demaerel P, Coolen J, Demedts M, Marchal G, Baert AL. Case report. Rounded atelectasis of the lung: MR appearance. *AJR* 1989;152:965–966.

123. Leff A, Hopewell PC, Costello J. Pleural effusion from malignancy. *Ann Intern Med* 1978;88:532–537.

124. Chernow B, Sahn SA. Carcinomatous involvement of the pleura: an analysis of 96 patients. *Am J Med* 1977;63:695–702.

125. Meyer PC. Metastatic carcinoma of the pleura. *Thorax* 1966;21:437–443.

126. Salyer WR, Eggleston JC, Erozan YS. The efficacy of pleural needle biopsy and of pleural fluid cytology in the diagnosis of malignant neoplasm involving the pleura. *Chest* 1975;67:5.

127. Scerbo J, Keltz H, Stone DJ. A prospective study of closed pleural biopsies. *JAMA* 1971;218:377–380.

128. Ryan CJ, Rodgers RF, Unni KK, Hepper NGG. The outcome of patients with pleural effusion of indeterminate cause at thoracotomy. *Mayo Clin Proc* 1981;56:145–149.

129. Tattersall MHN, Boyer MJ. Management of malignant effusions [Editorial]. *Thorax* 1990;45:81–82.

130. Martini N, Bains MS, Beattie EJ. Indications for pleurectomy in malignant effusion. *Cancer* 1975;35:734–738.

131. Heitzman ER, Markarian B, Raasch GN, Carsky EW, Lane EJ, Berlow ME. Annual oration. Pathways of tumor spread through the lung: radiologic correlations with anatomy and pathology. *Radiology* 1982;144:3–14.

132. Webb WR, Jeffrey RB, Godwin JD. Thoracic computed tomography in superior sulcus tumors. *J Comput Assist Tomogr* 1981;5:361–365.

133. Glazer HS, Duncan-Meyer J, Aronberg DJ, et al. Pleural and chest wall invasion in bronchogenic carcinoma: CT evaluation. *Radiology* 1985;157:191.

134. Pennes DR, Glazer GM, Wimbish KJ, et al. Chest wall invasion by lung cancer: limitations of CT evaluation. *AJR* 1985;144:507.

135. Shin MS, Anderson SD, Myers J, Ho KJ. Case report. Pitfalls in CT evaluation of chest wall invasion by lung cancer. *J Comput Assist Tomogr* 1986;10:136–138.

136. Pearlberg JL, Sandler MA, Beute GH, Lewis JW Jr, Madrazo BL. Limitations of CT in evaluation of neoplasms involving chest wall. *J Comput Assist Tomogr* 1987;11:290–293.

137. Glazer HS, Kaiser LR, Anderson DJ, Molina PL, Emami B, Roper CL, Sagel SS. Indeterminate mediastinal invasion in bronchogenic carcinoma: CT evaluation. *Radiology* 1989; 173:37.

138. Grenier P, Dubray B, Carette MF, Frija G, Musset D, Chastan GC. Preoperative thoracic staging of lung cancer: CT and MR evaluation. *Diagn Inter Radiol* 1989;173(P):69.

139. Heelan RT, Demas BE, Caravelli JF, Martini N, Bains MS, McCormack PM, Burt M, Panicek DM, Mitzner A. Superior sulcus tumors: CT and MR imaging. *Radiology* 1989;170:637.

140. McLoud TC, Filion RB, Edelman RR, Shepard JO. MR imaging of superior sulcus carcinoma. *J Comput Assist Tomogr* 1989;13:233–239.

141. Webb WR, Jensen BJ, Sollitto R, et al. Bronchogenic carcinoma: staging with MR compared with staging with CT and surgery. *Radiology* 1985;156:117.

142. Haggar AM, Pearlberg JL, Froelich JW, et al. Chest wall invasion by carcinoma of the lung: detection by MR imaging. *AJR* 1987;148:1075–1087.

143. Webb RW, Gatsonis C, Zerhouni EA, Heelan RT, Glazer GM, Francis IR, McNeil BJ. CT and MR in staging non-small cell bronchogenic carcinoma: Report of the Radiological Diagnostic Oncology Group. *Radiology* 1989;173(P):69.

144. Adams VI, Unni KK, Muhm JR, Jett JR, Ilstrup DM, Bernatz PE. Diffuse malignant mesothelioma of pleura. Diagnosis and survival in 92 cases. *Cancer* 1986;58:1540–1551.

145. Martini N, McCormack PM, Bains MS, Kaiser LR, Burt ME, Hilaris BS. Current review. Pleural mesothelioma. *Ann Thorac Surg* 1987;43:113–120.

146. Dunn MM. Asbestos and the lung. *Chest* 1989;95:1304–1308.

147. Butchart EE, Ashcroft T, Barnely NC, et al. The role of surgery in diffuse malignant mesothelioma of the pleura. *Semin Oncol* 1981;8:321.

148. Dedrick CG, McLoud TC, Shepard JO, Shipley RT. Computed tomography of localized pleural mesothelioma. *AJR* 1985;144:275–280.

149. Spizarny DL, Gross BH, Shepard J-A O. CT findings in localized fibrous mesothelioma of the pleural fissure. *J Comput Assist Tomogr* 1986;10:942–944.

150. Kreel L. Computed tomography in mesothelioma. *Semin Oncol* 1981;8:302–312.

151. Alexander E, Clark RA, Colley DP, Mitchell SE. CT of malignant pleural mesothelioma. *AJR* 1981;137:287–291.

152. Rabinowitz JG, Efremidis SC, Cohen B, Dan S, Efremidis A, Chakinian AP, Tierstein AS. A comparative study of mesothelioma and asbestosis using computed tomography and conventional chest radiography. *Radiology* 1982;144:453–460.

153. Grant DC, Seltzer SE, Antman KH, Finberg HJ, Koster K. Computed tomography of malignant pleural mesothelioma. *J Comput Assist Tomogr* 1983;7:626–632.

154. Mirvis S, Cutcher JP, Haney PJ, Whitley NO, Aisner J. CT of malignant pleural mesothelioma. *AJR* 1983;140:665–670.

155. Salonen O, Kivisaari L, Standertskjold-Nordenstam C-G, Somer K, Mattson K, Tammilehto L. Computed tomography of pleural lesions with special reference to the mediastinal pleura. *Acta Radiol [Diagn] (Stockh)* 1986;27:527–531.

156. Rusch VW, Godwin JD, Shuman WP. The role of computed tomography scanning in the initial assessment and the follow-up of malignant pleural mesothelioma. *J Thorac Cardiovasc Surg* 1988;96:171–177.

157. Kawashima A, Libshitz HI. Malignant pleural mesothelioma: CT manifestations in 50 cases. *AJR* 1990;155:965–969.

158. Shin MS, Berland LL, Ho K-J. Case report. Postoperative malignant seroma: CT demonstration of its formation mechanism. *J Comput Assist Tomogr* 1984;8:1001–1004.

159. Uri AJ, Schulman ES, Steiner RM, Scot RD, Rose LJ. Diffuse

contralateral pulmonary metastases in malignant mesothelioma. An unusual radiographic presentation. *Chest* 1988;93:433–434.

160. Taylor RD, Page W, Hughes D, Vargese G. Metastatic renal cell carcinoma mimicking pleural mesothelioma. *Thorax* 1987;42:901–902.

161. Reifsnyder AC, Smith HJ, Mullhollan TJ, Lee EL. Case report. Malignant fibrous histiocytoma of the lung in a patient with a history of asbestos exposure. *AJR* 1990;154:65–66.

162. Zerhouni EA, Scott WW, Baker RR, Wharam MO, Siegelman SS. Invasive thymomas: diagnosis and evaluation by computed tomography. *J Comput Assist Tomogr* 1982;6:92–100.

163. Scatariage JC, Fishman EK, Zerhouni EA, Siegelman SS. Transdiaphragmatic extension of invasive thymoma. *AJR* 1985;144:31–35.

164. Blank N, Castellino RA. The intrathoracic manifestations of the malignant lymphomas and leukemia. *Semin Roentgenol* 1980;15:227–245.

165. Xaubet A, Diumenjo MC, Marin A, et al. Characteristics and prognostic value of pleural effusions in non-Hodgkin's lymphomas. *Eur J Respir Dis* 1985;66:135–140.

166. Fisher AMH, Kendall B, Van Leuven BD. Hodgkin's disease: a radiologic survey. *Clin Radiol* 1962;13:115–127.

167. Stolberg HO, Patt NL, MacEwan KF, Warwick OH, Brown TC. Hodgkin's disease of the lung: radiologic-pathologic correlation. *AJR* 1964;192:96–115.

168. Ellert J, Kreel L. The role of computed tomography in the initial staging and subsequent management of the lymphomas. *J Comput Assist Tomogr* 1980;4:368–391.

169. Burgener FH, Hamlin DJ. Intrathoracic histiocytic lymphoma. *AJR* 1981;136:499–504.

170. Shuman LS, Libshitz HI. Pictorial essay. Solid pleural manifestations of lymphoma. *AJR* 1984;142:269–273.

171. Bernadreschi P, Bonechi I, Urbano U. Recurrent pleural effusion as manifesting feature of primitive chest wall Hodgkin's disease. *Chest* 1988;94:424–426.

172. Biondetti PR, Fiore D, Sartori F, Colognato A, Ravaseni S. Evaluation of the post-pneumonectomy space by computed tomography. *J Comput Assist Tomogr* 1982;6:238–242.

173. Peters JC, Desai KK. CT demonstration of postpneumonectomy tumor recurrence. *AJR* 1983;141:259–262.

174. Glazer HS, Aronberg DJ, Sagel SS, Bahman E. Utility of CT in detecting postpneumonectomy carcinoma recurrence. *AJR* 1984;142:487–494.

175. Heater K, Revzani L, Rubin JM. CT evaluation of empyema in the postpneumonectomy space. *AJR* 1985;145:39–40.

176. Shepard J-A O, Grillo HC, McLoud TC, Dedrick CG, Spirzarny DL. Right-pneumonectomy syndrome: radiologic findings and CT correlation. *Radiology* 1986;161:661–664.

177. Laissy J-P, Rebibo G, Iba-Zizen M-T, Cabanis EA, Benozio M. MR appearance of the normal chest after pneumonectomy. *J Comput Assist Tomogr* 1989;13:248–252.

178. Munk PL, Muller NL. Pleural liposarcoma: CT diagnosis. *J Comput Assist Tomogr* 1988;12:709–710.

179. Paling MR, Hyams DM. Computed tomography in malignant fibrous histiocytoma. *J Comput Assist Tomogr* 1982;6:765–788.

180. Leung AN, Muller NL, Miller RR. CT in differential diagnosis of diffuse pleural disease. *AJR* 1990;154:487–492.

181. Gouliamos AD, Carter BL, Emami B. Computed tomography of the chest wall. *Radiology* 1980;134:433–436.

182. Kirks DR, Korobkin M. Computed tomography of the chest wall, pleura, and pulmonary parenchyma in infants and children. *Radiol Clin North Am* 1981;19:421–429.

183. Leitman BS, Firoozna H, McCauley DI, Ettenger NA, Reede E, Golimbu CN, Rafii M, Naidich DP. The use of computed tomography in the evaluation of chest wall pathology. *J Comput Tomogr* 1983;7:399–405.

184. Gautard R, Dussault RG, Chahlaoui J, Duranceau A, Sylvestre J. Contribution of CT in thoracic bony lesions. *J Can Assoc Radiol* 1981;32:39–41.

185. Destouet JM, Gilula LA, Murphy WA, Sagel SS. Computed tomography of the sternoclavicular joint and sternum. *Radiology* 1981;138:123–128.

186. Goodman LR, Teplick SK, Kay H. Computed tomography of the normal sternum. *AJR* 1983;141:219–223.

187. Hatfield MK, Gross BH, Glazer GM, Martel W. Computed tomography of the sternum and its articulations. *Skeletal Radiol* 1984;11:197–203.

188. Stark P, Jaramillo D. Pictorial essay. CT of the sternum. *AJR* 1986;147:72–77.

189. Stark P, Watkins GE, Hildebrandt-Stark HE, Dunbar RD. Episternal ossicles. *Radiology* 1987;165:143–144.

190. Jafri SZ, Roberts JL, Bree RL, Tubor HD. Computed tomography of chest wall masses. *Radiographics* 1989;9:51–68.

191. Goodman LR, Kay HR, Teplick SK, Mundth ED. Complications of median sternotomy: computed tomographic evaluation. *AJR* 1983;141:225–230.

192. Carter AR, Sostman HD, Curtis AM, Swett HA. Thoracic alterations after cardiac surgery. *AJR* 1983;140:475–481.

193. Leitman BS, Naidich DP, McCauley DI. Computed tomography of pectoral flaps. *J Comput Assist Tomogr* 1988;12:392–393.

194. Aoki J, Moser RP, Kransdork MJ. Chondrosarcoma of the sternum: CT features. *J Comput Assist Tomogr* 1989;13:806–810.

195. Levinsohn EM, Bunnell WP, Wuan HA. Computed tomography in the diagnosis of dislocations of the sternoclavicular joint. *Clin Orthop* 1979;140:12–16.

196. Burnstein MI, Pozniak A. Case report. Computed tomography with stress maneuver to demonstrate sternoclavicular joint dislocation. *J Comput Assist Tomogr* 1990;14:159–160.

197. Sartoris DJ, Schreiman JS, Kerr R, Resnick CS, Resnick D. Sternoclavicular hyperostosis: a review and report of 11 cases. *Radiology* 1986;158:125–128.

198. Rafii M, Firooznia H, Golimbu C. Computed tomography of septic joints. *CT* 1985;9:51–60.

199. Alexander PW, Shin MS. CT manifestations of sternoclavicular pyarthrosis in patients with intravenous drug abuse. *J Comput Assist Tomogr* 1990;14:104–106.

200. Pollack MS. Staphylococcal mediastinitis due to sternoclavicular pyarthrosis: CT appearance. *J Comput Assist Tomogr* 1990;14:924–928.

201. Edelstein G, Levitt RG, Slaker DP, Murphy W. CT observation of rib abnormalities: spectrum of findings. *J Comput Assist Tomogr* 1985;9:65–72.

202. Edelstein G, Levitt RG, Slaker DP, Murphy WA. Computed tomography of Tietze syndrome. *J Comput Assist Tomogr* 1984;8:20–23.

203. Levine E, Levine C. Ewings tumor of rib: radiologic findings and computed tomography contribution. *Skeletal Radiol* 1983;8:227–233.

204. Moser RP, Davis MJ, Gilkey FW, Kransdorf MJ, Rosado de Christenson ML, Kumar R, Bloem JL, Stull MA. Primary Ewing sarcoma of rib. *Radiographics* 1990;10:899–914.

205. Ortega W, Mahboubi S, Dalinka MK, Robinson T. Computed tomography of rib hemangiomas. *J Comput Assist Tomogr* 1986;10:945–947.

206. Bhalla M, McCauley DI, Golimbu C, Leitman BS, Naidich DP. Counting ribs on chest CT. *J Comput Assist Tomogr* 1990;14:590–594.

207. Stark P, Lawrence DD. Intrathoracic rib. CT features of a rare chest wall anomaly. *Comput Radiol* 1984;8:365–367.

208. Trigaux J-P P, Sibille Y, Van Beers B. Case report. Intrathoracic rib: CT features. *J Comput Assist Tomogr* 1990;14:133–135.

209. Wechsler RJ. *Cross-Sectional Analysis of the Chest and Abdominal Wall*. St. Louis: CV Mosby, 1989.

210. Fishman EK, Zinreich ES, Jacobs CG, Rostock REA, Siegelman SS. CT of the axilla: normal anatomy and pathology. *Radiographics* 1986;6:475–502.

211. Goldberg RP, Austin RM. Computed tomography of axillary and supraclavicular adenopathy. *Clin Radiol* 1985;36:593–596.

212. Holbert BL, Holbert JM, Libshitz HI. CT of interpectoral lymph nodes. *AJR* 1987;149:687–688.

213. Meyer JE, Munzenrider JE. Computed tomographic demonstration of internal mammary lymph node metastasis in patients with locally recurrent breast carcinoma. *Radiology* 1981;139:661–664.

214. Munzenrider JE, Tchakarova I, Castro M, Carter BL. Computerized body tomography in breast cancer: internal mammary nodes and radiation treatment planning. *Cancer* 1979;43:137–150.

215. Lindfors KK, Meyer JE, Busse PM, Kopans DB, Munzenrider

JE, Sawicka JM. Evaluation of local and regional breast cancer recurrence. *AJR* 1985;145:833–837.

216. Shea WJ, de Geer G, Webb WR. Chest wall after mastectomy. Part 1. CT appearance of normal postoperative anatomy, postirradiation changes and optimal scanning techniques. *Radiology* 1987;162:157–161.

217. Shea WJ, de Geer G, Webb WR. Chest wall after mastectomy. Part 2. CT appearance of tumor recurrence. *Radiology* 1987;162:162–164.

218. Scatarige JC, Fishman EK, Zinreich ES, Brem RF, Almaraz R. Internal mammary lymphadenopathy in breast carcinoma: CT appraisal of anatomic distribution. *Radiology* 1988;167:89–91.

219. Scatarige JC, Boxen I, Smathers RL. Internal mammary lymphadenopathy: imaging of a vital lymphatic pathway in breast cancer. *Radiographics* 1990;10:857–870.

220. Hudson TM, et al. Aggressive fibromatosis: evaluation by computed tomography and angiography. *Radiology* 1984;150:495.

221. Berthoty DP, Shulman HS, Miller HAB. Elastofibroma: chest wall pseudotumor. *Radiology* 1986;160:341–342.

222. Marin ML, Austin JHM, Markowitz AM. Elastofibroma dorsi: CT demonstration. *J Comput Assist Tomogr* 1987;11:675–677.

223. Faer MJ, Burnam RE, Beck CL. Transmural thoracic lipoma: demonstration by computed tomography. *AJR* 1978;130:161–163.

224. Sullivan WT. Extrapleural fat prolapse mimicking recurrent bronchogenic carcinoma. *CT* 1986;10:277–279.

225. Buxton RC, Tan CS, Khine NM, Cuasay NS, Shor MJ, Spigos DG. Atypical transmural thoracic lipoma: CT diagnosis. *J Comput Assist Tomogr* 1988;12:196–198.

226. Biondetti PR, Fiore D, Perin B, Ravasini R. Infiltrative angiolipoma of the thoracoabdominal wall. *J Comput Assist Tomogr* 1982;6:847.

227. Wilinsky J, Costello P, Clouse ME. Liposarcoma involving the scapula. *CT* 1984;8:341–343.

228. Whalen MA, Naidich DP, Post JD, Chase NE. Computed tomography of spinal tuberculosis. *J Comput Assist Tomogr* 1983;7:25–30.

229. Webb WR, Sagel SS. Actinomycosis involving the chest wall: CT findings. *AJR* 1982;139:1007–1009.

230. Allen HA, Scatarige JC, Kim MH. Actinomycosis: CT findings in six patients. *AJR* 1987;149:1255–1258.

231. James R, Heneghan MA, Lipansky V. Thoracic actinomycosis. *Chest* 1985;87:536–537.

232. Trigaux J-P, Beers BV. Thoracic collateral venous channels: normal and pathologic CT findings. *J Comput Assist Tomogr* 1990;14:769–773.

233. Yedlicka JW, Schultz K, Moncada R, Flisak M. CT findings in superior vena cava obstruction. *Semin Roentgenol* 1989;24:84–90.

234. Moncada R, Cardella R, Demos TC, et al. Evaluation of superior vena cava syndrome by axial CT and CT phlebography. *AJR* 1984;143:731–736.

235. Bechtold RE, Wolfman NT, Karstaedt N, Choplin RH. Superior vena cava obstruction: detection using CT. *Radiology* 1985;157:485–487.

236. Gerard PS, Lefkovitz Z, Golbey SH, Bryk D. Transient thoracic venous collaterals: an incidental CT finding. *J Comput Assist Tomogr* 1986;10:75–77.

237. Toombs BD, Sandler LM, Lester RG. Computed tomography of chest trauma. *Radiology* 1981;140:733–738.

238. Wall SD, Federle MP, Jeffrey RB, Brett CM. CT diagnosis of unsuspected pneumothorax after blunt abdominal trauma. *AJR* 1983;141:919–921.

239. Tocino IM, Miller WH, Freerick PR, Bahr AL, Thomas F. CT detection of occult pneumothorax in head trauma. *AJR* 1984;143:987–990.

240. Murphy FB, Small WC, Wichman RD, Chalif M, Bernardino ME. CT and chest radiography are equally sensitive in the detection of pneumothorax after CT-guided pulmonary interventional procedures. *AJR* 1990;154:45–46.

241. Vargas FC, Vas W, Carlin B, Morris L, Salimi Z. Case report. Radiographic and CT demonstration of mammary emphysema. *J Comput Assist Tomogr* 1985;9:560–562.

242. Wagner RB, Crawford WO Jr, Schimpf PP. Classification of parenchymal injuries of the lung. *Radiology* 1988;167:77–82.

243. Mirvis SE, Rodriguez A, Whitley NO, Tarr RJ. CT evaluation of thoracic infections after major trauma. *AJR* 1985;144:1183–1187.

244. Sivit CJ, Taylor GA, Eichelberger MR. Chest injury in children with blunt abdominal trauma: evaluation with CT. *Radiology* 1989;171:815–818.

245. Kerns SR, Gay SB. Pictorial essay. CT of blunt chest trauma. *AJR* 1990;154:55–60.

246. Fernandez GG, Coblentz CL, Cooper C, Sallee DS. Hickman nodule: a mimic of metastatic disease. *Radiology* 1989;171:401–402.

247. Nguyen TH, Hoang T-A, Dash N, Christlieb I, Lupetin AR, Beckman I, et al. Latissimus dorsi cardiomyoplasty: radiographic findings. *AJR* 1988;150:545–547.

248. Seibel DG, Hopper KD, Ghaed N. Case report. Mammographic and CT detection of extrathoracic lung herniation. *J Comput Assist Tomogr* 1987;11:537–538.

249. Bhalla M, Leitman BS, Forcade C, Stern E, Naidich DP, McCauley DI. Lung hernia: radiographic features. *AJR* 1990;154:51–53.

250. Brown JJ, van Sonnenberg E, Gerber KH, Strich G, Wittich GR, Slutsky RA. Magnetic resonance relaxation times of percutaneously obtained normal and abnormal body fluids. *Radiology* 1985;154:727–731.

251. Terrier F, Revel D, Pajannen H, Richardson M, Hricak H, Higgins CB. MR imaging of body fluid collections. *J Comput Assist Tomogr* 1986;10:953–962.

252. Vock P, Hedlund LW, Herfkens RJ, Effmann EL, Brown MA, Putman CE. Work in progress: In vitro analysis of pleural fluid analogs by proton magnetic resonance. Preliminary studies at 1.5T. *Invest Radiol* 1987;22:382–387.

253. Davis SD, Henschke CI, Yankelevitz DF, Cahill PT, Yi Y. MR imaging of pleural effusions. *J Comput Assist Tomogr* 1990;14:192–198.

254. Lorigan JG, Libshitz HI. MR imaging of malignant pleural mesothelioma. *J Comput Assist Tomogr* 1989;13:617–620.

255. Vogel HJPh, Wondergem JHM, Falke THM. Mesothelioma of the pericardium: CT and MR findings. *J Comput Assist Tomogr* 1989;13:543–546.

256. Bergin CJ, Healy MJ, Zincone GE, Castellino RA. MR evaluation of chest wall involvement in malignant lymphoma. *J Comput Assist Tomogr* 1990;14:928–933.

257. Dooms GC, Hricak H, Solitto RA, Higgins CB. Lipomatous tumors and tumors with fatty component: MR imaging potential and comparison of MR and CT results. *Radiology* 1985;157:479–483.

258. Kaplan PA, Williams SM. Mucocutaneous and peripheral soft-tissue hemangiomas: MR imaging. *Radiology* 1987;163:163–166.

259. Bechtold RE, Karstaedt N, Wolfman NT. Case report. MR appearance of sternal hyperostosis. *J Comput Assist Tomogr* 1990;14:136–139.

260. Erickson SJ, Kneelan JB, Konorowsko RA, Knudson GJ, Carrera GF. Case report. Post-traumatic osteolysis of the clavicle: MR features. *J Comput Assist Tomogr* 1990;14:835–837.

261. Sharif HS, Clark DC, Aabed MY, Aideyan OA, Haddad MC, Mattson TA. MR imaging of thoracic and abdominal wall infections: comparison with other imaging procedures. *AJR* 1990;154:989–995.

262. Blari DN, Rapoport S, Sostman HD, Blair OC. Normal brachial plexus: MR imaging. *Radiology* 1987;165:763–767.

263. Castagno AA, Shuman WP. MR imaging in clinically suspected brachioplexus tumor. *AJR* 1987;149:1219–1222.

264. Rapoport S, Blair DN, McCarthy SM, Desser TS, Hammers LW, Sostman HD. Brachial plexus: correlation of MR imaging with CT and pathologic findings. *Radiology* 1988;167:161–165.

265. Kellman GM, Kneeland JB, Middleton WD, Cates JD, Pech P, Grist TM, Foley WD, Jesmanowicz A, Froncisz W, Hyde JS. Pictorial essay. MR imaging of the supraclavicular region: normal anatomy. *AJR* 1987;148:77–82.

266. Kneeland JB, Kellman GM, Middleton WD, Cates JD, Jesmanowicz A, Froncisz W, Hyde JS. Pictorial essay. Diagnosis of diseases of the supraclavicular region by use of MR imaging. *AJR* 1987;148:1149–1151.

Chapter 10

The Diaphragm

The diaphragm acts as a cone-shaped partition to separate the thoracic and abdominal cavities. Physiologically, the diaphragm is the chief muscle of inspiration. Anatomically, the diaphragm represents the interface, and, on occasion, the actual pathway for the spread of disease between the abdomen and thorax. In this chapter, the normal cross-sectional appearance of the diaphragm will be reviewed. How this knowledge can be applied to the diagnosis of peridiaphragmatic pathology will be illustrated extensively.

GENERAL PRINCIPLES AND ANATOMY

Essential to the accurate interpretation of cross-sectional images through the base of the lungs and upper abdomen is identification of the hemidiaphragms (1–6). This is made possible by appreciation of the following principles.

The actual position of the hemidiaphragms over most of its course must be inferred (Fig. 1). This is because visualization of the normally thin line of the diaphragm itself is impossible when the diaphragm abuts structures of similar density, such as the liver and spleen. The hemidiaphragms can be visualized as separate structures only when their inner aspect is marginated by intraperitoneal or retroperitoneal fat, their outer aspect is marginated by air within the lungs or extraperitoneal fat, or less commonly, when there is an alteration in the density of adjacent viscera, as may occur, for example, in patients with marked fatty infiltration of the liver (Figs. 1 and 2).

Despite this limitation, the position of the hemidiaphragms can be inferred from knowledge of characteristic anatomic relationships between the diaphragm and surrounding structures. Specifically, at all levels the lungs and pleura lie adjacent and peripheral to the dia-

phragm, whereas the abdominal viscera, fat, and retroperitoneal spaces lie adjacent and central to the hemidiaphragms (Fig. 1) (1).

Further analysis of the cross-sectional appearance of the diaphragm requires detailed knowledge of anatomy.

The diaphragm consists of a central tendon, with extensions to the right and left: the right and left leaflets (Fig. 3). Muscle fibers insert into the central tendon from all parts of the circumference of the inner aspect of the body wall (7,8). The pericardium is firmly attached to the upper surface of the central tendon.

Anatomically, the diaphragm consists of two parts: the lumbar diaphragm and the costal diaphragm. The posterior portion of the diaphragm is more properly referred to as the lumbar portion (1,7,8). It is composed, in part, of the two crura which arise from the anterolateral surfaces of the bodies of the first three lumbar vertebrae on the right and the first two lumbar vertebrae on the left, respectively (Fig. 3). The remainder of the lumbar portion of the diaphragm arises from the medial and lateral arcuate ligaments. These ligaments represent thickenings of the thoracolumbar fascia overlying the anterior surfaces of the psoas and quadratus lumborum muscles (1,7,8). The medial arcuate ligament arises from the lateral margin of the L1 vertebral body and inserts on the transverse process of L1. The lateral arcuate ligament arises from the transverse process of the L1 vertebral body and inserts on the 12th rib (Fig. 3).

Fibers arising from both the crura and arcuate ligaments arch forward to insert into the central tendon of the diaphragm and its extensions, the right and left leaflets. It is apparent from Fig. 3, as it is drawn, that there may be no clear line of demarcation between fibers arising from the crura and fibers arising from the arcuate ligaments. Furthermore, as a rule, no clear line of demarcation separates the costal from the lumbar portions of the diaphragm (Fig. 4).

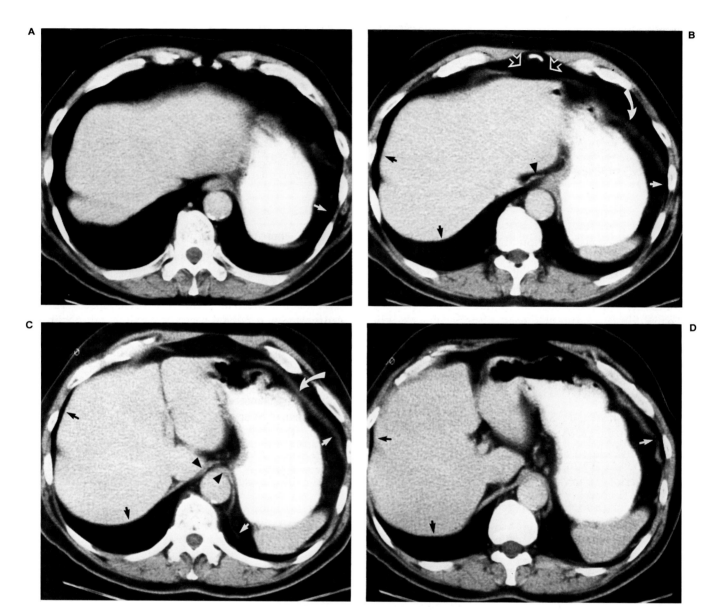

FIG. 1. Normal anatomy. **A–D:** Sequential 10-mm thick sections through the diaphragm at the level of the esophageal hiatus. The hemi-diaphragms can be visualized as separate structures only when marginated centrally by peritoneal or retroperitoneal fat (*white arrows* in A–D), or peripherally by air within the lungs, or by extraperitoneal fat (*curved arrows* in B and C). Visualization is lost when the diaphragms abut a structure of similar density (for example, the liver or spleen) (*straight black arrows* in B–D). The position of the diaphragm can still be inferred, however, from knowledge of characteristic anatomic relationships. At all levels, the lung and pleura lie adjacent and peripheral to the diaphragm; abdominal viscera, fat, and retroperitoneal structures lie adjacent and central to the hemidiaphragms. Note posteriorly the appearance of a normal esophageal hiatus defined by the medial margins of the crura, bilaterally (*arrowheads* in B and C). Anteriorly, note the subtle attachments of the diaphragm to the tip of the xiphoid.

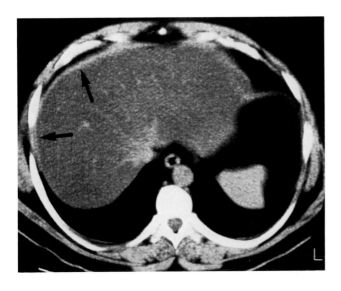

FIG. 2. Normal anatomy. CT section through the base of the lungs shows that the right hemidiaphragm can be visualized almost along its entire course due to marked fatty infiltration of the liver (*arrows*).

The most cephalad section in which the crura can be identified is at the level of the esophageal hiatus (Figs. 1 and 4). Typically, at this level the anteromedial margin of the right crus can be identified because of retroperitoneal fat within the posterior pararenal space (Fig. 1). Fat within this space has been identified in approximately 80% of normal subjects (1). More inferiorly, the right adrenal gland can be recognized within the perirenal space (Fig. 4). At this level, differentiation between perirenal fat and posterior pararenal fat can rarely be made.

On the left side, the anatomy appears less constant at the level of the esophageal hiatus. This is probably due to variability in the shape and position of the spleen. Analogous to the right side, retroperitoneal fat within the posterior pararenal space typically marginates the

anteromedial aspect of the left hemidiaphragm as well (Figs. 1 and 4). Fat in this same space marginates the spleen, accounting for the so-called "bare area" of the spleen (Fig. 1) (9). As on the right side, inferiorly, a clear distinction between fat in the left perirenal space and the left posterior pararenal space generally is not possible. As will be discussed later, differentiation between the retroperitoneal fat and peritoneal fat around the spleen is also difficult unless fluid is present in one or the other space.

The significance of identifying this fat as being retroperitoneal is of special consequence on the right side because the most lateral extension of retroperitoneal fat along the posterior border of the right lobe of the liver serves as a marker identifying the right coronary ligament (10). As will be discussed, identification of the

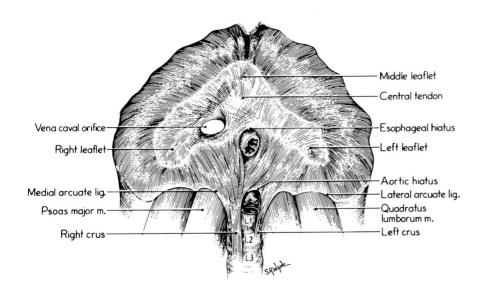

Vena caval orifice
Right leaflet
Medial arcuate lig.
Psoas major m.
Right crus

Middle leaflet
Central tendon
Esophageal hiatus
Left leaflet
Aortic hiatus
Lateral arcuate lig.
Quadratus lumborum m.
Left crus

FIG. 3. Schematic diagram of the lumbar portion of the diaphragm, as viewed from below. This portion is composed of the crura, which arise from the anterolateral surfaces of the first three lumbar vertebrae on the right and the first two lumbar vertebrae on the left, respectively, and fibers that arise from the medial and lateral arcuate ligaments. These ligaments represent thickenings of the thoracolumbar fascia overlying the anterior surface of the psoas and quadratus muscles. Note that as drawn, no clear line of demarcation separates the crura from the remainder of the posterior portions of the diaphragm.

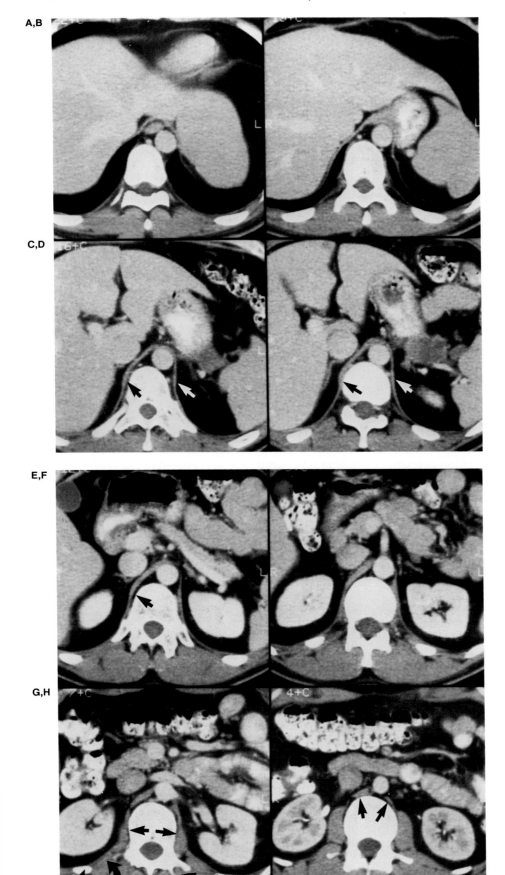

FIG. 4. Normal anatomy. **A–H:** Sequential 10-mm thick sections from the level of the esophageal hiatus to the inferior portions of the crura. The medial and lateral arcuate ligaments lie anterior to the uppermost portions of the psoas (*arrows* in G) and quadratus muscles (*curved arrows* in G). The lateral arcuate ligaments insert into the 12th rib (*arrowheads* in G). Note that the crura at all levels bilaterally merge imperceptibly with the remainder of the posterior portions of the diaphragms (*arrows* in C–E), and that the crura themselves are thin, smooth structures. In its inferior-most extent, the crura are all that remain of the diaphragm, and should not be mistaken for adenopathy (*arrows* in H).

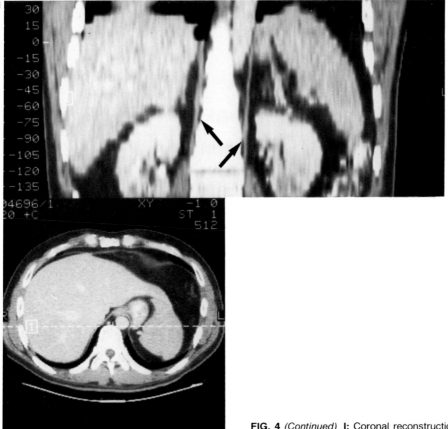

FIG. 4 *(Continued)* I: Coronal reconstruction through the crura in the same case as is shown in A–H. The full extent of the crura is easily visualized bilaterally (*arrows*).

right coronary ligament may be of particular value when attempting to differentiate intraperitoneal from pleural fluid.

As pointed out in Fig. 1, only those portions of the hemidiaphragms outlined centrally by fat will be identifiable as discrete lines. When the diaphragm abuts structures of similar density, such as the liver or spleen, the line of the diaphragm is lost. Intra-abdominal and retroperitoneal fat vary from patient to patient. In some cases, an unusual quantity of fat may be present anteriorly under the diaphragm. This appearance has been mistaken on liver-lung scintigraphy as subdiaphragmatic fluid (11). Computed tomography (CT) is especially efficacious in defining this apparent abnormality as a normal variant (Fig. 5).

Although the crura can be identified in their preaortic positions, laterally they merge with fibers from the medial arcuate ligaments. Variations in the cross-sectional appearance of the crura have been defined (1,4,6). The crura can be divided into two classes: those in which there is a smooth transition between the crura and the remainder of the lumbar portions of the diaphragms (that is, fibers arising from the medial arcuate ligaments) (Figs. 1 and 4) and those in which the transition is

abrupt (Fig. 6). A smooth transition can be seen in as many as 90% of individuals (1). Characteristically, the right crus appears thicker than the left crus. On occa-

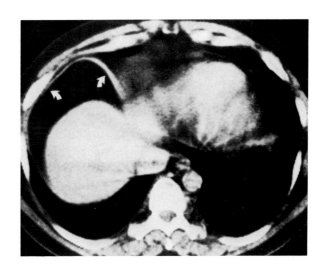

FIG. 5. Normal variant. Abundant fat is present under the anterior aspect of the right hemidiaphragm (*arrows*). This appearance on routine radiographs and scintigrams has been mistaken for pathology in the right upper quadrant.

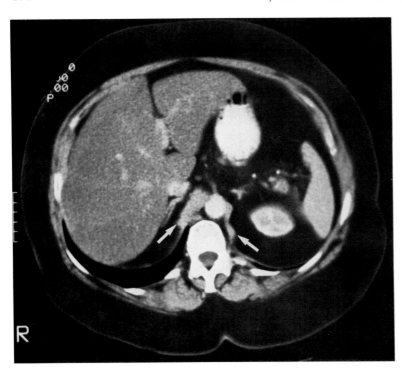

FIG. 6. Diaphragmatic crura: normal variant. CT section through the base of the lungs shows typical appearance of marked nodularity of the crura, which is especially prominent on the right side (*arrows*). Note that there is an abrupt transition between the crura bilaterally and the remainder of the lateral portions of the diaphragms. This appearance should not be mistaken for retroperitoneal adenopathy.

sion, actual separation between the various components of the lumbar portions of the diaphragms can be seen.

Inferiorly, the lumbar portion of the diaphragm extends to the arcuate ligament. As previously noted, the arcuate ligaments represent thickenings of the thoracolumbar fascia overlying the anterior surfaces of the psoas major and quadratus lumborum muscles. In cross-section, these muscles will lie just posterior and medial to the arcuate ligaments. Characteristically, sections obtained below the arcuate ligaments show that the only portions of the diaphragm that remain visible are the crura, which can be seen individually (Fig. 4). The psoas and quadratus muscles can also be defined; they are no longer in contact with the hemidiaphragms.

The anterior or costal portion of the diaphragm arises from the posterior surfaces of the lower six costal cartilages, interdigitating with the slips of origin of the transversus abdominis muscle and inserting into the anterolateral border of the central tendon (7,8,12–14). Additionally, the middle leaflet is attached anteriorly by muscles fibers to the xiphoid process of the sternum, which represents the most cephalic of all bony attachments. The costal portion of the diaphragm is usually more difficult to identify than the lumbar portion, especially on the right side. In a study of 102 normal adults, Patterson and Teates could identify portions of the anterior diaphragm on the right side in only 13 patients, while portions of the anterior diaphragm on the left side were identified in 82 individuals (13). Similar results have been published by Gale who noted that the anterior diaphragmatic muscle could be identified in 87% of 176 scans (14).

As described by Gale, the diaphragm anteriorly characteristically assumes one of three appearances, depending on the cephalocaudal relationship between the xiphoid and the central tendon of the diaphragm (14). In those individuals in whom the middle leaflet lies superior to the xiphoid, the anterior diaphragm appears as a smooth or slightly undulating line that is continuous across the midline with the lateral diaphragmatic attachments (Fig. 7). This appearance is present in nearly 50% of individuals. In distinction, if the apex of the middle leaflet of the central tendon lies inferior to the xiphoid, the anterior muscle fibers will be oriented opposite to muscle fibers in the lateral portion of the diaphragm; this results in apparent discontinuity of the costal diaphragm, with the lateral portion of the diaphragm diverging, opening anteriorly toward the sternum (Fig. 1). This appearance occurs in approximately 30% of individuals. Finally, if the dome of the central tendon and the xiphoid are at the same level, the anterior muscle fibers lie almost entirely within the scan plane; as a consequence, these appear as broad, poorly defined bands.

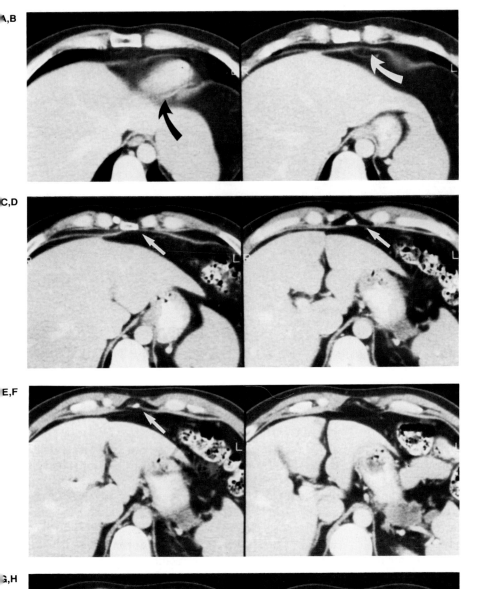

FIG. 7. The costal diaphragm: normal anatomy. **A–H:** Enlargements of sequential 10-mm thick sections through the costal diaphragm. This portion of the diaphragm arises from the posterior surfaces of the lower six costal cartilages and inserts into the anterolateral border of the central tendon. Additionally, fibers attach the middle leaflet to the xiphoid (*arrows* in C–E). Note the close association between the inferior portion of the pericardium and the central tendon (*curved arrow* in A). Most commonly, the costal portion of the diaphragm appears as a continuous, slightly undulating line that is continuous across the midline with the lateral diaphragmatic attachments (*curved arrow* in B). This results when the middle leaflet lies superior to the xiphoid.

NORMAL VARIANTS

A number of normal variants have been described (1,14–19). The significance of these lies primarily in their not being confused with more significant pathology.

Changes with Respiration

As first described by Rosen et al., variations in the degree of inspiration may have a profound effect on the cross-sectional appearance of the diaphragm (15). Specifically on scans obtained in deep inspiration, the dia-

A

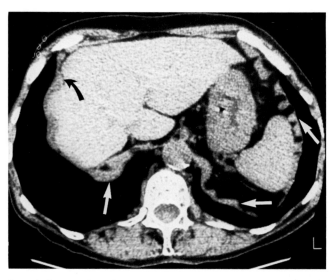

B

FIG. 8. Diaphragmatic pseudo-tumors. **A, B:** Ten-mm thick CT sections through the costal and lumbar portions of the diaphragm, respectively. Note the marked lobularity of the diaphragmatic surfaces both anteriorly (*curved arrows* in A and B), and posterolaterally (*arrows* in B). This appearance is due to infoldings of contracted and foreshortened muscle fibers resulting from a deep inspiratory effort. This phenomenon appears at least in part to be age related.

phragm often assumes an extremely nodular configuration, an appearance that can superficially mimic tumor implants (Fig. 8) (15–19). Presumably, this appearance is caused by infoldings or invaginations of contracted and foreshortened muscle fibers. This explanation is strongly supported by the finding that these changes are reversible when expiratory scans are obtained, and are accentuated on the left side when scans are obtained with patients in the right lateral decubitus position. As reported by Rosen et al., in a series of 150 consecutive scans, focal nodules could be identified involving the left hemidiaphragm in nearly 25% of cases and the crura in approximately 30% of cases, while nodules on the right were identified in only 5% of cases, presumably secondary to pressure exerted on the diaphragm by the adjacent liver (15). Importantly, these changes appear to be related to the patients' age: again as noted by Rosen et al., diaphragmatic pseudo-tumors occurred in 60% of patients older than 70 years, in 27% of patients between 50 and 69 years old, and in only 5% of those under age 50 (15).

Caskey et al. have also studied age-related changes in the appearance of the hemidiaphragms (19). In a study of 120 individuals evaluated by CT, these authors failed to note any appreciable change in the thickness of the diaphragm with age, even when the appearance was correlated with other indicators of physical condition, including skeletal muscle status, obesity, pulmonary emphysema, and the presence of an esophageal hiatal hernia. In agreement with Rosen et al., however, these authors also noted a generalized increase in nodularity and irregularity, especially of the left hemidiaphragm in older patients.

Retrocrural Air

Occasionally, air within the most medial and inferior portions of the lower lobes, in apparent isolation from the remainder of the lung, can be seen in cross-section. This normal variant has been described by Silverman et al. who have designated this as "retrocrural air" (20). As shown in Fig. 9, this represents air within lung posterior to the medial aspect of the right hemidiaphragm, marginated posteriorly by visceral and parietal pleura. This finding is present in approximately 1% of normal subjects. The only significance of this is that it is a normal

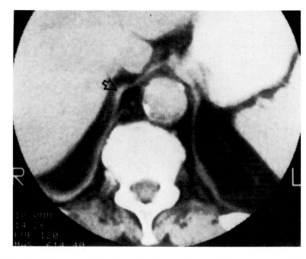

FIG. 9. Retrocrural air. Air within the medial and inferior portion of the right lower lobe can be identified; it is marginated anteriorly by the medial portion of the right hemidiaphragm (*arrow*) and posteriorly by visceral and parietal pleura.

variant not to be confused with true retrocrural (that is, retroperitoneal and/or posterior mediastinal) air.

DIAPHRAGMATIC DEFECTS

The most common pathways that allow communication between the abdomen and thorax are the aortic and esophageal hiatuses (see discussion of esophageal hiatal hernias in Chapter 2). Another potential pathway for spread of disease between the abdomen and thorax is focal defects in the hemidiaphragms. Posteriorly, the most common of these defects is caused by persistence of the embryonic pleuroperitoneal canal (so-called Bochdalek's hernia) (Figs. 10–13). Although it has been

reported that these defects occur in up to 90% of cases on the left side, it has, in fact, been shown that right-sided defects are also common (Figs. 11 and 12) (21). In an evaluation of 940 patients studied with CT, Gale identified 60 Bochdalek's hernias in 52 patients for a surprisingly high prevalence of 6% (22). As surprising, left-sided hernias proved only twice as common as right-sided hernias. Herniation of abdominal structures through this defect may occur, and may simulate intrathoracic masses (21–25). Herniation is presumably facilitated by lower intrathoracic viscera, as opposed to intra-abdominal pressure on the undersurface of the diaphragms, forcing them up into the thorax.

Recently, the precise nature of these posterior defects has been questioned. In an attempt to correlate the ap-

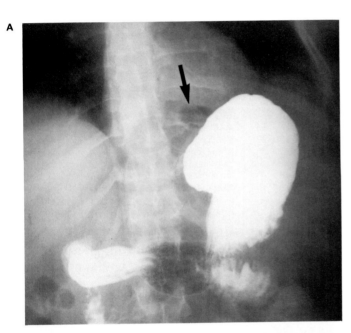

A

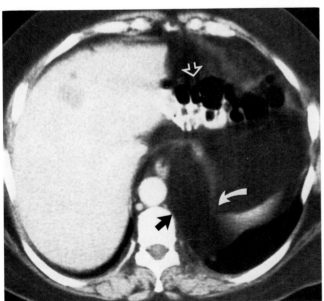

B

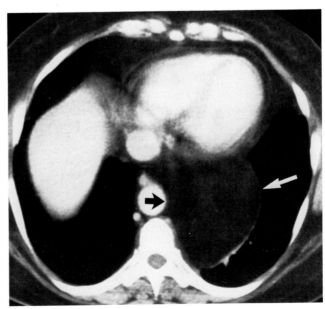

C

FIG. 10. Posterior diaphragmatic defect. **A:** Coned-down view from an upper GI series. Superior to the barium-filled stomach there is a focal area of soft-tissue density within which air can be identified (*arrow*). Findings suggest possible diaphragmatic hernia. **B, C:** Ten-mm thick CT sections through the base of the lungs and the lower mediastinum, respectively. Note that there is a defect present in the posterior aspect of the left hemidiaphragm (*curved arrow* in B) through which considerable intra-abdominal fat has protruded (*straight arrows* in B and C). Barium is present within the transverse colon anteriorly (*open arrow* in B), which lies superior to the stomach, accounting for the air seen on the barium study shown in A. Despite its unusual location, this portion of the transverse colon has not actually herniated through the diaphragm. Incidental area of low density in right lobe of liver subsequently proved to be a liver metastasis.

A,B

C,D

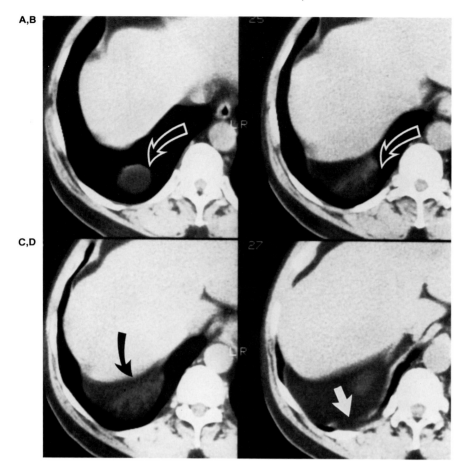

FIG. 11. Posterior diaphragmatic defect. A–D: Enlargements of sequential 10-mm thick sections through the right hemidiaphragm show that there is discontinuity in the posterior portion of the right hemidiaphragm (*arrow* in D) through which intra-abdominal fat has protruded (*curved arrows* in A–C).

pearance of the diaphragms with age, Caskey et al. described three types of diaphragmatic defects: Type 1, in which a localized defect can be identified in the thickness of the diaphragm without loss of diaphragmatic continuity; Type 2, in which an apparent defect can be identified where muscle fibers appear to separate into layers parallel to the diaphragmatic contour; and Type

3, any defect in which a portion of the diaphragm appears absent, typically associated with protrusion of omental fat (Figs. 10 and 11) (19). As shown by these authors, the appearance of diaphragmatic defects appears related to both age and the presence of pulmonary emphysema. In a review of 120 scans, these authors found that none of their patients in their 20s or 30s

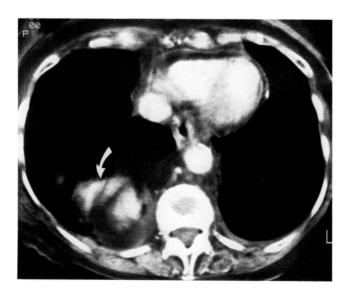

FIG. 12. Bilateral posterior diaphragmatic defects. A–C: Sequential 10-mm thick sections from above-downward through the diaphragm. Note that both kidneys have herniated into the thorax (*straight arrows* in B and C) accompanied by contrast-filled loops of bowel (*curved arrows* in A–C) as well as retroperitoneal fat. Findings are diagnostic of bilateral Bochdalek hernias.

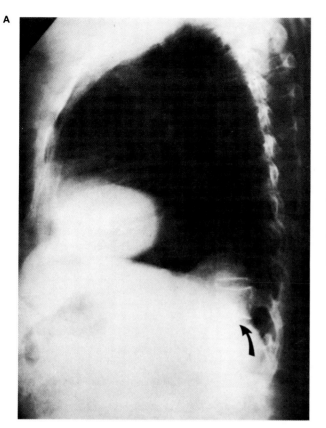

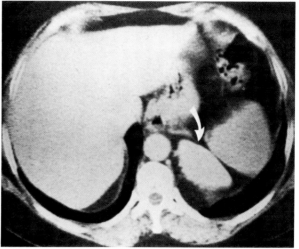

FIG. 13. Intrathoracic kidney. **A:** Lateral radiograph, following an intravenous pyelogram. A mass can be seen posteriorly. Contrast is faintly present in the collecting system of the left kidney (*arrow*). **B:** Section through the left hemidiaphragm. There is a diaphragmatic defect through which the left kidney has herniated from the retroperitoneum into the left hemithorax (*arrow*).

demonstrated defects of any type, whereas 56% of patients in their 60s and 70s proved to have defects. A significant association between diaphragmatic defects and pulmonary emphysema was also noted, especially in men. Based on these findings, these authors have suggested that many of the diaphragmatic defects identified, especially posteriorly in older patients, represent acquired defects occurring in areas of structural weakness, perhaps themselves embryologic in origin.

Regardless of their origin, diaphragmatic defects are easily identified with CT (Figs. 10–13) (1–3,21–24). Commonly identified on plain chest radiographs as areas of eventration, these defects characteristically are associated with protrusion of omental or even retroperitoneal fat. Care must be taken not to confuse these focal protrusions of intraperitoneal fat with intrapulmonary masses, especially when images are viewed sequentially through the lower thorax (Fig. 11).

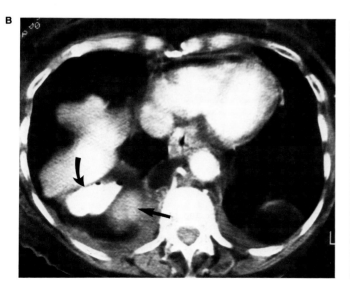

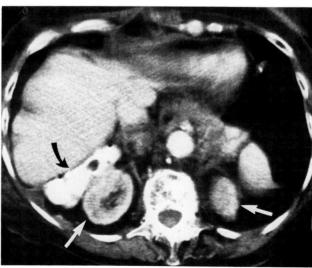

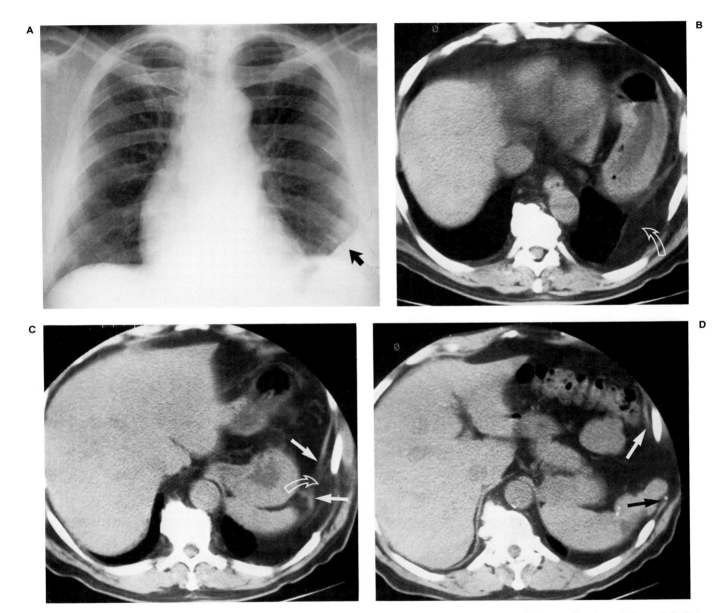

FIG. 14. Traumatic diaphragmatic rupture. **A:** Posteroanterior radiograph shows ill-defined density at the left costophrenic angle (*arrow*). **B–D:** Sequential 10-mm thick CT sections through the left hemidiaphragm. The left hemidiaphragm is discontinuous: there is wide separation of the diaphragmatic margins (*arrows* in C and D) through which considerable intra-abdominal fat has herniated (*curved arrows* in B and C).

A
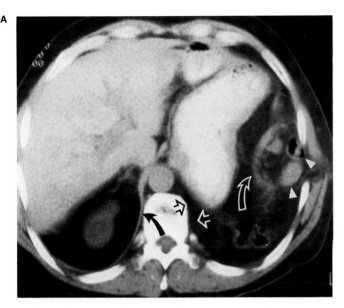

B
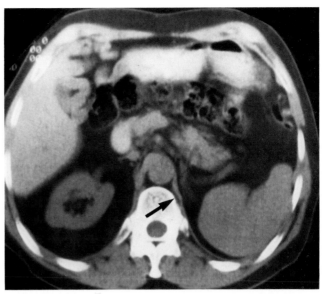

FIG. 15. Traumatic diaphragmatic rupture: the absent diaphragm sign. **A, B:** Ten-mm thick CT sections from above-downward through the left hemidiaphragm. Note that in A, in the location in which the left hemidiaphragm is usually seen, no distinct line is identifiable (*arrows* in A) as compared to the normal appearance of the right hemidiaphragm (*black curved arrow* in A). A portion of the left hemidiaphragm at this level is identifiable more medially (*open curved arrow* in A). There has been some herniation of both fat and a portion of colon into the lower left hemithorax (*arrowheads*). Note that inferiorly, the left hemidiaphragm is easily recognized in its usual position (*arrow* in B). This apparent loss of the diaphragm has proven to be an especially valuable sign for diagnosing traumatic diaphragmatic rupture.

Less commonly, abdominal viscera, especially the kidney, may be displaced into the thorax (24,25) (Figs. 12 and 13). CT is of obvious diagnostic value in such cases. In our experience, interpretation of complex pathology at the level of the diaphragm, especially when attempting to identify diaphragmatic rupture or intrathoracic herniation of abdominal contents, is often facilitated by evaluating images in an anterior-to-posterior direction, since this is the general direction of herniation (Fig. 13).

Herniation of intra-abdominal fat and/or viscera may also occur in the anterior portions (costal portions) of the diaphragms, resulting in a paracardiac mass (so-called Morgagni's hernia) (see Fig. 36, Chapter 2) (26). CT is efficacious, first, in defining such masses as fatty, and second, in demonstrating continuity between this fat and abdominal fat (see Fig. 2, Chapter 3). The actual point of the diaphragmatic defect may be definable using parasagittal reconstructions.

Diaphragmatic Rupture

In addition to congenital abnormalities, defects in the diaphragm may also be the result of trauma (27–34). Traumatic herniation following diaphragmatic rupture is another mechanism by which abdominal and thoracic pathology overlap. The appearance on CT of traumatic diaphragmatic rupture has been described (Figs. 14–17)

(30–34). This frequently occurs secondary to blunt trauma and may go undiagnosed for years. Diaphragmatic rupture following blunt trauma usually occurs on the left side (in up to 95% of patients) (27,28). As pointed out by Heiberg et al., radiologic diagnosis of diaphragmatic rupture may be difficult (31); this entity is frequently misdiagnosed as an elevated hemidiaphragm, left lower lobe atelectasis, left pleural effusion, or left subphrenic fluid collections and/or abscess (Fig. 14). Unfortunately, despite the long time interval, chronic traumatic diaphragmatic rupture may eventuate in patients presenting with symptoms of acute intestinal obstruction secondary to infarction and/or strangulation of herniated bowel or viscera (35,36). CT can identify discontinuities in the course of the diaphragm, especially along the posterolateral aspect, an appearance which when severe can be referred to as the "absent diaphragm sign" (Fig. 15). Superiorly, near the dome of the diaphragm, CT identification of diaphragmatic discontinuity is considerably more difficult: in these cases, recognition of diaphragmatic rupture usually necessitates identification of intrathoracic herniation of fat or abdominal contents (Fig. 17).

PERIDIAPHRAGMATIC FLUID COLLECTIONS

Accurate localization of peridiaphragmatic fluid requires detailed knowledge of normal cross-sectional

A

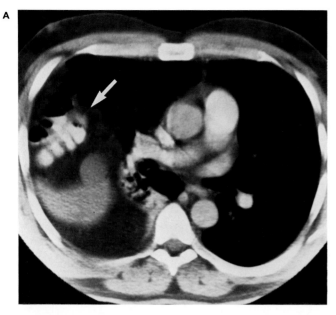

C

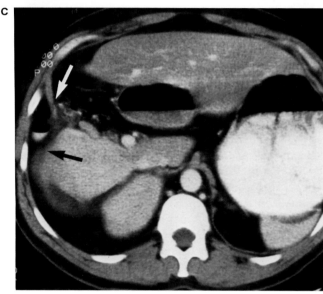

B

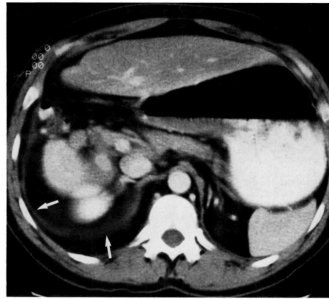

FIG. 16. Right-sided traumatic diaphragmatic rupture. **A–C:** Ten-mm thick CT sections through the right upper quadrant from above-downward show characteristic appearance of herniation of bowel and fat into the right hemithorax (*arrow* in A) secondary to traumatic rupture of the right hemidiaphragm. The right hemidiaphragm itself can be identified in B (*arrows*), appearing somewhat thickened and displaced medially. Diaphragmatic discontinuity can be identified in C (*arrows*).

anatomy through the lung bases and upper abdomen. The key to accurate localization of peridiaphragmatic fluid is identification of the hemidiaphragms, because these represent the interface between the thorax and the abdomen (1). In principle, at all levels the lungs and pleura lie adjacent and peripheral to the diaphragm while the abdominal viscera, fat, and intraperitoneal spaces lie adjacent and central to the diaphragm. Precise anatomic localization of the diaphragm depends on awareness of these anatomic relationships.

As shown in Fig. 18, a schematic drawing of a sagittal section through the diaphragm at the level of the lateral arcuate ligament and upper portion of the quadratus muscle, the lungs and pleura always lie peripheral to the diaphragm. The lung is invested with visceral pleura.

Just below the most inferior portion of the lung there is a space—generally a potential space—referred to as the posterior pleural recess. This space is defined anteriorly and posteriorly by layers of parietal pleura. Fibers of the lumbar portion of the diaphragm extend below the posterior pleural recess, ending at the lateral arcuate ligament at the level of the 12th rib.

Identification of the posterior pleural recesses is critical when evaluating peridiaphragmatic fluid collections, as this space represents the most inferior, dependent recess of the pleural space: it is this space that will be filled first by free pleural fluid (37). Although the posterior pleural recess is usually a potential space, on occasion it can be identified with CT in normal individuals (Fig. 19).

A

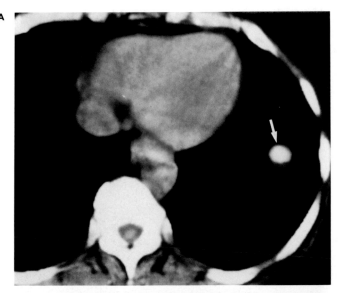

B

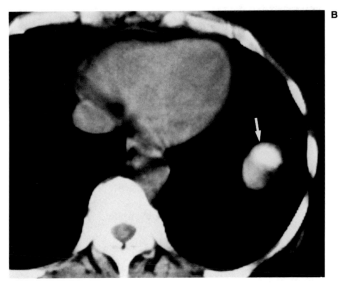

C

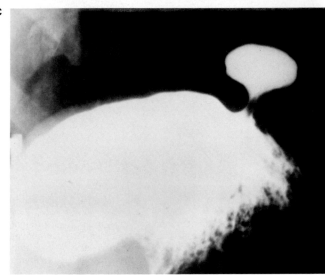

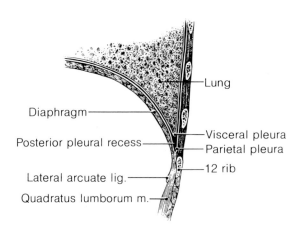

FIG. 17. Traumatic diaphragmatic rupture. **A, B:** Sequential 10-mm thick sections through the left lung base show a focal area of contrast on the left side (*arrows* in A and B). The exact relationship between bowel and the left hemidiaphragm is difficult to determine. **C:** Coned-down view from an accompanying upper GI series shows barium contrast in the stomach: a tiny rent in the apex of the left hemidiaphragm has resulted in herniation of a small portion of the stomach into the chest. Focal tears of the diaphragm, especially when they involve the dome, may be extremely difficult to diagnose with CT.

Lung

Diaphragm

Posterior pleural recess

Lateral arcuate lig.

Quadratus lumborum m.

Visceral pleura

Parietal pleura

12 rib

FIG. 18. Schematic diagram of a sagittal section through the lateral arcuate ligament. The lung is invested with visceral pleura. Below the inferior edge of the lung there is a potential space, the posterior pleural recess, which is defined anteriorly and posteriorly by layers of parietal pleura. The diaphragm always lies central to the lung and pleura when seen in cross-section.

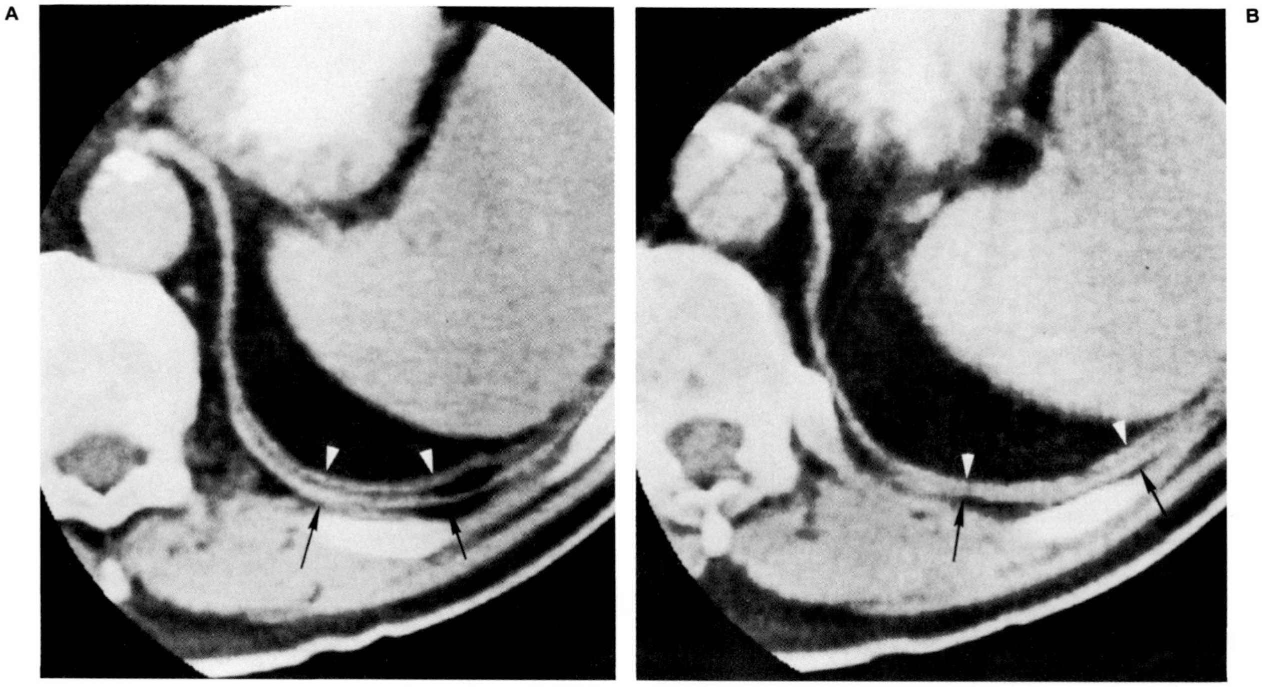

A
B

FIG. 19. A: Enlargement of a section through the left lung base. The lung is bordered anteriorly by the left hemidiaphragm and anterior parietal and visceral pleura (*arrowheads*). Posteriorly, the lung is bordered by posterior visceral and parietal pleura (*arrows*). **B:** Magnification of a section through the posterior pleural recess, 5 mm below A. Visceral pleura is no longer present at this level. This space is bordered anteriorly by the left hemidiaphragm and anterior parietal pleura, which are indistinguishable (*arrowheads*). Posteriorly, this space is defined by the posterior parietal pleura (*arrows*).

As illustrated in Fig. 20, peridiaphragmatic fluid can be localized to one of four potential spaces: the pleural cavity, the lung, the peritoneum, or the retroperitoneum.

Four main criteria have been proposed to differentiate pleural from peritoneal fluid (37–41): (a) The "diaphragm sign": as already discussed, direct visualization of the diaphragm itself allows accurate localization of peridiaphragmatic fluid collections, as fluid peripheral to the diaphragm is intrathoracic while fluid central to

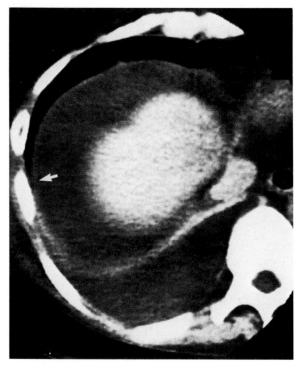

FIG. 21. Enlargement of a section through the right side near the dome of the liver in a patient with both ascites and pleural fluid. In this case the line of the diaphragm can be seen distinctly. Notice that the middle lobe interface with the chest wall laterally remains sharply defined despite the presence of pleural fluid (*arrow*).

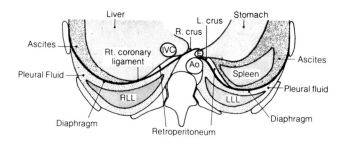

FIG. 20. Schematic drawing of the potential spaces in which peridiaphragmatic fluid may collect. Accurate identification of the diaphragm is critical. Fluid within the pleural spaces or lung lies peripheral to the hemidiaphragms; intraperitoneal or retroperitoneal fluid lies central to the hemidiaphragms. On the right side intraperitoneal fluid is restricted medially at the level of the right coronary ligament. Ao, aorta; E, esophagus; IVC, inferior vena cava; LLL, left lower lobe; RLL, right lower lobe.

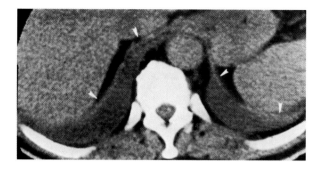

FIG. 22. Magnified section through the posterior pleural recesses, which are distended by bilateral subpulmonic effusions. The hemidiaphragms (*arrowheads*) can be identified bilaterally, outlined centrally by retroperitoneal and intraperitoneal fat, displaced anterolaterally, accounting for the "displaced crura sign."

the diaphragm is intra-abdominal (Fig. 21). (b) The "displaced crura sign": this sign results from the interposition of pleural fluid between the crus and adjacent vertebra, with resultant anterior displacement of the crus (Fig. 22). (c) The "interface sign": first described by Teplick et al., this sign is based on the nature of the interface between the liver and adjacent fluid (39). This interface is hazy in the case of pleural fluid, but distinct in the case of ascites (Fig. 23). (d) The "bare area sign": this sign is based on recognition that identification of the bare area of the liver indicates fluid within the peritoneum (Fig. 24).

As documented by Halvorsen et al., familiarity with each of these signs usually allows accurate localization of peridiaphragmatic fluid collections (42,43). Applying the above-mentioned four criteria to 52 cases with ascites (n = 13), right pleural effusions (n = 25), or both

ascites and right pleural effusions (n = 14), retrospectively, these authors found that although none of the four criteria proved entirely reliable by itself, together these signs allowed accurate localization of peridiaphragmatic fluid collections in all cases (42). For differentiating between ascites and pleural effusions, the diaphragm sign proved to have the highest sensitivity (97%) but was frequently indeterminate, while the bare area sign proved most accurate (92%) but was of little value in patients with pleural effusions. The displaced crura sign, while relatively specific, is contingent on pleural fluid extending medially and was therefore inaccurate in patients with loculated effusions, proving to be indeterminate in almost 25% of cases. In cases in which both ascites and pleural fluid were present, the interface sign proved most valuable, although its accuracy was only 75% (42).

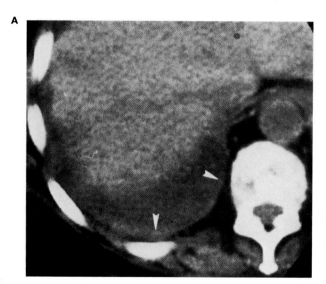
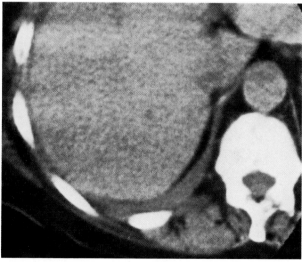

FIG. 23. A: Enlargement of a section on the right side shows a large pleural fluid collection. The "interface" between the fluid and the posterior aspect of the liver is indistinct. The posterior parietal pleura should not be confused with the right hemidiaphragm (*arrowheads*). **B:** Magnification of a section 2 cm below that shown in A, at the level of the right posterior pleural recess. Fluid lies posterior to the right hemidiaphragm. Compare with Fig. 24.

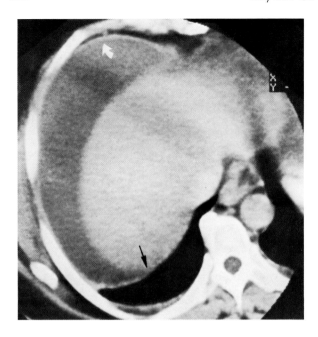

FIG. 24. Enlargement of a section through the right lung base in a patient with ascites. Medially, ascites taper to a point, where they are restricted by the coronary ligaments (*arrow*). Note that the intraperitoneal fluid lies central to the diaphragm, even anteriorly (*white arrow*).

Additional CT findings have been described as potential pitfalls in differentiating pleural from peritoneal fluid. Silverman et al. have noted that a combination of atelectasis and subpulmonic pleural fluid in particular may be misleading because subsegmental atelectasis may result in a curvilinear band at the lung base that superficially may simulate the hemidiaphragm (Fig. 25) (44). Similar findings have been reported by Federle et al. (45). In these cases, variability in the appearance of pleural fluid at the lung base probably reflects differences in the anatomy of the pulmonary ligaments (46,47). If there are incomplete attachments of these

ligaments, the lower lobes are free to float on pleural fluid provided the lung is not stiffened by disease and there are no adhesions between the lung and the adjacent pleura. In distinction, when these attachments are complete, the base of the lung may become tethered inferiorly, despite the presence of even sizable pleural effusions; the result may be the appearance of a "pseudo-diaphragm sign" (Fig. 25).

Potential difficulty may also be encountered in identifying basilar lung consolidation and/or atelectasis with or without associated pleural fluid (Figs. 26 and 27) (37). Superficially, areas of dense parenchymal consolidation

A,B

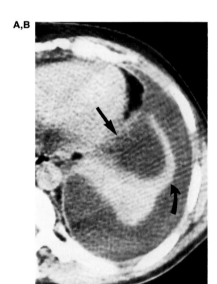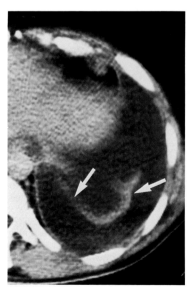

FIG. 25. Subpulmonic pleural fluid. **A, B:** Sequential 10-mm thick sections through the left lung base show a large pleural fluid collection associated with atelectasis of the left lower lobe. In this case, fluid lies both anterior (*arrow* in A) and posterior to the collapsed left lower lobe, which in cross-section has a curvilinear appearance, especially laterally (*curved arrow* in A). This appearance is still more accentuated inferiorly (*arrows* in B). The key to the diagnosis here is recognition that these scans are obtained through the base of a consolidated and collapsed left lower lobe: in this setting, fluid may accumulate anterior to the lung, superficially mimicking the appearance of fluid within the abdomen.

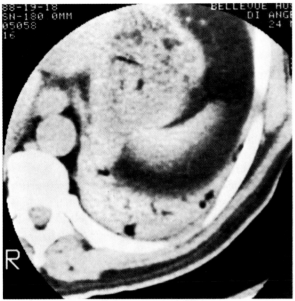

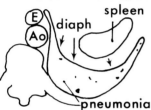

FIG. 26. Enlargement of a section through the base of the left lung. There is consolidation as well as air-bronchograms within the lower lobe. The consolidation conforms to the shape of the left lung base and lies peripheral to the left hemidiaphragm. Note that there is evidence of enhancement within consolidated lung following administration of i.v. contrast media.

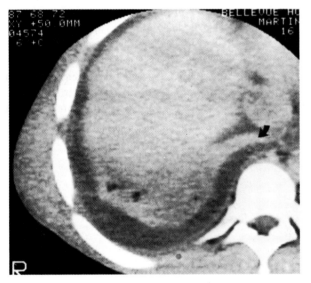

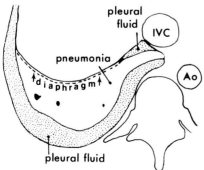

FIG. 27. Magnification of a section through the right lung base in a patient with right lower lobe volume loss and infiltrate and a right pleural effusion. There are a few scattered areas of residual aeration within the lower lobe. Note that despite volume loss and the presence of pleural fluid, the right lower lobe has retained its general configuration because of fixation by the pulmonary ligament (arrow) (compare with Fig. 26). Peripheral and anteromedial to the consolidated lower lobe there is pleural fluid. Significantly, the density of the consolidated lung is intermediate between the liver anteriorly and the pleural fluid posteriorly. This helps to define the position of the right hemidiaphragm.

may appear to have fluid density, and hence may be mistaken for pleural or even intra-abdominal fluid. In fact, consolidated lung almost never has a pure fluid density, representing instead an averaging of fluid and pulmonary parenchyma. Identification of areas of consolidated lung is facilitated by the following: as is true with pleural fluid collections, consolidated lung always lies peripheral to the hemidiaphragms; in addition, consolidated lung usually conforms to the expected shape of the lower lobes. The medial portions of the lower lobes extend in close proximity to the descending aorta and esophagus, as do the pleural reflections. Typically, residual areas of parenchymal aeration or air-bronchograms may be discernible to further aid in identification. Finally, in problematic cases, a bolus of intravenous contrast may be of value because consolidated lung enhances markedly, unlike pleural or peritoneal fluid (Fig. 26) (48).

Underneath the diaphragm, both peritoneal and retroperitoneal fluid may abut the diaphragm (10,49,50). Retroperitoneal fluid will conform to the anatomic space and/or structures involved, e.g., posterior pararenal versus perirenal spaces. The psoas muscles are also retroperitoneal, and, as discussed above, are intimately related to the arcuate ligaments. Generally, differentiation between retroperitoneal and intraperitoneal fluid is not difficult. This is especially true in cases where retroperitoneal fluid accumulates secondary to a leaking abdominal aortic aneurysm (Fig. 28) (51,52).

In distinction, intraperitoneal fluid will collect in the peritoneal spaces and will therefore be restricted by the peritoneal reflections (Fig. 29). On the right side, peritoneal fluid is restricted posteromedially by the right coronary ligament. This results in a characteristic medial tapering of intraperitoneal fluid (the "bare area sign") (Fig. 24). It should be remembered, however, that supe-

A

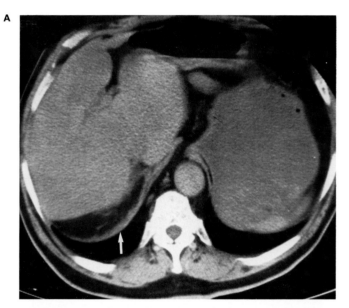

B

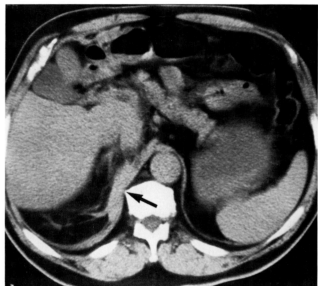

C

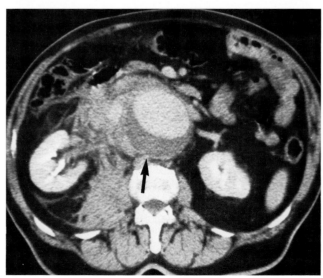

FIG. 28. Retroperitoneal fluid localization. A–C: Ten-mm thick CT sections from above-downward show apparent thickening of the right hemidiaphragm superiorly (*arrow* in A). Inferiorly, a high-density retroperitoneal fluid collection can be identified (*arrow* in B), the result of hemorrhage into the retroperitoneum from a leaking abdominal aortic aneurysm (*arrow* in C).

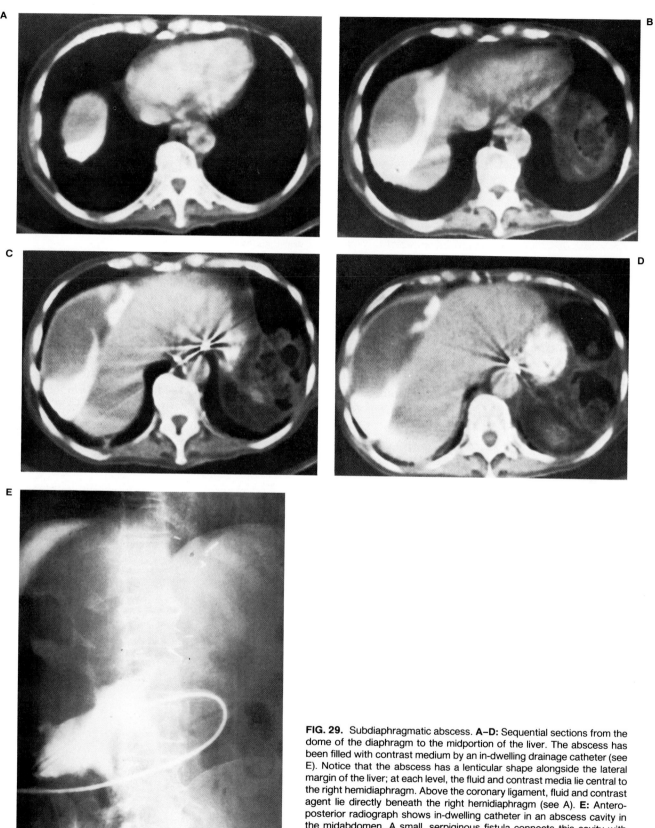

FIG. 29. Subdiaphragmatic abscess. **A–D:** Sequential sections from the dome of the diaphragm to the midportion of the liver. The abscess has been filled with contrast medium by an in-dwelling drainage catheter (see E). Notice that the abscess has a lenticular shape alongside the lateral margin of the liver; at each level, the fluid and contrast media lie central to the right hemidiaphragm. Above the coronary ligament, fluid and contrast agent lie directly beneath the right hemidiaphragm (see A). **E:** Antero-posterior radiograph shows in-dwelling catheter in an abscess cavity in the midabdomen. A small, serpiginous fistula connects this cavity with the subdiaphragmatic collection. These fistulae may be difficult to detect in cross-sectional images. Any patient with a subdiaphragmatic fluid collection-abscess should have scans of the entire abdomen.

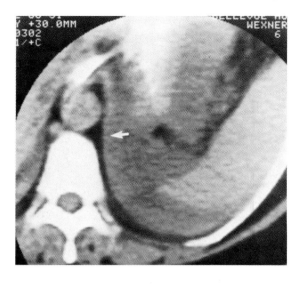

FIG. 30. A: Section through the upper abdomen shows intraperitoneal fluid surrounding the spleen. The fluid lies central to the left hemidiaphragm (*arrow*). There is also a small quantity of fluid in the lesser sac displacing the stomach medially.

riorly, ascites, when massive, may collect under the domes of the diaphragm on both the left and right sides (i.e., above the level of the coronary ligaments), thereby limiting considerably the value of the bare-area sign (Fig. 21). On the left side, intra-abdominal (intraperitoneal) fluid is easy to identify because it will characteristically be central to the left hemidiaphragm and, additionally, will surround the spleen (Fig. 30). As noted

previously, identification of intraperitoneal fluid around the spleen is facilitated by recognition of a bare area, analogous to that of the liver (9).

As already discussed, the medial aspect of the left hemidiaphragm is generally outlined by retroperitoneal fat in the upper portion of the left posterior pararenal space. Unlike the right side, the configuration of this portion of the posterior pararenal space and its relation-

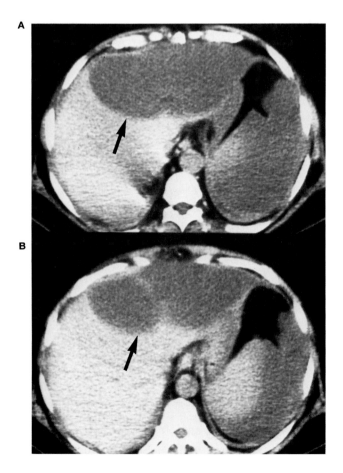

FIG. 31. Anterior subphrenic fluid. **A, B:** Sequential 10-mm thick CT sections through the upper abdomen show characteristic appearance of intraperitoneal fluid in the anterior subphrenic space, defined on the right by the falciform ligament and superiorly by the anterior aspect of the left hemidiaphragm. Additionally, fluid in this space lies adjacent to the left lobe of the liver (*arrows* in A and B).

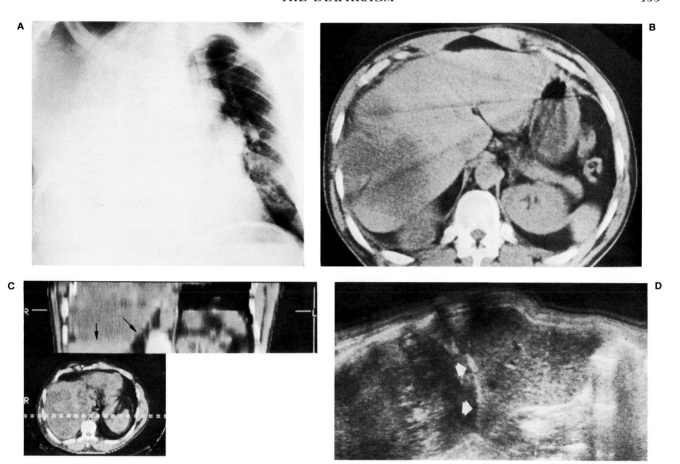

FIG. 32. A: Posteroanterior radiograph shows total opacification of the right hemithorax. This patient is status-post pneumonectomy. **B:** Section through the right lobe of the liver. There are ill-defined areas of decreased density in the lateral aspect of the liver. **C:** Coronal reconstruction through the midportion of the right lobe of the liver. There is a massive pleural fluid collection inverting the diaphragm (*arrows*). The liver is displaced inferiorly. There is no evidence of subdiaphragmatic fluid. **D:** Longitudinal ultrasonic section through the right lobe of the liver. Inversion of the right diaphragm is apparent (*arrows*). In cases of diaphragmatic inversion the usual rules of a peridiaphragmatic fluid localization are reversed: intrathoracic fluid collections now will appear central to the hemidiaphragms instead of peripheral (B). This problem is usually easily resolved by analysis of sequential sections, or by use of perisagittal reconstruction (C).

ship to the diaphragm may be variable. This variability should not cause confusion since in both cases, intra-abdominal fluid can be localized central to the left hemidiaphragm.

Anterior subdiaphragmatic fluid collections also are characteristic in appearance. As shown by Halvorsen et al., fluid may become confined to the anterior left subphrenic space (53). This space is defined on the right side by the falciform ligament and on the left by the left coronary ligament, which extends from the dorsal aspect of the liver posteriorly to the diaphragm (Fig. 31). The anterior subphrenic space extends superiorly to the dome of the diaphragm. Importantly, this fluid lies central to the anterior aspect of the left hemidiaphragm; additionally, fluid in this space will lie adjacent to the left lobe of the liver in a manner analogous to that of free intraperitoneal fluid, which surrounds the spleen posteriorly.

Despite clarification of normal cross-sectional anat-

omy of the pleural, peritoneal, and retroperitoneal spaces, certain cases remain difficult to evaluate. This is especially true when pleural fluid is sufficiently massive to cause inversion of the hemidiaphragms, since pleural fluid may then simulate the appearance of intra-abdominal fluid (54,55). In these cases, parasagittal reconstruction may prove helpful (Fig. 32) (37).

THE DIAPHRAGM AS PATHWAY FOR THE SPREAD OF DISEASE

The diaphragm usually serves to localize disease in either the thorax or abdomen. However, extension through the diaphragm can occur via several pathways. Direct contiguous spread most commonly occurs through the pre-existing normal channels of communication, that is, the aortic and esophageal hiatuses.

As discussed in detail in Chapter 2, the esophageal hiatus is an elliptical opening just to the left of the midline and is formed by the decussation of muscle fibers originating from the diaphragm around the lower esophagus. The margins of the hiatus are formed by the medial portions of the diaphragmatic crura (1,4,56). As the esophagus passes through the upper margin of the hiatus, it assumes an oblique orientation; the gastroesophageal junction itself lies just below the diaphragm. On cross-section the abdominal or submerged portion of the esophagus typically appears cone-shaped with its base at the junction of the gastric fundus (57).

Sliding hiatal hernias typically are manifest as widening of the esophageal hiatus on cross-section (Fig. 33: see also Figs. 37, 113, and 114 in Chapter 2). Measurements of the standard width of the esophageal hiatus, defined as the distance between the medial margins of the crura, have been reported (19,58). As documented by Caskey et al., the width of the esophageal hiatus clearly enlarges with age, especially in men (19). Measuring an average 1.25 cm in individuals in their 20s, the esophageal hiatus progressively widens each decade, measuring greater than 3 cm on average in individuals in their 70s. Hiatal hernias typically present little difficulty in diagnosis. They are frequently associated with an apparent increase in mediastinal fat surrounding the distal esophagus, secondary to herniation of omentum through the phrenicoesophageal ligament. Fluid within herniated peritoneum anterior to the contrast-filled stomach may occasionally be identified as well (see Fig. 114, Chapter 2) (59).

In addition to hiatal hernias, the esophageal hiatus serves as a passage for the spread of malignancy, especially that arising in the esophagus as well as the stomach (see Fig. 112, Chapter 2). Esophageal varices also may traverse the esophageal hiatus (60,61); in these cases, CT is especially valuable in detecting para-esophageal varices (see Fig. 112, Chapter 2). Frequently these present as nonspecific mediastinal soft-tissue masses, necessitating differentiation from enlarged periesophageal lymph nodes or other posterior mediastinal masses. Despite the accuracy of endoscopy and esophagography to detect esophageal varices, para-esophageal varices have previously required angiography for definite diagnosis.

CT has proven particularly valuable in diagnosing esophageal perforation (see Fig. 115, Chapter 2). This potentially lethal condition frequently results in peridiaphragmatic fluid collections both above and below the diaphragm. Unfortunately, as documented by Han et al., chest radiographs may be normal in up to 12% of patients (62). In select cases, CT may prove invaluable by delineating the extent of associated mediastinal, pleural, parenchymal disease, and subdiaphragmatic disease (63,64).

More rarely, the esophageal hiatus serves as the pathway for the spread of pancreatic fluid collections (Fig. 34). The key to evaluating these fluid collections is analysis of contiguous sections from the lung bases to the upper abdomen. It should be noted that fluid in the lesser sac may appear to extend past the crural margins, occasionally even mimicking the appearance of thrombosis of the inferior vena cava (65). This appearance

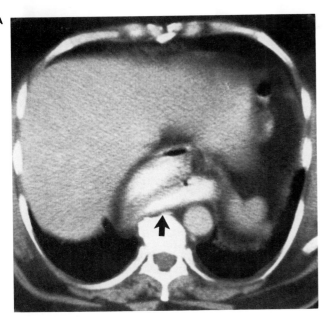
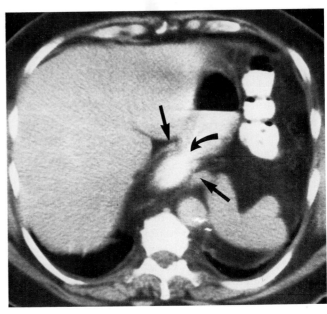

FIG. 33. Sliding hiatal hernia. **A, B:** Sequential 10-mm thick CT sections through the esophageal hiatus following oral administration of contrast media. A large sliding hiatal hernia can be identified (*arrow* in A). Note that there is wide separation of the crural margins (*arrows* in B), through which the stomach clearly passes (*curved arrow* in B).

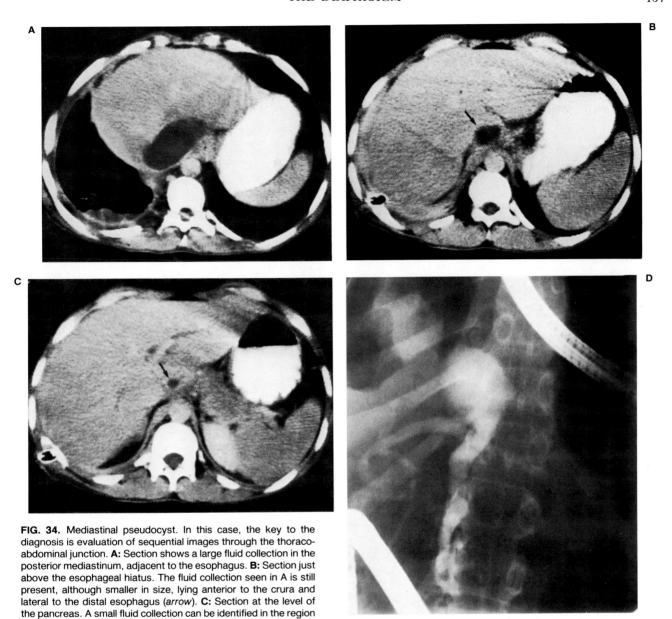

FIG. 34. Mediastinal pseudocyst. In this case, the key to the diagnosis is evaluation of sequential images through the thoraco-abdominal junction. **A:** Section shows a large fluid collection in the posterior mediastinum, adjacent to the esophagus. **B:** Section just above the esophageal hiatus. The fluid collection seen in A is still present, although smaller in size, lying anterior to the crura and lateral to the distal esophagus (*arrow*). **C:** Section at the level of the pancreas. A small fluid collection can be identified in the region of the head of the pancreas (*arrow*). In this case fluid has tracked from the retroperitoneum, through the esophageal hiatus, to localize in the posterior mediastinum. Communication of these fluid collections could be established by reviewing sequential images (not all are shown). **D:** Oblique view from an endoscopic retrograde cholangiopancreatogram confirming the diagnosis.

should not be confused with true mediastinal extension of disease.

The aortic hiatus is another important path for the spread of disease. As shown by Zerhouni et al. (66), malignant thoracic neoplasms, especially those involving the pleura, can extend into the retroperitoneum by this route. The propensity for tumor spread through the aortic hiatus is related to two anatomic features. First, the phrenicoesophageal membrane affixes the esophagus to the crura in most individuals. This may preferentially direct tumor spread through the aortic hiatus. Second, the thoracic duct traverses the aortic hiatus providing a direct lymphatic pathway between the

thorax and abdomen. These facts explain the frequent finding of retrocrural adenopathy as a clue to the simultaneous presence of intrathorax and abdominal malignancy. Less frequently, the aortic hiatus serves as the pathway for fluid spread between the thorax and abdomen (see Fig. 85, Chapter 2).

Although disease usually spreads between the abdomen and thorax by means of a diaphragmatic defect—either congenital or acquired—the diaphragm itself, on occasion, may actually serve as a pathway for disease, both inflammatory and malignant (67–69). This is most typically encountered in patients with diffuse malignant pleural disease, especially mesotheliomas (see Figs.

A
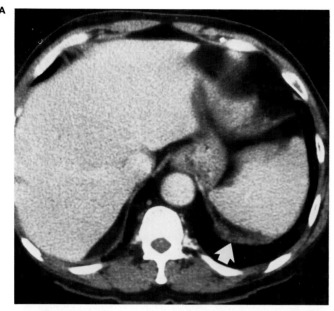

B
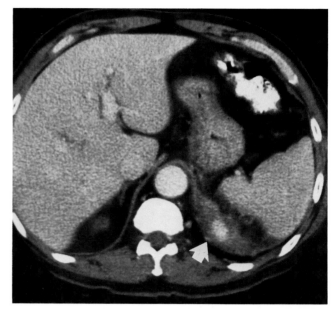

C
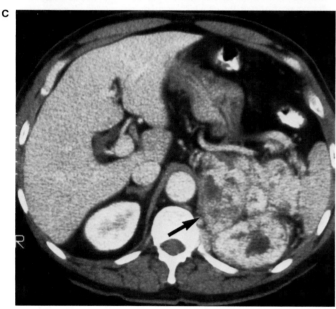

FIG. 35. Metastatic renal cell carcinoma. **A–C:** Sequential 10-mm thick CT sections through the left upper quadrant from above downward show a large renal cell carcinoma arising in the left kidney (*arrow* in C), clearly extending to and invading the left hemidiaphragm (*arrows* in A and B).

45–47, Chapter 9). In this setting, the diaphragm may become involved by tumor; the result is that tumor tracks along the diaphragm to gain entry into the abdomen. A similar appearance has been described in patients with invasive thymomas and lymphomas, and may be expected to be seen in any tumor that originates in viscera adjacent to the diaphragms (Fig. 35; see also Figs. 85 and 86, Chapter 2 and Fig. 53, Chapter 9) (67,68).

Analogous to the spread of tumor, the diaphragm may also serve as a means of extension of infection. In our experience this is most frequently secondary to tuberculosis, although a similar appearance may be seen with other infections including actinomycosis (Fig. 36).

Finally, tumors may arise within the diaphragm (70). This is exceptionally rare, and frequently presents diagnostic dilemmas. An example of a surgically confirmed hemangiopericytoma arising in the diaphragm is shown in Fig. 37. The intimate relationship between the tumor and the diaphragm is obvious, but the appearance should not be considered characteristic. Such cases invariably require surgery to actually confirm the precise origin of the lesion.

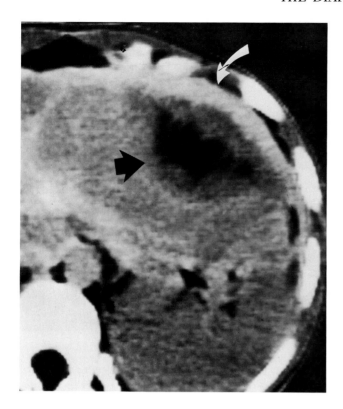

FIG. 36. Actinomycosis. Contrast-enhanced CT section through the left upper quadrant shows a well-defined, thick-walled abscess anteriorly (*arrow*), abutting the left hemidiaphragm. In this case, the diaphragm is markedly thickened (*curved arrow*) and shows considerable contrast enhancement, presumably as a result of hyperemia. At surgery, this abscess proved to be secondary to actinomycosis which involved the diaphragm directly.

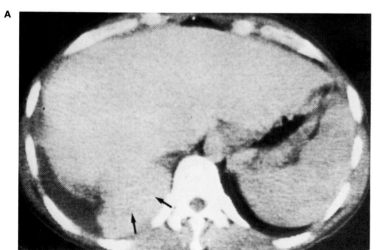

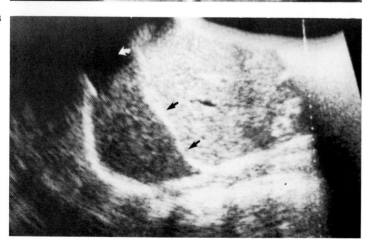

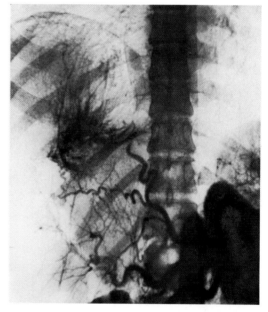

FIG. 37. Hemangiopericytoma (right diagram). **A:** Section through the inferior portion of the right pleural space. There is considerable pleural fluid, as well as a large oval soft-tissue mass, clearly peripheral to the hemidiaphragm (*arrows*). **B:** Longitudinal sonogram through the liver. The diaphragm is well-defined (*arrows*). Superior and adjacent to the diaphragm is an echogenic mass, above which pleural fluid can be identified (*white arrow*). **C:** Coned-down view from a celiac angiogram shows a markedly hypervascular mass being fed by a hypertrophied phrenic artery. Biopsy proven hemangiopericytoma arising in the right diaphragm. (Case courtesy of B. Nagesh Raghavendra, M.D., University Hospital, New York University Medical Center.)

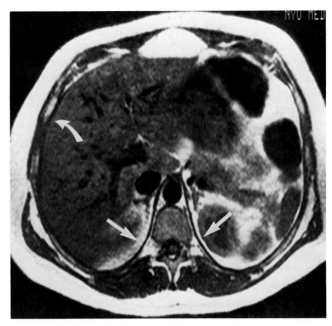

FIG. 38. Normal diaphragm: MR evaluation. **A, B:** Sequential T1-weighted axial spin-echo scans through the upper abdomen show typical appearance of the diaphragms, recognizable as a distinctly low signal intensity line, marginated centrally and peripherally by high signal intensity fat (*arrows* in A and B). Note that due to increased contrast resolution, the line of the diaphragm can also be appreciated marginating the lateral aspect of the liver (*curved arrows* in A and B) (compare with Fig. 1).

CONCLUSION

Various disease processes affect the diaphragm either directly or by contiguity. Delineation of disease is con-tingent on a thorough knowledge of the normal cross-sectional appearance of the diaphragm. Analysis is made difficult because of the overall oblique configuration of the diaphragm. In general, the exact position of the dia-

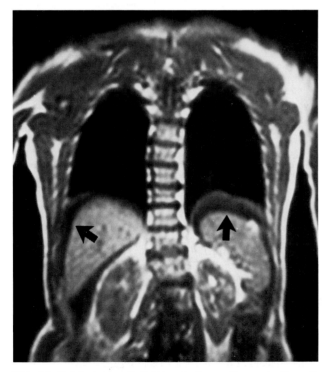

FIG. 39. Peridiaphragmatic fluid localization-ascites: evaluation with MR. Coronal T1-weighted MR scan clearly shows the presence of ascites surrounding both the liver and spleen (*arrows*), recognizable as a low signal intensity fluid collection.

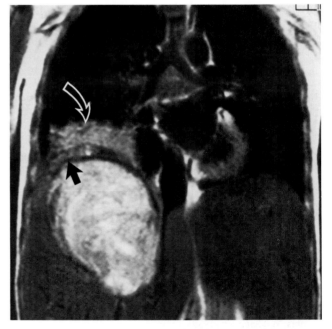

FIG. 40. Diaphragmatic tumor invasion: MR evaluation. Coronal T1-weighted scan through the liver shows a large, necrotic tumor mass in the liver extending superiorly to involve the diaphragm (*arrow*). Note the presence of basilar consolidation, as well, in the right lower lobe (*curved arrow*). Given the inherent advantages of multi-planar imaging and superior contrast resolution, MR should be of benefit in difficult cases for defining the true extent of peridiaphragmatic tumor.

phragm can only be inferred; it is visualized as an identifiable structure only when it is marginated by fat. Despite this limitation, the location of the diaphragm can be precisely defined, as illustrated throughout this chapter, by knowledge of the normal anatomic relationships between the diaphragm and surrounding structures.

Once the diaphragm has been localized, differentiation between intrathoracic and intra-abdominal disease, especially fluid collections, is facilitated. This is true even when fluid is present simultaneously in the chest and abdomen.

The diaphragm also can serve as a pathway for the spread of disease. This concept unifies evaluation of sections through the thoraco-abdominal interface, and further reinforces the necessity of overall familiarity with the cross-sectional appearance of diseases within both the thorax and abdomen.

To date, the role of magnetic resonance (MR) in evaluating disease in and around the diaphragm has been quite limited. Although isolated reports have shown the efficacy of MR in evaluating thoracic and abdominal wall infections, diaphragmatic rupture, Morgagni hernias, mediastinal pseudo-cysts, and even diaphragmatic endometriosis, no large series has ever been reported comparing MR with CT in the evaluation of peridiaphragmatic fluid collections (71–75). Given the superior contrast resolution of MR and advantages that accrue from coronal and sagittal imaging, it may be anticipated that at least in select cases, MR may ultimately prove of value in the assessment of peridiaphragmatic disease (Figs. 37–40).

REFERENCES

1. Naidich DP, Megibow AJ, Ross CR, Beranbaum ER, Siegelman SS. Computed tomography of the diaphragm: normal anatomy and variants. *J Comput Assist Tomogr* 1983;7:633–640.
2. Traver RD, Godwin JD, Putman CE. The diaphragm. *Radiol Clin North Am* 1984;22:618.
3. Panicek DM, Benson CB, Gottlieb RH, Heitzman ER. The diaphragm: anatomic, pathologic, and radiologic considerations. *Radiographics* 1988;8:385–425.
4. Callen PW, Filly RA, Korobkin M. Computed tomographic evaluation of the diaphragmatic crura. *Radiology* 1978;126:413–416.
5. Callen PW, Korobkin M, Isherwood I. Computed tomographic evaluation of the retrocrural pre-vertebral space. *AJR* 1977;129:907–910.
6. Shin MS, Berland LL. Computed tomography of retrocrural spaces: normal anatomic variants and pathologic conditions. *AJR* 1985;145:81–86.
7. Romanes GJ, ed. *Cunninghams textbook of anatomy,* 12th ed. New York: Oxford University Press, 1981;352–354.
8. Williams PL, Warwick R, eds. *Gray's anatomy,* 36th ed. Philadelphia: WB Saunders, 1980.
9. Vibhakar SD, Bellon EM. The bare area of the spleen: a constant CT feature of the ascitic abdomen. *AJR* 1984;141:953–955.
10. Meyers MA. *Dynamic radiology of the abdomen: normal and pathologic anatomy,* 2nd ed. New York: Springer-Verlag, 1982.
11. Pozderac R, Borlaza G, Green RA. Radiographic exhibit: subdiaphragmatic adiposity mimicking ascites by liver-lung scintigraphy. *Radiology* 1979;132:154.
12. Kleinman PK, Raptopoulos V. The anterior diaphragmatic attachments: an anatomic and radiologic study with clinical correlates. *Radiology* 1985;155:289–293.
13. Patterson NW, Teates CD. CT measurements of the anterior portions of the diaphragm with illustrative abnormal cases. *Comput Radiol* 1985;9:61–65.
14. Gale EM. Anterior diaphragm: variations in the CT appearance. *Radiology* 1986;161:635–639.
15. Rosen A, Auh YH, Rubenstein WA, Engel I, Whalen JP, Kazam E. CT appearance of diaphragmatic pseudotumors. *J Comput Assist Tomogr* 1983;995–999.
16. Anda S, Roysland P, Fougner R, Stovring J. CT appearance of the diaphragm varying with respiratory phase and muscular tension. *J Comput Assist Tomogr* 1986;10:744–745.
17. Nightingale RC, Dixon AK. Crural change with respiration: a potential mimic of disease. *Br J Radiol* 1984;57:101–102.
18. Williamson BRJ, Gouse JC, Rohrer DG, Teates CD. Variation in the thickness of the diaphragmatic crura with respiration. *Radiology* 1987;163:683–684.
19. Caskey CI, Zerhouni EA, Fishman EK, Rahmouni AD. Aging of the diaphragm: a CT study. *Radiology* 1989;171:385–389.
20. Silverman PM, Godwin JD, Korobkin M. Computed tomographic detection of retrocrural air. *AJR* 1982;138:824–827.
21. Demartini WJ, House AJS. Partial Bochdalek's herniation: computerized tomographic evaluation. *Chest* 1980;77:702–704.
22. Gale ME. Bochdalek hernia: prevalence and CT characteristics. *Radiology* 1985;156:449–452.
23. Curley FJ, Hubmayr RD, Raptopoulos V. Bilateral diaphragmatic densities in a 72-year-old woman. *Chest* 1984;86:915–917.
24. Weinshelbaum AM, Weinshelbaum EI. Incarcerated adult Bochdalek hernia with splenic infarction. *Gastrointest Radiol* 1982;7:287–289.
25. Coral A, Jones SN, Lees WR. Case report. Dorsal pancreas presenting as a mass in the chest. *AJR* 1987;149:718–720.
26. Fagelman D, Caridi JG. CT diagnosis of hernia of Morgagni. *Gastroinest Radiol* 1984;9:153–155.
27. Wiencek RG, Wilson RF, Steiger Z. Acute injuries of the diaphragm. An analysis of 165 cases. *J Thorac Cardiovasc Surg* 1986;92:989–993.
28. Hegarty MM, Bryer JV, Angorn IB, Baker LW. Delayed presentation of traumatic diaphragmatic hernia. *Ann Surg* 1978;188:229–233.
29. Ball T, McCrory R, Smith JO, Clements JL Jr. Traumatic diaphragmatic hernia: errors in diagnosis. *AJR* 1982;138:633–637.
30. Fagan CJ, Schreiber MH, Amparo EG, Wysong CB. Traumatic diaphragmatic hernia into the pericardium: verification of diagnosis by computed tomography. *J Comput Assist Tomogr* 1979;3:404–408.
31. Heiberg E, Wolverson MK, Hurd RN, Jagannad-Larad B, Sundaram M. Case report: CT recognition of traumatic rupture of the diaphragm. *AJR* 1980;135:369–392.
32. Demos TC, Solomon C, Posniak HV, Flisak MJ. Computed tomography in traumatic defects of the diaphragm. *Clin Imag* 1989;13:62–67.
33. Leekam RN, Ilves R, Shankar L. Case report. Inversion of gallbladder secondary to traumatic herniation of liver: CT findings. *J Comput Assist Tomogr* 1987;11:163–164.
34. Gurney J, Harrison WL, Anderson JC. Omental fat simulating pleural fluid in traumatic diaphragmatic hernia: CT characteristics. *J Comput Assist Tomogr* 1985;9:1112–1114.
35. Aronchick JM, Epstein DM, Gefter WB, Miller WT. Chronic traumatic diaphragmatic hernia: the significance of pleural effusion. *Radiology* 1988;168:675–678.
36. Radin DR, Ray MJ, Halls JM. Strangulated diaphragmatic hernia with pneumothorax due to colopleural fistula. *AJR* 1986;146:321–322.
37. Naidich DP, Megibow AJ, Hilton S, Hulnick DH, Siegelman SS. Computed tomography of the diaphragm: peridiaphragmatic fluid localization. *J Comput Assist Tomogr* 1983;7:641–649.
38. Dwyer A. The displaced crus: a sign for distinguishing between pleural fluid and ascites on computed tomography. *J Comput Assist Tomogr* 1978;2:598–599.
39. Teplick JG, Teplick SK, Goodman L, Haskin ME. The interface

sign: a computed tomographic sign for distinguishing pleural and intraabdominal fluid. *Radiology* 1982;144:359–362.

40. Alexander ES, Proto AU, Clark RA. CT differentiation of subphrenic abscess and pleural effusion. *AJR* 1983;140:47–51.

41. Griffin DJ, Gross BH, McCracken S, Glazer GM. Observations on CT differentiation of pleural and peritoneal fluid. *J Comput Assist Tomogr* 1984;8:24–28.

42. Halvorsen RA, Fedyshin PJ, Korobkin M, Thompson WM. CT differentiation of pleural effusion from ascites. An evaluation of four signs using blinded analysis of 52 cases. *Invest Radiol* 1986;21:391–395.

43. Halvorsen RA, Fedyshin PJ, Korobkin M, Foster WL Jr, Thompson WM. Ascites or pleural effusion? CT differentiation: four useful criteria. *Radiographics* 1986;6:135–149.

44. Silverman PM, Baker ME, Mahoney BS. Atelectasis and subpulmonic fluid: a CT pitfall in distinguishing pleural from peritoneal fluid. *J Comput Assist Tomogr* 1985;9:763–766.

45. Federle MP, Mark AS, Guillaumin ES. CT of subpulmonic pleural effusions and atelectasis: criteria for differentiation from subphrenic fluid. *AJR* 1986;146:685–689.

46. Friedman PJ. Case report. CT demonstration of tethering of the lung by the pulmonary ligament. *J Comput Assist Tomogr* 1985;9:947–948.

47. Berkmen YM, Davis SD, Kazam E, Auh YH, Yankelevitz D, Girgis FG. Right phrenic nerve: anatomy, CT appearance, and differentiation from the pulmonary ligament. *Radiology* 1989;173:43–46.

48. Bressler EL, Francis IR, Glazer GM, Gross BH. Bolus contrast medium enhancement for distinguishing pleural from parenchymal lung disease: CT features. *J Comput Assist Tomogr* 1987;11:436–440.

49. Rubenstein WA, Auh YH, Whalen JP, Kazam E. The perihepatic spaces: computed tomographic and ultrasound imaging. *Radiology* 1985;149:231–239.

50. Dodds WJ, Foley WD, Lawson TL, Stewart ET, Taylor A. Anatomy and imaging of the lesser peritoneal sac. *AJR* 1985;14:567–575.

51. Rosen A, Korobkin M, Silverman P, Moore AJ Jr, Dunnick NR. CT diagnosis of ruptured abdominal aortic aneurysms. *AJR* 1984;143:262–268.

52. Hopper KD, Sherman JL, Ghaed N. Aortic rupture into retroperitoneum (letter). *AJR* 1985;145:435–437.

53. Halvorsen RA, Jones MA, Rice RP, Thompson WM. Anterior left subphrenic abscess: characteristic plain film and CT appearance. *AJR* 1982;139:283–289.

54. Katzen BT, Choi WS, Friedman MH, Green IJ, Hindle WV, Zellis A. Pseudo-mass of the liver due to pleural effusion and inversion of the diaphragm. *AJR* 1978;131:1077–1078.

55. Dallemand S, Twersky J, Gordon DH. Pseudomass of the left upper quadrant from inversion of the left hemidiaphragm: CT diagnosis. *Gastrointest Radiol* 1982;7:57–59.

56. Thompson WM, Halvorsen RA, Williford ME, Foster WL, Korobkin M. Computed tomography of the gastroesophageal junction. *Radiographics* 1982;2:179–193.

57. Govoni AF, Whalen JP, Kazam E. Hiatal hernia: a relook. *Radiographics* 1983;3:612–644.

58. Ginalski JM, Schnyder P, Moss AA. Incidence and significance of a widened esophageal hiatus at CT scan. *J Clin Gastroenterol* 1984;6:467–470.

59. Godwin JD, MacGregor JM. Case report. Extension of ascites into the chest with hiatal hernia: visualization on CT. *AJR* 1987;148:31–32.

60. Clark KE, Foley WD, Lawson TL, Berland LL, Maddison FE. CT evaluation of esophageal and upper abdominal varices. *J Comput Assist Tomogr* 1980;4:510–515.

61. Balthazar EJ, Naidich DP, Megibow AJ, Lefleur RS. CT evaluation of esophageal varices. *AJR* 1987;148:131–135.

62. Han SY, McElvein RB, Aldrete JS. Perforation of the esophagus: correlation of site and cause with plain film findings. *AJR* 1985;145:537–540.

63. Glenny RW, Fulkerson WJ, Ravin CE. Occult spontaneous esophageal perforation. Unusual clinical and radiographic presentation. *Chest* 1987;92:562–565.

64. Pezzulli FA, Aronson D, Goldberg N. Case report. Computed tomography of mediastinal hematoma secondary to unusual esophageal laceration: a Boerhaave variant. *J Comput Assist Tomogr* 1989;13:129–131.

65. Raval B, Hall JT, Jackson H. Case report. CT diagnosis of fluid in the lesser sac mimicking thrombosis of inferior vena cava. *J Comput Assist Tomogr* 1985;9:956–958.

66. Zerhouni EA, Scott W, Baker R, Wharam MD, Siegelman SS. Invasive thymomas: diagnosis and evaluation by computed tomography. *J Comput Assist Tomogr* 1982;6:92–100.

67. Scatariage JC, Fishman EK, Zerhouni EA, Siegelman SS. Transdiaphragmatic extension of invasive thymoma. *AJR* 1985;144:31–35.

68. Shuman LS, Libshitz HI. Pictorial essay. Solid pleural manifestations of lymphoma. *AJR* 1984;142:269–273.

69. Peterson MW, Austin JHM, Yip CK, McManus RP, Jaretzki A. Case report. CT findings in transdiaphragmatic empyema necessitates due to tuberculosis. *J Comput Assist Tomogr* 1987;11:704–706.

70. Muller NL. Case report. CT features of cystic teratoma of the diaphragm. *J Comput Assist Tomogr* 1986;10:325–326.

71. Sharif HS, Clark DC, Aabed MY, Aideyan OA, Haddad MC, Mattson TA. MR imaging of thoracic and abdominal wall infections: comparison with other imaging procedures. *AJR* 1990;154:989–995.

72. Mirvis SE, Keramati B, Buckman R, Rodriguez A. Case report. MR imaging of traumatic diaphragmatic rupture. *J Comput Assist Tomogr* 1988;12:147–149.

73. Yeager BA, Guglielmi GE, Schiebler ML, Gefter WB, Kressel HY. Magnetic resonance imaging of Morgagni hernia. *Gastrointest Radiol* 1987;12:296–298.

74. Winsett MZ, Amparo EG, Fagan CJ, Bedi DG, Gallagher P, Nealon WH. Case report. MR imaging of mediastinal pseudocyst. *J Comput Assist Tomogr* 1988;12:320–322.

75. Posniak HV, Keshavarzian A, Jabamoni R. Diaphragmatic endometriosis: CT and MR findings. *Gastrointest Radiol* 1990;15:349–351.

Chapter 11

Pediatric Thorax

INDICATIONS

When evaluating disorders of the pediatric thorax, computed tomography (CT) and magnetic resonance (MR) should be used only as second- or perhaps third-order imaging procedures because plain chest films are satisfactory for evaluation of most common abnormalities. Even though CT and MR are not often indicated for investigation of diseases of the pediatric thorax, when they are necessary the diagnostic stakes are often high and the radiologist and the department staff may be somewhat uncomfortable dealing with a small, ill, or uncooperative child.

TECHNIQUE

CT and MR are expensive, time-consuming procedures that deserve to be performed optimally so that the information obtained is maximized. Previous studies and the history should be carefully reviewed. Take the time to call the clinician if you are not sure about just what it is you are after in a particular situation. Often the examination needs to be tailored, especially with MR. Be aware of what pulse sequences and planes will best show the suspected pathology. For CT, if contrast enhancement is likely to be needed, it is helpful to place an intravenous (i.v.) line before you start scanning so that the child does not cry during a venipuncture and ruin the contrast-enhanced scans.

Sedation will be necessary for optimal studies in many children. We have found that under the age of 8 or 9 years it is difficult for even a cooperative child to hold still long enough to assure completion of the MR study without patient motion. If sedation is needed, the child must be screened to make certain that he or she is a suitable candidate. A fever, upper respiratory infection, upper airway obstruction, and the presence of hepatic disease are all signals for caution. The child should have fasted for at least 3 and preferably 4 hours before the examination.

Although many different approaches to sedation have been suggested (1–3), I believe that if the radiology staff or the hospital personnel are not experienced in dealing with children, probably the safest sedation regimen is chloral hydrate (Noctec Syrup) given orally in a dose of 50–75 mg/kg ~30 min before the examination. A repeat dose, half of the original, may be used if the child does not fall asleep. In our department, we use this approach primarily in children younger than 6 months of age, especially if the examination is likely to be short and painless.

If no i.v. line is available or if no i.v. injection is contemplated, intramuscular Nembutal in a dose of 5–6 mg/kg may be used. The drawbacks are a somewhat unpredictable time of onset and relatively prolonged grogginess and irritability following the examination.

Our preferred method of sedation is the i.v. route using the drugs and dosages listed in Table 1. The advantages of this approach are that the time of onset is rapid and predictable, and the dose of drug can be accurately titrated to the patient's response.

TABLE 1. *Intravenous sedation in patients over 6 months of age*

Give drugs slowly and in divided doses.

Patients must be carefully monitored.

Nembutal (pentobarbital sodium), 1–2 mg/kg/dose. Wait at least 2–3 min for full effect of i.v. dose. If necessary to give additional sedation, use boluses of 1–2 mg/kg. Usually unnecessary to exceed 6 mg/kg total dose.

Sublimaze (fentanyl citrate), 1–2 µg/kg/dose. Then titrate with additional dose of 1 µg/kg i.v. PRN. Usually will not exceed total of 4–5 µg/kg. At higher doses, noticeable nasofacial itching occurs which keeps the older child awake. Very effective after Nembutal, if child almost asleep. Caution: Give slowly, since rapid administration can cause chest wall rigidity.

Valium (diazepam), 0.05–0.1 mg/kg/dose. Very effective in children with behavior problems. Give i.v. over a 2-min period. May be used alone or in combination with Sublimaze. Do not mix with other medications or dilute with dextrose solutions.

Regardless of what form of sedation is used, careful monitoring of the patient is necessary. The minimum requirement is to monitor the heart rate; an expired CO_2 apnea monitor is a valuable addition, but the ideal seems to be a pulse oximeter, which allows assessment of oxygen saturation as well as heart rate. Monitoring may be especially difficult in the MR environment. Discussions with the vendor, other users, and trial and error may be necessary to find the ideal solution.

When the patient is an infant, some system for maintaining body temperature is imperative. Wrapping the baby in blankets may be adequate, or it may be necessary to resort to using warming lamps or heating blankets, depending on the environment. All patients should be comfortably immobilized using a combination of ace bandages, Velcro straps, blankets, etc. Tape may be used but, of course, should not be placed directly on the child's sensitive skin. A sedated child should not have a pacifier taped in his mouth; should he happen to vomit, the risk of aspiration would increase (1).

CT

Exact technique will vary with the indication for the exam and the equipment available to the radiologist (1,4). The child will be prepared as discussed above. He should be positioned in the center of the scan circle, supine, with his arms over his head. The exam should be done using the shortest scan time available. The smallest field of view possible should be used to enhance spatial resolution; if the lung parenchyma is the primary region of interest, scans should be reconstructed using an edge enhancement algorithm. Thin-slice collimation (1.5–5 mm) may be necessary in infants and young children or if maximal pulmonary detail is sought; 1-cm collimation is used for most exams in older children.

Ultrafast computed tomography (UFCT) (Imatron, South San Francisco, CA) or "cine CT" offers a major improvement over conventional CT in examining the pediatric chest and mediastinum. By using electron gun technology rather than a conventional x-ray tube, it is possible to obtain a single image in 0.05 sec (5). This very short exposure time essentially stops respiratory motion in infants and children who are unable to cooperate (6). In the 0.05-sec mode, a distance of 8 cm can be covered utilizing 0.8-cm thick transaxial sections without moving the table. It requires only 0.224 sec to obtain a single set of eight images, and up to 17 images can be produced in 1 sec. These relatively low-resolution images have been used primarily to study cardiac anatomy and function, as well as for evaluation of dynamics of the airway. Single or multiple levels can be studied at one or more times and displayed as a CT movie (7–9).

By doubling the scan time to 0.1 sec and doubling the number of detectors sampled, high-resolution images comparable or superior to those obtained by conventional CT scanners can be obtained. Because of the very short scan time, 0.1 sec, motion artifact is markedly reduced and images of very good diagnostic quality are obtained even in the smallest of infants. Slice thickness in this mode may be varied between 3 mm and 1 cm. Rapid table incrementation, 17 cm/sec, allows scanning the entire thorax of a child in ~20 sec.

Regardless of the type of scanner available, i.v. contrast enhancement is necessary for most pediatric mediastinal studies and should be used for many pulmonary parenchymal and pleural lesions as well. As in adults, contrast enhancement is not needed for evaluation of pulmonary metastatic disease unless there is concern over mediastinal or hilar lymphadenopathy. In the past, we have used 60% methylglucamine diatrizoate in a dose of 2 cc/kg given as rapidly as possible as a bolus during the initiation of scanning, but the newer nonionic contrast agents are more satisfactory because of their lower incidence of side effects. Children are less likely to awaken and become agitated during the bolus injection with the result that studies of better quality are obtained.

Most children do not follow breath-holding instructions well; we perform most of our examinations either with the child breathing quietly, making no attempt at breath holding, or at the end of a quiet respiration. With UFCT, it is possible to scan most of the pediatric thorax in the time of a single breath-hold, and this is the technique we prefer if the child is able to cooperate.

Radiation exposure is a necessary hazard of CT examination, and every effort must be made to minimize the exposure. For chest CT, conventional scanners produce an exposure of 2.5–2.7 rad to the skin; the breast tissue of the young girl and the thyroid gland are the organs of greatest concern (10,11). UFCT can be performed for any pediatric thoracic condition at an exposure time of 0.1 sec with an entrance dose to the skin of the back of about 500 mrad and a much lower dose to the anterior structures (6,12).

MR

As with CT, exact MR technique will vary depending on the clinical question to be answered and the equipment available to the radiologist. We have used a 0.35-T superconducting unit (Diasonics, Milpitas, CA), and the following comments are based primarily on our experience with that unit. The smallest coil possible should be used; most children can be studied in the adult head coil. We prefer to use electrocardiographic (ECG) gating for most thoracic studies to limit motion artifact; for most conditions, we start with a 10-mm axial study and then employ one or two additional planes depending on the clinical situation. Conventional T1 and T2 spin-echo sequences can be used if characterization of a lesion is desired, although in our experience measurement of the actual T1 and T2 relaxation times has been of limited value. Because we could not cardiac gate them on our equipment, partial flip angle techniques with gradient refocused echoes have not been useful in the pediatric chest, although a spin-echo technique using short TR (0.25 sec) and short TE (15 msec), and multiple acquisitions has been helpful to reduce motion artifacts especially in the upper mediastinum.

Our experience with gadopentate dimeglumine is limited, but in a few selected mediastinal cases, it has not been dramatically helpful.

MEDIASTINUM

The anatomy of the child's mediastinum is in most respects similar to that of the adult described in detail elsewhere in this volume. Two important differences are the relative paucity of mediastinal fat and the prominence of the normal thymus. The lack of fat means that contrast enhancement is required in nearly all children for adequate CT delineation of mediastinal anatomy. The thymus is an important source of confusion and concern since it is so variable in size and shape throughout childhood.

The major indication for CT or MR investigation of the mediastinum is the presence of a mediastinal mass; which technique is superior is as yet unproven, although it appears likely MR will be the procedure of choice for evaluation of many abnormalities, especially in the posterior mediastinum.

Mediastinal lesions can be classified according to the organ of origin, their usual anatomic location, or, as detailed in chapter 2, by their CT or MR characteristics. For the purpose of pediatric evaluation, this section will be based on the more traditional concept of the organ of origin and the region of the mediastinum affected.

Anterior Mediastinal Abnormalities

Thymus

The normal thymus is seen as a soft-tissue density in the anterior superior mediastinum. The thymus is relatively soft and insinuates itself behind the sternum and along the cardiac margins (13). It normally lies anterior to the great vessels, although its left lobe often extends posteriorly and laterally along the arch of the aorta to the plane of the descending aorta (14). On MR studies, in ~10% of children we have seen a small nubbin of what appears to be normal thymus posterior to the superior vena cava; although this could be a retrocaval lymph node, the appearance on the sagittal MR scan suggests that this is a tongue of thymic tissue (Fig. 1). Superiorly, the thymus may extend as high as the thyroid gland (15). It extends an average of 1.7 cm superior to the innominate vein (Fig. 1C), where it may simulate adenopathy when seen on axial imaging (16). Its inferior extention is variable. In infancy, it is commonly seen to the level of the pulmonary arteries or below, but as the thorax elongates faster than the thymus, its relative inferior extention decreases with age (15).

In the axial plane, the gland is of quadrilateral shape in infants and younger children, becoming more triangular as the child grows. Its margins are sharp and smooth, convex in infants, and become straight or concave in older children (13,17,18).

The size of the gland is variable and has been measured with both CT (13,17) and MR (15,19,19a). Cranial-caudal measurements (length) increase with age; the width, and anteroposterior (AP) and transverse diameter show little change. On CT, the average thickness of the thymus appears to decrease with advancing age, diminishing from an average of 1.4 cm in children aged 0–5 years to 1.0 cm in children aged 10–19 years (19). In 59 children studied with MR, slightly different findings were noted (Table 2) (15). There was a slight but definite increase in the transverse dimension of the thymus but a marked decrease in the ratio of the size of the thymus relative to both the transverse and cranial-caudal measurements of the thorax, accounting for the thymus appearing relatively less prominent with advancing age. The width of the left lobe increased, but MR failed to reveal any age-related change in the thickness of the thymus. On MR, the thymus had slightly greater thickness than was noted by CT, with an average of 1.8 cm for the right lobe and 2.1 cm for the left lobe. The cra-

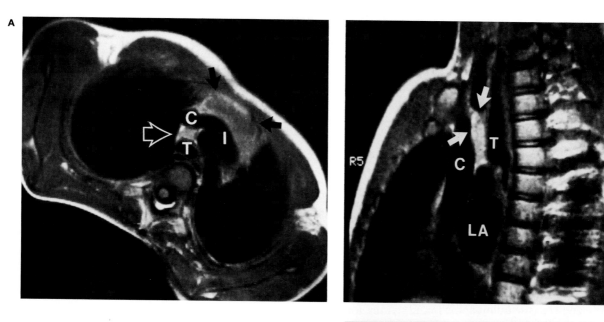

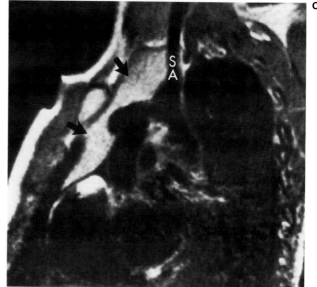

FIG. 1. Probable retrocaval thymic tissue in an 18-month-old child. **A:** Gated transaxial 5-mm section at the level of the innominate vein (I) reveals the thymus (*arrows*) to be of intermediate signal intensity. A nubbin of tissue with similar signal intensity (*open arrow*) is seen to lie posterior to the superior vena cava (C) and in front of the trachea (T). **B:** Oblique sagittal section, same patient, shows presumed retrocaval thymus (*arrows*) between the superior vena cava (C) and the trachea (T). LA, left atrium. **C:** Oblique section, 1 cm farther left, same patient, shows the thymus (*arrows*) to extend well cephalad past the level of the innominate vein seen posterior to the manubrium. Note the normal, tapered inferior margin. SA, subclavian artery.

TABLE 2. *MR measurements of thymic dimensions in 59 children*

	(0–1)	(2–4)	(5–9)	(10–14)	(15–19)	(0–19)	sd
				Age (in years)			
Max. trans. width (T)	4.9	5.0	5.4	6.3	5.8	5.4	(1.1)
Thymic/thoracic ratio	.51	.41	.34	.35	.28	.41	(.11)
A.P. in midline	1.7	1.7	1.6	1.7	2.0	1.7	(.5)
A.P. max left	3.5	4.1	4.2	4.5	5.0	4.1	(1.0)
A.P. max rt	2.8	2.7	2.6	2.8	3.1	2.7	(.9)
R. lobe width	2.5	2.4	2.8	3.0	3.0	2.7	(.6)
L. lobe width	2.9	3.3	3.6	4.2	4.4	3.5	(1.0)
R. lobe thickness	1.9	1.7	1.8	1.8	1.6	1.8	(.06)
L. lobe thickness	2.2	2.1	1.8	2.2	1.9	2.1	(.5)
Length (sagittal proj.)	5.6	6.6	7.6	8.0	8.5	7.2	(1.9)
Number of subjects	18	12	10	10	9	59	

Above first column is a diagrammatic representation of points at which MR thymus measurements were taken.

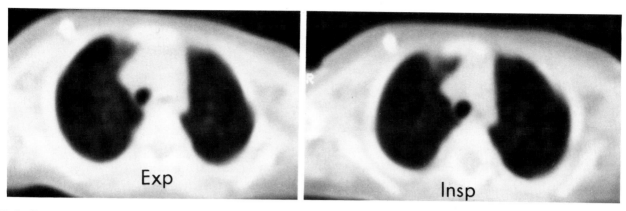

FIG. 2. Change in thymic shape with respiration demonstrated in an infant by UFCT. Images taken from a 0.05 cine sequence reveal the thymus to appear thicker and wider on expiration (Exp).

nial-caudad length of the thymus was found to increase from an average of 5.6 cm to 8.5 cm for children aged 0–1 year, compared with the age group of 15–19 years. It is likely that the differing measurements reflect the fact that the MR scans were made during quiet breathing, whereas CT, especially in older children, was commonly performed at inspiration (19), possibly producing some flattening of the thymus. Using UFCT, we have demonstrated this change in thymic shape with respiration (Fig. 2).

On CT, the thymus is of soft-tissue density, slightly more dense than the vessels, but approximately the same density as muscle tissue. The mean Hounsfield units (HU) of the thymus have been found to be 36 (18).

A

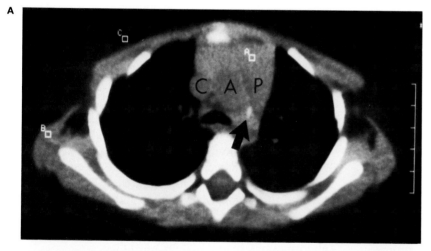

B

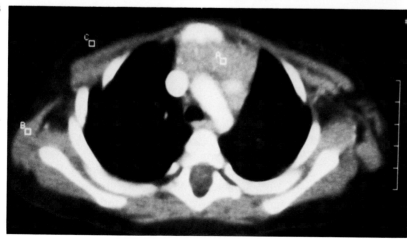

FIG. 3. Normal CT appearance of the thymus in a 10-month-old child. **A:** Thymus ("A" cursor) measures 56 hounsfield units (HU) and is seen to be denser than the superior vena cava (C), aorta (A), and pulmonary artery (P). A small linear calcification is incidently noted in the ductus (*arrow*). Muscle ("B" cursor) measures 49 HU; fat ("C" cursor) measures −106 HU. **B:** After contrast enhancement, the thymus ("A" cursor) is more easily distinguished from the great vessels; its attenuation has increased from 56 HU to 81 HU. Following i.v. contrast, muscle ("B" cursor) measures 62 HU; fat ("C" cursor) still measures −106 HU.

A

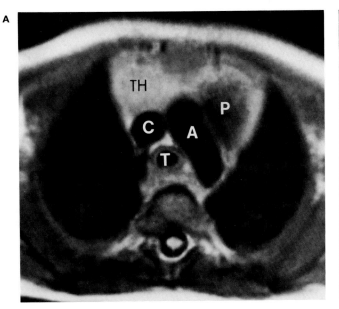

B

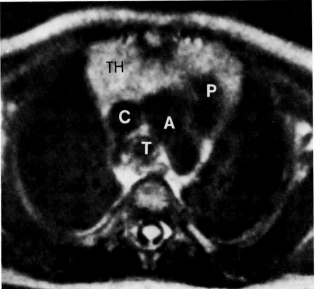

FIG. 4. MR appearance of normal thymus in a 10-month-old child. **A:** Intermediate weighted, gated transaxial image reveals the thymus (TH) to be slightly brighter than the muscle tissue but less bright than the subcutaneous fat. **B:** Non-gated T-2 weighted image (TR = 2 secs; TE = 80 msec) is less sharp than the gated image. The thymus is now slightly brighter than the subcutaneous fat and has considerably greater signal intensity than the skeletal muscle. A, aorta; C, superior vena cava; P, pulmonary artery; T, trachea.

Using UFCT, it is possible to distinguish between thymus and vessels even without contrast enhancement, but contrast enhancement is required to optimally delineate the gland, which shows homogeneous enhancement of 20–30 HU after bolus injection (Fig. 3). MR clearly distinguishes the thymus from the vascular structures in the mediastinum (20). On T1-weighted images, the signal intensity of the thymus is slightly brighter than muscle; on intermediate, gated sequences, it appears slightly less intense than fatty tissue; and on T2 images, it becomes brighter than both the surrounding fat and muscle (Fig. 4).

Congenital Abnormalities and Normal Variants

The thymus is absent in the DiGeorge syndrome in which absence of the parathyroid glands and congenital heart disease are other important features. These infants suffer from hypocalcemia and immune deficiency due to T-cell abnormalities (14).

Absence or hypoplasia of the thymus may be suggested from plain film findings, but CT or MR will often reveal that the thymus is present. There are no known reliable criteria for diagnosis of thymic hypoplasia as the gland is known to decrease in size as a normal response to stress.

A variant of normal thymic position and size is the retrocaval or ectopic thymus. As mentioned above, a small amount of what appears to be thymic tissue is seen posterior to the superior vena cava in some normal infants, but on occasion this portion of thymus is disproportionately enlarged and is perceived on plain film as a

possible mediastinal mass, leading to further investigation (21). CT or MR reveal tissue with characteristics identical to normal thymus that extends contiguously into the middle and even the posterior mediastinum, extending posterior to the superior vena cava when the enlargement is on the right side (Fig. 5) (22,23). On the left side, direct extension posteriorly, parallel to the aortic arch, may occur with the gland extending all the way into the posterior mediastinum. Although no imaging procedure can provide a histologic diagnosis, this appearance is so characteristic that in the absence of any atypical clinical or imaging features, it appears to be justified to observe this condition rather than resorting to biopsy. If there is evidence of airway or vascular compression or if the child has other significant clinical abnormalities, biopsy may be warranted.

Bizarre forms of thymic enlargement are seen as a rebound phenomenon after severe stress. This most commonly occurs in infants who have had severe respiratory distress syndrome or its complications; severe congenital heart disease is another common predisposing cause. Usually, despite the bizarre size and shape of the thymus, there is little, if any, difficulty in establishing the correct diagnosis of rebound thymic enlargement (Fig. 6). These children only need CT or MR examination in unusual circumstances. Greater diagnostic difficulty occurs when thymic enlargement occurs as a rebound phenomenon following therapy for malignancy. If imaging characteristics are all consistent with normal thymus, it may be possible to follow the patient, but biopsy is the only certain way of establishing the correct diagnosis (Fig. 7).

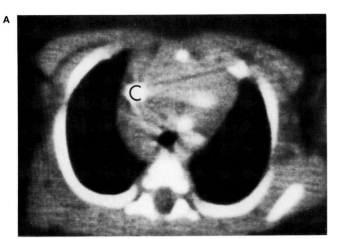 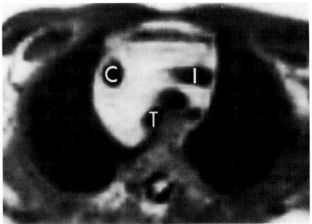

FIG. 5. Ectopic (retrocaval) thymus in a 2-month-old child. **A:** Contrast-enhanced CT scan reveals soft tissue contiguous with normal thymus extending posterior to the superior vena cava. **B:** Transaxial gated MR scan reveals the tissue to have signal characteristics identical with normal thymus. C, superior vena cava; I, innominate vein; T, trachea.

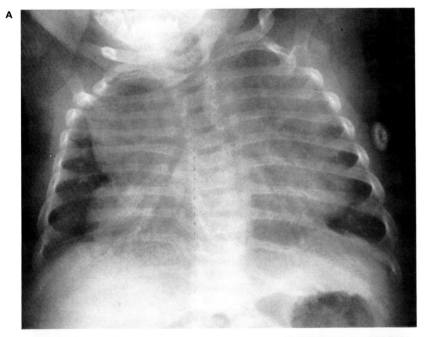

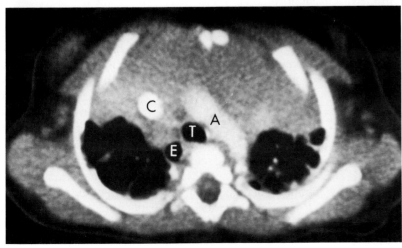

FIG. 6. Rebound thymic enlargement. **A:** Six-month-old ex-premature infant with bronchopulmonary dysplasia presented with a bizarre cardiomediastinal silhouette. **B:** Contrast enhanced UFCT (0.1 sec), reveals marked enlargement of the thymus filling the anterior-superior mediastinum. A, aorta; C, superior vena cava; E, esophagus; T, trachea.

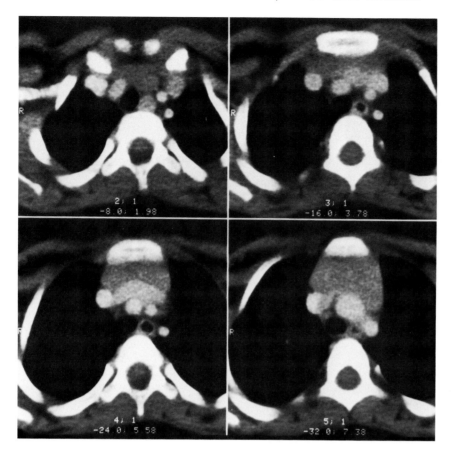

FIG. 7. Rebound thymic hypertrophy following chemotherapy for Wilms' tumor in a 7-year-old patient presenting with an upper mediastinal fullness. Four images from UFCT examination reveal normal vascular anatomy and a prominent thymus for age. However, the homogeneous appearance and smooth contours of the thymus suggest that it probably is normal thymus. MR examination was also normal. One-year follow-up has failed to reveal any abnormality.

Thymic Hyperplasia

Thymic hyperplasia may occur in association with hyperthyroidism or therapy for hypothyroidism. It may also be seen in association with myasthenia gravis and red cell aplasia. A true thymoma in association with myasthenia gravis is uncommon in childhood (14).

Pathologic Causes of Thymic Enlargement

In the newborn, acute thymic enlargement, particularly if associated with pleural effusion, should suggest acute thymic hemorrhage. Thymic cysts are relatively unusual causes of thymic enlargement; they probably are of developmental origin, representing persistent tu-

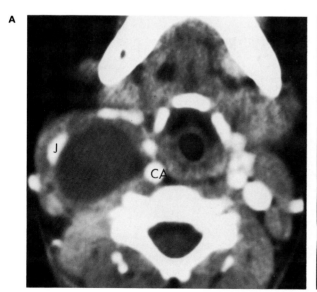
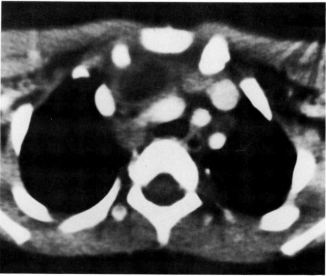

FIG. 8. Thymic cyst. Two-year-old female presented with a mass in the right side of the neck. A: Contrast enhanced CT scan reveals an avascular mass in the carotid sheath, separating the carotid artery (CA) and jugular vein (J). B: The mass extends contiguously into the thymus and the upper mediastinum. At surgery a congenital thymic cyst was removed.

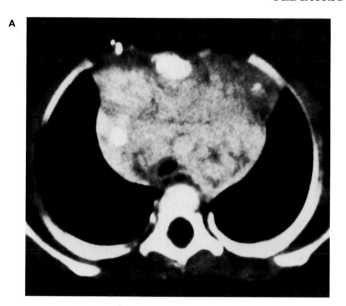

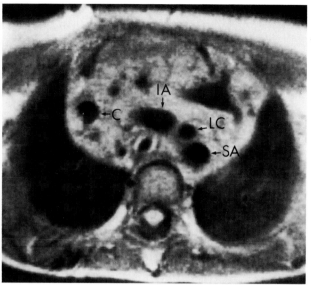

FIG. 9. Thymic hemangioma. One-year-old child with respiratory distress and a large mediastinal mass. CT scan (**A**) and gated MR image (**B**) reveal diffuse thymic enlargement with multiple vascular channels. At surgery a thymic hemangioma was partially resected. C, superior vena cava; IA, innominate artery; LC, left carotid artery; SA, subclavian artery.

bular remnants of the third pharyngeal pouch. The cysts may vary in size from microscopic to several centimeters, and they may be unilocular or multilocular. Ultrasound and CT have been used in diagnosis; contrast enhancement is necessary for CT. The cyst may present in the neck, mediastinum or in both regions (Fig. 8) (24). Thymic cysts are more frequent in children with various forms of bone marrow aplasia; acute hemorrhage into a thymic cyst has been reported in children with aplastic anemia (25).

Thymic enlargement may also occur as a result of a thymic hemangioma, the nature of which can be strongly suggested from the CT and MR studies that show abnormal vessels in the thymus (Fig. 9).

Thymic Neoplasms

Thymomas are rare in infancy and childhood. There appears to be little association between thymomas and myasthenia gravis in children. Radiographic features resemble those of lymphoma. Calcification is seen somewhat more commonly in thymoma than in untreated lymphoma, but this alone is not a reliable differential point; biopsy is required.

Lymphoma is the most common cause of an anterior mediastinal mass in children. Hodgkin lymphoma is three to four times more frequent than non-Hodgkin lymphoma. Differentiation of normal thymus from thymus involved by lymphoma is usually quite simple,

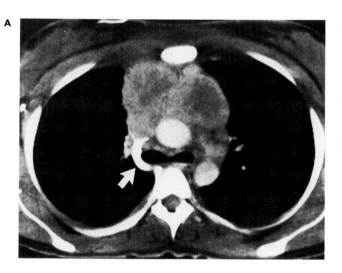

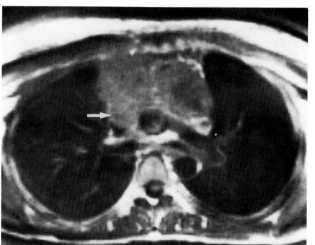

FIG. 10. Biopsy proven Hodgkin lymphoma affecting the thymus in a 14-year-old girl. **A:** Contrast-enhanced CT scan reveals superior vena caval obstruction and dilation of the azygos vein (*arrow*). The region of the thymus is markedly enlarged with nodular, irregular borders in areas of homogeneous contrast enhancement. **B:** Transaxial cardiac-gated MR image reveals a mass within the superior vena cava (*arrow*); the thymus is replaced by tissue of inhomogeneous signal intensity. Biopsy proven Hodgkin lymphoma.

but difficult cases require biopsy. With lymphomatous involvement, the thymus is usually grossly enlarged; its margins are lobular instead of smooth, and nodularity is often evident; contrast enhancement is inhomogenous, and large areas of necrosis are commonly seen (19,26,27). T2-weighted MR scans may show areas of inhomogeneity in the mass. There may be narrowing of the airway and compression of vascular structures (Fig. 10). Moreover, detection of enlarged hilar or supraclavicular nodes often give valuable clues to the true nature of the pathology.

Other Anterior Mediastinal Abnormalities

By far, the most common cause of an anterior mediastinal mass in a child is lymphoma, which often also affects the middle mediastinum and will be discussed in the section relating to that area; other conditions are all uncommon (Table 3). Cystic hygromas (lymphangiomas) are classified as being simple, cavernous, or cystic (28). Most arise in the neck, but ~10% arise in the mediastinum. Rarely, the lesion may present in the mediastinum without cervical involvement. Hygromas are found most commonly in the anterior superior mediastinum but may extend posteriorly and inferiorly; rarely, they may arise in the posterior mediastinum. In infancy, airway compression is common, but most children over the age of 2 years are asymptomatic. CT reveals a well-

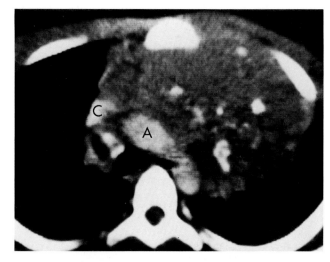

FIG. 11. Mediastinal seminoma with calcification. Contrast-enhanced CT scan reveals a large, irregular, anterior mediastinal mass containing several coarse areas of calcification. Pathologic diagnosis is mediastinal seminoma. A, aorta; C, superior vena cava.

circumscribed lesion of low attenuation molding to the mediastial contours and enveloping the great vessels. Contrast enhancement is minimal and, if present, suggests a hemangiomatous component. Venous malformations have been described (Fig. 62) (28a). MR shows a mass with morphologic characteristics similar to that seen on CT. T2 is prolonged; T1 may be either prolonged or shortened, depending on the makeup of the cyst fluid.

Lymph node enlargement due to histiocytosis X may occur and, interestingly, may cavitate; at times, it is difficult to know if these cysts are in the mediastinum or are pleural based parenchymal cysts (29). Teratomas are diagnosed by seeing a mass of mixed density—fat, fluid, and bone; they may be recognized either on CT or MR. Germ cell tumors are indistinguishable from other malignancies (30,31); calcification is said to be more common than in untreated lymphoma (Fig. 11). Abscesses can occur in the anterior mediastinum; the clinical picture usually suggests the correct diagnosis. CT and MR appearances are those of abscesses elsewhere in the body. An enlarged thyroid is quite uncommon as a cause of a mediastinal mass in children; marked contrast enhancement is typical.

Middle Mediastinal Abnormalities

Table 4 lists the CT characteristics of middle mediastinal masses that are most commonly encountered in children.

Lymphadenopathy

Normal lymph nodes are rarely visible on CT examination in infants and young children; in older teenagers,

TABLE 3. *CT characteristics of anterior mediastinal masses*

Solid
  Thymus
    Normal
    Thymic enlargement
      Physiologic
      Pathologic
  Lymphadenopathy
    Lymphoma
    Histiocytosis
    Sarcoidosis
    Infectious mononucleosis
    Mediastinitis/abscess
  Germ cell tumor/teratoma (may contain fat/fluid)
  Thyroid (may enhance)
  Chest wall tumor
  Morgagni hernia (liver)
Cystic/avascular
  Cystic hygroma
  Thymic cyst
  Abscess
Vascular
  Aneurysm of sinus of Valsalva
Fatty
  Lipoma, thymolipoma, lipoblastoma
  Teratoma
Calcified
  Granulomatous infection
  Teratoma, germ cell tumor
  Seminoma

TABLE 4. *CT characteristics of middle mediastinal masses*

Solid
  Lymph node enlargement
    Malignant
      Lymphoma
        Hodgkin
        Non-Hodgkin
      Leukemic
      Metastatic
    Benign inflammatory
      Bacterial infection
      Viral infection
        Infectious mononucleosis
        Pertussis
        Viral pneumonia
      Mycoplasma infection
      Granulomatous infection
        Tuberculosis
        Histoplasmosis
        Other granulomatous infections
    Miscellany
      Histiocytosis X
      Sarcoid
    Reactive
      Castleman's disease
      Sinus histiocytosis
Cystic
  Bronchogenic cyst
  Pericardial cyst
  Foregut cyst
  Pancreatic pseudocyst
  Intrapericardial teratoma (multi-cystic)
Vascular
  Venous
    Azygos
    Superior vena cava
    Total anomalous pulmonary venous return
    Arteriovenous malformations
  Arterial
    Aortic aneurysm
      Mycotic
      Connective tissue
    Coronary artery aneurysm
    Pulmonary artery aneurysm
Miscellaneous
  Esophagus
    Hiatal hernia
    Achalasia
  Neurofibromatosis

when mediastinal fat is somewhat more extensive, small normal nodes may occasionally be seen. Nodal groups that may enlarge include anterior mediastinal, paratracheal, hilar, subcarinal, peribronchial, anterior pericardial, and posterior mediastinal.

Adenopathy may be caused by any pulmonary infection but is most marked in tuberculosis and histoplasmosis. Sarcoidosis, a common cause of adenopathy in adults, is infrequent in children. Children with cystic fibrosis, in our experience, frequently have extensive adenopathy. The most common causes of marked lymphadenopathy are lymphoma and leukemia. Lymph node enlargement also occurs in infectious mononucleosis

and histiocytosis X. Castleman's disease is a rare cause of massive mediastinal adenopathy. Neoplasms such as neuroblastoma in the younger child and testicular carcinoma in the teenager metastasize to mediastinal nodes.

Because there is so little mediastinal fat in most children, if one wishes to visualize nodes on CT it is nearly always necessary to use bolus contrast enhancement to separate mediastinal nodes from the other soft tissue structures. Non–contrast-enhanced CT is indicated prior to contrast-enhanced CT to detect calcified nodes that would suggest granulomatous disease. Nodes are seen as discrete or confluent rounded masses of soft-tissue density. As in adults, discrimination between normal and abnormal nodes is made by criteria of visibility (present where none are usually seen), size (>1 cm), and abnormalities of enhancement. MR more readily separates nodes from vessels than does CT. On T1-weighted images, nodes are similar in intensity to muscle; on T2, they are brighter than muscle and become similar in signal intensity to surrounding fat. Their MR signal characteristics are quite similar to those of normal thymus. Regardless of the pulse sequence used, they are clearly distinguished from vessels that show no signal.

Evaluation of possible anterior mediastinal adenopathy in children, especially infants, is complicated by the presence of the thymus. There is considerable variation in the size and shape of the normal thymus, and it can be difficult at times to distinguish an anterior mediastinal nodal mass from normal thymus. Usually, however, lymphoma and other diseases associated with marked nodal enlargement occur in older children in whom the thymus is relatively smaller and the abnormal findings are quite apparent either because of the size of the mass, its multiple irregular nodular densities, or a pattern of uneven contrast enhancement (Fig. 10). Anterior mediastinal nodes can be seen to be in continuity with enlarged nodes in the neck or the lower mediastinum, thus aiding differentiation from the normal thymus.

Retrocaval and paratracheal adenopathy is frequent in lymphoma, granulomatous infection, and sarcoidosis. A small amount of soft tissue can be seen normally in some children posterior to the superior vena cava (Fig. 1); some of the time this represents "ectopic thymus," but distinction from adenopathy cannot always be made.

Hilar adenopathy has similar appearances in children and adults. Diagnosis is readily apparent on MR. Without UFCT, the diagnosis in children is sometimes difficult even with good bolus enhancement because of motion artifact; with UFCT, the diagnosis of hilar adenopathy is equal to that of MR; even peribronchial node enlargement is readily apparent with this technique (Fig. 12).

In children, slight convexity in the azygoesophageal recess is normal due to the azygous vein; despite this common normal variation, subcarinal adenopathy can

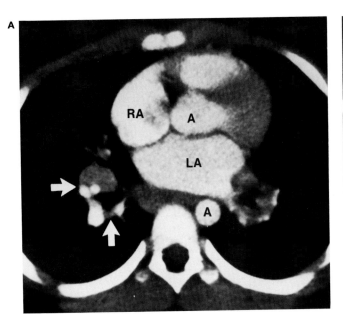
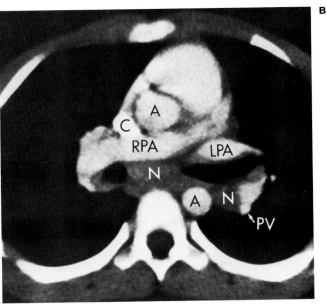

FIG. 12. A: Bilateral hilar and subcarinal adenopathy in a 10-year-old patient with asthma and chronic recurrent infection. Contrast-enhanced UFCT (0.1 sec), reveals bilateral hilar adenopathy, more prominent in the right (*arrows*). A, aorta; LA, left atrium; RA, right atrium. **B:** UFCT section, 16 mm. superior to **A,** reveals subcarinal adenopathy as well as bilateral hilar adenopathy, more prominent in the left side in this patient with recurring infections. N, peribronchial nodes; C, superior vena cava; LPA, left pulmonary artery; PV, pulmonary vein; RPA, right pulmonary artery.

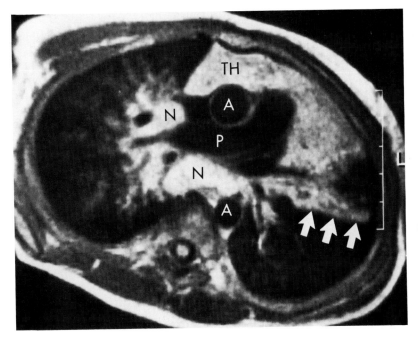

FIG. 13. Hilar and subcarinal adenopathy in a 9-month-old patient examined with MR for a vascular ring and recurrent pulmonary infections. Gated T1-weighted axial MR image reveals extensive subcarinal and right hilar adenopathy. Lingular atelectasis is present but is difficult to separate from the thymus (TH) because of similar signal intensity. A, aorta; N, nodes; P, pulmonary artery; *arrows,* lingular atelectasis.

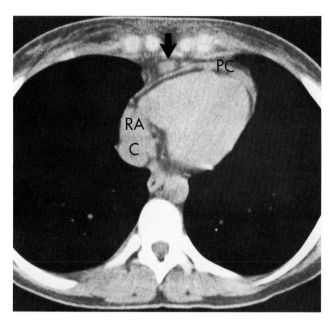

FIG. 14. UFCT in a 16-year-old girl with Hodgkin lymphoma. Small, anterior pericardiac nodes (*arrow*) are present. C, superior vena cava; PC, pericardium; RA, right atrium.

still be accurately diagnosed by either contrast-enhanced CT or MR. In addition to being a common site for adenopathy associated with lymphoma, we have seen several children with pulmonary infections who have had a moderate amount of subcarinal adenopathy (Figs. 12 and 13).

Anterior pericardiac nodes (cardiophrenic angle nodes) can be involved with lymphoma, and they may be clearly seen either by CT or MR (Fig. 14).

Posterior mediastinal nodes can be enlarged in chronic infection, particularly reflux esophagitis (32),

but they are much more frequently enlarged by metastatic retroperitoneal malignancy, most commonly neuroblastoma. They are retrocrural in location and displace the crura laterally and anteriorly and produce widening of the paraspinal line on chest roentgenogram (Fig. 15).

Lymphomas

Lymphomas are the third most common malignant group of diseases of childhood after leukemia and CNS tumors. The Hodgkin group of lymphomas are divided into the nodular sclerosing, mixed cellularity, lymphocyte depletion, and lymphocyte predominant types, with the first two groups accounting for >90% of cases. Non-Hodgkin lymphoma is a more heterogeneous group of diseases but includes T-cell, histiocytic, mixed cell, and B-cell type (including Burkitt's). The distinction between acute lymphoblastic leukemia with thymic and or nodal involvement and malignant lymphoma cannot be made by CT or MR. Hodgkin lymphoma is approximately three to four times more frequent than lymphomas of the non-Hodgkin group in children.

Lymphoma is the most common cause of a mediastinal mass in childhood. Approximately one-third of children with Hodgkin lymphoma have mediastinal involvement at the time of diagnosis (33). The mass tends to be bilateral but asymmetric. Anterior mediastinal nodes are the most frequently involved.

CT is indicated for differential diagnosis, staging, and radiation therapy planning (34). In patients with cervical adenopathy, mediastinal adenopathy will decrease the survival rate by ~10% according to North et al. (35). CT can be positive with a normal chest roentgenogram

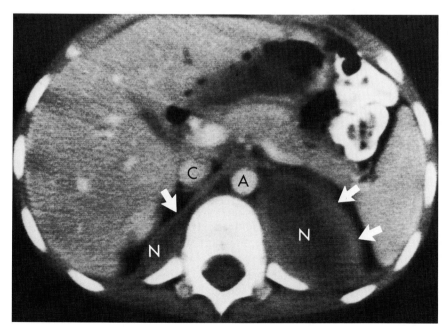

FIG. 15. Retrocrural adenopathy secondary to rhabdomyosarcoma in a 10-year-old boy. Contrast-enhanced CT scan reveals bilateral retrocrural nodal masses (N) displacing the crus (*arrows*) laterally. A, aorta; C, superior vena cava.

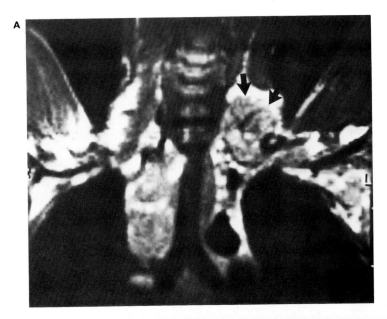

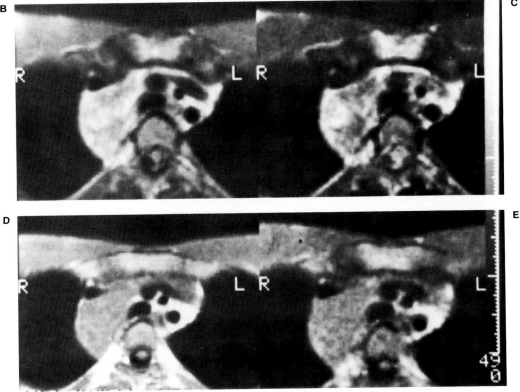

FIG. 16. Fifteen-year-old with Hodgkin lymphoma. **A:** T1-weighted coronal MR image reveals right paratracheal adenopathy with extension into the left supraclavicular region (*arrows*). **B–E:** Same patient as in **A. B** and **C:** Axial images acquired with progressively greater T2-weighting (TR = 2.0 sec; TE = 40 and 80 msec, respectively). **D** and **E:** Axial, T1-weighted images (TR = 0.25 sec; TE = 15 msec; TR = 0.5 sec, TE = 30 msec, respectively). Note that the right paratracheal mass becomes progressively brighter in relation to the muscle tissue with increasing T2-weighting; it also becomes less homogeneous.

and may add information about extent of nodal, chest wall, and pulmonary parenchymal involvement (34,36). CT is less important for staging of non-Hodgkin lymphoma (37) but may still give important information about vascular and tracheobronchial compression.

CT findings of lymphoma are those of lymph node enlargement, usually in the anterior mediastinum, but involvement of hilar and middle mediastinal nodes is common. Nodes may range in size from a centimeter to huge masses filling the mediastinum. Nodes may be seen as discrete nodular masses or as confluent masses of tumor. Calcification is rare in untreated cases (38); areas of necrosis are commonly seen, particularly following contrast enhancement. In our experience, approximately one case in four shows a homogeneous mass of tumor that could be mistaken for normal thymus except for its abnormal size; usually, other areas of disease are noted, commonly adenopathy in the neck or elsewhere in the mediastinum, simplifying the differential diagnosis (39). Morphology of the nodal masses on MR (Fig. 16) is similar to that seen with CT, although the coronal view gives a clearer idea of the cephalocaudad extent of disease. Signal characteristics tend to be similar, if not identical, to normal thymus on all pulse sequences. The relative roles of CT and MR in diagnosis and staging of lymphoma are not yet clear, although in many instances the anatomy is shown more clearly by MR.

Complications

Tracheobronchial compression of some degree occurred in 55% of the children with Hodgkin disease reported by Mandell et al. (40). This complication is seen better by CT than by airway films. Superior vena cava obstruction is readily diagnosed by CT or MR; findings include extensive collateral flow and failure to visualize the superior vena cava (Fig. 17).

Pulmonary involvement is rarely seen as the sole manifestation of disease. Typically, it tends to occur as the disease spreads contiguously from the mediastinal nodes, to the hilar nodes, to the lung parenchyma. A nodular or infiltrative pattern may be seen, and pleural masses may also be present. These findings are better demonstrated by CT than by conventional roentgenogram studies.

Residual masses are often seen in the mediastinum following therapy, and it is difficult to know if they represent fibrotic areas or residual tumor. Calcifications seen on CT suggest fibrosis as do areas of shortened T2 on MR. Gallium-67 citrate scanning can be helpful in some of these patients, particularly if the tumor has previously shown gallium avidity.

Non-Hodgkin Lymphoma

"Non-Hodgkin lymphoma" does not refer to a single disease entity, but rather to a more heterogeneous group of diseases generally having a more aggressive course and a worse prognosis than Hodgkin lymphoma.

The Burkitt type of non-Hodgkin lymphoma is characterized by abdominal involvement with relatively infrequent involvement of the mediastinum. The poorly differentiated lymphocytic variety of non-Hodgkin lymphoma has a high association of leukemic transformation and may, in fact, be part of the same disease process.

Findings on CT and MR are nonspecific and cannot be differentiated from Hodgkin disease. The masses may be larger, and airway and vascular compression tend to be more frequent and more severe; pulmonary parenchymal involvement is reported in only 2% of cases, but pleural effusion is seen in approximately 1 in 7 children (33).

Bronchogenic Cysts

Bronchogenic cysts, thought to result from an abnormal budding of the ventral diverticulum of the foregut, may present in the pulmonary parenchyma or the mediastinum (41). They are thin-walled cysts lined with respiratory epithelium and filled with mucoid material. Usually, there is no direct communication with the tracheobronchial tree, but if they become secondarily infected, communication may occur.

Most mediastinal bronchogenic cysts are situated near the carina and are often attached by a stalk to one of the major airways. Radiographic examination shows a round or oval mass of homogeneous density with clearly defined margins. The mass varies in size and often ex-

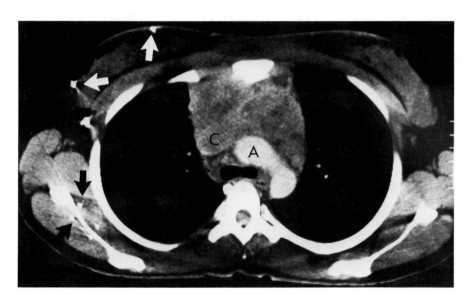

FIG. 17. Hodgkin lymphoma with superior vena cava obstruction. Contrast enhanced CT reveals inhomogeneous enhancement of a large anterior mediastinal mass. There is absence of visualization of the superior vena cava (C) and extensive collateral circulation is noted over the anterior chest wall and scapula (*arrows*). A, aorta.

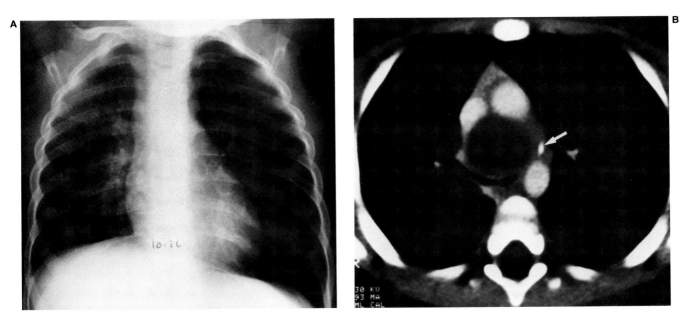

FIG. 18. Bronchogenic cyst. **A:** Frontal chest radiograph shows air trapping in the left lung with no other obvious abnormality. The patient was bronchoscoped because of a suspected foreign body. No foreign body was found but extrinsic tracheobronchial compression was apparent. **B:** Contrast enhanced CT scan at the level of the aortic pulmonary window reveals a 2-cm sharply defined avascular lesion anterior to the carina and extending inferiorly to it on other sections. Other findings include increased volume of the left lung and incidental calcification in the ligamentum arteriosum (*arrow*).

tends slightly to the right side. In infants, the masses are usually discovered because associated airway compression causes signs such as wheezing, stridor, and cough. Unilateral airway obstruction may be present. Usually, the cyst is obvious on a radiographic examination, although subcarinal cysts may be hidden and difficult to diagnose (Fig. 18). The esophagus may be deviated by the subcarinal mass.

CT is helpful to determine the nature and extent of a bronchogenic cyst (42). Although usually not frankly calcified on plain radiographic examination, some cysts have CT numbers much higher than water. Although

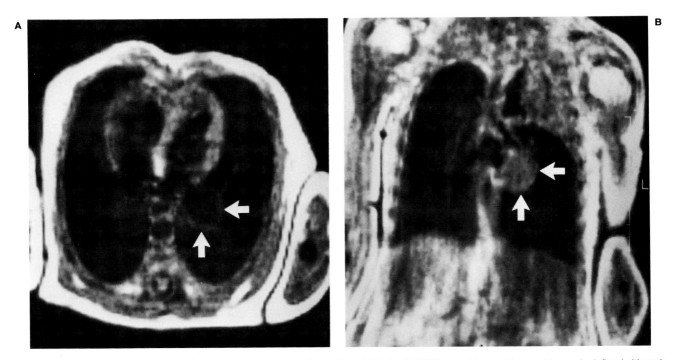

FIG. 19. MR evaluation of a bronchogenic cyst in a 2-day-old male. **A:** T1-weighted axial MR image. The cyst (*arrows*) is poorly defined although its wall is faintly visible. **B:** T2-weighted coronal image. The signal intensity of the cyst fluid (*arrows*) is now increased, and it is more clearly delineated from the lung parenchyma.

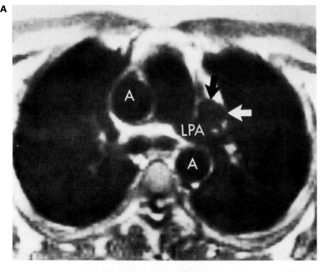

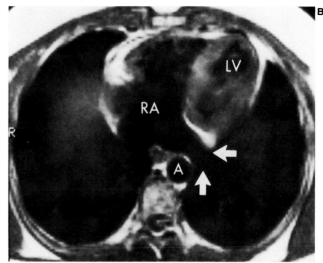

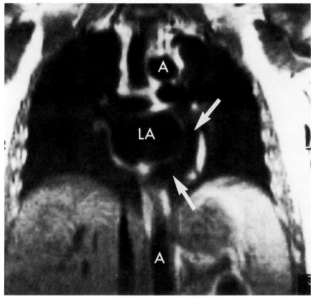

FIG. 20. Persistent left superior vena cava in a 12-year-old boy. **A:** Gated transaxial image reveals the anomalous vein (*arrows*) to lie anterior and lateral to the left pulmonary artery (LPA). **B:** The vessel is seen to drain into the coronary sinus (*arrows*). **C:** Coronal gated MR image reveals the curvilinear course of the abnormal left superior vena cava as it empties into the coronary sinus (*arrows*). A, aorta; LV, left ventricle; RA, right atrium; LA, left atrium.

the high numbers suggest the possibility of a solid mass, contrast enhancement reveals the true avascular, cystic nature of the mass. Airway obstruction, not apparent on plain radiography, is obvious on CT examination (Fig. 18). MR demonstrates the anatomy well in additional planes. Fluid-filled masses tend to have prolonged T1 and T2 relaxation times; on T1-weighted images, the mass may blend with the pulmonary parenchyma, but T2-weighted images reveal increased signal from the cyst fluid (Fig. 19). Sagittal and coronal sections are helpful in establishing the geography of the mass; airway obstruction and air trapping are less well visualized than on CT.

Vascular Lesions: Venous Anomalies

Intrahepatic absence or interruption of the inferior vena cava is associated with congenital heart disease and causes an increase in the size of the azygos and often the hemiazygos veins. These dilated vessels may simulate a mediastinal or paravertebral mass, but their true nature is revealed by contrast enhancement. The superior vena cava may be present bilaterally or be persistent on the left and absent on the right; the persistent left vena cava is anterolateral to the aortic arch and anterior to the left pulmonary artery, and drains into the coronary sinus (Fig. 20). Anomalous pulmonary venous return of the supracardiac type can result in an enlargement of the upper mediastinum. In the scimitar syndrome (pulmonary venolobar syndrome), an anomalous right pulmonary vein may drain into the right atrium or may extend below the diaphragm and insert into the inferior vena cava, or the hepatic or portal veins.

All of these conditions can be diagnosed by CT (43) but probably are better visualized by MR because of the availability of the sagittal and coronal views.

Arterial Anomalies

Pulmonary Arteries

The pulmonary arteries are well seen by MR in three views and can also be well demonstrated by CT in the transaxial plane with the use of bolus contrast enhancement, particularly if UFCT is available. There is no significant difference in the anatomy of the pulmonary arteries in children from that detailed elsewhere in this volume in adults. The left and right pulmonary arteries are approximately equal in size, but there is a lack of normal CT standards for size in the pediatric patient.

Either of the pulmonary arteries may be absent or "interrupted" with the artery present in the lung, but atretic centrally. The absent pulmonary artery tends to occur on the side opposite the aortic arch; when absence of the left pulmonary artery occurs, there is a high incidence of associated congenital cardiovascular anomalies, especially tetralogy of Fallot. Hypoplasia of the ipsilateral pulmonary artery is common in patients with pulmonary hypoplasia.

Enlargement of the pulmonary arteries occurs with pulmonary hypertension or with large left-to-right shunts. Ready recognition of pulmonary artery enlargement and separation from questionable hilar adenopathy is easily performed with either CT or MR.

Rarely, the pulmonary arteries may be aneurysmally dilated in the neonate. This usually occurs with congenital absence of the pulmonary valve, associated with a variant of the tetralogy of Fallot. The enlarged pulmonary artery may cause bronchial compression and either delayed clearance of neonatal lung liquid or, in older life, segmental or lobar air trapping.

The pulmonary artery sling or anomalous left pulmonary artery is a congenital condition in which the left pulmonary artery arises from the right pulmonary artery, passing across the mediastinum and between the esophagus and trachea. The lesion is associated with varying forms of obstructive emphysema as well as with congenital tracheal stenosis due to complete cartilage rings. It is clearly demonstrated by either CT or MR.

A tumor thrombus and pulmonary thromboembolism of any etiology is rare in children, but the pulmonary artery may, on occasion, be compressed by a mediastinal mass, most commonly, lymphoma.

Although a discussion of congenital heart disease is not in the scope of this chapter, familiarity with the various types of shunting procedures that may affect the pulmonary artery will be considered since MR is often used to evaluate their size and patency. In general, these shunts are used in congenital cyanotic heart disease where there is pulmonary valvular stenosis or atresia or tricuspid atresia (44).

A Blalock-Taussig shunt is used primarily in tetralogy of Fallot. It consists of direct anastomosis of the subcla-

vian artery to the pulmonary artery on the side contralateral to the aortic arch. The Waterston shunt is a side-to-side shunt in which the ascending aorta is anastomosed to the ipsilateral pulmonary artery, usually on the right side. The Potts is another central shunt similar to the Waterston in that it is a side-to-side anastomosis, but it is between the descending aorta and the ipsilateral pulmonary artery, usually on the left side. The Glenn procedure, which anastomoses the superior vena cava to the right pulmonary artery, is used in cases of tricuspid atresia. There are procedures in which direct conduits are made for correction of tricuspid atresia, including the Fontan procedure, where right atrial to pulmonary artery communication is made. A direct conduit can also be established between the right ventricle and the pulmonary artery using a valved or nonvalved artificial conduit. This procedure is utilized in cases of transposition of the great arteries, with ventricular septal defect, and pulmonic stenosis, truncus arteriosis, or severe tetralogy.

Aortic Anomalies

Vascular rings are significant anomalies because they cause airway compression and frequently require surgical correction. They are described in more detail elsewhere in this volume, but the common types seen in children will be described briefly here. In infancy, a double aortic arch is likely to cause severe respiratory distress and can even be fatal. The affected baby has stridor and wheezing. Contrast-enhanced CT or MR reveal a larger right aortic arch that extends posterior to the trachea and a smaller, anterior left-sided arch. Both arches commonly give rise to their corresponding subclavian and carotid vessels (Fig. 21). The trachea is variably compressed. MR graphically depicts the anatomy in multiplanar projections (45). The second frequent type of ring that tends to present in slightly older children is a right aortic arch with an aortic diverticulum and an aberrant left subclavian artery. The ring is completed by a left ligamentum arteriosum that is not directly visualized by the imaging procedures. In either of these anomalies, the aorta may descend on either the right or the left side, although most commonly it crosses from the right to descend on the left. The carina, and in particular the left main bronchus, are frequently deviated anteriorly (Fig. 22). A right aortic arch with mirror image branching is seen in association with congenital heart disease, but is not a true vascular ring, nor is the commonly seen aberrant right subclavian artery with a left aortic arch. A diagnosis of vascular ring is frequently made on the basis of plain film findings and esophagram, but if further delineation of the anatomy is required by the cardiovascular surgeon, either MR or UFCT provides noninvasive evaluation of the anomaly. An enlarged aorta in

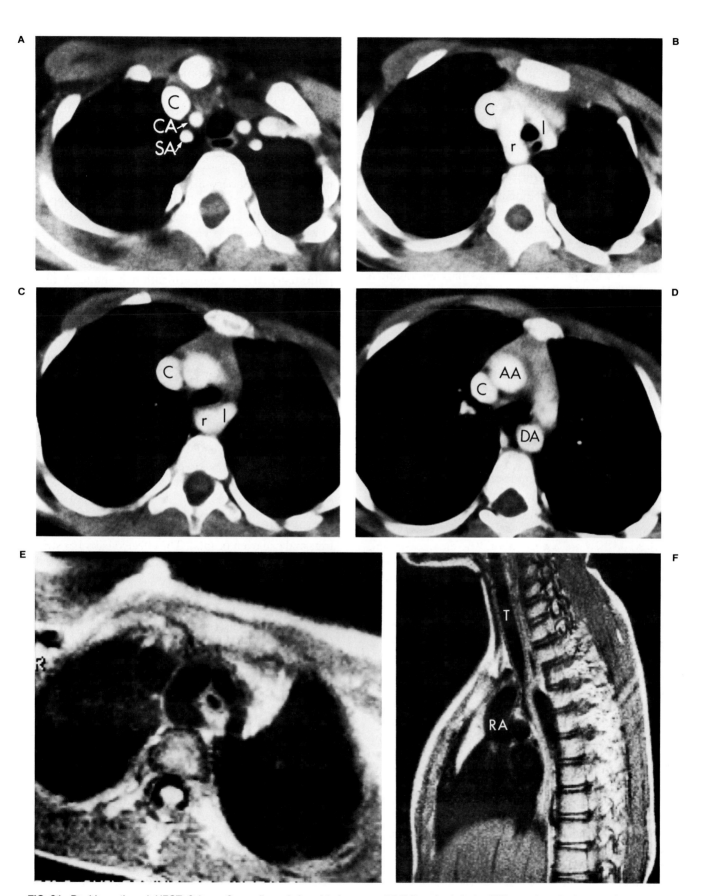

FIG. 21. Double aortic arch UFCT, 0.1 sec, 3 mm slices. **A:** Level 1 shows carotid (CA) and subclavian (SA) vessels on both sides of the trachea. **B:** Level 2, 6 mm inferior, shows a larger right aortic arch (r) and a smaller left aortic arch (l) giving rise to the great vessels. **C:** Level 3 shows the right aortic arch (r) crossing to the left of the midline and joining with the descending left aortic arch (l). Note that the trachea is not severely compressed at this level. **D:** Level 4 at the level of the aortic pulmonary window. The descending aorta (DA) is now to the left of the midline and the carina is displaced anteriorly. **E:** Transaxial gated MR image corresponds to level 2 of the CT scan. **F:** Sagittal MR image through the level of the right aortic arch reveals tracheal (T) compression. AA, ascending aorta; C, superior vena cava; RA, right aorta.

A
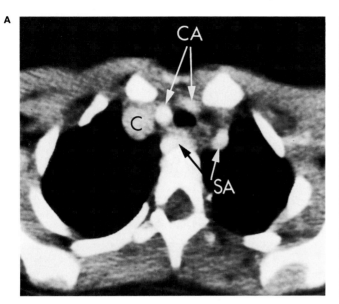
B
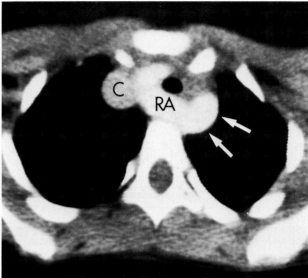

FIG. 22. Right aortic arch with an aortic diverticulum gives rise to the left subclavian artery. **A:** UFCT examination, level 1, reveals carotid (CA) and subclavian vessels (SA) on both sides of the trachea. C, superior vena cava. **B:** Level 2 shows a right aortic arch (RA) with a diverticulum giving rise to the left subclavian artery (*arrows*).

children with congenital heart disease can cause airway compression even in the absence of a vascular ring.

Coarctation of the Aorta

Coarctation of the aorta varies in severity from a mild indentation to a complete constriction. In the infant form, the periductal aortic isthmus and the transverse portion of the arch may be hypoplastic. The most common type is a short segment of membranous stenosis between the left subclavian artery and the ductus arteriosis. CT can delineate the narrowed segment of the artery as well as the poststenotic dilatation and collateral

A
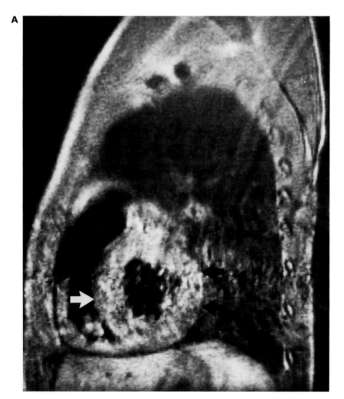
B
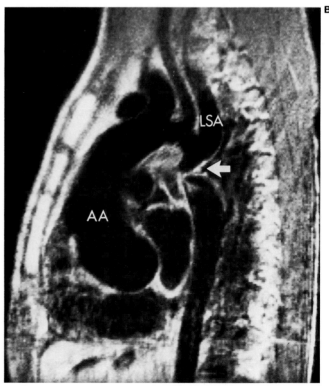

FIG. 23. Coarctation of the aorta and left ventricular hypertrophy in a 12-year-old boy. **A:** Left parasagittal gated image reveals marked left ventricular hypertrophy (*arrows*). Despite the use of cardiac gating, some cardiac and respiratory artifacts are still noted. **B:** Oblique parasagittal section reveals typical short segment coarctation just distal to the left subclavian artery that is dilated. AA, ascending aorta; LSA, left subclavian artery; *arrow,* coarctation.

arterial flow. The lesion is better evaluated with MR because of the availability of sagittal projections (Fig. 23). MR has the added advantage of assessing left ventricular hypertrophy and can be used in follow-up evaluation of previous coarctectomy. Both MR and CT are limited in their ability to define the presence of other anomalies such as bicuspid aortic valve.

Aneurysms of the thoracic aorta are rare in children. They may be seen following trauma, and septic aneurysms may develop in the neonate following umbilical arterial catheterization. In the older child, aneurysms are seen in patients with Marfan's syndrome, Ehlers-Danlos syndrome, cystinosis, polyarteritis nodosa, and Takayasu's arteritis. Aneurysms can be delineated with either CT or MR using the same diagnostic criteria as utilized in adults.

Mediastinal Calcification

Calcifications in the mediastinum are infrequent and usually are detected only by CT examination with which small linear or curvilinear calcification is seen in the ductus (ligamentum) arteriosum in ~5–10% of children (Fig. 24). Calcification, usually speck-like or rounded, occurs in mediastinal nodes in granulomatous infections. Mediastinal neoplasms that may contain calcifications include germ cell tumors, teratoma, neuroblastomas, ganglioneuroblastomas, and ganglioneuromas. Calcifications are very rare in untreated lymphoma, but may develop following radiation therapy.

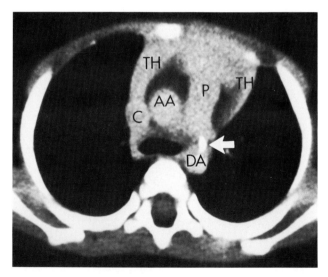

FIG. 24. Non-contrast enhanced UFCT, 0.1 sec. Calcification in the ligamentum arteriosum. UFCT examination in a 2-year-old infant reveals curvilinear calcification at the level of the aortic pulmonary window. AA, ascending aorta; C, superior vena cava; DA, descending aorta; P, pulmonary artery; TH, thymus; arrow, calcification. (Compare with Fig. 3A.)

TABLE 5. *CT characteristics of posterior mediastinal masses*

Solid
  Neurofibroma
  Ganglioneuroma
  Neuroblastoma (primary or metastatic)
  Lymphoma
  Ectopic thymus
  Chest wall tumor
  Paraspinal abscess/diskitis
  Hamartoma, mesenchymoma
  Extramedullary hematopoiesis
  Germ cell tumor
Cystic
  Neuroenteric cyst
  Gastroenteric cyst
  Meningocele
Vascular
  Descending aorta aneurysm
  Dilated azygos vein
Fatty
  Lipoblastoma
  Teratoma
Calcified
  Neuroblastoma (primary)
  Ganglioneuroma
Miscellaneous
  Bochdalek hernia

Posterior Mediastinal Masses

Posterior mediastinal masses that occur in children are listed in Table 5. Masses in the posterior mediastinum account for ~35–40% of all pediatric mediastinal masses, and neurogenic masses constitute ~95% of all posterior mediastinal masses (46).

Neoplasms of neural origin are divided into three groups: (a) those arising from sympathetic ganglia—neuroblastoma, ganglioneuroblastoma, and ganglioneuroma; (b) those arising from peripheral nerves—neurofibromas and neurolemmomas; and (c) those arising from paraganglion cells; these are rarely seen in children and will not be discussed here.

Neurogenic Tumors of Sympathetic Nervous System Origin

Included in this group are neuroblastoma, ganglioneuroblastoma, and ganglioneuroma. Approximately 15% of all neuroblastomas are of mediastinal origin; these nearly always are in the posterior mediastinum. Forty percent of neuroblastomas are in children younger than 2 years old, and most of the rest occur in preschool age children. A posterior mediastinal mass found in this age group should be considered a neuroblastoma until proven otherwise. Ganglioneuroblastoma and ganglioneuroma are most commonly found in somewhat older children. The ganglioneuroma is a benign tumor that may represent a maturing neuroblastoma. Although many neurogenic tumors are discovered incidentally, the neuroblastoma may present with a wide variety of signs and symptoms including fever, malaise, pain, anemia, and other nonspecific findings. Horner syndrome may be present in apical lesions, and extremity weakness may be present in lesions with intraspinal extension. A few children present with a bizarre neurologic syndrome (dancing eyes, dancing feet), the opsoclonus cerebellar ataxia syndrome.

On CT, neuroblastomas are soft-tissue masses, ~40% of which may contain speckled or curvilinear calcification. The masses show variable, usually inhomogeneous enhancement following contrast medium injection.

They are located in the paravertebral region where they may extend superiorly and inferiorly for several centimeters. Extradural extension is frequent, even in the absence of neurologic signs and symptoms; one of the important aims of the imaging procedure is to diagnose or exclude such spread (46,47). In the past, this has been achieved by the use of CT metrizamide myelography. Our experience has been that a high-quality, bolus i.v. CECT provides equivalent information, as the dural spread of tumor nearly always enhances (Fig. 25). Even though MR fails to demonstrate the calcification often associated with neuroblastoma, it is likely that MR will become the modality of choice for staging because of the

A

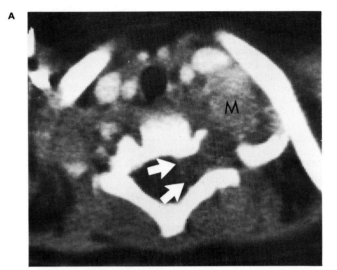

B

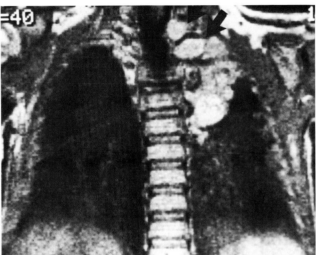

C

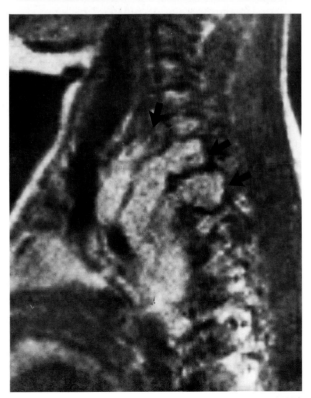

FIG. 25. Posterior mediastinal and cervical neuroblastoma in an 8-month-old child. **A:** Intravenous contrast-enhanced CT section reveals a cervical mass (M) with intraspinal extension (*arrows*). Widening of the neural foramina is noted and contrast enhanced tumor is clearly seen. Coronal (**B**) and sagittal (**C**) MR images in the same patient. Intraspinal extension of tumor along the nerve roots is seen at three levels (*arrows*).

accuracy with which this modality demonstrates intraspinal spread of tumor. In sagittal and coronal views, tumor spread along nerves can be seen extending into neural foramina (Fig. 25). On T2-weighted images, the tumor has bright signal because of a prolonged T2. MR has the additional benefits of separating tumor from other surrounding soft tissues more readily than CT, as well as being more accurate in the recognition of bone marrow involvement, which is seen as areas of shortened T1.

Though intraspinal spread and marrow involvement are more frequent, neuroblastoma can also extend directly into the mediastinum and even into the hilar vessels. Either CT or MR can document this extension. Neuroblastoma may extend from a primary site in the abdomen into the thorax. Most commonly, this occurs by direct invasion through the retrocrural space and into the lower paravertebral regions, often bilaterally. Metastatic spread to lung parenchyma or pleura tends to be a late complication; the metastases can, on occasion, be large enough to be recognized on CT but frequently are microscopic.

Ganglioneuroblastomas are regarded as malignant neuroblastomas that have partially matured. Their imaging characteristics are indistinguishable from neuroblastoma. Ganglioneuromas are benign tumors that may be the end result of the maturation process. They present either as a large, smooth spherical mass or as a small, elongated sausage-shaped mass. Some of the large ones are of low, homogenous density and show little, if any, contrast enhancement; neuroblastoma tends to appear more inhomogenous following contrast enhancement, but these masses cannot be reliably distinguished from one another by CT. Experience with MR is limited, but it seems unlikely that there will be enough difference in signal characteristics to allow confident differentiation of a benign from a malignant mass.

Neurogenic Tumors of Peripheral Nervous System Origin: Neurofibromas

Neurofibromas occur predominantly in patients with systemic neurofibromatosis rather than as isolated lesions. These tumors arise most often in the superior and posterior mediastinum; they are more often bilateral than other neurogenic lesions. In addition to revealing the mass, a chest radiograph is often diagnostic because of the presence of other stigmata of neurofibromatosis such as scoliosis or typical rib deformities. On CT, the masses are smooth and typically homogeneous, of slightly lower density than muscle (48). Little contrast enhancement is usually present. In addition to dumbbell extension, extension into the neck has been present in several of our cases and airway compression has occurred. Involvement of the middle mediastinum sug-

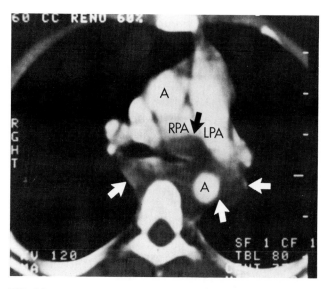

FIG. 26. Middle and posterior mediastinal neurofibromatosis in a 12-year-old male with prominent hilar shadows noted on chest radiography; family history of neurofibromatosis. Contrast-enhanced CT scan reveals a low-density infiltrative mass (*arrows*) in the middle and posterior mediastinum surrounding the aorta (A) and left pulmonary artery (LPA). RPA, right pulmonary artery.

gesting lymphoma has been seen (Fig. 26). It has been suggested that detection of an area of low density in the mass may indicate fibrosarcomatous degeneration, but fat in the tumor may cause an identical appearance on CT, although it should be possible to make the distinction on MR examination.

Other Posterior Mediastinal Lesions

Cystic duplications, either of enteric or foregut origin, are the second most common type of posterior mediastinal mass. Neurenteric cysts contain both neural and gastrointestinal elements. The cyst is connected by a stalk to the meninges and is associated with a vertebral anomaly as part of the so-called split notochord syndrome. Vertebral anomalies include hemivertebrae, fusion anomalies, and spina bifida (49).

A gastroenteric foregut cyst, or an intramural esophageal duplication cyst, can present as either a middle or posterior mediastinal mass that varies in size but can be quite large. The cyst is lined by gastrointestinal mucosa, is round or oval, and of homogeneous density. It often indents the esophagus but rarely communicates with it. Technetium pertechnetate scanning can demonstrate gastric mucosa in the cyst, aiding in preoperative diagnosis. The lesions are cystic and avascular on CT; MR shows a prolonged T2 relaxation time and clearly separates the mass from the aorta (Fig. 27).

Lymphangiomas can occur in the posterior mediastinum, although they are more commonly found anteriorly. Their avascular nature and extent can be nicely

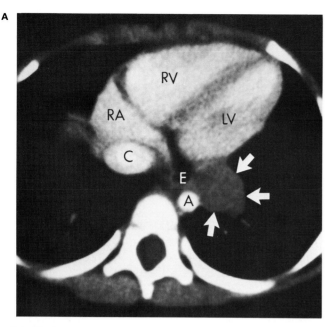

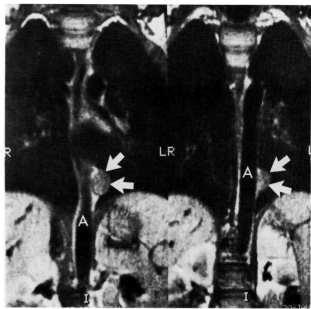

FIG. 27. Esophageal duplication cyst. **A:** UFCT in a 2-year-old female reveals an avascular mass anterolateral to the descending aorta closely related to the esophagus (E). A, aorta; C, superior vena cava; LV, left ventricle; RA, right atrium; RV, right ventricle. **B:** Different patient. Esophageal duplication cyst in a 6-year-old male. Coronal T1-weighted MR images reveal an oval mass (*arrows*) with intermediate signal intensity separated from the aorta (A) by fat plane. On T2-weighted images (not shown) the signal intensity of the mass increased.

demonstrated on contrast-enhanced CT. These lesions may extend across the midline (Fig. 28).

Lymphoma, metastatic neuroblastoma, and, rarely, other metastatic malignancy can involve the posterior mediastinal and retrocrural nodes. These lesions present with paraspinal widening, suggesting disease both above and below the diaphragm.

Siegel et al. (50) described two cases of posterior mediastinal mass due to inflammatory lymphadenopathy secondary to severe esophagitis and gastroesophageal reflux. Probably more common is an inflammatory

mass due to diskitis or spondylitis. The mass is often relatively small and may be associated with disk space narrowing and vertebral body destruction, which is well demonstrated by either CT or MR. Spondylitis with a paravertebral mass from tuberculosis is now rarely seen in children in the United States.

Vascular lesions can present as posterior mediastinal masses. These occur less commonly in children than in adults, but aortic aneurysms of either mycotic or connective tissue origin can be seen (51). Dilatation of the azygos and hemiazygos veins serving as collateral channels can be seen if the inferior vena cava is congenitally absent or obstructed.

Posteriorly situated pneumonias can simulate mediastinal masses. The clinical picture or follow-up radiographs usually establish the diagnosis. A sequestration of the lung may appear on chest radiography to arise in the mediastinum. CT is helpful in these cases.

Chest wall masses may be due to benign or malignant tumors as well as to inflammatory lesions. They may simulate mediastinal lesions if they arise either anteriorly or posteriorly; when they are more lateral, an intrapulmonary process may be mimicked. Lipomas, lipoblastomas, and benign or malignant mesenchymal tumors occur. Ewing sarcoma and rhabdosarcoma are the malignant lesions that occur most frequently. Actinomycosis may extend to the chest wall from a pulmonary lesion, and primary osteomyelitis of the rib can also be seen. Plain film findings are usually limited to visualization of the mass itself; bone destruction may be noted in either the malignant or inflammatory lesions. Fatty

FIG. 28. Posterior mediastinal lymphangioma in a 7-year-old male. The mass (*arrows*) is well circumscribed, of relatively homogeneous low intensity, envelops the aorta (a) and crosses the midline. Biopsy revealed a cystic lymphangioma that could not be completely removed surgically.

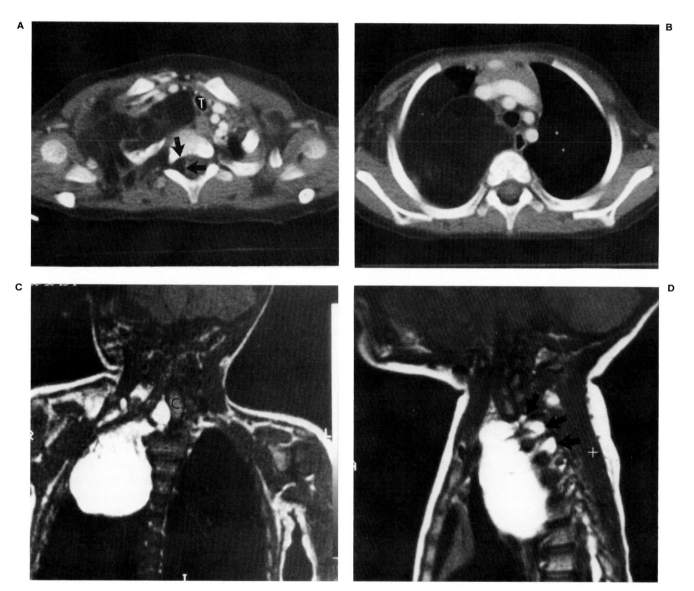

FIG. 29. Lipoblastoma in an 18-year-old male who presented with a right cervical mass and mediastinal mass on chest roentgenogram. **A:** UFCT at the level of the thoracic inlet reveals a low density multi-septated mass that is infiltrating the soft tissues of the neck and displacing the trachea (T). Intraspinal extension (*arrows*) is also noted. **B:** Lower section through the upper thorax reveals a huge multi-septated mass of fat density infiltrating the mediastinum. No intraspinal extension is present at this level. **C:** T1-weighted 2.5-mm coronal MR image reveals intraspinal extension with slight displacement of the cord (C). **D:** T1-weighted sagittal image to the right of the midline reveals intraspinal extension at three levels (*arrows*). Note the pattern of extension along the nerve roots similar to that seen in the patient with neuroblastoma (Fig. 26).

A

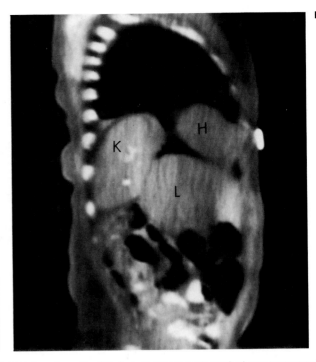

B

FIG. 30. Ectopic thoracic kidney herniating through the Foramen of Bochdalek in a 4-month-old infant. **A:** Chest radiograph shows an unusual density at the left lung base initially misinterpreted as pneumonia. **B:** Direct sagittal CT image following intravenous contrast enhancement reveals the left kidney to be intrathoracic. H, heart; K, kidney; L, liver.

tumors may be recognized on CT by their low density, and on MR by their short T1, but the other lesions cannot be distinguished from one another, although cross-sectional imaging is of value in determining location and extent of disease (Fig. 29).

Extramedullary hematopoiesis should be considered a possible cause for a mediastinal mass in any patient with severe anemia. The characteristic radiographic findings are multiple smooth or lobulated paravertebral masses (52).

Meningoceles are rare mediastinal masses due to spinal canal anomalies in which the leptomeninges herniate through the neural foramina. These lesions occur mostly in patients with neurofibromatosis, usually in conjunction with kyphoscoliosis, with the meningocele at the convex apex of the curve. MR is probably the diagnostic method of choice.

Organs extending through the diaphragm in a posterior Bochdalek hernia, such as ectopic kidney (53), liver, or spleen, may simulate mediastinal masses or pulmonary lesions (Fig. 30). A large hiatal hernia may project either as a middle or posterior mediastinal mass.

HEART AND PERICARDIUM

The availability of MR and UFCT has made intracardiac anatomy and pathology easily visible. Despite this, echocardiography and angiography remain the pri-

mary diagnostic methods for diagnostic evaluation of congenital heart disease, which will not be considered in this section because of space constraints.

Cardiac masses are relatively rare in infancy and childhood. They may be intracardiac or arise from the pericardium and be primary or metastatic in origin (54).

The most common intracardiac tumor of infancy and childhood is the rhabdomyoma, which accounts for ~45% of cardiac neoplasms in children. This may be a true hamartoma and is found most frequently in children with tuberous sclerosis. The mass tends to be relatively small (<1 cm) and presents as a circumscribed mass projecting through the epicardium. Cardiac fibroma is probably the next most frequent tumor. Fifty percent of these are discovered before 1 year of age. They may arise from the intraventricular septum or the free wall of either ventricle and tend to be a single larger mass.

Pericardiac tumors constitute ~20% of cardiac tumors. The most common, the intrapericardiac teratoma, is usually diagnosed in the first year of life, often in infancy. The patient presents with cardiomegaly and massive pericardial effusion. Surgery reveals a septated multicystic mass attached by a broad pedicle to the aorta. The mass usually presents on the right side of the heart (Fig. 31) (55).

Metastatic disease can affect either the pericardium or the heart itself. The most common lesions are non-

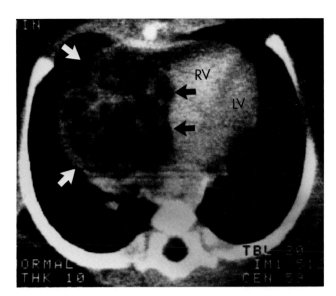

FIG. 31. Intrapericardiac teratoma in a 20-day-old female. Contrast-enhanced CT scan performed following pericardiocentesis for massive pericardial effusion reveals a multi-cystic septated mass which is intrapericardiac. At surgery, a teratoma was removed. LV, left ventricle; RV, right ventricle; *arrows*, teratoma.

Hodgkin's lymphoma, neuroblastoma, and osteosarcoma. Wilms' tumor and, occasionally, adrenal carcinoma may extend directly through the inferior vena cava into the right atrium.

Pericardial effusion is relatively uncommon in childhood. It is usually diagnosed by ultrasonography but can be recognized either by MR or UFCT. The density and signal characteristics of the fluid vary with its etiology—transudate, exudate, or hemorrhage. Smaller effusions are visible first posterior and lateral to the left ventricle; as the fluid collection becomes larger, it extends ventrally in front of the right ventricle and right atrium until it eventually encircles the heart in an asymmetric fashion, and the heart appears to be floating in a bath of fluid. Fluid may be seen as high as the level of the aortic arch.

Congenital defects affecting the pericardium include total absence, left-sided absence, and partial absence on the left side (56). Total agenesis of the pericardium is least common. Partial agenesis of the pericardium can occur in association with absence of the septum transversum of the diaphragm. There is an anterior-median diaphragmatic defect, and the liver and heart are contained in a common cavity. Cardiomegaly, a mediastinal mass, or pericardial effusion may be simulated. With left-sided absence of the pericardium, CT or MR reveals that the left pericardium is not visualized, there is a change in axis of the heart and great vessels, and the heart extends freely to the left lateral chest wall in decubitus position. Cardiac levoposition and direct contact of the lung with the great vessels are other findings.

Pericardial cysts may be either acquired or congenital but seem more common in adults than in children. These appear as smooth, thin-walled, round or oval, water-density masses usually in the cardiophrenic angle.

MAJOR AIRWAYS

Trachea

Radiographic evaluation of pediatric airway abnormalities begins with chest radiography and high Kv films of the tracheobronchial tree (57). Chest fluoroscopy with a barium esophagram is frequently employed as the next diagnostic step. CT and MR are usually reserved for problem cases.

How one evaluates the trachea with CT varies with the pathology suspected and the equipment available. In general, one should employ contiguous slices; if sagittal or coronal reconstruction is to be performed, overlapping, thinner slices provide somewhat better images but at a cost of higher radiation exposure. Although not yet widely available, UFCT promises to be a valuable technique for evaluation of the pediatric airway, because in addition to producing high quality conventional CT images in scan times of 0.1 sec, UFCT is capable of recording dynamic alterations in airway morphology. It is possible using the electron beam technology of this scanner to obtain a single slice in 50 msec or eight 0.8-cm thick slices in 0.224 sec. Moreover, by obtaining multiple images at up to 10 different levels, it is possible to obtain a cine-CT study of the entire trachea in small infants and children (58–61).

Preliminary work has suggested that MR may be of value in the assessment of airway abnormalities in children (62). MR clearly reveals the signal void of the trachea in three imaging planes as well as revealing surrounding vessels or mass lesions. The use of cardiac-gated pulse sequences provides images with less artifacts. Partial volume averaging is a problem in smaller children, especially when using the sagittal or coronal views, as the thinnest slice generally available is 5 mm.

Although normal standards for the size and shape of the airway in infants and young children are not yet available, it is apparent from UFCT studies that the trachea is round and of normally relatively uniform caliber from the thoracic inlet to the carina. It may appear elongated at the thoracic inlet because it angles from anterior to posterior and the plane of the axial section may not be perpendicular to the long axis of the trachea. UFCT shows that the normal trachea changes very little in size or shape during quiet breathing (61,63). Griscom (64) and Effman et al. (65) have reported normal values for tracheal cross-sectional areas in children that appear to correlate with increases in body height. Our experience has suggested that tracheal narrowing is usually quite obvious either in relation to the subglottic area or in comparison to another, unaffected area of the trachea. It has been suggested that a decrease in cross-sectional area of about one-third is necessary before the airway is compromised.

Congenital Anomalies

Tracheoesophageal fistula, the most common anomaly of tracheal development, is not usually studied by CT. The fistula is better demonstrated by an esophagram, and the upper level of the blind tracheal pouch is well seen by plain films when filled by either air or barium. Children with tracheoesophageal fistula commonly

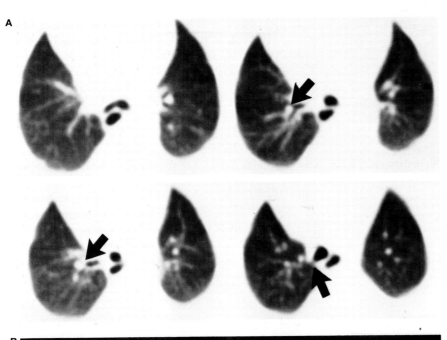

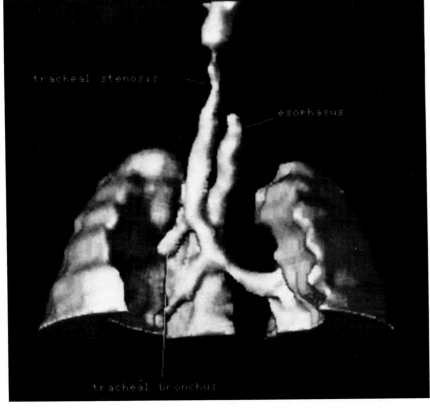

FIG. 32. Tracheal bronchus and tracheal stenosis in a neonate. **A:** Serial 3-mm UFCT images from a neonate with congenital stridor reveal the right upper lobe bronchus to be ectopic and originate from the posterior lateral wall of the trachea cephalad to the carina. *Arrow,* tracheal bronchus. **B:** Same patient, three-dimensional reconstruction of the airway, esophagus, and lungs dramatically reveals the tracheal stenosis as well as the ectopic tracheal bronchus.

have tracheomalacia, which becomes symptomatic following surgical repair of the primary lesion, and UFCT evaluation may be useful to demonstrate this lesion.

Tracheal bronchus occurs predominantly on the right side; it may be due to duplication of the right upper lobe bronchus but more commonly is due to an ectopic or displaced right upper lobe bronchus. It may be demonstrated by CT even in infants if contiguous thin sections are employed. It is often associated with tracheal stenosis (Fig. 32) (66).

Tracheobronchomegaly

Tracheobronchomegaly (Mounier-Riley syndrome) is rarely seen in childhood. Acquired tracheal enlargement occurs in cases of bronchopulmonary dysplasia due to respiratory therapy and is also seen commonly in longstanding cases of cystic fibrosis.

Tracheomalacia is a condition in which there is abnormal collapse of the trachea due to weakness of the tracheal wall. Increased intrathoracic pressure, such as occurs with asthma or bronchiolitis, commonly causes some decrease in the caliber of the trachea during expiration. This does not represent true "tracheomalacia." Although tracheomalacia may be a primary entity, usually it is secondary to other conditions (67). Tra-

cheomalacia most commonly is seen following prolonged intubation or in children who have esophageal atresia with or without associated tracheoesophageal fistula. UFCT is the diagnostic method of choice for demonstration of tracheomalacia, which is considered to be present if there is tracheal collapse of >50% on expiration. The segment of collapse is usually focal (Fig. 33). For accurate diagnosis, dynamic study is necessary because tracheal caliber may be normal on static studies. Focal tracheal collapse is usually caused by an abnormality in the tracheal wall or by extrinsic pressure from adjacent vessels or masses. The offending vessel or mass is well demonstrated by either CT or MR. The subject of innominate artery compression of the upper trachea as a cause of symptoms of cough, stridor, dyspnea, and apnea remains a controversial one. Many asymptomatic children have an area of tracheal narrowing at the thoracic inlet, and it is difficult to be certain if innominate artery compression of the trachea may be responsible for the narrowing and/or the symptoms. The relationship of the artery to the trachea can be well established by CT or MR. A recent study by Fletcher and Cohn (62) using MR showed that the innominate artery was anterior and to the left of the trachea both in symptomatic and asymptomatic patients, and there was no evidence of mediastinal crowding. They felt that the tracheal narrowing seen was not due to an anomalous position of the

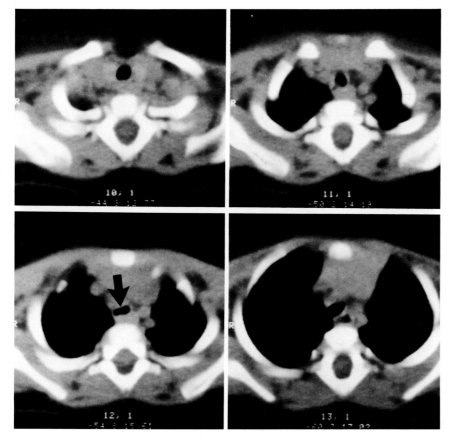

FIG. 33. Two-month-old with stridor and endoscopic diagnosis of tracheomalacia. Serial UFCT images, 0.5 sec, reveal focal tracheal narrowing (*arrow*). A change in diameter of >50% was noted on serial images at the same level.

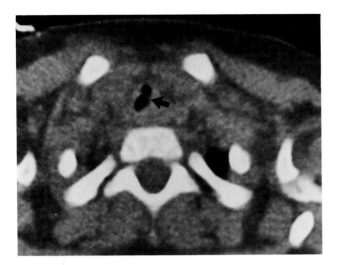

FIG. 34. Tracheal stenosis UFCT image, 0.1 sec. An area of 3-mm tracheal stenosis is noted (*arrow*). A small band interpreted as a tracheal web is present. At endoscopy, stenosis but no web was found. It is not known with certainty if the apparent web was ruptured at endoscopy or if it may have been a mucous strand.

innominate artery but that the narrowing was probably due to an intrinsic deficiency of tracheal cartilage.

Tracheal stenosis is defined as a fixed area of tracheal narrowing. This, too, is probably best evaluated by UFCT. UFCT can determine the exact cross-sectional caliber of the trachea and determine the degree of change, if any, that occurs with respiration. We prefer to do 0.1-sec, high-resolution scans in addition to the dynamic study to obtain optimal anatomic detail (Fig. 34).

Conventional CT has been used in the diagnosis of congenital tracheal stenosis that is associated with increased incidence of congenital thoracic and vascular anomalies. The stenosis is due to the presence of complete cartilaginous rings replacing the normally posterior membranous portion of the tracheal wall. Tracheal caliber is markedly reduced and is smaller in diameter than the immediate subglottic portion of the trachea. The trachea remains round in shape; often, a long length is affected.

The most common cause of tracheal stenosis in children today is chronic trauma to the tracheal wall from intubation. In these patients, CT is of value because it accurately demonstrates the cross-sectional area and the length of the affected segment. UFCT has the added advantage of determining the degree of fixation of the narrowed segment.

Intratracheal Lesions

Primary tracheal neoplasms are rare in children. They may present with symptoms suggestive of asthma. CT characteristics are identical to those in adults. Intratracheal thymus is a rare cause of tracheal obstruction that

may simulate subglottic hemangioma (68). Papillomatosis primarily affects the larynx, although the lesions may seed down the trachea and be detected as discrete intratracheal masses, although frequently they are too small to be reliably seen. The presence of a suspected tracheal foreign body can be confirmed or excluded by CT if thin, contiguous slices are performed.

Extrinsic masses causing tracheal obstruction are discussed in the mediastinal section; vascular rings, bronchogenic cysts, lymphoma, neurofibromas, and mediastinal abscesses are the usual causes. All are clearly demonstrated with either CT or MR.

Bronchi

Using thin (1.5–3 mm), contiguous slices, it is possible in children to reliably demonstrate all the major segmental bronchi. The anatomy is identical to that seen in adults and detailed elsewhere in this volume. Because of the speed of the examination, UFCT, if available, is the CT method of choice. MR can reliably demonstrate the main-stem bronchi but does not demonstrate the bronchi well distal to the hilar region, and even in the hilum there can be some confusion between the signal void of the bronchus and nearby vessels. There are two major reasons to do cross-sectional imaging of the bronchi in children: suspected partial or complete bronchial obstruction, and bronchiectasis. CT is presently preferred to MR, although MR has proven of value in some cases.

Bronchial obstruction can cause localized fluid retention in the neonate. This subject is discussed in this section under lobar and segmental opacities. Both in

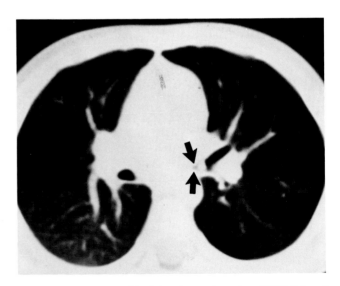

FIG. 35. Foreign body of the left mainstem bronchus. UFCT (0.1 sec) in an 18-month-old with equivocal plain film examination. A mass (*arrows*) is present within the left mainstem bronchus. Slight hyperinflation of the left lung is noted. Subsequently proven aspirated foreign body.

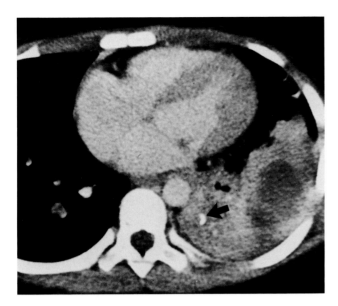

FIG. 36. Persistent left lower lobe atelectasis due to an aspirated chicken bone. UFCT examination reveals a high density curvilinear density within an atelectatic left lower lobe (*arrow*). Although nonspecific, in the pediatric age group the appearance of an otherwise unexplained calcific density either within the airways or associated with collapse should suggest the diagnosis of a possible aspirated foreign body.

neonates and in older children, bronchial obstruction can cause either focal air trapping, atelectasis, or pneumonia and bronchiectasis, depending on the completeness and severity of the obstruction.

Obstruction may be due to congenital bronchial atresia. The most commonly affected segment is the posterior apical branch of the left upper lobe. Absence of the bronchial segment can be suspected on good quality CT examination. In the older child, a bronchial mucocele and focal hyperinflation are additional findings.

Lymph nodes, either inflammatory or malignant, can

cause extrinsic bronchial obstruction as can other mediastinal masses. These are all well demonstrated by CT or MR. In more chronic cases, when atelectasis or pneumonia is present, CT can demonstrate whether the segmental or lobar bronchus is patent or occluded.

In *suspected foreign bodies,* inspiration/expiration frontal chest films are all that are usually required for diagnosis, although if findings are subtle or if the studies appear normal and the history is strong, we prefer UFCT as the next test as it is more sensitive and more specific than chest fluoroscopy in our experience. A recent study suggests plain film radiology alone is not sufficiently sensitive or specific for the diagnosis of foreign body aspiration. Using UFCT, it is nearly always possible to directly demonstrate the foreign body in a mainstem bronchus (Fig. 35); even with conventional CT, using contiguous slices, this is usually possible. Either technique will clearly demonstrate air trapping on the affected side, even when plain films are normal. Persistent or recurrent atelectasis should raise the possibility of a foreign body (Fig. 36). In a teenage child, although foreign bodies may occur, a bronchial adenoma should be considered as a possible cause of intrabronchial obstruction. This, too, can be directly visualized by CT and/or even with MR (Fig. 37).

The other major indication for cross-sectional imaging of the bronchi is for the evaluation of suspected bronchiectasis. A common indication for CT in our experience is a child with chronic or recurrent atelectasis in whom an endobronchial lesion or bronchiectasis is usually suspected. A normal CT scan probably obviates the need for bronchography, but bronchoscopy may still be indicated in many cases for diagnostic or therapeutic reasons.

As discussed in detail elsewhere in this volume, CT has been successfully used in adults for evaluation of bronchiectasis, and using similar diagnostic criteria in

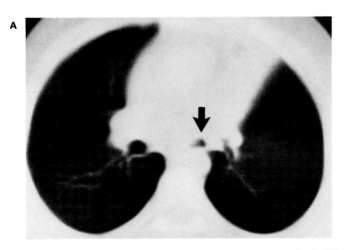

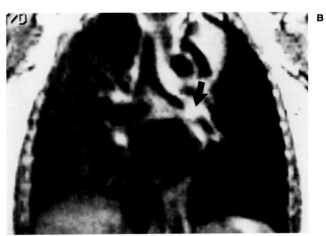

FIG. 37. Teenage girl with persistent left upper lobe atelectasis. **A:** CT scan reveals soft tissue (*arrow*) in the left mainstem bronchus. **B:** Coronal T1-weighted MR image reveals an area of increased signal intensity (*arrow*) in the left mainstem bronchus. Bronchial adenoma was partially removed at surgery.

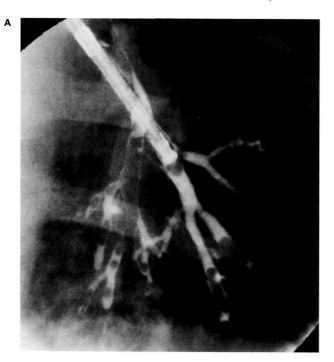
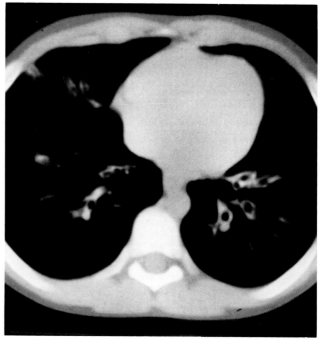

FIG. 38. Mild cylindric bronchiectasis in a 10-year-old child with asthma and recurrent atelectasis. **A:** Left lower lobe bronchogram reveals mild cylindric bronchiectasis. **B:** UFCT reveals left lower lobe bronchi larger than their corresponding pulmonary arterial branches. Note also the mild cylindric bronchiectasis in the right lower and right middle lobes.

children, Kuhn et al. (63) demonstrated sensitivity and specificity exceeding 90% in children. Cylindric bronchiectasis was diagnosed by the presence of bronchial wall thickening (bronchi visible where none usually are seen) and mild bronchial dilatation diagnosed by seeing a bronchus larger than its accompanying pulmonary artery or by direct demonstration of lack of tapering in a bronchus seen parallel to the axis of the slice (Fig. 38).

Varicose or saccular bronchiectasis is diagnosed most easily if the long axis of the bronchus is in the plane of the slice; a dilated, beaded appearance is seen, and this can be inferred in the transaxial plane as well (Fig. 39). Severe, cystic bronchiectasis, is rarely seen in children except in those patients with cystic fibrosis; its diagnosis on CT is usually obvious, as multiple air-, or air- and fluid-filled cysts are demonstrated.

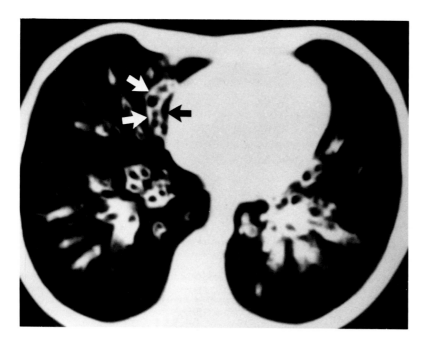

FIG. 39. Fifteen-year-old girl with chronic pulmonary disease of unknown etiology manifested by bronchiectasis. UFCT reveals bilateral cylindric and saccular bronchiectasis. Note the beaded appearance in the medial segment of the right middle lobe (*arrows*).

LUNG PARENCHYMAL ABNORMALITIES

If a plain radiograph is not diagnostic, CT is the method of choice for evaluation of many pediatric pulmonary parenchymal problems. Although there has been some interest in using MR for evaluation of lung parenchymal diseases (69), it currently is of limited usefulness because of the long examination times and its inferior spatial resolution as compared with CT.

The CT appearance of the child's lungs is not significantly different from the adult. The lungs are of low attenuation, ranging from −500 to −900 HU, depending on position and phase of respiration with the dependent portions of the lower lobes being normally the most opaque regions. Branching pulmonary vessels can be followed to the pleural surface even in young infants using UFCT. Fissures are only occasionally visible as fine lines, but their location is inferred from the presence of avascular areas. The anatomy of the bronchi and the hilar regions is discussed in detail elsewhere in this volume.

Indications for CT of the pediatric lung include evaluation of the unilaterally small lung, opaque hemithorax, pulmonary cysts and masses, pulmonary nodules, segmental and lobar densities, and some diffuse lung diseases.

Unilaterally Small Lung

The radiographic findings are those of volume loss on the affected side; the abnormal lung usually is more radiolucent and may or may not show evidence of normal ventilation. The history and age of the patient are helpful in differential diagnosis (70).

Pulmonary Hypoplasia and the Hypogenetic Lung Syndrome

In simple unilateral *pulmonary hypoplasia,* CECT or MR are valuable to study the pulmonary arterial supply to the affected lung; usually the vessel is small (Fig. 40), but if it is absent, this can be documented by the noninvasive modalities.

In the *hypogenetic lung syndrome* (pulmonary venolobar syndrome, scimitar syndrome), the right lung is nearly always the affected side. It is hypoplastic, and either its lower half or the entire lung is drained by an anomalous vein that typically inserts in the inferior vena cava, the portal vein, or a hepatic vein. Arterial supply to the hypoplastic lung is usually from a small pulmonary artery, but systemic arterial supply may be present as well. Anomalies of bronchial branching are frequent. Radiographs typically show dextroposition of the heart, a small right lung, and the scimitar sign of the abnormal vein extending inferiorly. There is usually a prominent retrosternal soft tissue density noted on the lateral radiograph, which has been thought to be due to "loose areolar connective tissue." However, CT has shown in several cases that the density is due to mediastinal shift secondary to the loss of normal pulmonary volume. CT is valuable for demonstration of hypoplasia of the pulmonary artery (71), anomalies of pulmonary venous return (72), and bronchial abnormalities. Less common related disorders include horseshoe lung and the accessory diaphragm syndrome. The latter probably requires surgery for definitive diagnosis; horseshoe lung is diagnosed on CT by seeing retrocardiac lung without a dividing pleural surface.

Pulmonary hypoplasia may be acquired following radiation therapy, ligation of the pulmonary artery, and

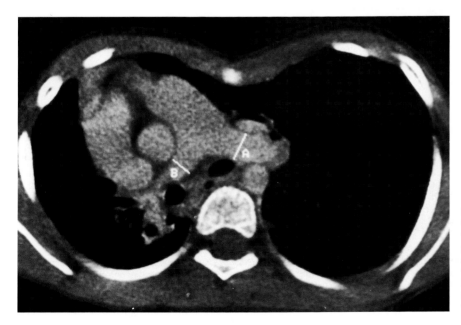

FIG. 40. Pulmonary hypoplasia secondary to congenital diaphragmatic hernia in an 8-year-old female. Contrast-enhanced UFCT reveals a hypoplastic right lung with marked shift of the heart and mediastinum from left to right. The right pulmonary artery (cursor labelled "B") is smaller than the left (cursor labelled "A") measuring 9 mm as compared to 12 mm.

infection. The Swyer-James-Macleod (SJM) syndrome is a form of pulmonary hypoplasia that is probably caused by a postinflammatory obliterative bronchiolitis. The SJM syndrome is distinguished from other causes of pulmonary hypoplasia by the presence of expiratory air-trapping. The bronchogram shows a failure of distal filling (pruned tree appearance), and the CT scan will show cylindric bronchiectasis, a paucity of vessels and an abnormally radiolucent lung or segment of lung (72a).

Opaque Hemithorax

Opaque hemithorax is initially assessed by the history, physical examination, and plain film findings. If there is loss of volume, the likely diagnoses are absence of the lung, either congenital or postsurgical, or massive total atelectasis. CT is useful in problem cases to assess the bronchial tree and to exclude an intrabronchial lesion or a mass causing extrinsic bronchial obstruction. More common is an opaque hemithorax with shift away from the abnormal side. In this situation, usually there is a pleural effusion or empyema secondary to pneumonia, but occasionally the effusion is of malignant origin. Rarely, there may be a malignant mass filling the thorax without associated fluid. Lymphoma can be responsible, although often there is obvious adenopathy in the opposite thorax; undifferentiated sarcomas and huge metastases rarely can produce these findings. Contrast-enhanced CT is usually necessary in evaluation of the opaque thorax to distinguish pleural, parenchymal, and, if present, neoplastic components. Fluid or fibrinous pleural collections fail to enhance; consolidated and at-

electatic lung markedly enhance (Fig. 41); (73,74) and neoplasms typically show variable, inhomogenous enhancement.

Air- and Fluid-Filled Cysts and Masses

Air- and fluid-filled cysts and masses represent the largest and most complex group of pulmonary parenchymal abnormalities that are evaluated by CT and MR. These lesions may be of congenital, inflammatory, neoplastic, or traumatic origin.

Congenital Anomalies of the Lungs

It has been postulated that congenital pulmonary anomalies are part of a developmental continuum known as the "sequestration spectrum." At one end is normal lung tissue supplied by abnormal vessels (arteriovenous malformation) and at the other end abnormal lung supplied by normal vessels (lobar emphysema, bronchial atresia). Considerable overlap exists from one group of anomalies to the next, and exact categorization of a single case may often be difficult (75). Congenital lesions may be seen at birth but can be discovered either incidentally or because of associated infection in the older child. Many times, the anomalous portion of lung is cystic or multicystic, and differentiation from a post-inflammatory pneumatocele may be difficult or impossible. If entirely fluid-filled, the cyst may appear to be a mass. CT and MR are useful in the delineation of some anomalies. The goals of the imaging investigation are to assess the parenchymal component, determine the pres-

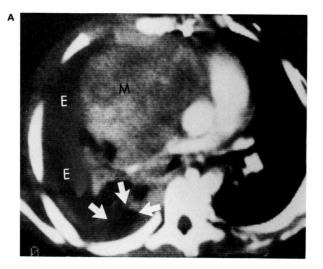
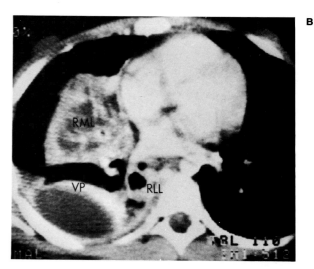

FIG. 41. **A:** Opaque thorax due to tumor, effusion, and atelectasis in a 7-year-old male treated for pneumonia for four days. Contrast enhanced CT scan reveals a large mediastinal mass (M) showing irregular enhancement, a homogeneously low-density effusion (E) and collapsed right lower lobe (*arrows*). **B:** Opaque lower right thorax in a 12-year-old male. Contrast-enhanced CT reveals an aerated right upper lobe, atelectatic right lower lobe (RLL), and loculated pleural fluid with thickened visceral pleura (VP) consistent with an empyema. The right middle lobe (RML) is of increased volume showing peripheral enhancement in a relatively low-density center. The infection was treated medically, and the patient recovered without incident.

ence or absence of normal bronchial supply, and, when possible, determine arterial supply and venous drainage.

Bronchogenic cysts probably result from defective growth of the lung bud and may be either intrapulmonary or mediastinal. They are lined with respiratory epithelium and may be filled with clear or mucoid material or they may be air-filled (76). If the cyst is air-filled, CT reveals a unilocular cyst with a nonenhancing, thin wall, no apparent feeding bronchus, and normal vascular anatomy. If the cyst is entirely fluid-filled, it may, as with mediastinal bronchogenic cysts, have Hounsfield numbers greater than water values, but contrast enhancement will confirm its avascular, cystic nature. In the case of air- and fluid-filled cysts, CT may be of value in distinguishing bronchogenic cysts (usually unilocular) from congenital cystic adenomatoid malformation (CCAM) (usually multilocular). MR demonstrates fluid-filled cysts well, but is less helpful in evaluation of the air-filled ones as discrimination from adjacent pulmonary parenchyma is difficult.

CCAM is defined as a multicystic mass of pulmonary tissue in which there is a proliferation of bronchial structures at the expense of normal alveolar development. The bronchial structures are disorganized, but communication with the normal tracheobronchial tree may be present. Although there are three pathologic types, the only one usually compatible with life past the neonatal period is Type 1 in which multiple cysts of varying sizes are present (77). Some of the cysts are partially fluid-filled, and their walls are of variable thickness. The lesion occurs equally in both lungs, but there is a slight tendency for upper lobe predominance. The affected lobe is of increased volume. In the neonate,

CCAM may cause severe respiratory distress. The lesion may be cystic, fluid-filled, or mixed, and significant mediastinal shift may be present. Anasarca or pleural effusion are often present. In the older child, air-filled cysts tend to be more evident. CT clearly shows the morphology of the lesion and can demonstrate the lack of normal bronchial anatomy and should demonstrate any associated vascular abnormalities. CCAM is distinguished from bronchogenic cyst by the presence of a multicystic pattern (Fig. 42) (78); other entities in the differential diagnosis include lobar emphysema in which the lung is hyperexpanded but not multicystic, and lobar pulmonary interstitial emphysema (Fig. 43) (79), which typically shows no fluid levels and a normal bronchial supply. If CCAM occurs in the lower lobes, it may simulate sequestration of the lung. CCAM usually is larger, contains more cysts, and tends not to be supplied by a large vessel from the abdominal aorta. Nonetheless, in some cases, the correct diagnosis is not made until pathologic examination is performed.

Bronchopulmonary sequestration is a congenital mass of nonfunctioning pulmonary tissue that has no normal connection with the bronchial tree or the pulmonary artery. Its arterial supply is usually from the abdominal aorta, and its venous drainage may be via the pulmonary veins, the inferior vena cava, or the azygos system (80). Many authors consider intra- and extralobar forms of sequestration to be different entities. Intralobar sequestration is contiguous to normal lung parenchyma and lies within the pleural covering of the normal lung; extralobar sequestration has its own pleural covering. Table 6 summarizes the classical separation of intra- and extralobar sequestration.

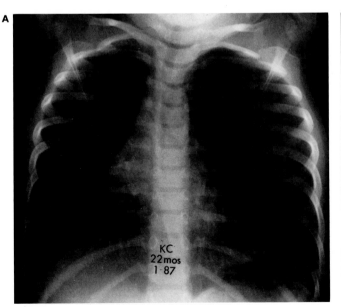
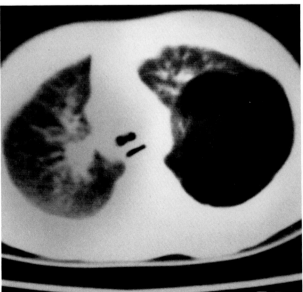

FIG. 42. Congenital cystic adenomatoid malformation in a 22-month-old girl. **A:** Chest radiograph shows a hyperlucent expanded left upper lobe with mediastinal shift. **B:** CT scan at the level of the carina reveals a somewhat lobulated multi-septated cystic mass actually arising in the left lower lobe.

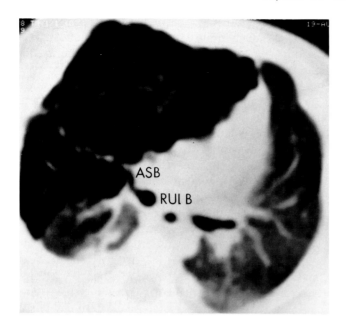

FIG. 43. Interstitial pulmonary emphysema of the right upper lobe in a 24-day-old infant. UFCT (0.1 sec), reveals hyperinflation of the right upper lobe. The lung has a somewhat irregular multi-cystic appearance due to stretching of the intrapulmonary vessels. Note that there is a patent segmental bronchus of the right upper lobe supplying the affected segment. The interstitial emphysema resolved spontaneously several days after this image was made. ASB, anterior segmental bronchus; RULB, right upper lobe bronchus.

Intralobar sequestration occurs in the left paravertebral gutter about two-thirds of the time, and in the corresponding location on the right side most of the rest of the time. Upper lobe involvement (81) and bilateral cases (Fig. 44) have been reported but are very rare. The radiographic appearance depends on the degree of aeration and the presence or absence of associated infection. The lesion may present as a water density mass and be mistaken for pneumonia, atelectasis, bronchogenic cyst, or neoplasm. Alternatively it may be an air-containing multicystic mass simulating CCAM.

CT (82) and MR are useful in noninvasive evaluation of sequestration. Lesions simulating sequestration such as chronic pneumonia or atelectasis can be diagnosed by the finding of an air bronchogram serving the affected segment. If sequestration is present, CT or MR more

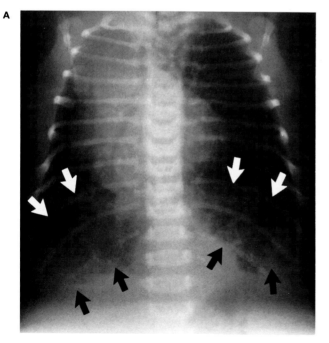
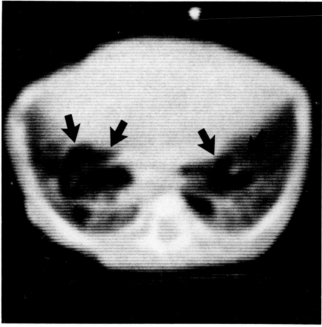

FIG. 44. Unusual bilateral intralobar sequestration in a neonate with respiratory distress. **A:** Chest radiograph reveals marked pulmonary hyperinflation and multicystic appearing parenchymal densities at both bases best visualized through the hemidiaphragms (*arrows*). **B:** Nonenhanced conventional CT scan reveals medial basilar cystic masses (*arrows*). Arteriography (not shown) revealed vessels arising from the abdominal aorta supplying both basilar masses. The pathologic diagnosis was intralobar sequestration.

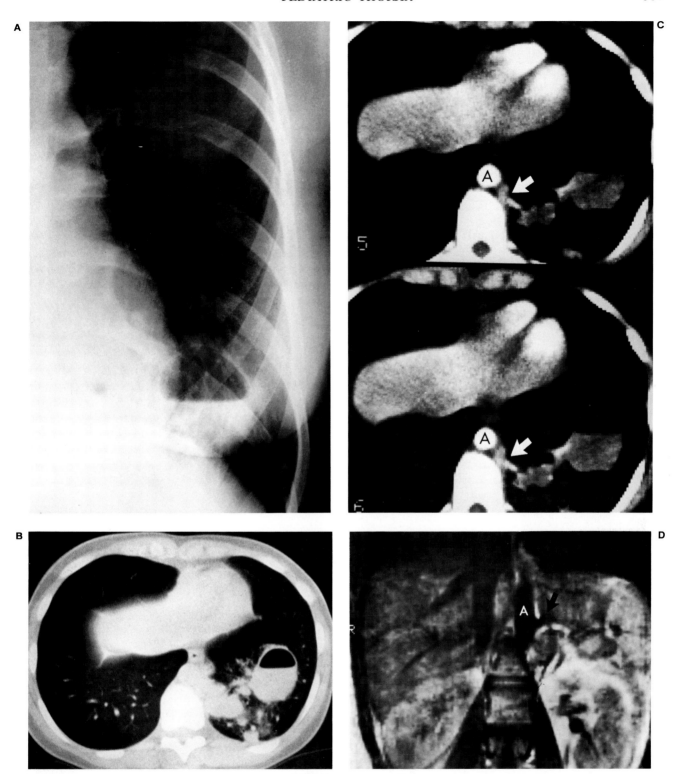

FIG. 45. Intralobar sequestration. **A:** Chest radiograph of a 12-year-old female reveals an air fluid level in a cystic cavity at the left lung base. **B:** UFCT (0.1 sec) reveals a cystic mass in the left lower lobe containing fluid. Surrounding irregular parenchymal density is noted extending toward the aorta. **C:** Two images from UFCT (0.05 sec) show a vessel (*arrow*) arising directly from the aorta (A) supplying the left lower lobe mass. With each systolic contraction, contrast could be seen entering the pulmonary malformation. **D:** Coronal MR image does not show the intrapulmonary pathology as clearly but nicely demonstrates the abnormal vessel (*arrow*) arising from the aorta (A) which was later confirmed by aortography.

clearly reveal the anatomy and its location than does plain film examination (Fig. 45). The abnormal systemic artery is dramatically shown in coronal MR;

UFCT with bolus enhancement is capable of detection of the abnormal blood supply, and it, too, shows the venous drainage that typically is via the inferior pulmo-

TABLE 6. *Pulmonary sequestration*

	Sequestration	
Characteristic	Intralobar	Extralobar
Location of bronchopulmonary malformation	Posterior basilar segments, left 60%	Above or below diaphragm; left 90%
Arterial supply	Large vessel of aorta	Small, variable pulmonary or systemic artery
Venous drainage	To pulmonary vein	To azygos vein
Connection with foregut	Very rare	Sometimes
Associated anomalies	None	Frequent
Found in neonates	Rare	Often
Pleural covering	Shared with lung	Own
Femalt to male ratio	Equal	Higher incidence in males

nary vein to the left atrium. CT with its superior spatial resolution shows details of the bronchial anatomy and the pulmonary parenchymal lesion better than does MR, but MR more clearly reveals the associated vascular anomalies. Either technique clearly visualizes any

associated transdiaphragmatic extension. An esophagram is warranted to exclude any communication with the esophagus or stomach, the bronchopulmonary foregut malformation (83). Both of these latter findings are more frequent with extralobar sequestration in which

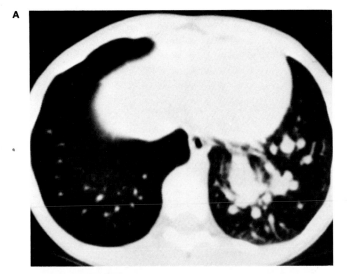

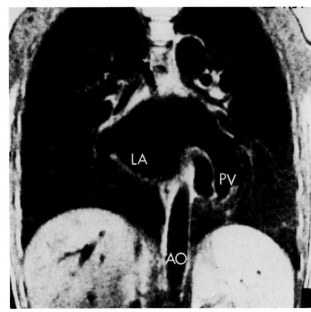

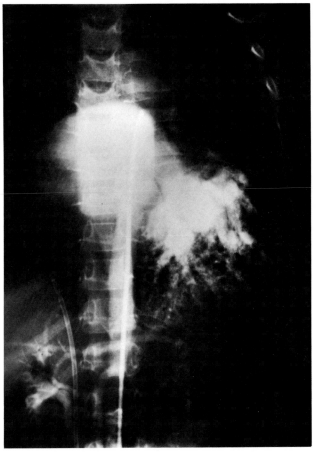

FIG. 46. Six-year-old male with systemic arterial supply to normal lung. Chest radiograph (not shown) showed left lower lobe density thought to be pneumonia. **A:** Nonenhanced CT scan reveals large vessels in the left lower lobe. **B:** Coronal MR image reveals a markedly enlarged pulmonary vein entering the left atrium (LA). A dilated vessel supplying the malformation is shown between the pulmonary vein and aorta on this 5-mm coronal slice (*arrow*). PV, pulmonary vein; AO, abdominal aorta. **C:** Confirmatory angiogram (late phase) reveals large draining veins from the malformation as visualized on the MR scan.

the aberrant lung tissue has its own pleural covering. This lesion is usually seen as a left-sided paravertebral, water density mass.

Systemic arterial supply to normal lung may present as a lower lobe mass lesion or be mistaken for an area of chronic pneumonia (84). Bronchial supply and venous drainage are normal, and the lesion can be dramatically demonstrated by either CT or MR (Fig. 46). The feeding vessel is often huge and may arise from the thoracic aorta rather than from the abdominal aorta as occurs in sequestration.

Other congenital abnormalities that may be mistaken for intrapulmonary cysts or masses by plain radiography include diaphragmatic hernia and intrathoracic kidney (Fig. 31). These are usually diagnosed on conventional studies, and CT or MR are rarely needed. Either of these conditions can occur with sequestration.

Trauma can cause intrapulmonary hematoma and laceration and produce cysts or masses, but the history usually establishes the diagnosis. CT may be helpful in assessing the extent of pulmonary injury. Posttraumatic cysts usually arise in an area of previous hematoma.

Inflammatory Cysts and Masses

Infection is the most common cause of pulmonary cysts and pseudotumors. Most pediatric pulmonary in-

fections are of viral etiology and resolve without sequelae except for the unusual SJM syndrome discussed above. Bacterial pneumonia is usually readily diagnosed clinically and with routine radiography, but unusual presentations or complications may occur, prompting the use of CT.

Bacterial infection may produce a rounded area of consolidation, simulating a mass lesion, the "round pneumonia." This diagnosis is usually not difficult because the child has signs and symptoms of infection, not neoplasm, but the radiographic appearance can be disturbing (85). Typically, a solitary rounded mass density is present in the superior segment of the lower lobe. The density may have surprisingly sharp borders, and it may be difficult to see an air-bronchogram. A follow-up radiograph is indicated to make certain the lesion is inflammatory and does resolve. If it is elected to do CT, the margins of the lesion will be seen to be less sharp than suggested on the radiograph and nearly invariably an air bronchogram will be noted (Fig. 47). Contrast enhancement may demonstrate pulmonary vessels in the opacity, which nearly always shows some degree of enhancement. Rim enhancement suggests an empyema loculated in a fissure (Fig. 41). Pneumatoceles may develop following some bacterial pneumonias of childhood, usually staphylococcal, but pneumococcus and *Escherichia coli* also are etiologic agents. Whether these cystic lesions are localized areas of interstitial emphy-

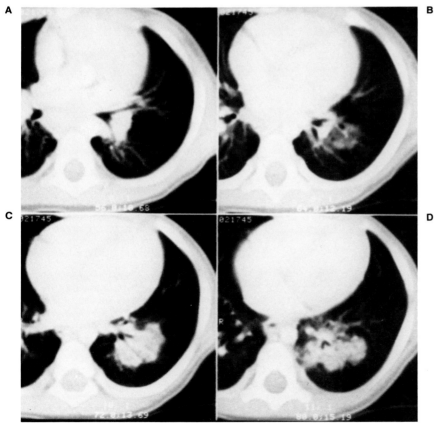

FIG. 47. Round pneumonia in a 1-year-old child with leukemia. A round mass was seen in the left lower lobe on chest roentgenogram. Four serial sections (**A–D**) from UFCT examination reveal an enhancing area of consolidation containing air bronchogram and indistinct margins typical of pneumonic pulmonary consolidation.

sema or whether they are due to ball valve obstruction and/or alveolar wall necrosis is not clear in all cases (86). They may be single or multiple and can contain fluid, making distinction from lung abscess or infection of a congenital cystic lesion difficult (Fig. 48). They usually resolve without sequelae, but if they enlarge or persist, surgery may be warranted. CT may aid in the differential diagnosis in some cases by demonstrating a thick, irregular wall suggesting an abscess, or features of some

of the congenital cystic lesions described above may be apparent. Empyema and loculated pyopneumothorax are also complications of bacterial infection, usually due to pneumococcus, staphylococcus, or *Hemophilus influenza.*

Invasive aspergillosis occurs in children who are immunocompromised, often those being treated for malignancy; its appearance is similar to the descriptions in adults with an intracavitary fungus ball often present.

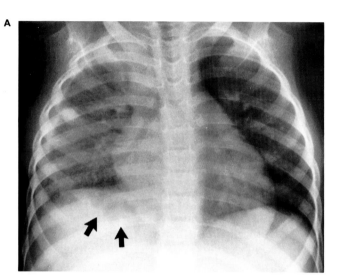
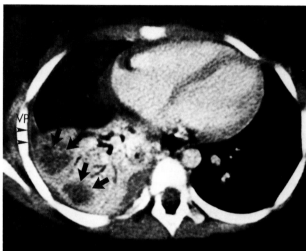
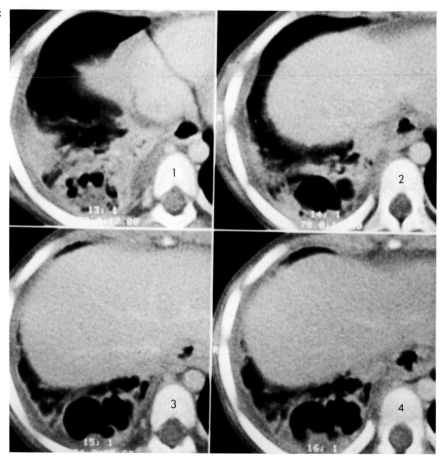

FIG. 48. Three-year-old female with pneumococcal pneumonia. **A:** Chest radiograph shows pleural thickening, pleural effusion and a cystic lesion in the right lower lobe (*arrows*). **B:** Contrast-enhanced UFCT scan reveals right lower lobe consolidation. Air bronchogram and enhancement of the affected lobe is noted as are two large round low-density areas in the lower lobe (*arrows*). Slight thickening (*arrowheads*) of the visceral pleura (VP) is also evident. The low-density lesions are thought to represent areas of pulmonary necrosis that may or may not go on to become pneumatoceles. **C:** Serial sections (1–4) inferior to **B** reveal multiple air-containing cavities in the inferior portion of the right lower lobe representing pneumatocele formation.

Coccidiomycosis can also occur in children and produce a thin-walled cavity simulating a congenital cystic lesion.

Plasma cell granulomas are probably postinflammatory pseudotumors. They vary in size from 1 to 12 cm and are uncommon lesions, but, because they are sharply marginated and can increase in size, they can be mistaken for neoplasms. Approximately 10% show evidence of calcification that may be detected on CT (87). Plasma cell granulomas may be detected incidentally or following a documented bout of pneumonia.

Neoplastic Masses

Primary pulmonary neoplasms are rare in children, but they must be excluded if a mass lesion is noted on a chest radiograph. Most commonly, the "mass" will prove to be one of the congenital or inflammatory lesions discussed above, but unfortunately some malignancies do occur. Bronchial adenomas are low-grade malignancies of the tracheobronchial tree and usually present with findings of partial or complete bronchial obstruction. A persistently atelectatic lobe in a child too old for foreign body aspiration should suggest the diagnosis. If intrapulmonary, the lesion can present as a pulmonary mass.

Sarcomas usually are undifferentiated, although rhabdomyosarcomas may occur in the lung. The mass may be small or grow to fill the whole thorax. Extension through the chest wall may occur. CT is useful in staging the disease and in the search for metastases, but there are no differentiating features that give reliable clues to the pathology.

A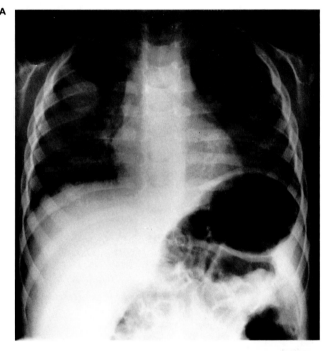

B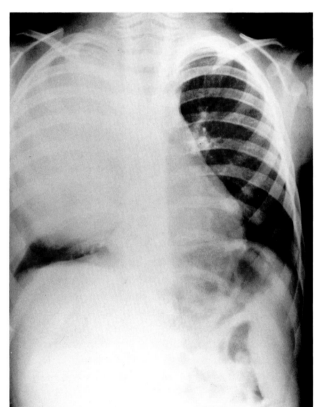

C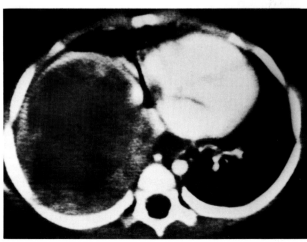

FIG. 49. Pulmonary blastoma. **A:** Chest radiograph reveals a round mass lesion in the right upper lobe thought to represent a round pneumonia. Follow-up radiograph was suggested. **B:** One month later, a huge mass is present. **C:** Contrast-enhanced CT reveals a mass with an enhancing rim and irregular center. The CT appearance is somewhat similar to that seen in a classic Wilms' tumor. At surgery, a pulmonary blastoma was resected.

Pulmonary blastoma, another rare primary neoplasm of lung, is a primitive tumor with features resembling a nephroblastoma. It can vary greatly in size. CT shows a complex mass (Fig. 49). Both rhabdosarcomas and blastomas have been reported as arising in the wall of a pulmonary cyst or at the site of a previously resected cyst (88,89). Moreover, a rhabdomyosarcoma may be multicystic and resemble a CCAM. For this reason, pediatric pulmonary cysts should be carefully evaluated and probably surgically removed unless they can clearly be shown to be postinflammatory pneumatoceles.

When seen on chest roentgenogram, malignant lesions arising from the chest wall may simulate pneumonia, or a pulmonary or mediastinal mass depending on their size and location. CT is valuable in suggesting the correct diagnosis. Most of these lesions are sarcomas; they are discussed in the chest wall section of this chapter.

Pulmonary Nodules

Rarely, a metastatic lesion may be large enough to suggest that it is a primary pulmonary mass, but, much more commonly, metastatic lesions are multiple and range in size, in my experience, from a few millimeters to several centimeters. The pediatric tumors that most frequently metastasize to the lungs are listed in Table 7.

CT is indicated for the detection of pulmonary metastases if knowledge of their presence, size, or number affects staging or therapy. Metastatic tumor is by far the most common cause of malignant disease in the pediatric thorax.

CT examination should not be performed under general anesthesia or even heavy sedation because the associated atelectasis can obscure or simulate metastatic disease. Contiguous 5- to 10-mm slices should be made throughout the lungs. Contrast enhancement is necessary only if the tumor being searched for is likely to be associated with mediastinal or hilar adenopathy. Using UFCT, the entire thorax can be scanned in one breathhold, but when using a conventional scanner it is important to have the child either breathing very quietly if

TABLE 7. *Tumors that can metastasize to the lungs*

Wilms' tumor
Ewing sarcoma
Osteosarcoma
Lymphoma
Thyroid carcinoma
Rhabdomyosarcoma
Ovarian tumors
Hepatocarcinoma
Yolk sac carcinoma
Leukemia
Melanoma
Neuroblastoma
Pheochromocytoma

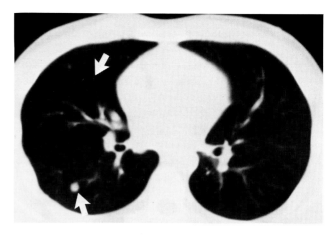

FIG. 50. Typical pulmonary metastases of hematogenous origin in a teenage boy with metastatic pheochromocytoma (*arrows*).

breath-holding is not feasible or, if it is, to have the patient hold her or his breath at the same level of inspiration for each scan to minimize the chance that an area of lung will be missed by falling between slices. If an equivocal area is seen, additional thinner slices through the area in question and prone or decubitus positioning may help to determine the significance of the suspected nodular density. Metastic lesions are most frequent in a subpleural location and often can be seen to be at the end of a vessel, confirming their hematogenous origin (Fig. 50). Differentiation of a nodule from a vessel can usually be made with high-resolution CT, by changing the position of the patient, or, if all else fails, by a follow-up examination. MR theoretically should be of value in this differentiation as metastatic lesions are brighter in signal intensity than the lung parenchyma or the pulmonary vessels, but the long examination time and relatively poor spatial resolution have thus far pre-

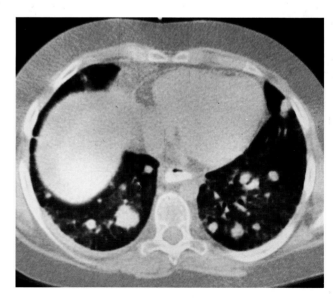

FIG. 51. Candida pneumonia with multiple septic emboli in a patient with brain tumor. The round lesions superficially simulate metastatic disease.

cluded its routine use. On CT examination, metastatic lesions are usually rounded and homogenous in attenuation. Cavitation is unusual, but may occur especially following therapy. Metastatic osteosarcoma nodules frequently ossify, but otherwise the appearance of the nodule yields no clue as to its site of origin.

Nodules other than ones due to metastatic neoplasms are uncommon in children. Granulomatous lesions can occur and are often associated either with calcification in one or more nodules or in a mediastinal node. Multiple small arteriovenous malformations may simulate metastases, and multiple nodular densities that can cavitate can be seen if laryngeal papillomatosis seeds to the lung parenchyma. Multiple septic emboli can simulate metastatic lesions; often, they are relatively larger, and knowledge of the clinical course is often helpful in arriving at a correct diagnosis (Fig. 51).

Other causes of errors in diagnosis include mistaking the anterior end of a rib or an exostosis arising from a rib for a nodule; peripheral rounded atelectasis in a sedated child can simulate a metastasis, as can the azygos vein if there is an azygos lobe.

LOBAR AND SEGMENTAL OPACITIES

Most lobar or segmental opacities result from inflammation, atelectasis, or in the neonate retention of normal fetal lung liquid. CT/MR may be indicated for evaluation of such opacities if the diagnosis remains unclear after plain film evaluation.

In the fetus, the lungs are filled with fluid; normally, at birth, aeration occurs with the first breaths of life. If there is a bronchial obstruction or a primary pulmonary abnormality, a delay in clearance of fluid can occur. Lesions that have been described as causing this abnormality include bronchogenic cyst, bronchial atresia, pulmonary artery aneurysms associated with the tetralogy of Fallot, and congenital lobar emphysema (90). In evaluation of these conditions, one should use the thinnest slice selection possible for optimal delineation of bronchial anatomy and i.v. contrast enhancement to allow optimal visualization of vascular anatomy and to allow delineation of a possible mediastinal mass. An opacity can be recognized as being of pulmonary origin if an air bronchogram can be seen or if vessels can be identified in the "mass" (Fig. 52).

Bronchogenic cyst, accounting for these findings, may be in either the subcarinal or hilar region and will be recognized as an avascular round or oval mass. In the few cases in which MR has been used to date, the mass has had prolonged T1 and T2 relaxation times. On T1 images it may be difficult to distinguish the mass from the normal lung parenchyma, but on T2 the brighter signal from the mass makes its presence obvious.

Bronchial atresia, a rare condition, usually involves the posterior apical segmental branch to the left upper lobe. CT findings are those of a pulmonary opacity without an air bronchogram but with a demonstrable blood supply. Careful evaluation of the airway will reveal the missing segmental or lobar branch (Fig. 52).

Tetralogy of Fallot, with absent pulmonary valve, may cause bronchial obstruction and fluid retention, most commonly in the right middle or left lower lobe (90). The diagnosis should be suspected if the infant has cyanosis and a to-and-fro heart murmur. The lateral chest radiograph is particularly helpful as the large pulmonary arteries are often seen more clearly in this projection. These findings are more obvious on CT.

Congenital lobar emphysema has a variety of causes and, in cases seen early, may present with a fluid-filled, rather than an enlarged air-filled lung. CT can exclude a primary bronchial obstructing lesion. When the lung becomes air filled, it is seen on CT to be emphysematous but not multi-cystic, differentiating congenital lobar emphysema from CCAM.

Atelectasis

The patterns of atelectasis occurring in children are essentially the same as those described elsewhere in this volume in adult patients. The major differences are in etiology. In children, infection, asthma, cystic fibrosis, and foreign body are the major causes; neoplasms and masses are relatively rare. CT is used in cases of chronic atelectasis to exclude the possibility of extrinsic obstruction and to evaluate possible bronchiectasis, both in the affected segment as well as in the remaining more normal-appearing lung. The right middle and left lower are the most commonly affected lobes; in both regions, atelectasis due to pulmonary disease is more common than bronchial compression or obstruction. It was once thought that the "right middle lobe syndrome" was most commonly due to a ring of lymph nodes causing pressure on the right middle lobe bronchus, but our experience with UFCT in children with chronic right middle lobe atelectasis has shown the right middle lobe bronchus to be patent in most such cases. It is assumed the atelectasis is due to peripheral parenchymal disease (91).

In addition to parenchymal and airway causes of atelectasis, volume loss can result from compression, by large effusions or neoplasms, and from postinflammatory or radiation scarring. In the former situation, CT can be helpful in sorting out the plain film findings by clearly separating the collapsed lung from the surrounding fluid or neoplasm (Fig. 41). In the latter situation, CT can assess the size of the atelectatic segment, determine bronchial patency, and may aid in determining the extent of bronchiectasis. An unusual form of "peripheral atelectasis" in either upper lobe can simulate pleural effusion on chest roentgenogram (92). CT shows the anatomy, suggesting the correct diagnosis (Fig. 53). Atelectasis of the right upper lobe or the azygos lobe can

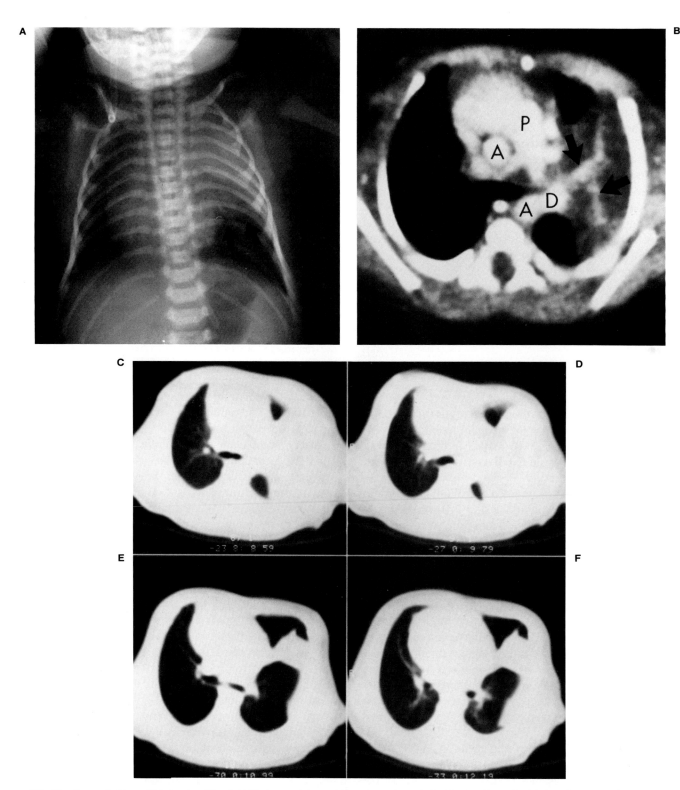

FIG. 52. Congenital bronchial atresia with a fluid-filled upper lobe and bronchogenic cyst. **A:** Chest radiograph at 1 day of age reveals an opaque left upper lobe with slight mediastinal shift from left to right. There is a suggestion of a round opacity inferior to the opaque upper lobe (*arrows*). **B:** Contrast-enhanced UFCT at the aortic pulmonary window. The aorta (A), pulmonary artery (P), and ductus arteriosus (D) are all well delineated. The opaque left upper lobe is seen to have pulmonary vascular supply (*arrows*) but is entirely airless. **C–F:** Serial 3-mm UFCT sections viewed at a lung window fail to reveal any evidence of a left upper lobe bronchus. This is the same patient illustrated in Fig. 19 who also had a mediastinal bronchogenic cyst. At surgery, the bronchogenic cyst was removed, and atresia of the left upper lobe segmental bronchus was confirmed.

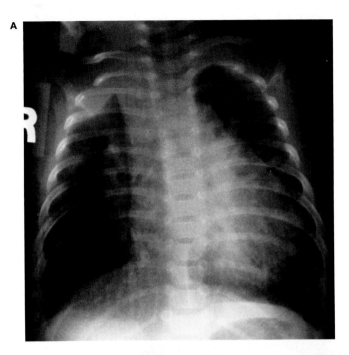

FIG. 53. Peripheral atelectasis. Three-month-old infant with left-to-right shunt who developed increasing respiratory distress. **A:** Chest radiograph reveals cardiomegaly, hyperinflation, increased lung vascularity, and right apical peripheral opacities stimulating pleural effusion suggesting a loculated pleural effusion. **B–E:** Contiguous 3-mm contrast-enhanced CT images reveal right upper lobe atelectasis. The atelectatic lung typically enhances and shows an air bronchogram and triangular configuration. There is no evidence of pleural effusion. Note the enlarged pulmonary outflow tract and right pulmonary artery in a patient who had a large ventricular septal defect (VSD).

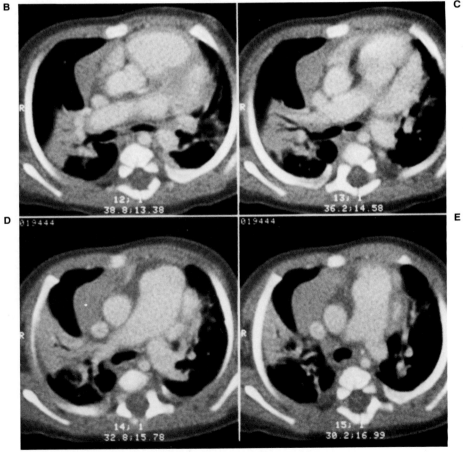

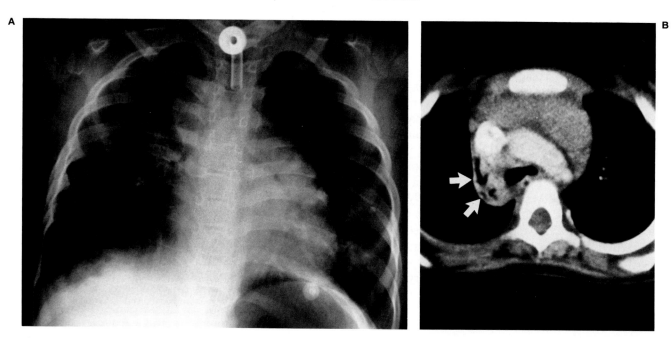

FIG. 54. Consolidation and atelectasis of the azygos lobe simulating a mediastinal mass in a 5-year-old with chronic lung disease. **A:** Chest radiograph. **B:** Contrast enhanced CT scan reveals consolidation and atelectasis of the azygos lobe (*arrows*).

simulate a mediastinal mass and prompt a CT examination (Fig. 54).

Pneumonia

The use of CT in the differential diagnosis of a "round pneumonia" simulating a pulmonary neoplasm has been discussed above. CT is rarely used in other pediatric pneumonias except when complications ensue, such as failure of resolution, development of pneumatoceles and empyemas, or when the radiographs become confusing in trying to differentiate between pneumonia, atelectasis, lung abscess, pneumatocele, and empyema. CECT can be very useful in sorting out these often confusing findings and can aid in the clinical decision as to

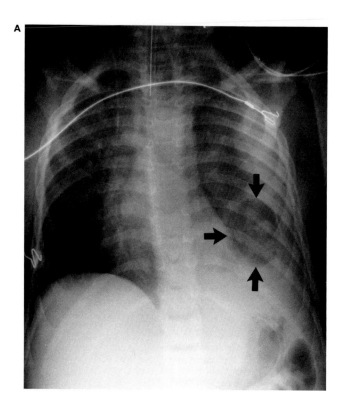

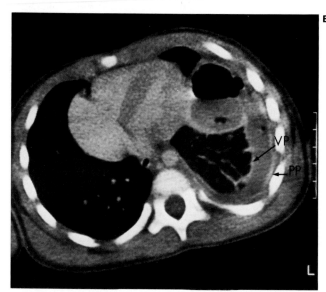

FIG. 55. Pyopneumothorax simulating lung abscess. **A:** Chest radiograph reveals a large pleural density and a radiolucency (*arrows*), suggesting a possible lung abscess. **B:** Contrast-enhanced UFCT reveals a characteristic "split-pleura" sign. Note the separation of the parietal (PP) and visceral pleura (VP). The air fluid cavity is clearly in the pleural space.

whether to continue with antibiotic therapy or to consider chest tube placement.

We have seen children with lobar pneumonia in whom CECT showed a hypovascular area in an otherwise enhancing, consolidated segment of lung; these patients' pneumonias have resolved uneventfully, but whether or not these regions may have represented incipient lung abscesses aborted by successful antibiotic therapy is not known (Figs. 41 and 48).

Differentiation of lung abscess from pyopneumothorax or bronchopleural fistula with empyema can be difficult on plain radiography but is relatively easily accomplished with CT using the same criteria as are used in adult patients. CECT provides optimal delineation of the pleural collection as manifest by the "split pleura" sign which definitely localizes a collection to the pleura (Fig. 55). If consolidation is intrapulmonary, enhancement usually occurs and often intrapulmonary vessels may be recognized.

Diffuse Lung Disease

The use of CT to evaluate diffuse lung disease in children has received virtually no attention as compared to the widespread interest this technique has received in adult patients. This is probably due in part to the difficulties in getting high-quality chest CT in many children who cannot cooperate by breath-holding, concerns over cost and radiation exposure, and the relative rarity of many kinds of diffuse lung disease in children. The pulmonary acinus enlarges throughout childhood from 1 mm at 1 month to 6 mm at 12 years and, therefore,

should be visible on CT scans made without motion artifact (93).

In the 2 years during which we have had access to UFCT, we have been exploring the use of this technology in the assessment of diffuse lung diseases in children. It seems feasible to try to divide abnormalities into those caused predominantly by airspace, interstitial, vascular, and airway abnormalities; of course, as in adults, there are many cases of overlapping findings. The diseases we are studying in an attempt to determine the role of CT include cystic fibrosis (94), asthma, and bronchopulmonary dysplasia.

In a series of 30 patients with cystic fibrosis, we compared the findings on chest CT with plain chest film (Brasfield) score and a clinical scoring system (Schwachmann) and found very good correlation of the CT findings with the clinical score. Not surprisingly, CT was more sensitive than plain films in detecting early disease (95) and more accurately depicted extensive disease than did plain films. Early changes included increased lung volume, marked bronchial wall thickening, often quite focal; progressively severe bronchiectasis, usually most severe in the upper lobes; and mucoid bronchial impactions that were much more extensive on CT than on conventional chest roentgenograms (Figs. 56 and 57).

In children with asthma, CT can be used to evaluate areas of persistent atelectasis and determine bronchial patency and exclude significant bronchiectasis. We have observed extensive regions of irregular aeration in some asthmatic children and cylindric bronchiectasis in others (Figs. 58 and 59); the clinical utility of these findings is the subject of an on-going study.

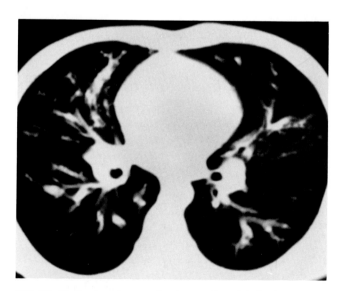

FIG. 56. Moderate pulmonary involvement in cystic fibrosis in a 13-year-old male. UFCT shows increased lung volumes, extensive bronchial wall thickening, and mucoid impaction in the medial segment of the right middle lobe as well as mucoid impactions in the left lower lobe and multiple other areas of peribronchial thickening.

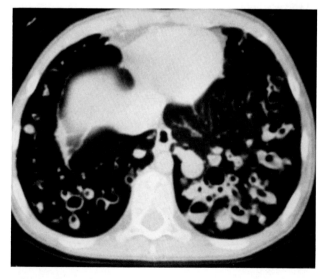

FIG. 57. Severe cystic fibrosis in an 11-year-old male. UFCT reveals bilateral severe cystic bronchiectasis especially posteriorly. Many of the areas of cystic bronchiectasis contain fluid. Marked peribronchial thickening is present, but some areas of lung, notably the anterior portion of the left lower lobe, appear completely uninvolved.

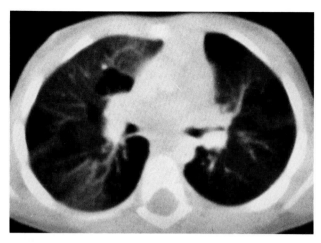

FIG. 58. Two-year-old male with history of reactive airway disease and recurrent left lower lobe atelectasis. UFCT section reveals triangular areas of increased density in the periphery of the right lung and in the lingula on the left, interspersed with areas of relative hyperinflation.

Preliminary observations on a group of children with bronchopulmonary dysplasia has suggested that CT may be of benefit by more accurately detecting the extent of disease. Atelectasis and bands of fibrosis are clearly localized; tracheal enlargement and abnormal tracheal dynamics are other findings observed frequently.

Other diffuse lung diseases that occur in children have findings similar to those reported in adult patients; included in this group are histiocytosis X in which a reticulonodular pattern may progress to cystic lung lesions, lymphoid interstitial pneumonia in children with AIDS, radiation pneumonia, acute granulomatous infections, sarcoid, and extrinsic allergic alveolitis.

Early diagnosis of infection is important in immunocompromised children. The use of CT can clarify equiv-ocal plain film chest radiographic findings, prompting early therapy, and can direct the lung biopsy if one is needed for diagnosis.

DISEASES OF THE PLEURA AND CHEST WALLS

There are no significant differences in the appearance of the pleura between children and adults. The fissures may be visualized as fine lines when their plane intersects the CT plane at a right angle (major fissure), and their location is inferred by seeing a relatively avascular area when they are parallel to the CT axis (right minor fissure).

The most common indication for CT in pleural abnormalities is the plain film finding of an opaque thorax, usually with no mediastinal shift, or an increase in volume on the affected side. CT is required to clearly delineate the underlying anatomy. Most commonly, the abnormality is due to a combination of effusion and compressive atelectasis, but occasionally a malignancy, usually lymphoma, will be found. CECT is essential for accurate differentiation between pleural and parenchymal densities. Parenchymal abnormalities virtually always show some enhancement (Figs. 48 and 54) and, except for enhancement of the pleural surfaces themselves, pleural densities are avascular (Figs. 41 and 55). We have not found CT of pleural fluid collections to reliably differentiate between different types of fluid collections (i.e., transudate versus exudate). The differentiation of fluid from fibrinous pleural collections is also difficult by CT.

Small, free pleural effusions are seen as water-density, curvilinear collections posteriorly located that follow the configuration of the chest wall. They are medial and posterior to the diaphragmatic crus. Effusions typically

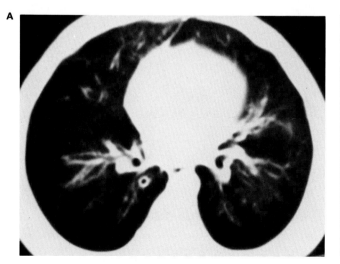

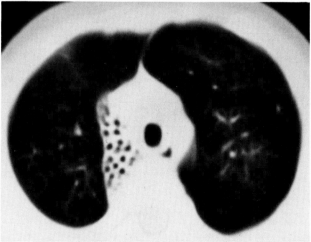

FIG. 59. Two-year-old male with history of reactive airway disease. **A:** Ultrafast CT scan reveals marked increase in lung volumes and extensive cylindric bronchiectasis bilaterally. **B:** Clinically unsuspected total atelectasis of the right upper lobe with apparent cylindric bronchiectasis.

TABLE 8. *Causes of pleural effusion*

Cardiac
  Congestive heart failure
Renal
  Acute glomerulonephritis (AGN)
  Nephrotic syndrome
  Renal failure
Inflammatory
  Infection
  Pleuritis
  Subphrenic abscess
Traumatic
  Hemothorax
  Malpositioned intravascular catheter
  Surgical sequelae
  Chylothorax
Neoplastic
  Mediastinal mass (especially lymphoma)
  Malignant effusion
  Hemangiomatosis
  Leukemia
Other
  Ascites
  Collagen vascular disease
  Hypoproteinemia
  Fluid overload
  Ventriculopleural shunt

move freely when the patient's position is changed. Failure to do so implies loculation and often means an empyema is present. The normal parietal and visceral pleura are too thin to be discriminated from the collection of pleural fluid by either CT or MR, but when an empyema is present, thickening of both the parietal and visceral pleura is readily recognized on CECT. Thicken-

ing of the parietal pleura inferiorly and medially can simulate the diaphragmatic crus, leading to confusion between pleural effusion and ascites.

Causes of pleural effusion seen in children are listed in Table 8.

Empyema is a common complication of bacterial pneumonia in childhood. Imaging is not usually necessary but is used primarily when there is uncertainty as to the etiology of a large pleural or parenchymal density (opaque hemithorax), or when the empyema is complicated by the development of a bronchopleural fistula or a pyopneumothorax, suggesting a lung abscess or pneumatocele. It is usually possible using CECT to successfully distinguish these complications from that of a lung abscess. Characteristically, a lung abscess has a thick wall, has shaggy outer margins, and is round; empyema is lenticular, has a thin, smooth wall, has a sharper interface with lung, and has the "split pleura" sign on CECT that results from enhancement of the thickened parietal and visceral pleural layers surrounding the avascular fibrinopurulent exudate (Fig. 55).

Pleural neoplasms are rare in children with the exception of pleural-based metastatic lesions. The pleural surfaces can be involved in lymphoma and neuroblastoma, usually quite late in the course of the disease.

Abnormalities of the soft tissues of the chest wall are studied by CT or MR to aid in the differential diagnosis but, more importantly, to determine the extent of the lesion before surgery. If extension into the thorax itself can be demonstrated, the surgical approach may be altered. Lesions may extend into the pleural cavity and suggest an intrapulmonary or mediastinal mass on plain

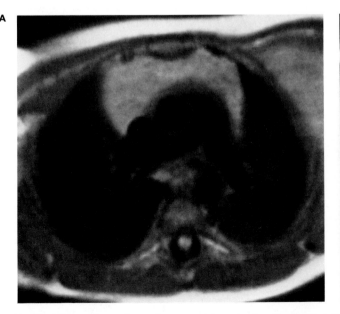
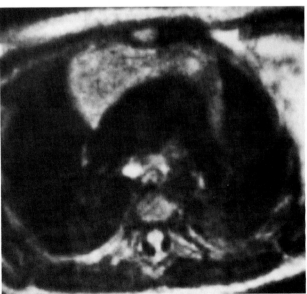

FIG. 60. Inflammatory adenopathy present in a chest wall mass in a 9-month-old female. **A:** Gated transaxial MR image reveals a relatively homogeneous appearing soft-tissue mass in the left axillary region. The mass is entirely extrathoracic, displaces the pectoralis major muscle anteriorly, and is of approximately the same signal intensity as the thymus. **B:** On the T2-weighted image, the mass is somewhat more inhomogeneous and becomes of brighter signal intensity than the thymus.

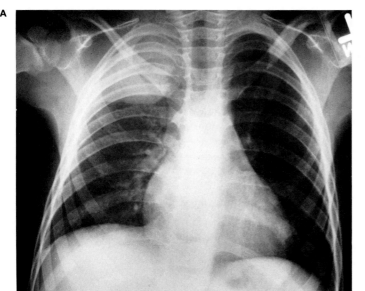

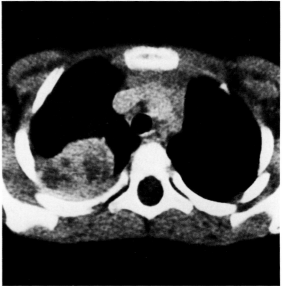

FIG. 61. Four-year-old girl with cough, fever and chest pain, and pathologic diagnosis of small cell sarcoma. **A:** Chest radiograph shows a right upper parenchymal density which was initially interpreted as pneumonia. In retrospect, an extrapleural sign is present and no air bronchogram is noted. The margins are also unusually sharp even for a round pneumonia. **B:** CT scan reveals a large mass with irregular inhomogeneous enhancement following administration of i.v. contrast.

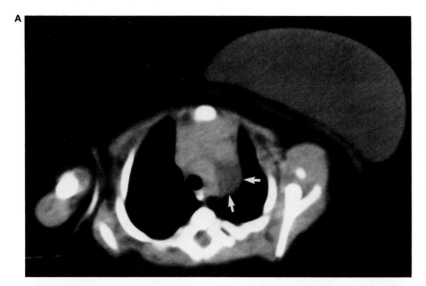

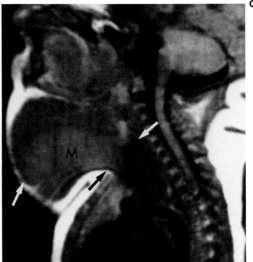

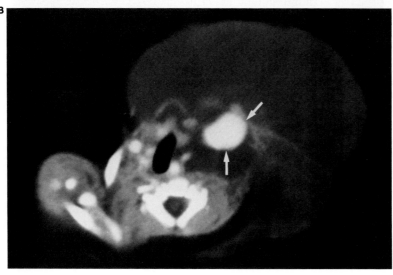

FIG. 62. Cystic hygroma of the neck, anterior chest wall and mediastinum associated with venous aneurysm. Two-day-old infant with a huge cervical mass. **A:** Non-enhanced CT reveals a water-density mass extending down over the left anterior chest wall from the cervical region. Also noted is extension of the mass into the upper middle mediastinum posterior to the thymus and lateral to the aortic arch (*arrows*). **B:** Contrast enhanced CT scan reveals aneurysmal enlargement of the left jugular vein (*arrows*). The rest of the mass remains primarily avascular except for a few enhancing septi. **C:** Sagittal MR scan, T1-weighted, shows the cervical mass (M) extending posterior to the thymus into the upper mediastinum (*arrow*).

film examination, or they may present as obvious, visible, and palpable masses. The most common conditions responsible for chest wall masses are benign—lymphangiomas (cystic hygroma), hemangiomas, neurofibromas, lipomas, and lymph node masses that may be either inflammatory or malignant in origin (Fig. 60). Some inflammatory lesions may extend to the chest wall from the lung parenchyma; most commonly seen are actinomycosis and, in children with chronic granulomatous disease, aspergillosis. Aggressive fibromatosis is a locally recurrent condition although not a true malignancy. Rhabdomyosarcoma and nonosseous Ewing sarcoma are the most commonly encountered malignant lesions.

As elsewhere in the body, malignant lesions require biopsy for diagnosis; CT or MR can neither exclude nor classify malignancy. Features commonly seen suggesting malignancy are a large mass, bone destruction, violation of soft-tissue planes, and irregular contrast enhancement (Fig. 61). Some rhabdomyosarcomas we have seen have shown marked ring enhancement suggestive of an abscess. The Askin tumor is a primitive neuroectodermal tumor arising from the chest wall and having imaging characteristics identical to Ewing sarcoma.

Lipomas are readily recognized either on CT, by hypodensity, or on MR by their bright signal on T1-weighted images. Lipoblastoma may be suspected if a fatty lesion is large and infiltrative, but biopsy is needed for definitive diagnosis. Liposarcomas are very rare in children. Hemangiomas show intense contrast enhancement on CT and may also be bright on T1-weighted images. Calcifications may be seen on CT, and, in some cases, vascular channels may be detected as areas of signal void on the MR study.

Cystic hygromas have variable appearances on CT and MR depending on their histologic nature. They may be avascular or show irregular contrast enhancement, depending on the extent of the hemangiomatous component of the lesion. They may have either a bright signal on T1 or, less commonly, a prolonged T1 (Fig. 62).

Neurofibromas are usually of soft-tissue density on CT, although larger lesions may be hypodense and relatively avascular; they may occur in the chest wall along the course of the ribs, and in the neck or mediastinum. On MR examination, the lesions usually have a prolonged T1 and T2. The lesions of fibromatosis often arise in the muscles, and biopsy is required to distinguish them from sarcomas. On CT, these lesions often show irregular margins and contrast enhancement; on MR, they have prolonged T1 and T2 compared to muscle.

Bony Thorax

Focal lesions of the bony thorax that may be investigated by CT or MR include infection, neoplasm, congenital, and, occasionally, traumatic lesions.

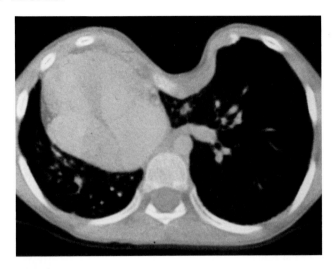

FIG. 63. Severe pectus excavatum deformity in a patient with hypoplastic right lung. The pectus index is 5.7.

Although MR does not show cortical bone well and its spatial resolution is less than CT, its greater soft tissue contrast and sagittal and coronal views are helpful in the assessment of marrow abnormalities in the pediatric thorax.

A bifid anterior rib is often suddenly noticed by an anxious parent who is convinced that it is a new finding and most likely something sinister. Usually plain film examination will resolve the issue, but we have had a few occasions in which the attending physician could not be convinced that there was not an associated mass; CT was, therefore, helpful. A similar situation exists with a solitary rib exostosis when it may be more difficult to be certain of the findings on plain film study alone, and CT may be used. Other neoplasms of the ribs are uncommon in children, although either Ewing sarcoma or osteosarcoma may arise there; Ewing sarcoma is also seen in the scapula; neither neoplasm is common in the clavicle. The sternum is well seen on CT and MR; infection following thoracotomy is the most common nontraumatic lesion of this bone. Sternoclavicular dislocations are well shown by CT. Posterior rib fractures in different stages of healing, especially those showing internal callus formation, are suggestive of child abuse.

Among the few generalized thoracic bony abnormalities prompting CT examination in children is evaluation of a severe pectus excavatum deformity (Fig. 63). The cross-sectional imaging technique provides an accurate assessment of the severity of the deformity and its effect on the cardiopulmonary structures. The deformity appears to involve primarily the cartilaginous portion of the ribs. The use of a pectus index, derived from dividing the transverse diameter by the anteroposterior diameter on a CT scan has been suggested as a possible objective assessment of the degree of deformity. An index of >3.25 was found in those children requiring surgery

(96). Three-dimensional reconstruction of the CT images may prove to give even more information. Severe scoliosis can also produce thoracic deformities that can be well studied by CT. CT can be of use in studying lung volume abnormalities in patients with chondrodystrophies.

REFERENCES

1. Berger PE, Kuhn JP, Brusehaber J. Technique for computed tomography in infants and children. *Radiol Clin North Am* 1981;19:399–408.
2. Strain JD, Campbell JB, Harvey LA, Foley LC. IV Nembutal: safe sedation for children undergoing CT. *AJR* 1988;151:975–979.
3. Thompson JR, Schneider S, Ashwal S, et al. The choice of sedation for computed tomography in children: a prospective evaluation. *Radiology* 1982;143:475–479.
4. Kirks DR. Practical techniques for pediatric chest computed tomography. *Pediatr Radiol* 1983;13:148–155.
5. Peschmann KR, Napel S, Couch JL, Rand RE, Alei R, Ackelsberg SM, Gould R, Boyd DP. High-speed computed tomography: systems and performance. *Allied Optics* 1985;24:4052–4060.
6. Brasch RC. Ultrafast computed tomography for infants and children. *Radiol Clin North Am* 1988;26:277–286.
7. Ell SR, Jolles H, Keyes WD, Galvin JR. Cine CT technique for dynamic airway studies. *AJR* 1985;145:35–36.
8. Lipton MJ, Higgins CB, Boyd DP. Computed tomography of the heart: evaluation of anatomy and function. *J Am Coll Cardiol* 1985;5(suppl 1):55S–69S.
9. Frey EE, Smith WL, Grandgeorge S, et al. Chronic airway obstruction in children: evaluation with cine-CT. *AJR* 1987;148:347–352.
10. Brasch RC, Cann CE. Computed tomographic scanning in children. II. An updated comparison of radiation dose and resolving power of commercial scanners. *AJR* 1982;138:127–133.
11. Fearon T, Vucich J. Pediatric patient exposures from CT examinations: GE CT/T 9800 scanner. *AJR* 1985;144:805–809.
12. ECRI: Scanner, computed axial tomography, full body. In: *Diagnostic imaging and radiology*. Pennsylvania: ECRI, Plymouth Meeting, 1988:13–22.
13. Heiberg E, Wolverson MK, Sundaram M, Nouri S. Normal thymus: CT characteristics in subjects under age 20. *AJR* 1982;138:491–494.
14. Day DL, Gedgaudas E. The thymus. *Radiol Clin North Am* 1984;22:519–538.
15. Kuhn JP, Neeson H. Magnetic resonance imaging of the normal thymus. *AJR* (submitted).
16. Cory DA, Cohen MD, Smith JA. Thymus in the superior mediastinum simulating adenopathy: appearance on CT. *Radiology* 1987;162:457–459.
17. Baron RL, Lee JKT, Sagel SS, Peterson RR. Computed tomography of the normal thymus. *Radiology* 1982;142:121–125.
18. Salonen OLM, Kivisaari ML, Somer JK. Computed tomography of the thymus of children under 10 years. *Pediatr Radiol* 1984;14:373–375.
19. St. Amour TE, Siegel MJ, Glazer HS, Nadel SN. CT appearances of the normal and abnormal thymus in childhood. *J Comput Assist Tomogr* 1987;11:645–650.
19a.Siegel MJ, Glazer HS, Wiener JI, Molina PL. Normal and abnormal thymus in childhood: MR imaging. *Radiology* 1989;172:367–371.
20. deGeer G, Webb WR, Gamsu G. Normal thymus: assessment with MR and CT. *Radiology* 1986;158:313–317.
21. Bar-Ziv J, Barki Y, Itzchak Y, Mares AJ. Posterior mediastinal accessory thymus. *Pediatr Radiol* 1984;14:165–167.
22. Cohen MD, Weber TR, Sequeira FW, Vane DW, King H. The diagnostic dilemma of the posterior mediastinal thymus: CT manifestations. *Radiology* 1983;146:691–692.
23. Rollins NK, Currarino G. MR imaging of posterior mediastinal thymus. *J Comput Assist Tomogr* 1988;12:518–520.
24. Levine C. Cervical presentation of a large thymic cyst: CT appearance. *J Comput Assist Tomogr* 1988;12:656–657.
25. Moscowitz PS, Noon MA, McAlister WH, Mark JBD. Thymic cyst hemorrhage: a cause of mediastinal widening in children with asplastic anemia. *AJR* 1980;134:832–836.
26. Baron RL, Lee JKT, Sagel SS, Levitt RG. Computed tomography of the abnormal thymus. *Radiology* 1982;142:127–134.
27. Heron CW, Husband JE, Williams MP. Hodgkin disease: CT of the thymus. *Radiology* 1988;167:647–651.
28. Pilla TJ, Wolverson MK, Sundaram M, Heiberg E, Shields JB. CT evaluation of cystic lymphangiomas of the mediastinum. *Radiology* 1982;144:841–842.
28a.Joseph AE, Donaldson JS, Reynolds M. Neck and thorax venous aneurysm: Association with cystic hygroma. *Radiology* 1989;170:109–112.
29. Sumner TE, Volbert FM, Kiser PE, Shaffner LS. Mediastinal cystic hygroma in children. *Pediatr Radiol* 1981;11:160–162.
30. Abramson SJ, Berdon WE, Reilly BJ, Kuhn JP. Cavitation of anterior mediastinal masses in children with histiocytosis-X: report of four cases with radiographic-pathologic findings and clinical follow-up. *Pediatr Radiol* 1987;17:10–14.
31. Levitt RG, Husband JE, Glazer HS. CT of primary germ-cell tumors of the mediastinum. *AJR* 1984;142:73–78.
32. Siegel MJ, Nadel SN, Glazer HS, Sagel SS. Mediastinal lesions in children: comparison of CT and MR. *Radiology* 1986;160:241–244.
33. Parker B, Castellino R. *Pediatric oncologic radiology*. St. Louis: C. V. Mosby Co., 1977.
34. Hopper KD, Diehl LF, Lesar M, et al. Hodgkin disease: clinical utility of CT in initial staging and treatment. *Radiology* 1988;169:17–22.
35. North LB, Fuller LM, Hagemeister FB, Rodgers RW, Butler JJ, Shullenberger CC. Importance of initial mediastinal adenopathy in Hodgkin disease. *AJR* 1982;138:229–235.
36. Castellino RA, Blank N, Hoppe RT, Cho C. Hodgkin disease: contributions of chest CT in the initial staging evaluation. *Radiology* 1986;160:603–605.
37. Khoury MB, Godwin JD, Halvorsen R, Hanun Y, Putman CE. Role of chest CT in non-Hodgkin lymphoma. *Radiology* 1986;158:659–662.
38. Panicek DM, Harty MP, Scicutella CJ, Carsky EW. Calcification in untreated mediastinal lymphoma. *Radiology* 1988;166:735–736.
39. Heron CW, Husband JE, Williams MP. Hodgkin disease: CT of the thymus. *Radiology* 1988;167:647–651.
40. Mandell GA, Lantieri R, Goodman LR. Tracheobronchial compression in Hodgkin lymphoma in children. *AJR* 1982;139:1167–1170.
41. Ramenofsky ML, Leape LL, McCauley RGK. Bronchogenic cyst. *J Pediatr Surg* 1979;14:219–224.
42. Hernandez RJ. Role of CT in the evaluation of children with foregut cyst. *Pediatr Radiol* 1987;17:265–268.
43. Kellman GM, Alpern MB, Sandler MA, et al. Computed tomography of vena caval anomalies with embryologic correlation. *Radiographics* 1988;8(3):533–556.
44. Fletcher B. *Magnetic resonance imaging of congenital heart disease*. St. Louis: C. V. Mosby, 1988.
45. Bissett GS III, Strife JL, Kirks DR, Bailey WW. Vascular rings: MR imaging. *AJR* 1987;149:251–256.
46. Kirks DR, Korobkin M. Computed tomography of the chest in infants and children: techniques and mediastinal evaluation. *Radiol Clin North Am* 1981;19:409–419.
47. Armstrong EA, Harwood-Nash DCF, Ritz CR, et al. CT of neuroblastomas and ganglioneuromas in children. *AJR* 1982;139:571–576.
48. Bourgouin PM, Shepard JO, Moore EH, McLoud TC. Plexiform neurofibromatosis of the mediastinum: CT appearance. *AJR* 1988;151:461–463.
49. Geremia GK, Russell EJ, Clasen RA. MR imaging characteristics of a neurenteric cyst. *AJNR* 1988;9:978–980.
50. Siegel MJ, Nadel SN, Glazer HS, Sagel SS. Mediastinal lesions in children: comparison of CT and MR. *Radiology* 1986;160:241–244.

51. Silverman F, ed. *Caffey's pediatric x-ray diagnosis.* Chicago: Year Book Medical Publishers, 1985:1342.
52. Silverman F, ed. *Caffey's pediatric x-ray diagnosis.* Chicago: Year Book Medical Publishers, 1985:1350.
53. Liddell RM, Rosenbaum DM, Blumhagen JD. Delayed radiologic appearance of bilateral thoracic ectopic kidneys. *AJR* 1989;12:120–122.
54. Dehner LP, ed. *Pediatric surgical pathology.* 2nd ed. Baltimore: Williams & Wilkins, 1987:304.
55. Arcinegas F, Hakimi M, Farooki ZQ, et al. Intrapericardial teratoma in infancy. *J Thorac Cardiovasc Surg* 1980;79:306–311.
56. Nassar WK. Congenital diseases of the pericardium. In: Spodich DH, ed. *Pericardial diseases.* Philadelphia: F. A. Davis Company, 1976:93–111,271–286.
57. Joseph PM, Berdon WE, Baker DH, et al. Upper airway obstruction in infants and small children: improved radiographic diagnosis by combining filtration, high kilovoltage and magnification. *Radiology* 1976;121:143–148.
58. Ell SR, Jolles H, Galvin JR. Cine CT demonstration of nonfixed upper airway obstruction. *AJR* 1986;146:669–677.
59. Ell SR, Jolles H, Keyes WD, Galvin JR. Cine CT technique for dynamic airway studies. *AJR* 1985;145:35–36.
60. Brasch RC. Ultrafast computed tomography for infants and children. *Radiol Clin North Am* 1988;26:277–286.
61. Brasch RC, Gooding CA, Gould RA, et al. Upper airway obstruction in infants and children evaluated with ultrafast CT. *Radiology* 1987;165:459–466.
62. Fletcher BD, Cohn RC. Tracheal compression and the innominate artery: MR evaluation in infants. *Radiology* 1989;170:103–107.
63. Kuhn JP, Brody AS, Afshani E. Ultrafast CT evaluation of pediatric bronchiectasis. *AJR* (submitted).
64. Griscom NT. Computed tomographic determination of tracheal dimensions in children and adolescents. *Radiology* 1982;145:361–364.
65. Effman EL, Fram EK, Vock P, Kirks DR. Tracheal cross-sectional area in children: CT determination. *Radiology* 1983;149:137–140.
66. Benjamin B, Pitkin Z, Cohen D. Tracheal stenosis. *Ann Otol Rhinol Laryngol* 1981;90:364–371.
67. Strife JL. Upper airway and tracheal obstruction in infants and children. *Radiol Clin North Am* 1988;26:309–322.
68. Martin KW, McAlister WH. Intratracheal thymus: a rare cause of airway obstruction. *AJR* 1987;149:1217–1218.
68a. Svedstrom E, Puhakka H, Kero P. How accurate is chest radiography in the diagnosis of tracheobronchial foreign bodies in children? *Pediatr Radiol* 1989;19:520–522.
69. Cohen MD, Eigen H, Scott PH, Tepper R, et al. Magnetic resonance imaging of inflammatory lung diseases: preliminary studies in children. *Pediatr Pulmonol* 1986;2:211–217.
70. Currarino G, Williams B. Causes of congenital unilateral pulmonary hypoplasia: a study of 33 cases. *Pediatr Radiol* 1985;15:15–24.
71. Gilman MJ, Somogyi J, Taber M. Hypoplastic right pulmonary artery in the hypogenetic lung syndrome. *J Comput Assist Tomogr* 1982;6:1015–1018.
72. Goldwin JD, Tarver RD. Scimitar syndrome: four new cases examined with CT. *Radiology* 1986;159:15–20.
72a. Marti-Bonmati L, Perales FR, Catala F, Mata JP, Calonge E. CT findings in Swyer-James syndrome. *Radiology* 1989;172:477–480.
73. Bressler EL, Francis IR, Glazer GM, Gross BH. Bolus contrast medium enhancement for distinguishing pleural from parenchy-

mal lung disease: CT features. *J Comput Assist Tomogr* 1987;11:436–440.
74. Cleveland RH, Foglia RP. CT in the evaluation of pleural versus pulmonary disease in children. *Pediatr Radiol* 1988;18:14–19.
75. Panicek DM, Heitzman ER, Randall PA, et al. The continuum of pulmonary developmental anomalies. *Radiographics* 1987; 7:747–772.
76. Rogers LF, Osmer JC. Bronchogenic cyst: a review of 46 cases. *AJR* 1964;91:273–283.
77. Stocker JT, Madewell JE, Drake RM. Congenital cystic adenomatoid malformation of the lung. *Hum Pathol* 1977;8:155–171.
78. Hulnick DH, Naidich DP, McCauley DI, et al. Late presentation of congenital cystic adenomatoid malformation of the lung. *Radiology* 1984;151:569–573.
79. Blane CE, Donn SM, Mori KW. Congenital cystic adenomatoid malformation of the lung. *J Comput Assist Tomogr* 1981;5:418–420.
80. Heithoff KB, Sane SM, Williams HJ, et al. Bronchopulmonary foregut malformations: a unifying etiological concept. *AJR* 1976;126:46–55.
81. Choplin RH, Siegel MJ. Pulmonary sequestration: Six unusual presentations. *AJR* 1980;134:695–700.
82. Buckwalter KA, Gross BH, Hernandez RJ. Bolus dynamic computed tomography in the evaluation of pulmonary sequestration. *J Comput Assist Tomogr* 1987;11:335–340.
83. Leithiser RE Jr, Capitanio MA, Macpherson RI, Wood BP. "Communicating" bronchopulmonary foregut malformations. *AJR* 1986;146:227–231.
84. Currarino G, Willis K, Miller W. Congenital fistula between an aberrant systemic artery and a pulmonary vein without sequestration. *J Pediatr* 1985;87:554–557.
85. Griscom NT. Pneumonia in children and some of its variants. *Radiology* 1988;167:297–302.
86. Quigley MJ, Fraser RS. Pulmonary pneumatocele: pathology and pathogenesis. *AJR* 1988;150:1275–1277.
87. Kaufman RA. Calcified postinflammatory pseudotumor of the lung: CT features. *J Comput Assist Tomogr* 1988;12:633–655.
88. Becroft DMO, Jagusch MF. Pulmonary sarcomas arising from mesenchymal cystic hamartomas. *Pediatr Pathol* 1987;7:477–498.
89. Weinberg AG, Currarino G, Moore GC, Votteler TP. Mesenchymal neoplasia and congenital pulmonary cysts. *Pediatr Radiol* 1980;9:179–182.
90. Strife JL, Towbin RB, Francis P, Kuhn JP. Retained fetal lung fluid in two neonates with congenital absence of the pulmonary valve and tetralogy of Fallot. *Radiology* 1981;141:675–677.
91. Livingston GL, Holinger LD, Luck SR. Right middle lobe syndrome in children. *Int J Pediatr Otorhinolaryngol* 1987;13:11–23.
92. Franken EA, Klatte EC. Atypical (peripheral) upper lobe collapse. *Ann Radiol (Paris)* 1977;28:87–93.
93. Osborne DRS, Effmann EL, Hedlund LW. Postnatal growth and size of the pulmonary acinus and secondary lobule in man. *AJR* 1983;140:449–454.
94. Jacobsen LE, Houston CS, Habbick BF, et al. Cystic fibrosis: a comparison of computed tomography and plain chest radiographs. *J Can Assoc Radiol* 1986;37:17–21.
95. Kuhn JP, Nathanson I, Afshani E, et al. UFCT in evaluation of cystic fibrosis. Society for Pediatric Radiology, Cincinnati, Ohio, April 1990.
96. Haller JA Jr, Kramer SS, Lietman SA. Use of CT scans in selection of patients for pectus excavatum surgery: a preliminary report. *J Pediatr Surg* 1987;22:904–906.

Chapter 12

The Heart and Pericardium

Conventional computed tomography (CT) has played a limited role in the evaluation of cardiac disease (1–11). Due to the generally poor definition of intracardiac structures with CT, evaluation of cardiac and pericardiac pathology has devolved to other modalities such as echocardiography, angiography, and radionuclide studies. With the advent of cine CT, studies of intracardiac anatomy and function have become feasible (12–17). However, CT requires the use of significant amounts of intravenous contrast medium. As a consequence its use has been limited to investigations of the pericardium, in particular, or the heart, especially in those cases for which two-dimensional echocardiography proves nondiagnostic.

With improved technology and newer pulse sequences, magnetic resonance (MR) has evolved to be an effective technique for imaging the heart and pericardium. Because thoracic MR studies are now uniformly performed using cardiac (ECG) gating, clear depiction of intracardiac structures is routinely achievable. The ability of MR to depict the cardiovascular system in multiple planes has made it an especially precise technique for evaluating relationships between mediastinal, pulmonary, and chest wall masses and adjacent cardiovascular structures. In addition, it can be anticipated that MR is likely to play a major role in the near future in the evaluation of a wide range of cardiovascular diseases (18). This chapter, then, will emphasize MR with the intent of providing the reader with a basis for interpretation of MR studies of the heart and pericardium. Emphasis will be placed on practical applications commonly encountered in daily practice.

GENERAL PRINCIPLES AND METHODOLOGY

CT

Although the role of CT in the evaluation of cardiac pathology is limited, a surprisingly wide range of pathologic changes can be identified with CT, provided care is taken to maximize technique. It cannot be overemphasized that every thoracic CT study involves imaging the heart. Not infrequently, unexpected pathologic changes can be recognized, especially following routine administration of intravenous contrast media. Accurate differentiation between paracardiac, pericardial, and intracardiac pathology requires thorough knowledge of cross-sectional cardiac anatomy. In select cases, CT can serve as a second-line imaging modality, following echocardiography, especially in those institutions in which MR is not presently available. Finally, cross-sectional CT anatomy is identical to that seen with axial MR, and therefore serves to reinforce an understanding of MR images.

Optimal visualization of cardiac anatomy requires the administration of a large bolus of i.v. contrast medium. CT technique is identical to that used to evaluate either the hila or the thoracic aorta. Images can be acquired at a single level, or incrementally through the entire heart (Fig. 1). The primary advantage of acquiring images at the same level is that the bolus of contrast can be traced sequentially from the right to the left side of the heart. This technique maximizes the likelihood of obtaining images with dense contrast opacification of the ventricular chambers, and is not dissimilar to the logic behind the use of multiple imaging planes when evaluating aor-

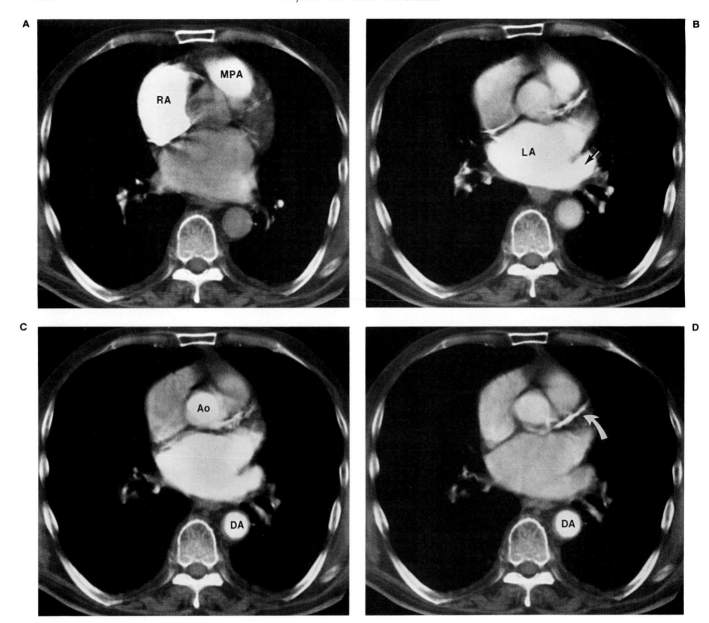

FIG. 1. Cardiac anatomy: CT evaluation. **A–D:** Sequential images at the same exact level acquired following the bolus administration of approximately 120 cc of intravenous contrast media. Note that initially, contrast appears within the right atrium (RA) and pulmonary outflow tract (MPA). This is followed first by dense opacification of the pulmonary veins (*arrow* in B) and left atrium (LA) and then of the ascending (Ao) and descending aorta (DA). Calcification of the left coronary artery is easily identified when present (*curved arrow* in D).

tic dissection (see Chapter 2, Fig. 57). The major disadvantage of this approach is that only one imaging plane is visualized, and is therefore of most value when the appropriate level to assess pathology is already known.

MR

As discussed in Chapter 1, ECG gating is an absolute requirement (19). For routine thoracic imaging, peripheral gating using sensors affixed to the fingers or toes is acceptable. However, optimal imaging of cardiac structures requires central gating with leads placed on the patient's thorax. The most reliable ECG landmark is the

QRS complex, and gating should be triggered by the upslope of the R wave. It should be emphasized that within the magnet, the ECG tracing typically is distorted: in fact, blood flow-related currents may generate larger voltages than the QRS complex. The major source of these extraneous currents is blood flowing in the thoracic aorta. To reduce this effect it is imperative to place at least two of the ECG leads in or near the left anterior oblique (LAO) plane intersecting the ascending and descending aortas. Based on the rules of electromagnetism, current will be minimal if the leads are parallel to the direction of blood flow. In practice, one should place the electrodes in a left posterior paraspinal location along the course of the descending aorta on the back of the patient near the medial aspect of the scapula. Sometimes this posterior location leads to receiving weak ECG signals. This is especially true in patients with emphysema or a deformed chest. In such cases, the electrodes can be placed along the course of the ascending aorta on the anterior chest wall in a right parasternal location. An important safety consideration is to always isolate the patient from direct contact with the ECG leads. Multiple reports of superficial burns due to induced currents in the ECG leads have appeared. Looping of ECG leads or cables also should carefully be avoided because this enhances current induction. Respiratory gating is not required for cardiac imaging. Other forms of respiratory motion compensation, such as respiratory-ordered phase encoding are, however, recommended (see Chapter 1).

IMAGING TECHNIQUES

The most reliable pulse sequence to image the heart is a T1-weighted spin-echo (SE) series with repetition-time (TR) equal to the RR interval and echo-times (TE) of 15–20 msec. This sequence provides excellent depiction of intracardiac structures contrasted against the null signal of flowing blood. To achieve the best cancellation of blood signal, presaturation of the inflowing blood is mandatory (20). In our experience, the best T1-weighted SE cardiac images are obtained during the systolic phase of the cardiac cycle. During this phase, flow velocity is at a maximum, thus enhancing the flow void effect. In addition, systole is the least variable portion of the cardiac cycle, ensuring spatial reproducibility. It is therefore not surprising that the quality of images obtained through the heart may not be uniform (see Chapter one, Fig. 17). It should be emphasized that with cardiac gating, each image is acquired at a different time in the cardiac cycle. Accordingly, cardiac structures are imaged at different points during their contraction. Although this is usually not an impediment to analysis of structural abnormalities, it is sometimes necessary to ensure that the best images are acquired at the location of suspected abnormalities. For example, when evaluating the heart for an intracardiac mass, it is important to acquire images in the area of suspected pathology early in the cardiac cycle, specifically between the QRS complex and the down slope of the T-wave of the ECG. To obtain images of different sections of the heart at multiple cardiac phases with a spin-echo T1-weighted sequence requires several acquisitions and consequently is time consuming. Therefore, whenever dynamic information is required, we prefer to use gated gradient echo recalled sequences in a cine mode in the areas of most interest as outlined by initial spin-echo sequences (21,22). These sequences are usually limited in the number of anatomic levels that can be examined in a reasonable amount of time. In summary, spin-echo T1-weighted sequences are used for anatomic information and gradient echo recalled cine sequences at selected levels are used for dynamic information.

The dependence of all current methods of cardiac MR imaging on proper ECG gating implies that patients should remain motionless and their cardiac rhythm should remain stable over many cardiac cycles. Obviously, this limits the use of cardiac MR in patients with arrhythmias. In such patients, high-quality images are not achievable. Non-gated sequences relying on the averaging of multiple excitations with a short TR can sometimes be valuable (23). The ultimate solution to this problem, however, lies in the recent development of subsecond imaging techniques based on extremely fast gradient echo sequences using short TR and TE times on the order of 7 and 3 msec, respectively, with a total of 300–700 ms per scan (24). Echoplanar imaging, which relies on the acquisition of a whole image with a single excitation and a train of multiple echoes, can produce a scan in 30–100 ms (25). These methods are capable of overcoming problems of cardiac motion.

IMAGING PLANES

The heart is a complicated anatomic structure which moves in a complex manner during contraction. More than any other organ in the body, a three-dimensional understanding of cardiac chambers and structures is a prerequisite for proper image interpretation. Unlike echocardiography, MR can image the heart in any plane regardless of the availability of acoustic windows. The appropriate combination of orthogonal planes provides the interpreter with an operator-independent three-dimensional canvas upon which cardiac structure can be precisely defined. In routine imaging, transverse, sagittal, and coronal planes are generally sufficient to solve most of the common clinical problems encountered. However, these standard planes are not orthogonal to the intrinsic axes of the heart. In fact, the heart is rotated leftward and caudally by about 30–45°. Because any arbitrary orientation of imaging planes is achievable with MR, views in the long or short axis of the heart can be easily obtained (26). However, these views can only be prescribed from preliminary pairs of axial and sagittal or coronal images. Long axis and short axis oblique images, therefore, are generally acquired only when precise intracardiac localization of a pathologic process is needed (27).

NORMAL ANATOMY

The natural contrast between blood and myocardium on MR images results in clear delineation of the ventric-

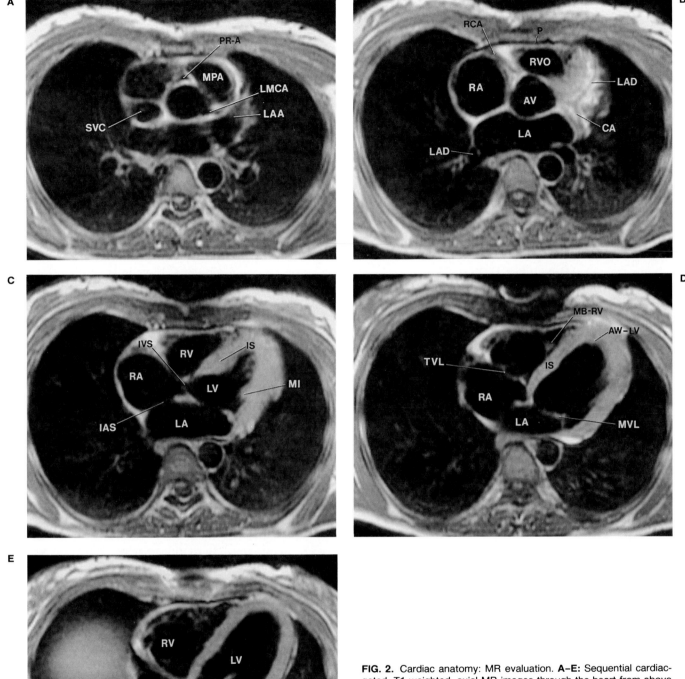

FIG. 2. Cardiac anatomy: MR evaluation. **A–E:** Sequential cardiac-gated, T1-weighted, axial MR images through the heart from above downward. SVC, superior vena cava; MPA, main pulmonary artery; LAA, left atrial appendage; LMCA, left main coronary artery; PR-A, pericardial recess; LA, left atrium; CA, circumflex artery; LAD, left anterior descending coronary artery; AV, aortic valve; RA, right atrium; RVO, right ventricular outflow tract; RCA, right coronary artery; P, pericardium; IAS, interatrial septum; RV, right ventricle; LV, left ventricle; MI, papillary muscle insertion; IS, intraventricular septum, muscular portion; IVS, membranous portion of intraventricular septum; TVL, tricuspid valve leaflet; MVL, mitral valve leaflet; MB-RV, moderator band of the right ventricle; AW-LV, anterior wall of the left ventricle; IVC, inferior vena cava; CS, coronary sinus.

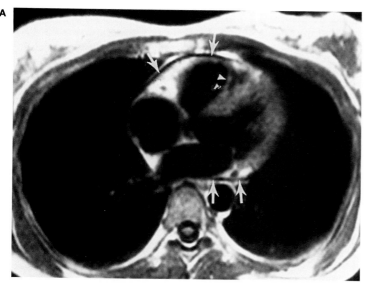

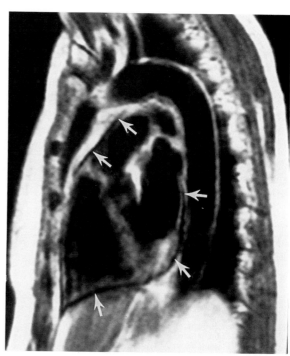

FIG. 3. A, B: Cardiac-gated, T1-weighted, axial and sagittal images, respectively, in a normal patient. The pericardium (*arrows* in A and B) is seen as a low signal band surrounding the heart. Fibrous composition and moving pericardial fluid are responsible for low signal intensity. Note moderator band in the right ventricle (*arrowheads*).

ular and atrial septa (see Fig. 2). Endocardial surfaces are well demonstrated, including the moderator band of the right ventricle and papillary muscles. Atrioventricular valves are so thin and mobile that they are not always visualized. These valves are most commonly depicted during the systolic phase of the cardiac cycle. During diastole, they lie against the endocardial surface of the ventricles and are not generally distinguishable. The epicardial surface of the heart is generally well-delineated by epicardial fat.

The pericardium is a double-layered fibroserous sac. The visceral layer is closely adherent to the heart, while the fibrous parietal layer is free. Normally, 20–25 ml of fluid can be present within the pericardial space. The pericardium normally appears as a thin band of reduced signal intensity. The appearance of the pericardium as a thin, low-signal band is due, in part, to its fibrous composition. In addition, the low signal intensity probably is related to motion of either fluid or of the position of the pericardial layers against each other during the cardiac cycle, resulting in dephasing of spins (28). In our experience, the pericardium and pericardial space are better visualized during systole. This suggests that circulating pericardial fluid, even though minimal in amount, is at least partially responsible for visualization of the pericardial space (Fig. 3).

CLINICAL APPLICATIONS

Intracardiac and Pericardiac Masses

MR has become an important clinical tool in the evaluation of cardiac and paracardiac masses. Two-

dimensional echocardiography is the initial procedure for evaluating suspected cardiac masses. Echocardiography is limited, however, by its field of view and by the availability of ultrasonic windows on the anterior chest wall. The origin or extension of tumors from neighboring mediastinal structures often cannot be appreciated. Multiple studies have shown that reliance on echocardiography for evaluating cardiac masses provides equivocal or false-positive results in a large number of patients. For example, the diagnostic sensitivity of echocardiography in detecting left atrial thrombus is poor (29). An area of particular difficulty is the left atrial appendage. The source of right atrial tumors which sometimes arise from beneath the diaphragm and extend into the right atrium via the inferior vena cava frequently cannot be visualized. Incomplete or inconclusive echocardiographic studies appear to be the most common indication for cardiac MR in clinical practice. In previous studies, MR has been found to be comparable to echocardiography, CT, and angiography combined in evaluating intracardiac, pericardiac, and paracardiac masses (30–32). In a recent comparative study, MR was found to be equivocal or erroneous in only 7% of patients as compared to 27% for two-dimensional echocardiography (33). In a series of 61 patients with cardiac masses studied by Lund et al., MR provided diagnostic information that affected clinical management or surgical planning in 87% of cases (34). Although echocardiography continues to be the primary imaging technique for detecting cardiac masses, it is apparent that MR can play a major complementary role by reducing diagnostic uncertainty and frequently providing critical information essential for adequate preoperative assessment (35).

Direct extension of intrathoracic tumors such as bronchogenic carcinoma, thymoma, malignant teratoma, and lymphoma have been described (Fig. 4). Clinically, this information may be critical to accurate preoperative assessment. Because of its exquisite delineation of cardiac and paracardiac anatomy without the need to administer i.v. contrast, MR often can document the full extent of myocardial involvement, and may consequently affect decisions regarding resectability (34). In our experience, the necessity for proper surgical planning in these difficult cases justifies the use of MR despite its cost (36).

Distant metastases via hematogenous seeding are also now more commonly appreciated with the increased use of MR (Fig. 5). Metastatic cardiac masses are 40 times more common than primary cardiac tumors (37,38).

Primary tumors of the heart and pericardium are found in less than 0.1% of autopsy series: two-thirds of these are benign. The most common benign tumors are myxomas, fibromas, rhabdomyomas, and lipomas. Left atrial myxomas make up approximately 50% of benign cardiac tumors in adults, while rhabdomyomas, fibromas, and lipomas are most common in younger patients. One-third of primary cardiac tumors are malignant. Of these, angiosarcomas comprise 33%, rhabdomyosarcomas 20%, mesotheliomas 15%, and fibrosarcomas or malignant fibrous histiocytomas 10% (39,40).

Few specific MR characteristics distinguishing cardiac masses have been described. Nonetheless, the combination of tumor location and MR appearance may be helpful. For example, although signal intensities within

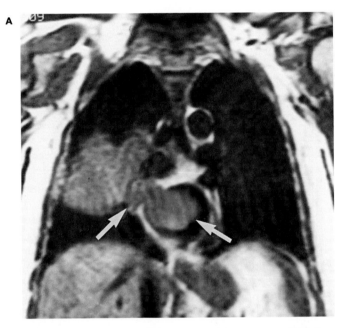

FIG. 4. Lung cancer invasion, left atrium. **A:** Coronal view shows a large pulmonary mass with evidence of extension into the left atrium via the right superior pulmonary vein (*arrows*). **B, C:** Sequential axial sections demonstrate growth of the tumor through the pulmonary vein (*arrows* in B) to form a large tumor thrombus in the left atrium (*arrow* in C).

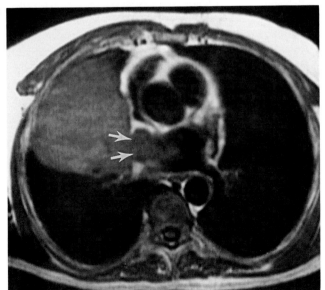

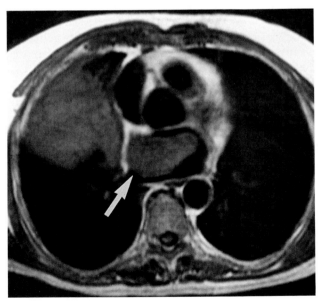

A

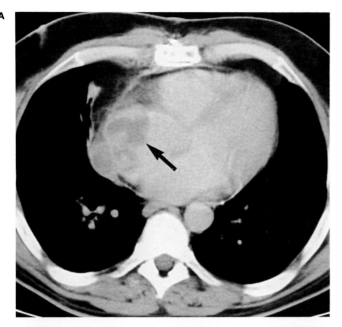

B

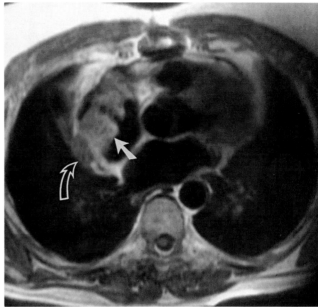

C

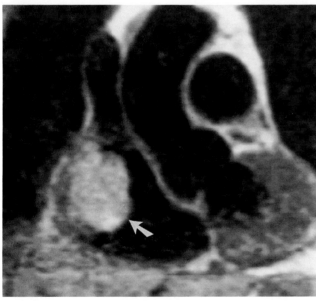

FIG. 5. Patient with a history of unexplained pulmonary nodules and infiltrates. **A:** Contrast-enhanced CT scan shows thickening of the pericardium with an abnormal filling defect in the right atrium (*arrow*). **B, C:** Cardiac-gated, T1-weighted, axial and coronal MR scans, respectively, demonstrate a large mass in the right atrium with high signal intensity (*arrow* in B and C). The mass appears to have transgressed the right atrial wall to extend into the pericardial space (*curved arrow* in B). Biopsy revealed metastatic melanoma to the right atrium. The high signal intensity of this lesion is related to a shortened T1 relaxation time typical of melanoma. Differential diagnosis in this case would necessarily include angiosarcoma, which can also demonstrate high signal intensities due to large, blood-filled spaces.

myxomas are variable, with some showing high intensity suggestive of fatty components while others show lower intensity, typically, these tumors are pedunculated and are found in the atrial chambers most commonly arising from the interatrial septum (Figs. 6–8). Additionally, while invasion and extension across the interatrial septum have been described, invasion of the atrial wall or annulus of the mitral valve is unusual and, when demonstrated, should suggest additional etiologies.

Cardiac lipomas can be specifically recognized by their high signal intensity on T1-weighted scans (Fig. 9). An important caveat in the diagnosis of lipoma is the frequent presence of small deposits of fat in the atrial septum which may mimic a small atrial mass on echo-

cardiography. This process, known as lipomatous hypertrophy of the atrial septum, is commonly mistaken for an interatrial myxoma by echocardiography. Lipomatous hypertrophy of the interatrial septum is a condition characterized pathologically by deposits of fat between cardiac muscle fibers. This is an unencapsulated infiltrative process frequently seen in overweight patients and is often associated with atrial fibrillation. This process is most often found at the junction of the interatrial septum and the membranous portion of the interventricular septum.

Benign masses involving the cardiac wall such as fibromas (Fig. 10) and rhabdomyomas are not discernible from normal surrounding myocardial muscle by virtue of signal intensity patterns. In some cases, signal inten-

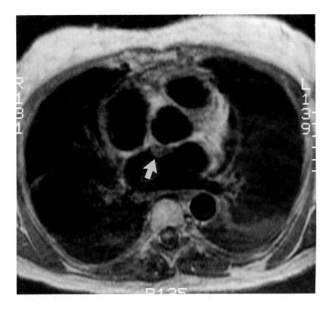

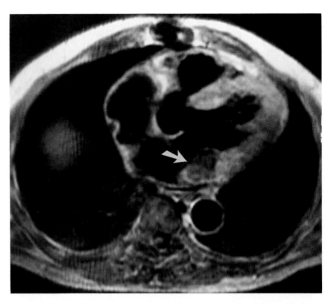

FIG. 6. Atrial myxoma, 47-year-old woman with a history of transient ischemic attacks. MR shows a small 2 cm mass in the anterior aspect of the left atrium near the aorta (*arrow*). No transgression of the atrial wall is seen.

FIG. 7. Atrial myxoma, 72-year-old patient with a history of unexplained syncope. Cardiac-gated, axial, T1-weighted MR scan shows a relatively low signal intensity mass in the left atrium immediately posterior to the mitral valve (*arrow*). There is no evidence of invasion.

A

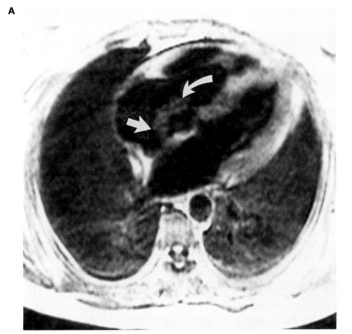

B

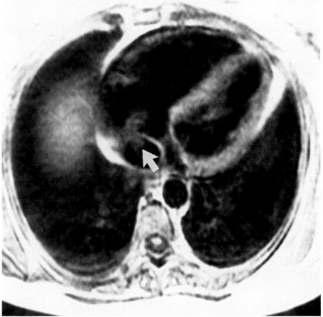

FIG. 8. Right atrial myxoma. **A, B:** Cardiac-gated, T1-weighted, axial MR images show a pedunculated mass arising from the interatrial septum (*arrow* in A). The mass was seen to move with blood flow during the cardiac cycle. Note that the mass protrudes across the tricuspid plane (*curved arrow* in A), and also lies adjacent to the insertion of the inferior vena cava (*arrow* in B).

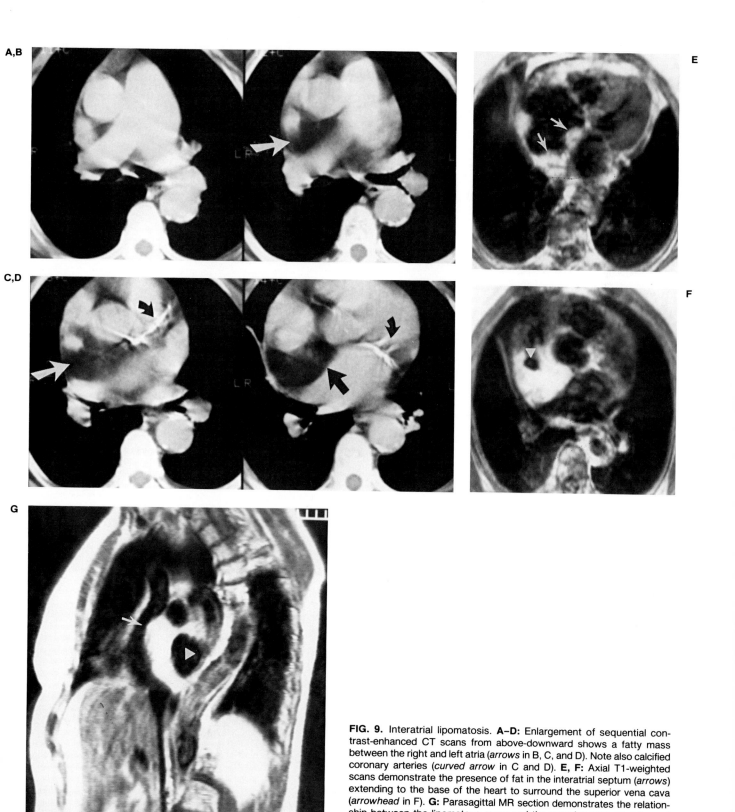

FIG. 9. Interatrial lipomatosis. **A–D:** Enlargement of sequential contrast-enhanced CT scans from above-downward shows a fatty mass between the right and left atria (*arrows* in B, C, and D). Note also calcified coronary arteries (*curved arrow* in C and D). **E, F:** Axial T1-weighted scans demonstrate the presence of fat in the interatrial septum (*arrows*) extending to the base of the heart to surround the superior vena cava (*arrowhead* in F). **G:** Parasagittal MR section demonstrates the relationship between the lipomatous mass and the superior vena cava (*arrow*) and left atria (*arrowhead*), respectively.

A

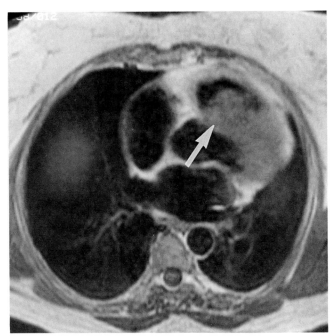

B

C

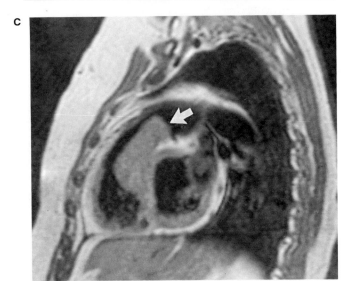

FIG. 10. Right ventricular fibroma. 60-year-old woman with a known mass in the right ventricle, stable for 4 years with biopsy diagnosis of right ventricular fibroma. **A, B:** Cardiac-gated, axial, T1-weighted MR images demonstrate the mass arising from the right ventricular aspect of the interventricular septum, and extending into and causing partial obstruction of the right ventricular outflow track (*arrows*). **C:** Coronal MR image demonstrates the full extent of the mass arising from the right ventricular septum and extending into the proximal pulmonary artery (*arrow*). Note that the signal intensity of the mass is equal to that of myocardium.

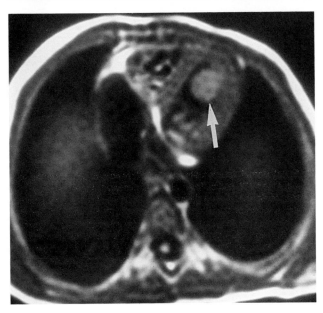

FIG. 11. Interventricular rhabdomyoma. Cardiac-gated, axial, T1-weighted MR scan shows a well-defined mass arising from the left ventricular wall (*arrow*) in a patient with tuberous sclerosis. Note that the slightly higher intensity of the mass relative to the myocardium is atypical. (Case courtesy of Dr. Nancy Genieser, New York University, NY.)

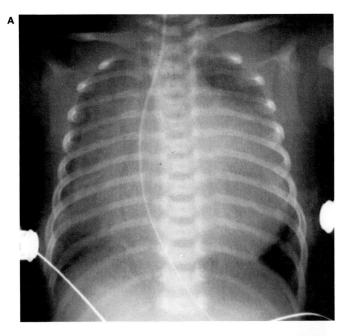

FIG. 12. Rhabdomyoma in a 3-day-old infant with a low Apgar score at birth. **A:** AP chest radiograph suggests the presence of a mediastinal or cardiac mass. **B:** Cardiac-gated MR scan obtained 4 ms after the QRS complex at end-diastole using a myocardial tagging technique demonstrates that the mass is intracardiac (*arrow*). The pericardium appears normal. Note that there is no significant displacement of the cardiac tags. **C:** Cardiac-gated MR scan obtained at end-systole. The tags seen within the ventricular mass do not appear deformed, even though they have moved globally in relation to the tags of the chest wall. However, the tag seen at 5 o'clock (*arrow*) demonstrates bowing due to ventricular contraction. The presence of tag distortion distinguishes the normal contracting myocardium from the mass in which no distortion of tags can be seen.

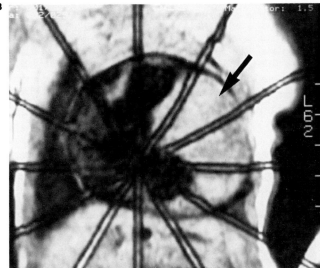

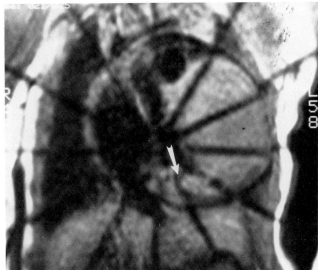

sity differences have been demonstrated (Fig. 11). Generally, however, unless special techniques are used such as cardiac tagging, it is not always possible to accurately separate viable myocardium from infiltrating benign tumors (Fig. 12).

In distinction to most benign masses, angiosarcomas often present with a very suggestive MR appearance. This has been related to their histologic appearance. Typically, angiosarcoma is characterized by variable amounts of spindle cells and collagen bordering blood-filled spaces. The presence of large, blood-filled spaces accounts for a "cauliflower" MR appearance with high signal intensity areas seen on both T1- and T2-weighted scans (41). Angiosarcomas occur predominantly in men between 20 and 50 years of age and has been associated with AIDS. Eighty percent of angiosarcomas arise in the right side of the heart or in the pericardium, often causing tamponade and/or inflow obstruction (Figs. 13–15). Cardiac hemangiomas also exhibit a high signal intensity on T2-weighted scans and, except for location, are difficult to distinguish from angiosarcomas (Fig. 16). In distinction, malignant fibrous histiocytoma, previously known as fibrosarcoma, typically arises in the left atrium of younger women. Rhabdomyosarcoma is more commonly found in children.

Defining the limits of myocardial invasion by malignant tumors is not always possible. The use of T2- or proton-weighted sequences can sometimes be helpful because these may demonstrate a different signal intensity for the tumor than for surrounding myocardium.

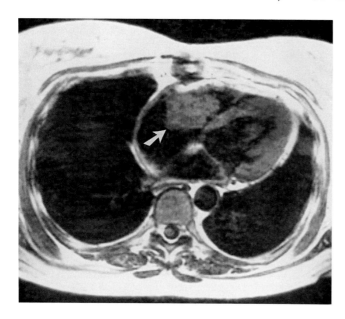

FIG. 13. Fifty-one-year-old woman with documented angiosarcoma of the heart involving the right atrium and tricuspid valve. Cardiac-gated, T1-weighted, axial MR scan shows the mass to good effect (*arrow*).

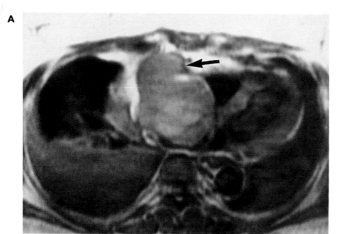

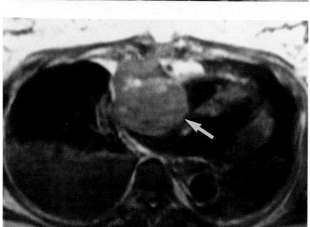

FIG. 14. Forty-six-year-old woman with documented angiosarcoma. **A, B:** Sequential, cardiac-gated, T1-weighted, axial MR scans show a large mass involving the right atrium (*arrows*) extending into the pericardium as well as the superior vena cava resulting in obstruction of inflow into the right heart.

However, this is variable depending on the composition of the tumor mass, and cannot be expected to be accurate enough to consistently define areas of invasion. Extension of tumors beyond the myocardium and into the pericardium is more easily demonstrated. Disruption of the thin band of decreased signal typical of normal pericardium can be demonstrated, and is a helpful sign in defining the presence of pericardial invasion (Figs. 5, 17, 18).

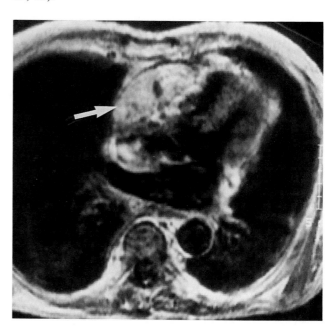

FIG. 15. Cardiac-gated, T1-weighted, axial MR scan in another patient with a documented angiosarcoma of the heart. In this case, tumor involves the right atrium (*arrow*). Note that the tumor demonstrates a high signal intensity more typical of angiosarcomas (compare with Figs. 13 and 14).

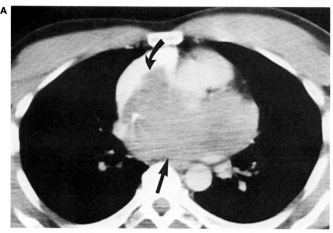

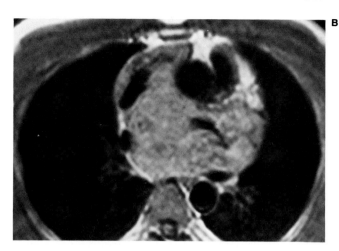

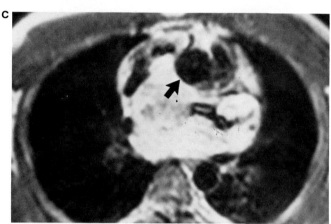

FIG. 16. Cardiac hemangioma. **A:** Contrast-enhanced CT scan demonstrates large, nonenhancing mass near the base of the heart (*arrow*). The mass is displacing the aorta anteriorly and distorts the right atrium (*curved arrow*). **B, C:** T1- and T2-weighted axial MR scans, respectively, demonstrate a mass of moderately high signal intensity on the T1-weighted scan and very high signal intensity on the T2-weighted scan. This high level of signal intensity is consistent with hemangioma. Note that the lesion is insinuating itself between the vascular structures at the base of the heart, but does not compress the aorta, (*arrow* in C) indicating that the tumor is relatively soft. These findings were subsequently verified surgically.

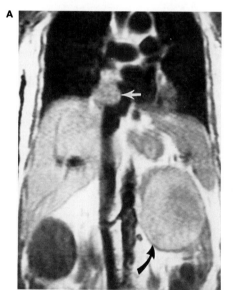

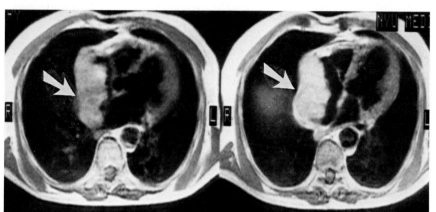

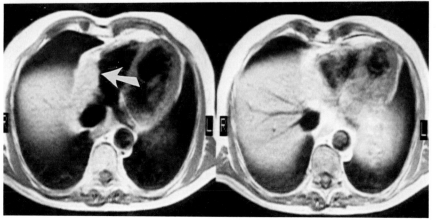

FIG. 17. Renal cell carcinoma metastatic to the pericardium. **A:** Cardiac-gated, T1-weighted, coronal MR scan demonstrates a large mass in the left kidney. Note that there is no evidence of direct extension into the inferior cava (*curved arrow*). A mass is present within the right atrium (*arrow*). **B–E:** Sequential axial views show tumor mass invading the wall of the right atrium and adjacent pericardium (*arrows* in B,C, and D). Note absence of normal, thin, pericardial, low intensity band in the area of the tumor.

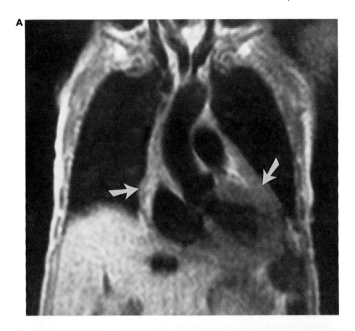

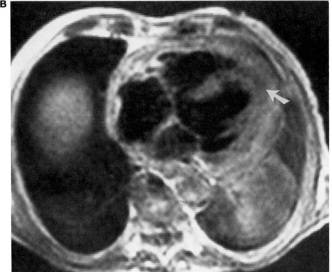

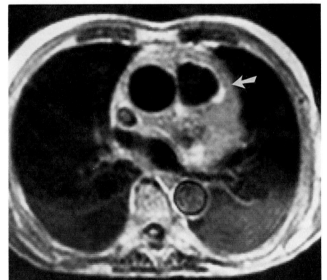

FIG. 18. Pericardial carcinomatosis. A–C: Cardiac-gated, T1-weighted, coronal and sequential axial MR scans, respectively, show absence of usual pericardial band of low signal intensity (*arrows* in A–C). The contours of the epicardium are blurred and the pericardium is thickened. Multiple pericardial implants of mestastatic adenocarcinoma were subsequently confirmed surgically.

Other Intracardiac Masses

Cardiac masses that are nonneoplastic in etiology are also common. Although vegetations from endocarditis have been demonstrated, MR has not proved as accurate as echocardiography in demonstrating valvular implants, especially when these are less than 5–10 mm in size. Motion of the valve leaflets often prevents adequate delineation. On the other hand, MR has proved quite effective for the detection of intracavitary thrombus

(42). The appearance of intracardiac thrombus varies with low to medium-high signal intensity noted on T1-weighted spin-echo scans. Thrombus, as well as most tumors, appears as a low intensity area on gradient echo recalled sequences. The differentiation of intracavitary thrombus from slow flow is sometimes a problem. However, in our experience, the combination of T1-weighted spin-echo and the acquisition of a dynamic cine gradient echo recalled sequence at the level of the suspected abnormality usually resolves this dilemma.

Pericardial Disease: CT/MR Correlations

The normal pericardial thickness on both CT and MR images is about 2 mm or less. Near the diaphragm, the thickness of the pericardium may reach 4 mm (43,44). Clinically, the assessment of pericardial effusion has been greatly facilitated by the use of two-dimensional echocardiography. CT remains the second-line modality of choice to evaluate the thickness of the pericardium and effusions in cases where echocardiography is ineffective. The CT appearance of both the normal and abnormal pericardium has been thoroughly described (45–58). In particular, CT is most efficacious in detecting pericardial fluid collections and calcifications, as is commonly seen in old tuberculous pericarditis (Fig. 19). In some cases, a deformed chest or interposition of air between the heart and the chest wall prevents pericardial evaluation with two-dimensional echocardiography. Herniation of intestinal structures into the thorax also can be confusing at echocardiography and may require CT for elucidation (Fig. 20). To some extent, CT can differentiate the type of pericardial effusion by virtue of density differences (Fig. 21) (59,60). CT is often required in the evaluation of potentially loculated pericardial effusions or abscesses for management as well as diagnostic purposes (Fig. 22).

MR is not indicated in primary pericardial disease even though it is capable of fully evaluating pericardial

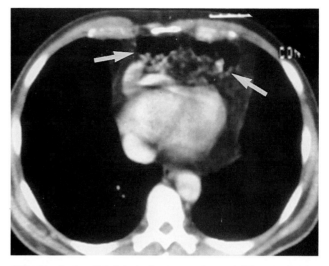

FIG. 20. Pericardial defect. Contrast-enhanced CT scan demonstrates that a portion of the transverse colon has herniated into the pericardial cavity (*arrows*), presumably caused by congenital deficiency in closure of the coelomic cavity. (Case courtesy of Dr. Barry Gross, Henry Ford Hospital, Detroit, MI.)

pathology. However, when combined pericardial and cardiac involvement is suspected, MR usually is superior to CT. With MR, intracardiac structures are demonstrated easily in both a static and dynamic mode, providing a more complete evaluation (Figs. 5, 17, 18). The MR appearance of both the normal and abnormal pericardium has been described (44,61,62–64). Pericar-

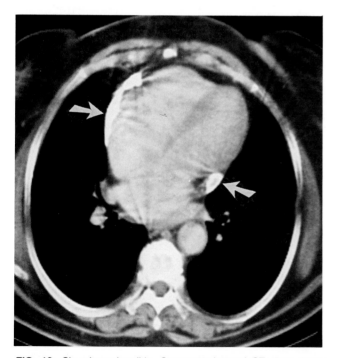

FIG. 19. Chronic pericarditis. Contrast-enhanced CT scan shows evidence of extensive, bilateral, pericardial calcifications presumed to be tuberculous in origin (*arrows*). Typically, calcifications are uncommon in patients with viral pericarditis. Despite extensive pericardial calcifications, this appearance does not necessarily correlate with clinical evidence of constrictive pericarditis.

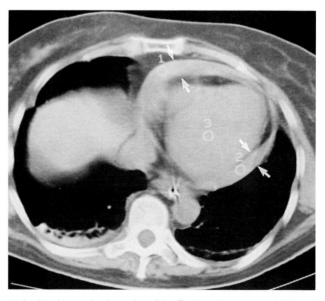

FIG. 21. Hemorrhagic pericardial effusion. Noncontrast-enhanced CT scan. Note that CT density is equal in regions 1, 2, and 3, the latter representing blood in the ventricular chamber. The effusion is recognizable because it is outlined by both mediastinal and epicardial fat (*arrows*). It should be noted that absence of fat around the heart may hamper detection of pericardial effusions.

A 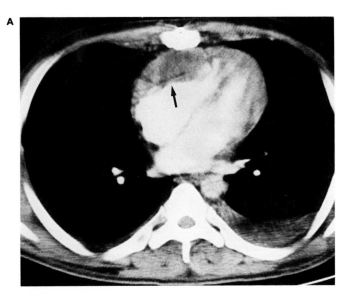 B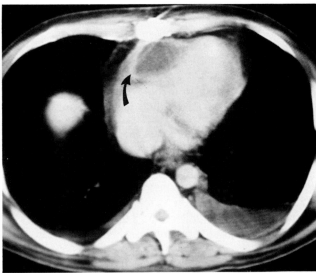

FIG. 22. Pericardial abscess. **A:** Contrast-enhanced CT scan shows an apparently loculated pericardial effusion anteriorly (*arrow*). **B:** Delayed CT image shows rim enhancement of the abscess (*curved arrow*).

dial effusions typically appear variable in signal intensity (28). Because of fluid movement during cardiac contraction, flow void effects are apparent which prevent, in most cases, accurate characterization of pericardial fluid as either transudative or exudative (Fig. 23). However, effusions with high proteinaceous or hemorrhagic content can be recognized by their high signal intensity on T1-weighted scans (Fig. 23) as well as by the presence of associated signs, such as an irregular pericardial surface suggestive of metastatic or inflammatory disease (Fig. 18). An increased amount of pericardial fluid may distend the pericardial recesses. The anterior and posterior pericardial recesses are located adjacent to the root of the aorta and may, for the unwary observer, simulate dissection (Fig. 24). MR is effective in characterizing pericardial cysts (Fig. 25).

An especially important clinical indication for MR in pericardial disease is to differentiate constrictive pericarditis from restrictive cardiomyopathy (61). In contrast to pericardial effusions, echocardiography is poor in diagnosing constrictive pericarditis because thickening due to fibrosis or calcification of the pericardium is difficult to diagnose. Today, most cases of constrictive pericarditis are a late sequela of viral pericarditis, whereas formerly, tuberculous pericarditis accounted for most cases. In viral pericarditis the pericardium is seldom calcified. Clinically, such patients present with evidence of depressed ventricular function with elevated diastolic filling pressures. In constrictive pericarditis, this is due to the constraining effect on diastolic filling of the scarred pericardium, while in restrictive myocardial disease, the heart muscle is thickened and exhibits decreased compliance. In the United States, the most common cause of restrictive cardiomyopathy is amyloid infiltration. MR is helpful because it can directly demonstrate the thickened pericardium in constrictive peri-

carditis as well as the dynamics of the cardiac chambers. Typically, the atria appear dilated whereas the ventricular cavities are normal or reduced in size, frequently associated with a characteristically funnel-shaped right ventricle. In restrictive cardiomyopathy, thickening of the myocardium may be present, but there is no evidence of pericardial thickening and little discrepancy between atrial and ventricular chamber size (Fig. 26).

Finally, MR is helpful in the postoperative evaluation of patients following cardiac surgery, especially when infection is suspected in the heart or pericardium. In this setting, MR provides the most comprehensive examination for evaluation of these frequently difficult cases (Fig. 27).

Despite initial enthusiasm, especially in the assessment of postcoronary artery bypass patients, CT has proven of limited value in assessing patients with ischemic heart disease (8,9). It has recently been suggested that CT may play a potential role in screening patients at risk by detecting coronary artery calcifications (Figs. 1 and 9), especially using ultrafast, cardiac-gated CT (11,12). Breen et al., in a prospective evaluation of 84 patients undergoing routine coronary artery angiography found a significant correlation (sensitivity = 100%) between the presence of coronary artery calcifications detected by ultrafast CT and significant coronary artery stenosis, defined as at least 50% narrowing of a major branch coronary artery (12). In fact, these findings have proven controversial. In a similar prospective study of 50 patients also evaluated by ultrafast CT, Bormann et al., using a CT-specific calcium scoring system, found no correlation between calcium scores and significant coronary artery stenosis, defined as at least 70% narrowing of a major branch artery (13). At present, accurate determination of the prognostic value of CT detection of coronary calcification must await further investigation.

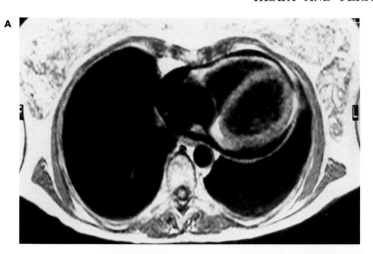

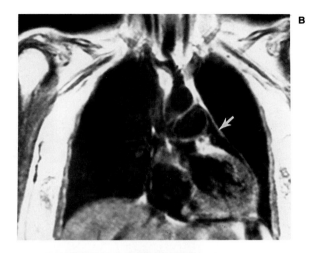

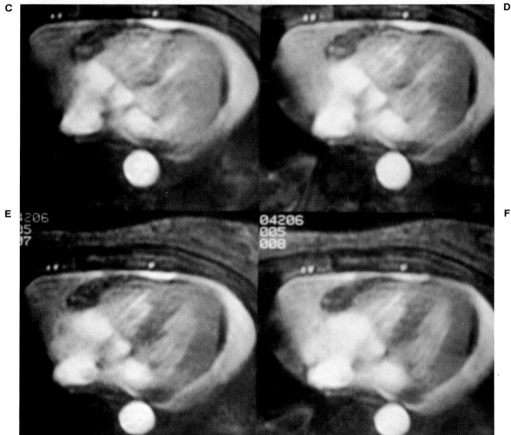

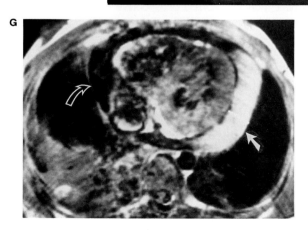

FIG. 23. Pericardial effusion: MR evaluation. **A, B:** Cardiac-gated, T1-weighted, axial and coronal MR scans, respectively, show a low signal intensity pericardial effusion around the heart extending into the superior recesses of the pericardium (*arrow* in B). Despite low signal intensity, one cannot infer a low protein content because extensive fluid motion during the cardiac cycle prevents accurate characterization. **C–F:** Cine sequence shows high signal intensity of moving effusion equal to that of moving blood. **G:** Hemorrhagic effusion in a different patient than shown in C–F, suffering from uremia. Note high signal intensity on the left side (*solid arrow*) consistent with hemorrhage on this T1-weighted MR scan. Low signal intensity noted within the pericardium anteriorly and on the right side (*open arrow*) presumably is secondary to a local flow void effect.

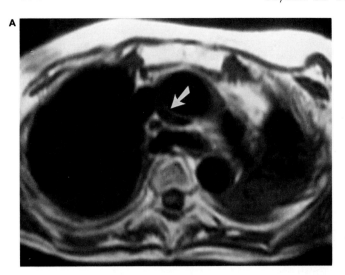
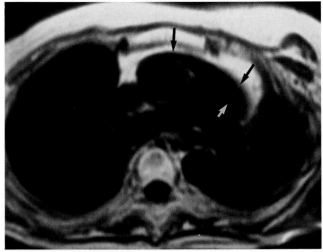

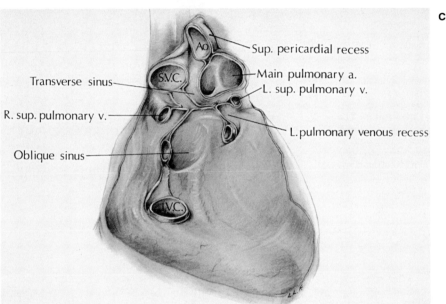

FIG. 24. Pericardial recesses, normal anatomy. **A:** Cardiac-gated, T1-weighted, axial MR scan at the level of the carina. A prominent superior pericardial recess (*arrow*) can be identified in a patient with a pericardial effusion. This appearance should not be mistaken for an intimal flap within the ascending aorta. **B:** Axial MR scan obtained approximately 1 cm below A. Note that the anterior superior pericardial recess often encompasses both the proximal aorta and pulmonary artery (*arrows*). **C:** Schematic representation of the pericardial recesses.

Ischemic Heart Disease

At the present time, MR plays a limited role in the evaluation of acute ischemic heart disease. Clinically, MR is most helpful in evaluating the delayed effects of myocardial infarction. In acute myocardial infarction, early studies demonstrated differences in signal intensi-ties on T2-weighted scans between the normal and infarcted myocardium (18,65,66). Clinically, however, this capability has not been useful because these findings develop relatively late in the course of the disease; additionally, multiple flow- and motion-related artifacts frequently occur which simulate abnormal high signal intensity in the myocardial wall.

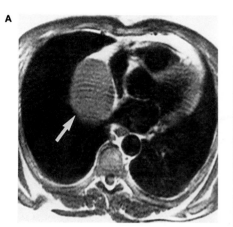

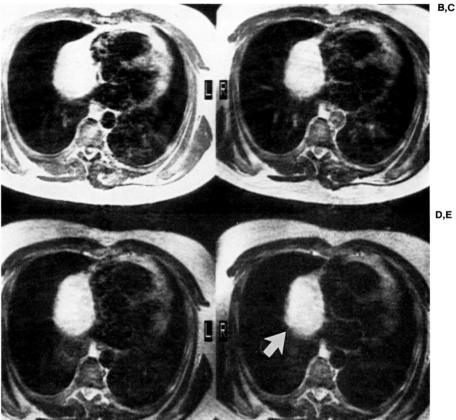

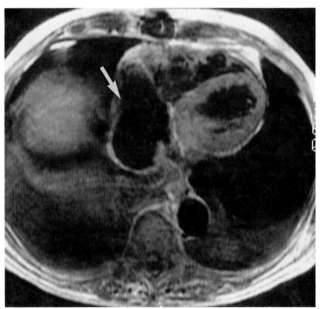

FIG. 25. Pericardial cyst. **A:** Cardiac-gated, T1-weighted, axial MR scan shows a sharply demarcated mass (*arrow*) which appears contained within pericardial fat. The signal intensity of this mass is equal to that of muscle. On a T1-weighted scan it is not possible to determine whether this mass is solid or cystic. **B–E:** Progressively T2-weighted, axial MR scans at the same level as in A demonstrate very high signal intensity (*arrow* in E) consistent with the diagnosis of a pericardial cyst.

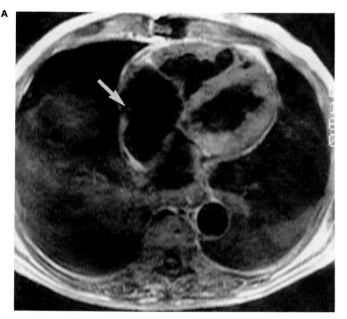

FIG. 26. Constrictive pericarditis. **A, B:** Sequential cardiac-gated, T1-weighted, axial MR scans in a 66-year-old man with a history of prior coronary artery bypass surgery presenting with shortness of breath and signs of increased right atrial pressure. Note that the normal pericardium anteriorly cannot be identified. There is dilatation of both the right atrium and the inferior vena cava (*arrows* in A and B), as well as large, bilateral pleural effusions. Although pericardial calcifications were noted on accompanying chest radiographs (not shown), these are inapparent on MR. A subsequent pericardiectomy was performed with resultant resolution of symptoms.

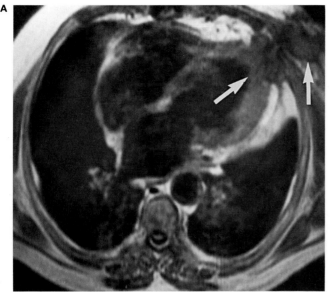

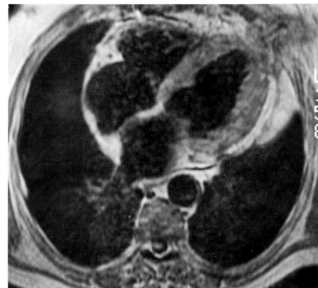

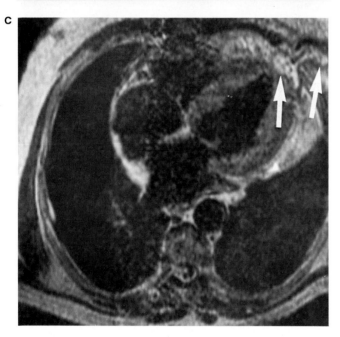

FIG. 27. Postoperative pericardial and chest wall abscesses. This patient presented with a fluctuant chest wall mass with evidence of transmitted pulsations several months following routine coronary artery bypass surgery. **A:** Cardiac-gated, T1-weighted, axial MR scan shows a subcutaneous mass which appears connected to a mass adjacent to the apex of the left ventricle (*arrows*). **B, C:** Proton density and T2-weighted MR scans, respectively, demonstrate a relatively high signal intensity mass suggestive of a fluid collection (*arrows* in C). Note that the ventricular chamber appears intact. Surgery confirmed a pericardial abscess with spontaneous drainage into the chest wall.

From the standpoint of clinical management, little is gained by visualizing the infarct itself. The ability to differentiate salvageable from necrosed myocardium is important because it could potentially play a role in directing early therapy; unfortunately, to date, MR has not proven useful in this regard. Work in progress using subsecond imaging with contrast agents and MR spectroscopy is attempting to address these issues (24,67).

Unlike myocardial assessment in acutely ill patients, MR is useful in assessing the extent of structural damage in patients with chronic myocardial infarction. Clinically, MR is indicated in patients whose recovery is slower than expected. Lack of functional recovery in the chronic phase of myocardial infarction can be related to (a) the extent of wall damage; (b) infarct expansion; and

(c) the development of ventricular aneurysms or pseudo-aneurysms (Fig. 28).

Prior myocardial infarctions appear as regions of wall thinning on MR images. Typically, there is an abrupt transition in thickness between normal and infarcted regions. The site of the infarction and its relationship to the vascular territories of the coronary arteries is easily determined. With dynamic cine images, dyskinetic segments of the thinned wall can be identified. It is possible to estimate the volume of muscle lost by infarction versus residual functional myocardium by estimating the spatial distribution of the infarct on multiple adjacent slices (68). It should be noted that relative stasis of ventricular blood commonly occurs adjacent to nonfunctional infarcted myocardium. High signal intensity

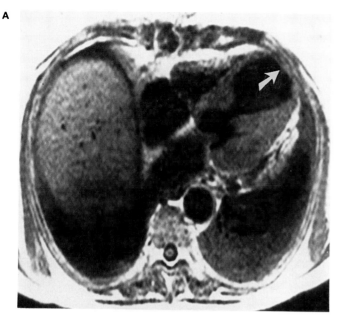

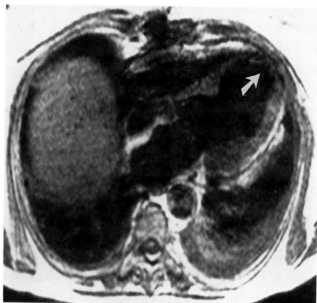

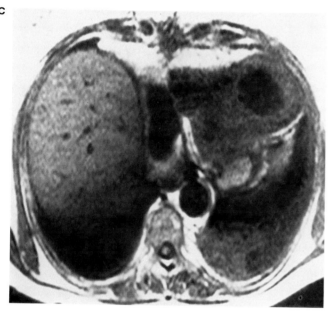

FIG. 28. Left ventricular aneurysm. **A–C:** Sequential cardiac-gated, T1-weighted, axial MR images performed in a patient several months following a documented myocardial infarction. Note marked thinning of the anterior septal and apical regions of the ventricle (*arrows* in A and B) with compensatory hypertrophy of the myocardium near the base of the heart. There is no evidence of intraventricular thrombus. The smooth transition between normal and thinned myocardium is typical of true ventricular aneurysms.

from slowly moving blood is often demonstrated and consequently may simulate an intraventricular thrombus. In most cases this problem is easily resolved by cine gradient echo images. Still more important is the depiction of false aneurysms and their effect on ventricular function. MR is an ideal method to assess the full extent and location of such aneurysms and pseudo-aneurysms for preoperative planning.

ASSESSMENT OF THE POSTOPERATIVE HEART

MR has been advocated for the postoperative assessment of bypass grafts (68–71). Although promising, early experience indicates that limited reliability, mostly due to technical limitations, hampers the widespread use of MR in assessing graft patency. An important advantage of MR is a lack of image distortion due to surgical hardware, including all types of modern heart valves. Detailed cardiac evaluation is thus still possible except in the immediate vicinity of the hardware. With the possible exception of the older Starr-Edwards type valve, MR is a safe means to assess postoperative myocardial status (72). Although still inadequate in assessing the patency of coronary bypass grafts, MR is excellent in detecting other complications such as false aneurysms (Fig. 29) and perigraft hematomas.

MR is adequate in assessing the function of various artificial grafts and shunts used in modern cardiovascular surgery, including composite valves (Fig. 30).

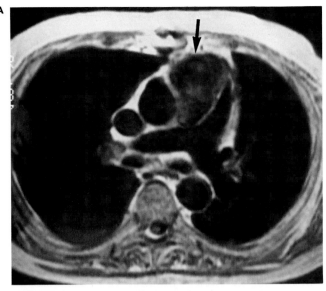

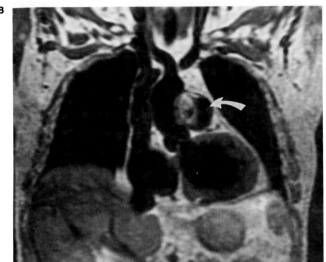

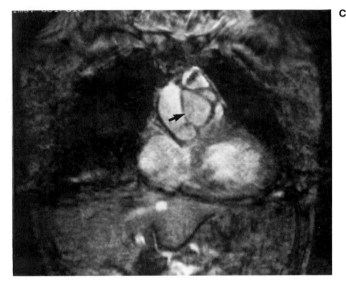

FIG. 29. Postoperative coronary artery bypass graft aneurysm. **A, B:** Cardiac-gated, T1-weighted, axial and coronal MR scans, respectively, show an abnormal structure with low signal intensity located between the aorta and the pulmonary artery (*arrows*). **C:** Cine MR study obtained in the coronal plane demonstrates flow within the abnormal structure (*arrow*) confirming it as vascular in etiology. This appearance suggested the preoperative diagnosis of an anastomotic pseudo-aneurysm. At surgery a mycotic aneurysm of the saphenous vein graft was subsequently documented.

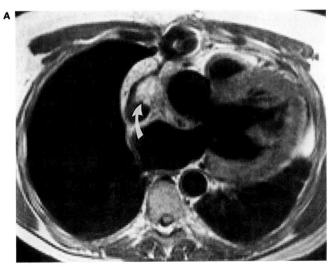

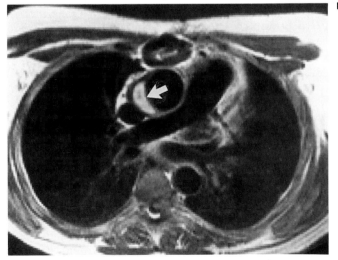

FIG. 30. Postoperative hematoma. **A, B:** Sequential cardiac-gated, T1-weighted, axial MR scans in a patient status-post composite aortic valve replacement. A high signal intensity mass can be identified (*arrows*) between the wall of the aortic graft and the wall of the native aorta. This appearance is typical of a subacute hematoma. Note the near total absence of image distortion despite the presence of a prosthetic aortic valve.

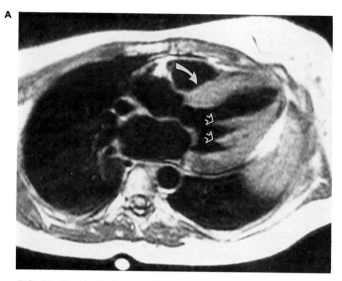

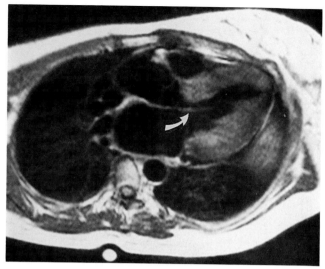

FIG. 31. Ventricular hypertrophy: MR evaluation. **A, B:** Sequential cardiac-gated, T1-weighted, axial MR scans performed in a patient in whom echocardiography had previously suggested the presence of a mass in the interventricular septum. Ventricular hypertrophy is slightly more prominent in the basal region of the septum (*curved arrow* in A) involving the papillary muscles as well (*arrows* in A). Slight prolapse of the anterior leaflet of the mitral valve can be identified as well (*curved arrow* in B). These findings are consistent with a diagnosis of asymmetric septal hypertrophy (ASH).

Cardiomyopathies

MR is most helpful in hypertrophic cardiomyopathies (73). Accurate definition of the extent, location, and severity of left ventricular hypertrophy can be achieved. Cine images in the areas of hypertrophy easily demonstrate the flow impairment and cardiac wall dynamics in these patients. It is important for radiologists to be familiar with the appearances of hypertrophic cardiomyopathies of various etiologies because they are commonly unsuspected and are often seen incidentally on routine thoracic MR studies (Figs. 31 and 32). The abnormal morphology of the ventricle is, to date, the only reliable sign of the presence or absence of a cardiomyopathy. No differences in relaxation times have been noted in patients with congestive cardiomyopathy compared to normal volunteers. Although metabolic data derived from MR spectroscopy may, in the future, play a role in this regard, final evaluation must await further developments.

Congenital Heart Disease

A detailed analysis of the MR manifestations of congenital heart disease is beyond the scope of this chapter (74). However, familiarity with the most common forms of congenital heart disease, including especially ventricular septal (VSD) and atrial septal (ASD) defects, is required in daily practice (75). Intraventricular septal defects are best recognized by a combination of morphologic and dynamic features (76). Often, the interventricular septum appears shortened at the level of the ventricular septal defect (Fig. 33). When small, VSDs may not be directly identifiable. Cine imaging,

however, will reveal the ventricular septal defect in most cases because of associated jet effects. The effect of a turbulent jet of blood across a VSD will be a zone of decreased signal intensity during systole. This corresponds to dephasing of spins related to the turbulence of

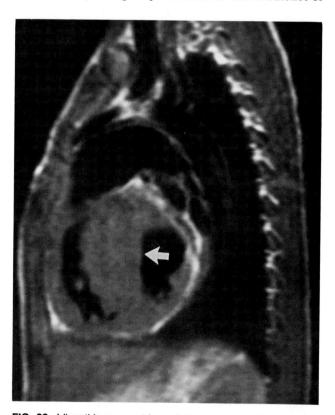

FIG. 32. Idiopathic asymmetric septal hypertrophy (ASH). Cardiac-gated, T1-weighted, coronal MR scan shows characteristic appearance of a markedly enlarged interventricular septum (*arrow*) characteristic of ASH.

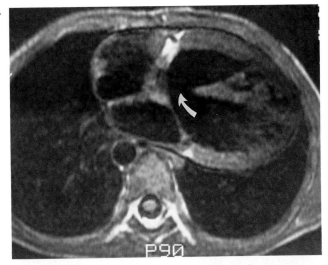

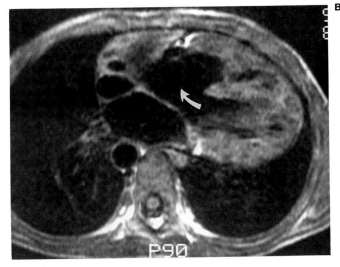

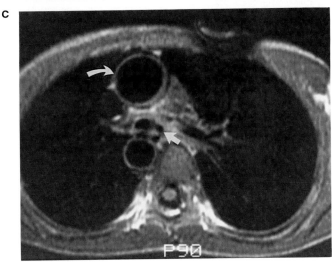

FIG. 33. Truncus arteriosus: MR evaluation. **A–C:** Sequential cardiac-gated, axial MR images from below-upward in a 4-year-old boy with truncus arteriosus type IV. Note that there is a large ventricular septal defect (*curved arrow* in A). The aorta is the only vessel arising from the ventricles and is right-sided (*curved arrows* in B and C). Note the absence of pulmonary arteries. The descending aorta is right-sided as well. Multiple small collateral vessels can be identified representing dilated bronchial arteries near the main-stem bronchi (*straight arrow* in C).

the jet. However, it should be emphasized that normal flow-void patterns can be seen during the ejection phase of the ventricle or emptying of the atria due to high velocity (77).

An interatrial septal defect can also be recognized by the presence of interatrial turbulence-related jets, but this is less common (Fig. 34). An important pitfall in the diagnosis of atrial septal defect is the frequent nonvisualization of the fossa ovalis of the interatrial septum, which is normally extremely thin. Thus, the diagnosis of atrial septal defect requires images of high quality and some evidence of distortion or transeptal flow to prove the presence of the defect (78).

Valvular Heart Disease

MR is not well-suited to the study of the rapid events associated with valvular function. Often, visualization of the valve leaflets is limited. Atrioventricular valves are best visualized during the systolic phase of the cardiac cycle, while the aortic and pulmonic valves are best seen during the diastolic phase of the cardiac cycle. With cine MR, disturbed flow effects due to pathologic valves

are visualized as areas of decreased signal intensity across regions of valvular stenosis or insufficiency (Fig. 35). Quantification of blood flow velocity across pathologic valves and assessment of the degree of valvular malfunction is possible with MR (79–82). However, while of scientific interest, to date these determinations do not play an important clinical role in patient management.

Bicuspid aortic valves are usually easy to recognize on static MR images. MR also has been useful in the diagnosis of complications related to bacterial endocarditis. Infectious implants on the annulus can be visualized without difficulty when larger than 5–10 mm in size. In addition, endocardiac abscesses, which typically occur at the margins of the annulus of the aortic valve and are frequently in communication with the vascular chambers, appear to be well-demonstrated by MR (83).

Pathology of the Proximal Aorta and Pulmonary Artery

As discussed in detail in Chapters 2 and 5, MR is effective in evaluating the proximal aorta and pulmo-

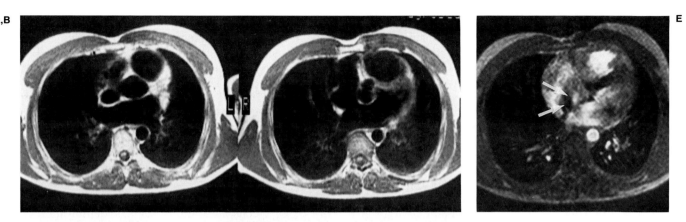

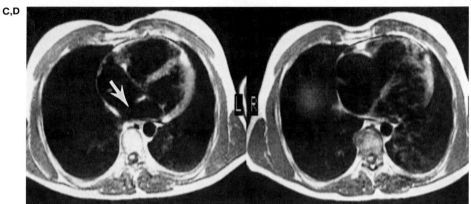

FIG. 34. Interatrial septal defect (ASD). **A–D:** Cardiac-gated, T1-weighted, axial MR scans from above-downward demonstrate partial absence of the interatrial septum (*arrow* in C) in this patient with a documented ASD. It should be emphasized that the interatrial septum is not always identifiable even in normal individuals, thereby necessitating cine confirmation whenever applicable. **E:** Cine MR study shows a transatrial jet effect as an area of low signal intensity extending from the left to the right atrium (*arrows*).

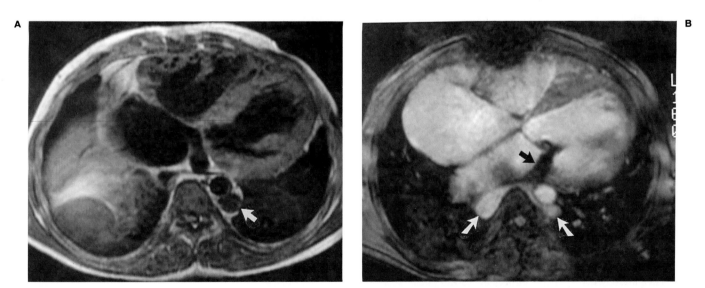

FIG. 35. Endocardial cushion defect with azygos continuation of the inferior vena cava and mitral regurgitation. **A:** Cardiac-gated, T1-weighted, axial MR scan in a 31-year-old patient status-post partial repair of a previously documented endocardial cushion defect. A large vessel can be identified parallel to the descending aorta representing a dilated azygos vein (*arrow*). **B:** Cine MR study confirms the presence of a large regurgitant jet between the left ventricle and the left atrium typical of mitral regurgitation (*black arrow*). Note again the presence of enlarged azygos and hemiazygos veins (*white arrows*).

nary arteries for acquired and congenital forms of pathology. MR is especially useful in the diagnosis and monitoring of patients with Marfan's syndrome. In addition to routine atherosclerotic aortic aneurysms, characteristically, patients with Marfan's syndrome develop enlarged valvular cusps as well as dilatation of the proximal portion of the ascending aorta (see Fig. 73, Chapter 2). As discussed in Chapter 2, MR has become a primary modality in the diagnosis and management of aortic dissection (Fig. 36; see also Figs. 67, 68, 70, 71, Chapter 2) (84,85). It should be noted that despite the reputed efficacy of MR to diagnose dissections, in a recent series, up to 25% of acute dissections presented in an atypical fashion with asymmetric thickening of the aorta as the only sign (86). Presumably due to a limited intramural hematoma with no flow in the false lumen or rupture of the intimal flap, asymmetric thickening is often seen in the root of the aorta immediately above the aortic valve (Fig. 37). Because in some cases the proper diagnosis can be made by the demonstration of a typical intimal flap in another region of the thoracic or abdominal aorta, it is imperative in these cases to scan the entire aorta for proper diagnosis.

Although image formation is hampered locally by the presence of aortic valves, MR plays an important role in follow-up of the postoperative aorta or pulmonary artery. Despite image distortion, the various shunts and conduits arising from or located near the aorta usually are easily assessed.

NEW DEVELOPMENTS IN CARDIAC MR

Even though MR has intrinsic advantages unequaled by other imaging techniques for evaluating the heart, it does not yet play a significant clinical role. MR is currently limited to serving primarily as a problem solving device for specific indications, such as identification of intracardiac and/or pericardiac masses, complex congenital anomalies, and constrictive pericarditis. In most instances, information provided by conventional MR appears redundant of information available from less costly techniques, such as radionuclide imaging, echocardiography, and CT. However, during the past few years, significant developments have occurred that offer the potential for a radically enlarged role for MR in cardiac imaging. Progress has taken place in several areas. Most important has been the development of ultrafast scanning techniques permitting imaging within a single cardiac cycle. This offers the possibility of myo-

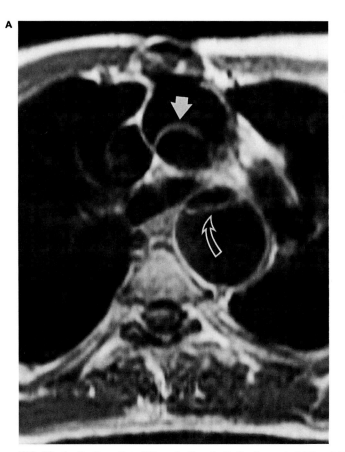
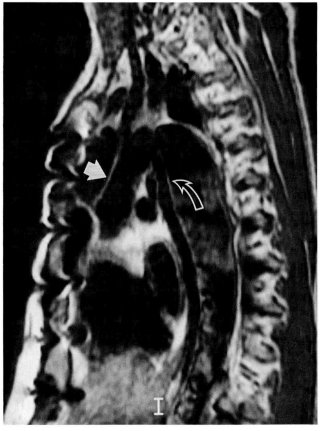

FIG. 36. Aortic dissection: MR evaluation. **A, B:** Cardiac-gated, T1-weighted, axial and left anterior oblique parasagittal MR images, respectively. An intimal flap is easily identifiable in both the ascending aorta (*arrows* in A and B) and the descending aorta (*open arrows* in A and B). Note that there is evidence of flow in both the true and false lumens. Distortion artifacts are due to the presence of sternal sutures.

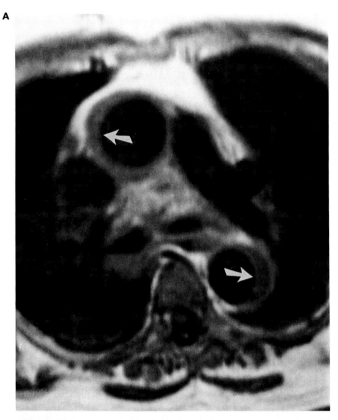

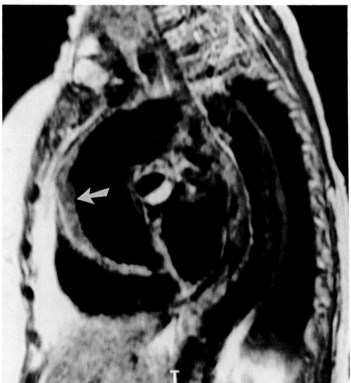

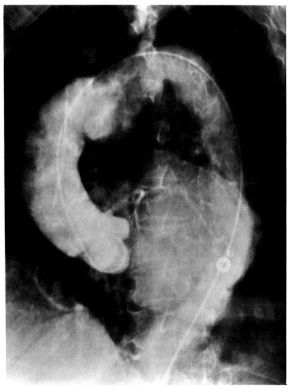

FIG. 37. Aortic dissection: atypical MR presentation. **A, B:** Cardiac-gated, T1-weighted, axial and sagittal MR scans, respectively, show asymmetric thickening along the lateral aspect of both the ascending and descending aortas (*arrows*), associated with minimal distortion of the aortic lumen. No obvious intimal flap can be identified. **C:** Corresponding aortogram. Note lack of evidence either of an intimal flap or distortion of the aortic lumen. At surgery, this patient proved to have a type A dissection involving both the ascending and descending aortas. This atypical form of dissection presumably represented an acute intramural hematoma which failed to evolve into a frank intimal tear. In our experience, these findings are not unusual.

A,B
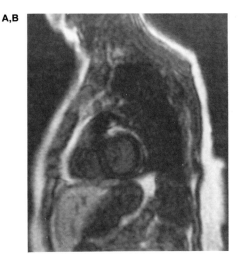
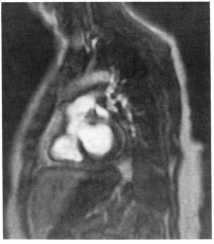
C
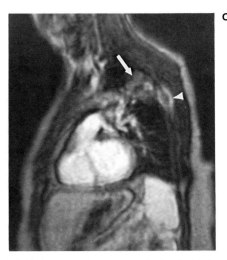

FIG. 38. Myocardial perfusion: contrast-enhanced subsecond MR evaluation using gadolinium-DTPA contrast enhancement. **A:** Sagittal MR scan. Using a subsecond gradient echo technique, images can be obtained in 400–700 ms. To enhance T1 contrast, the gradient echo sequence is preceded by a 180° inversion pulse. Note that there is low signal intensity within the myocardium due to the preinversion pulse. **B:** Sagittal MR scan at the same level as A, a few seconds after the i.v. injection of Gd-DTPA. Note high signal intensity within the ventricular chambers as well as the pulmonary vessels. **C:** Sagittal MR scan at same level as B obtained a few seconds later shows that the myocardial signal intensity has increased, reflecting the myocardial distribution of contrast media. A large tumor within the left upper lobe (*arrows*) can now be identified associated with enhancement of the adjacent chest wall due to metastatic involvement. (Case courtesy of Dr. Don Schnapf, Director, York Imaging Center, York, PA.)

cardial perfusion studies with contrast enhancement (Fig. 38). In addition, the active development of analysis software will provide comprehensive quantitative analyses of myocardial function. Finally, the development of new pulse sequences to better evaluate myocardial mechanics and visualize coronary arteries also promises an increased clinical role for utilization of MR.

These new developments have the potential for making MR the most comprehensive single-modality test for evaluating cardiac structure and function. In addition, MR may provide unique information not otherwise available. For example, a recently developed technique termed myocardial tagging modifies the magnetization of specific regions of the myocardium, permitting the tracking of myocardial muscle throughout the cardiac cycle (87). This in turn allows measurement of ventricular deformation in three dimensions, including analysis of shear and torsion from endocardium to epicardium.

A,B
C,D
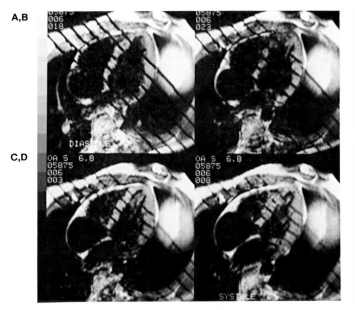
E,F
G,H
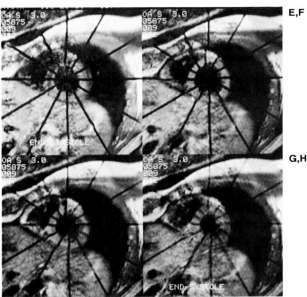

FIG. 39. Myocardial tagging. With this technique, thin bands of saturated (low-signal) myocardial tissue are generated during diastole that subsequently can be followed throughout the cardiac cycle. **A–D:** Parallel tagging. Six parallel lines are seen across the myocardium which is imaged in the long axis commencing with diastole (A) and extending through systole (D). Note that the tags near the apex of the heart undergo much less displacement than the tags near the base of the heart. **E–H:** Radial tagging. Six radially oriented tags centered in the left ventricle are generated, with images obtained through the short axis of the ventricle.

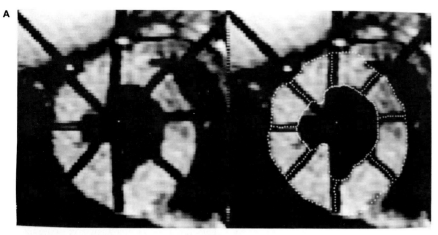

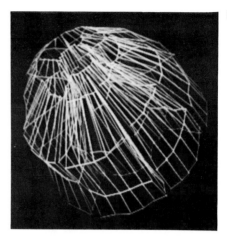

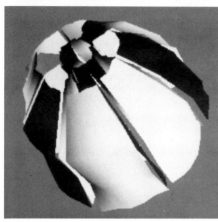

FIG. 40. Three-dimensional tagged myocardial images. **A:** With this technique, each image of the myocardium is first radially tagged (compare with Fig. 39E). **B:** Subsequently, using contoured points, a wire frame representation of the ventricle throughout its cycle can be reconstructed utilizing a dedicated computer. **C:** These results then serve as the basic data representing the beating ventricle in three dimensions. This display format offers the advantage of interactive user interchange. Additionally, each tagged region of the myocardium can be characterized by the nature of its deformation.

The ability to image these parameters solves a long-standing problem in cardiac imaging—the inability to track identical points in the myocardium from systole through diastole. The heart moves in an extremely complex fashion during its cycle. As demonstrated in Fig. 39, intrinsic myocardial deformation can be tracked using tagging methods. In addition, these methods can serve as the framework for true three-dimensional analysis of cardiac mechanics (Fig. 40).

SUMMARY

Expertise in analyzing the intracardiac structures made visible both by CT and especially MR is a prerequisite for a comprehensive evaluation of paracardiac, pericardiac, and intracardiac pathology. Familiarity with the anatomic detail of the cardiac region has become a demand which will undoubtedly increase in importance in the future. In our judgment, MR is indicated for all processes involving the paracardiac regions, especially in cases for which i.v. contrast cannot be administered. This is because of the documented precision with which MR can be used to evaluate the relationship of paracardiac disease to cardiovascular structures. MR is equally reliable in assessing space-occupying processes within the heart and in evaluating the extent of struc-

tural damage following myocardial infarction. Differentiation of restrictive cardiomyopathy versus constrictive pericarditis is an uncommon but important primary indication for pericardial imaging by MR. Finally, it may be anticipated that ongoing developments will eventuate in the emergence of a major role for MR in the primary evaluation of cardiac pathology in the near future (88).

REFERENCES

1. Guthaner DF, Wexler L, Harell G. CT demonstration of cardiac structures. *AJR* 1979;133:75–81.
2. Lackner K, Thurn P. Computed tomography of the heart: ECG-gated and continuous scans. *Radiology* 1981;140:413–420.
3. Farmer DW, Lipton MJ, Webb WR, Ringertz H, Higgins CB. Computed tomography in congenital heart disease. *J Comput Assist Tomogr* 1984;8:677–687.
4. Godwin JD, Herfkens RJ, Skioldebrand CG, Brundage BH, Schiller NB, Lipton MJ. Detection of intraventricular thrombi by computed tomography. *Radiology* 1981;138:717–721.
5. Gross BH, Glazer GM, Francis IR. CT of intracardiac and intrapericardial masses. *AJR* 1983;140:903–907.
6. Hidalgo H, Korobkin M, Breiman RS, Kisslo JR. CT of intracardiac tumor. *AJR* 1981;137:608–609.
7. Tsuchiya F, Kohno A, Saitoh R, Shigeta A. CT findings of atrial myxoma. *Radiology* 1984;151:139–143.
8. Albrechtsoson U, Stahl E, Tylen U. Evaluation of coronary artery bypass graft patency with computed tomography. *J Comput Assist Tomogr* 1981;5:822–826.
9. Engelstad BL, Wagner S, Herfkens R, Botvinick E, Brundage B,

Lipton M. Evaluation of the post-coronary artery bypass patient by myocardial perfusion scintigraphy and computed tomography. *AJR* 1983;141:507–512.

10. Stanford W, Galvin JR. The radiology of right heart dysfunction: chest roentgenogram and computed tomography. *J Thorac Imaging* 1989;4:7–19.

11. Moore EH, Greenberg, Merrick SH, Miller SW, McLoud TC, Sheparre JAO. Coronary artery calcifications: significance of incidental detection on CT scans. *Radiology* 1989;172:711–716.

12. Breen JF, Sheedy PF, Stanson AW, Rumberger J, Schwartz RS. Coronary calcification detected with fast CT as a marker of coronary artery disease. *Radiology* 1990;177:279.

13. Bormann JL, Stanford W, Stenberg R, Winniford M, Galvin JR, Berbaum KS, Talman C, Marcus M. Ultrafast CT detection of coronary artery stenosis. *Radiology* 1990;177:163.

14. Garret JS, Jaschke W, Aherne T, Botvinick EH, Higgins CB, Lipton MJ. Quantitation of intracardiac shunts by cine-CT. *J Comput Assist Tomogr* 1988;12:82–87.

15. Marcus ML, Rumberger JA, Stark CA. Cardiac applications of ultrafast computed tomography. *Am J Cardiac Imaging* 1988;2:116–121.

16. Flicker S, Neidich HJ, Altin RS, Eldgredge WJ, Carr KF. Ultrafast computed tomography techniques in cardiac disease. *J Thorac Imaging* 1989;4:42–49.

17. Diethelm L, Simonson JS, Dery R, Gould RG, Schiller NB, Lipton MJ. Determination of left ventricular mass with ultrafast CT and two-dimensional echocardiography. *Radiology* 1989;171:213–217.

18. Higgins CB. Malcolm Hanson memorial lecture. MR of the heart: anatomy, physiology, and metabolism. *AJR* 1988;151:239–248.

19. Westcott JL, Henschke CI, Berkmen Y. MR imaging of the hilum and mediastinum: effects of cardiac gating. *J Comput Assist Tomogr* 1985;9:1073–1078.

20. Felmlee JP, Ehman RL. Spatial presaturation: a method for suppressing flow artifacts and improving depiction of vascular anatomy in MR imaging. *Radiology* 1987;164:559–564.

21. Glover GH, Pelc NJ. A rapid-gated cine MRI technique [review]. Magn Reson Ann 1988;299–333.

22. Sechtem U, Pflugfelder PW, White RD, Gould RG, Holt W, Lipton MJ, Higgins CB. Cine MR imaging: potential for the evaluation of cardiovascular function. *AJR* 1987;148:239–246.

23. Stark DD, Hendrick RE, Hahn PF, Ferrucci JT, Jr. Motion artifact reduction with fast spin-echo imaging. *Radiology* 1987;164:183–191.

24. Edelman RR, Thompson R, Kantor H, Brady TJ, Leavitt M, Dinsmore R. Cardiac function: evaluation with fast-echo MR imaging. *Radiology* 1987;162:611–615.

25. Rzedzian RR, Pykett IL. Instant images of the human heart using a new, whole-body MR imaging system. *AJR* 1987;149:245–250.

26. Burbank F, Parish D, Wexler L. Echocardiographic-like angled views of the heart by MR imaging. *J Comput Assist Tomogr* 1988;12:181–195.

27. Akins EW, Hill JA, Fitzsimmons JR, Pepine CJ, Williams CM. Importance of imaging plane for magnetic resonance imaging of the normal left ventricle. *Am J Cardiol* 1985;56:366–372.

28. Sechtem U, Tscholakoff D, Higgins CB. MRI of the abnormal pericardium. *AJR* 1986;147:245–252.

29. Shapiro EP. Magnetic resonance imaging of the heart: a cardiologist's viewpoint [review]. Top Magn Reson Imaging 1990;2:1–12.

30. Winkler M, Higgins CB. Suspected intracardiac masses: evaluation with MR imaging. *Radiology* 1987;165:117–122.

31. Go RT, O'Donnell JK, Underwood DA, Feiglin DH, Salcedo EE, Pantoja M, MacIntyre WJ, Meaney TF. Comparison of gated cardiac MRI and 2D echocardiography of intracardiac neoplasms. *AJR* 1985;145:21–25.

32. Amparo EG, Higgins CB, Farmer D, Gamsu G, McNamara M. Gated MRI of cardiac and paracardiac masses: initial experience. *AJR* 1984;143:1151–1156.

33. Gomes AS, Lois JF, Child JS, Brown K, Batra P. Cardiac tumors and thrombus: evaluation with MR imaging. *AJR* 1987;149:895–899.

34. Lund JT, Ehman RL, Julsrud PR, Sinak LJ, Tajik AJ. Cardiac masses: assessment by MR imaging. *AJR* 1989;152:469–473.

35. Freedberg RS, Kronzon I, Rumancik WM, Liebeskind D. The contribution of magnetic resonance imaging to the evaluation of intracardiac tumors diagnosed by echocardiography. *Circulation* 1988;77:96–103.

36. Brown JJ, Barakos JA, Higgins CB. Magnetic resonance imaging of cardiac and paracardiac masses. *J Thorac Imaging* 1989;4:58–64.

37. Barakos JA, Brown JJ, Higgins CB. MR imaging of secondary cardiac and paracardiac lesions. *AJR* 1989;153:47–50.

38. Lee R, Fisher MR. MR imaging of cardiac metastases from malignant fibrous histiocytoma. *J Comput Assist Tomogr* 1989;13:126–128.

39. Mahajan H, Kim EE, Wallace S, Abello R, Benjamin R, Evans HL. Magnetic resonance imaging of malignant fibrous histiocytoma. *Magn Reson Imaging* 1989;7:283–288.

40. Watanabe AT, Teitelbaum GP, Henderson RW, Bradley WG, Jr. Magnetic resonance imaging of cardiac sarcomas. *J Thorac Imaging* 1989;4:90–92.

41. Kim EE, Wallace S, Abello R, Coan JD, Ewer MS, Salem PA, Ali MK. Malignant cardiac fibrous histiocytomas and angiosarcomas: MR features. *J Comput Assist Tomogr* 1989;13:627–632.

42. Dooms GC, Higgins CB. MR imaging of cardiac thrombi. *J Comput Assist Tomogr* 1986;10:415–420.

43. Stark DD, Higgins CB, Lanzer P, et al. Nuclear magnetic resonance imaging of the pericardium: normal and pathologic findings. *Radiology* 1984;150:469.

44. Sechtem U, Tscholakoff D, Higgins CB. MRI of the normal pericardium. *AJR* 1986;147:239–244.

45. Moncada R, Baker M, Salinas M, et al. Diagnostic role of computed tomography in pericardial disease: congenital defects, thickening, neoplasms, and effusions. *Am Heart J* 1982;103:263–282.

46. Aronberg DJ, Peterson RR, Glazer HS, Sagel SS. The superior sinus of the pericardium: CT appearance. *Radiology* 1984;153:489–492.

47. Levy-Ravetch M, Auh YH, Rubenstein WA, Whalen JP, Kazam E. CT of the pericardial recesses. *AJR* 1985;144:707–714.

48. Choe YH, Im J-G, Park JH, Han MC, Kim C-W. Pictorial essay. The anatomy of the pericardial space: a study in cadavers and patients. *AJR* 1987;149:693–697.

49. Paling MR, Williamson BRJ. Epicardial fat pad: CT findings. *Radiology* 1987;165:335–339.

50. Gale ME, Kiwak MG, Gale DR. Pericardial fluid distribution: CT analysis. *Radiology* 1987;162:171–174.

51. Takasugi JE, Godwin JD. Pictorial essay. Surgical defects of the pericardium: radiographic findings. *AJR* 1989;152:951–954.

52. Higgins CB, Mattrey RF, Shea P. Technical note. CT localization and aspiration of postoperative pericardial fluid collection. *J Comput Assist Tomogr* 1983;7:734–736.

53. Doppman JL, Rienmuller R, Lissner J, Cryan J, Bolte HD, Strauer BE, Hellwig H. Computed tomography in constrictive pericardial disease. *J Comput Assist Tomogr* 1981;5:1–11.

54. Rienmuller R, Doppman JL, Lissner J, Kemkes BM, Strauer BE. Constrictive pericardial disease: prognostic significance of a nonvisualized left ventricular wall. *Radiology* 1985;156:753–755.

55. Rees M, MacMillan R, Flicker S, Fender B, Clark C. Rapid-acquisition computed tomography demonstration of chronic calcified pericardial constriction. *CT* 1986;10:183–186.

56. Glazer GM, Gross BH, Orringer MB, Buda AJ, Francis IR, Shapiro B. Computed tomography of pericardial masses: further observations and comparison with echocardiography. *J Comput Assist Tomogr* 1984;8:895–899.

57. Pugatch RD, Brayer JM, Robbins AH, Spira R. CT diagnosis of pericardial cysts. *AJR* 1975;131:515–516.

58. Brunner DR, Whitley NO. A pericardial cyst with high CT numbers. *AJR* 1984;142:279–280.

59. Gouliamos A, Steriotis J, Kalovidouris A, Andreou J, Sandilos P, Michalis A, Papavasiliou C, Pontifex GR. Computed tomography of water-like densities mimicking pericardial effusion in a case of a pericardial tumor. *J Comput Assist Tomogr* 1984;8:343–345.

60. Goldstein L, Mirvis SE, Kostrubiak IS, Turney SZ. CT diagnosis of acute pericardial tamponade after blunt chest trauma. *AJR* 1989;152:739–741.

61. Soulen RL, Stark DD, Higgins CB. Magnetic resonance imaging of constrictive pericardial disease. *Am J Cardiol* 1985;55:480–484.

62. Im JG, Rosen A, Webb WR, Gamsu G. MR imaging of the transverse sinus of the pericardium. *AJR* 1988;150:79–84.

63. McMurdo KK, Webb WR, von Shulthess GK, Gamsu G. Magnetic resonance imaging of the superior pericardial recesses. *AJR* 1985;145:985–988.

64. Sechtem U, Tscholakoff D, Higgins CB. MRI of the abnormal pericardium. *AJR* 1986;147:245–252.

65. Fisher MR, McNamara MT, Higgins CB. TI acute myocardial infarction: MR evaluation in 29 patients. *AJR* 1987;148:247–251.

66. Pflugfelder PW, Wisenberg G, Prato FS, Carroll SE, Turner KL. Early detection of canine myocardial infarction by magnetic resonance imaging in vivo. *Circulation* 1985;71:587–594.

67. Van-Rossum AC, Visser FC, Van Eenige MJ, Sprenger M, Valk J, Verheugt FW, Roos JP. Value of gadolinium-diethylene-triamine pentaacetic acid dynamics in magnetic resonance imaging of acute myocardial infarction with occluded and reperfused coronary arteries after thrombolysis. *Am J Cardiol* 1990;65:845–851.

68. Shapiro EP, Rogers WJ, Beyar R, Soulen RL, Zerhouni EA, Lima JA, Weiss JL. Determination of left ventricular mass by magnetic resonance imaging in hearts deformed by acute infarction. *Circulation* 1989;79:706–711.

69. Stahlberg F, Mogelvang J, Thomsen C, Nordell B, Stubgaard M, Ericsson A, Sperber G, Greitz D, Larsson H, Henriksen O, et al. A method for MR quantification of flow velocities in blood and CSF using interleaved gradient-echo pulse sequences. *Magn Reson Imaging* 1989;7:655–667.

70. Rubinstein RI, Askenase AD, Thickman D, Feldman MS, Agarwal JB, Helfant RH. Magnetic resonance imaging to evaluate patency of aortocoronary bypass grafts. *Circulation* 1987;76:786–791.

71. White RD, Caputo GR, Mark AS, Modin GW, Higgins CB. Coronary artery bypass graft patency: noninvasive evaluation with MR imaging. *Radiology* 1987;164:681–686.

72. Soulen RL, Budinger TF, Higgins CB. Magnetic resonance imaging of prosthetic heart valves. *Radiology* 1985;154:705–707.

73. Doyoshita H, Murakami E, Takekoshi N, Matsui S, Nakato H, Enyama H. Differentiation of hypertrophic cardiomyopathy from left ventricular hypertrophy induced by essential hypertension using magnetic resonance imaging. *So J Cardiol* 1988;18:113–119.

74. Kersting-Sommerhoff BA, Diethelm L, Teitel DF, Sommerhoff CP, Higgins SS, Higashino SS, Higgins CB. Magnetic resonance imaging of congenital heart disease: sensitivity and specificity using receiver operating characteristic curve analysis. *Am Heart J* 1989;118:155–161.

75. Lowell DG, Turner DA, Smith SM, Bucheleres GH, Santucci BA, Gresick RJ Jr, Monson DO. The detection of atrial and ventricular septal defects with electrocardiographically synchronized magnetic resonance imaging. *Circulation* 1986;73:89–94.

76. Sechtem U, Pflugfelder P, Cassidy MC, Holt W, Wolfe C, Higgins CB. Ventricular septal defect: visualization of shunt flow and determination of shunt size by cine MR imaging. *AJR* 1987;149:689–692.

77. Mirowitz SA, Lee JK, Gutierrez FR, Brown JJ, Eilenberg SS. Normal signal-void patterns in cardiac cine MR images. *Radiology* 1990;176:49–55.

78. Nishimura T, Yamada N, Itoh A, Miyatake K. Cine MR imaging in valvular heart disease. *Rinsho Hoshasen* 1989;34:11–17.

79. Mitchell L, Jenkins JP, Watson Y, Rowlands DJ, Isherwood I. Diagnosis and assessment of mitral and aortic valve disease by cine-flow magnetic resonance imaging. *Magn Reson Med* 1989;12:181–197.

80. Wagner S, Auffermann W, Buser P, Lim TH, Kircher B, Pflugfelder P, Higgins CB. Diagnostic accuracy and estimation of the severity of valvular regurgitation from the signal void on cine magnetic resonance images. *Am Heart J* 1989;118:760–767.

81. Pflugfelder PW, Landzberg JS, Cassidy MM, Cheitlin MD, Schiller NB, Auffermann W, Higgins CB. Comparison of cine MR imaging with Doppler echocardiography for the evaluation of aortic regurgitation. *AJR* 1989;152:729–735.

82. Utz JA, Herfkens RJ, Heinsimer JA, Shimakawa A, Glover G, Pelc N. Valvular regurgitation: dynamic MR imaging. *Radiology* 1988;168:91–94.

83. Winkler ML, Higgins CB. MRI of perivalvular infectious pseudo-aneurysms. *AJR* 1986;147:253–256.

84. Hill JA, Lambert CR, Akins EW, Carmichael MJ. Ascending aortic dissection: detection by MRI. *Am Heart J* 1985;110:894–896.

85. Kersting-Sommerhoff BA, Higgins CB, White RD, Sommerhoff CP, Lipton MJ. Aortic dissection: sensitivity and specificity of MR imaging. *Radiology* 1988;166:651–655.

86. Wolff KA, Herold CJ, Tempany CMC, Parravano JJ, Zerhouni EA. Atypical patterns of aortic dissection with MR imaging [abstract]. *Radiology* 1990;177(P):201.

87. Zerhouni EA, Parish DM, Rogers WJ, Yang A, Shapiro EP. Human heart: tagging with MR imaging—a method for noninvasive assessment of myocardial motion. *Radiology* 1988;169:59–63.

88. Council on Scientific Affairs. Magnetic resonance imaging of the cardiovascular system. Present state of the art and future potential [review]. Report of the Magnetic Resonance Imaging Panel. *JAMA* 1988;259:253–259.

Subject Index